TEXTBOOK
of
ACQUIRED
HEART VALVE
DISEASE

VOLUME II

Jean Acar
Endre Bodnar

ICR Publishers

TEXTBOOK OF ACQUIRED HEART VALVE DISEASE
Published by ICR Publishers, London
First Edition, First Printing
ISBN: 1 872743 05 6

Printed in the United Kingdom
ISBN: 1 872743 05 6

CONTENTS

Volume I

Volume II

TEXTBOOK
of
ACQUIRED
HEART VALVE
DISEASE

ICR Publishers

Tricuspid Valve Disease
Tricuspid Insufficiency

Pierre-Louis Michel

Tricuspid insufficiency (TI) consists of an abnormal reflux of blood from the right ventricle into the right atrium during ventricular systole. It may be of organic origin, resulting from changes in the tricuspid valve apparatus, or more often functional, resulting from dilation of the tricuspid annulus. Its clinical and etiologic diagnosis and its quantification benefited greatly from the development of Doppler echocardiography.

HISTORICAL BACKGROUND

The first clinical description of tricuspid insufficiency was by Homberg in 1704, while an increased systolic murmur during inspiration was described by Rivero-Carvallo in 1946 (1), and hemodynamic assessment of this condition was provided by Cournand (1948), Gorlin (1951) and Soulie (1956). The introduction of Doppler echocardiography greatly increased the rate of detection and improved the quantitative determination of TI, while the development of repair surgery and valve replacements revolutionized the treatment of tricuspid insufficiency.

ANATOMIC LESIONS

The normal tricuspid orifice (2) consists of a fibrous annulus, 100-120 mm in diameter, enclosing three leaflets; the anterior, which is the largest, the posterior and septal leaflets. These three leaflets are separated by three commissures; the anteroseptal, the anteroposterior, or external, and the posteroseptal. The subvalvular apparatus comprises three papillary muscles, the pointed ends of which are attached to the chordae tendineae extending to the respective leaflet. The tricuspid annulus has a solid structure at its point of contact with the septal leaflet and the anteroseptal commissure, where it merges with the right fibrous trigone. On the other hand, it is much weaker in the area of the anterior and posterior leaflets and of the external and posteroseptal commissures.

Dilation of the annulus is the predominant pathologic process in functional tricuspid insufficiency (3,4). This dilation is asymmetrical due to the characteristic structure of the annulus; it affects the anterior leaflet and in particular the base of insertion of the posterior leaflet. The circumference of the dilated annulus may be as much as 150-170 mm.

In organic tricuspid insufficiency the nature of the lesions depends on the etiology (5); in the case of rheumatic origin, leaflet retraction is the dominant lesion, affecting mainly the posterior leaflet, the chordae tendineae are shortened to a varying degree, but the pathology is usually less severe than it is in the mitral valve, which is always affected simultaneously. Commissural fusion may also be present, causing mixed tricuspid disease. In addition, annular distension is always present.

In infective tricuspid insufficiency, the lesions are similar to those normally found in infective endocarditis. The vegetations may be located in the leaflets, on the chordae tendineae or even on the wall of the endocardium. They may be combined with leaflet mutilation or rupture of the chordae tendineae (6). Unlike the picture in the left heart, however, the lesions tend not to reach the site of insertion of the leaflets on the annulus, thus explaining the efficacy of tricuspid valvectomy for sterilization of the lesions (7).

In traumatic tricuspid insufficiency, the lesions affect the anterior subvalvular apparatus in the great majority of cases, generally involving rupture of the chordae tendineae and on occasion rupture of the papillary muscle or tearing of the leaflet. Other lesions may appear simultaneously, including aortic insufficiency, rupture of the ventricular septum (8) or right ventricular aneurysm (9). Ischemic rupture of the anterior papillary muscle has been described as an exceptional case, following inferior myocardial infarction (10).

In tricuspid lesions linked with a carcinoid syndrome, the characteristic features of the lesions are the retractile fibrous sheets which cover the endocardium of the leaflets, the subvalvular apparatus, the cardiac cavities and the intima of the veins and the coronary sinus (11).

ETIOLOGY

A fully competent tricuspid valve requires proper functioning of the complete valvular apparatus. Any abnormality affecting the function of one or more of its elements may involve regurgitation. A distinction has to be made between tricuspid insufficiency of functional or organic origin.

Functional tricuspid insufficiency

This condition is secondary to a dilation of the annulus associated with right ventricular dilation. The distension of the right ventricle is in turn the result of pulmonary arterial hypertension, irrespective of its specific cause (12). Although mitral or mitro-aortic valve diseases are the most frequent cause, ischemic or hypertensive heart diseases, primary or secondary myocardiopathies (13), or acute or chronic pulmonary heart disease may all be responsible for the tricuspid regurgitation.

Organic tricuspid insufficiency

Apart from congenital cases, which are outside the scope of the present work, the main causes of organic tricuspid insufficiency are acute rheumatic fever and infective endocarditis (4,5).

Rheumatic tricuspid valve disease

This condition never occurs in isolation; mitral valve involvement is always present and the aorta is involved in two cases out of three (5). The frequency of organic tricuspid valve disease during mitral valve disease varies from series to series; from 6% in the echocardiographic study by Daniels (14) to 33% in the Aceves autopsy series (15). The decreasing incidence of acute rheumatic arthritis has been accompanied by a parallel decrease in the frequency of rheumatic tricuspid valve disease. In the Mayo Clinic trial, in which 360 tricuspid valve replacements were followed over a period of 25 years, the incidence of rheumatic etiology fell from 79% for the 1963-1967 period to only 24% during the 1983-1987 period (5).

Tricuspid endocarditis

Previously regarded as rare - three cases reported by Ahn and Segal in 1966 (16) - the incidence of tricuspid endocarditis has increased considerably during recent years as a result of the progressive increase in drug addiction. This form of tricuspid insufficiency mainly affects intravenous drug users. The micro-organisms most frequently isolated in this case are *Staphylococcus aureus* and to a lesser extent gram-negative bacteria. Relapses are frequent in habitual and incurable drug addicts.

Other less frequent causes of tricuspid insufficiency

Tricuspid insufficiency of traumatic origin is in the great majority of cases a secondary condition accompanying a closed thoracic trauma (17,18). Two cases have been reported following external cardiac massage (19).

Although it may occur in isolation (20-22) or in conjunction with an atrial septal defect (23), tricuspid leaflet prolapse is mainly observed in patients with mitral leaflet prolapse. Its incidence in patients with Barlow's disease varies from 21% to 52% according to whether echocardiography (24-26) or angiography (27,28) is used for the investigation. The especially frequent association in patients with Marfan's syndrome (26) suggests a common dystrophic origin. This combined leaflet prolapse may also be associated with an aortic lesion of dystrophic origin, for example dilation of the ascending aorta and aortic leaflet prolapse in floppy valve syndrome (25,29). The incidence of tricuspid insufficiency in tricuspid valve prolapse has been estimated at 40%, based on echocardiography (30).

Tricuspid insufficiency may occur in the acute phase of myocardial infarction with bilateral ventricular extension. The clinical and hemodynamic picture is in this case more serious and the mortality figures are higher (31). It is linked with necrosis of the papillary muscle, which may rupture on occasion (10,32,33). It sometimes occurs as a secondary condition against a background of overall cardiac insufficiency (34,35).

Tricuspid disease as part of the carcinoid syndrome is covered in the chapter devoted to tricuspid stenosis (36-38).

Less common causes of tricuspid insufficiency include cardiac tumors, particularly right atrial myxoma, endomyocardial fibrosis (39), systemic lupus erythematosus (40), sinus of Valsalva aneurysm (41) and lesions induced by methysergide therapy (42). It should also be noted that an echocardiographic study in pregnant women revealed minor or moderate tricuspid regurgitation in more than 40% of patients (43).

PATHOPHYSIOLOGY

Dilation of the annulus plays a major part in the pathophysiology of functional tricuspid insufficiency (TI), the dilation apparently being proportional to the dimensions of the regurgitant jet (44-47). The surface area of the tricuspid leaflet is not a constant parameter but varies during the cardiac cycle (46,48); it is maximal during enddiastole after the P wave on the ECG, reaching a minimum during midsystole. The percentage shortening of the annulus is reduced in inverse proportion to the magnitude of the regurgitation (45,46).

In addition to the dilation of the annulus, right ventricular dilation predisposes the patient to tricuspid insufficiency by causing a misalignment of the papillary muscles with a consequent abnormal tensile stress on the chordae tendineae which interferes with normal leaflet function. Pathologic echocardiographic phenomena such as an anterior displacement of the site of valvular coaptation or unsatisfactory leaflet alignment have been described on occasion (47,49). Even though there is no close correlation between the level of pulmonary arterial hypertension and the degree of tricuspid insufficiency (11,50), pulmonary arterial hypertension is the main cause of functional TI. In the case of massive isolated tricuspid regurgitation, such as after tricuspidectomy for the treatment of bacterial endocarditis, the right ventricular volume overload gives rise, as a result of ventricular interdependence, to changes in the geometry of the left heart, a reduction in the left ventricular preload and a decrease in the left atrial contribution to left ventricular filling (51).

CLINICAL MANIFESTATIONS

Rheumatic tricuspid insufficiency

Functional signs

Since rheumatic tricuspid insufficiency never occurs in isolation, its characteristic clinical symptoms are often masked by those of the associated cardiopathy. The functional symptoms are in general clearly marked; effort dyspnea has been noted in more than 80% of the cases (52-54). It is frequently associated with decubitus dyspnea or even with attacks of paroxysmal dyspnea. On the other hand, these forms of dyspnea may be only minor or absent. The symptoms of dyspnea secondary to a left heart cardiopathy tend sometimes to become less frequent with the onset of tricuspid insufficiency, although many patients continue to suffer dyspnea as a result of pleural effusions or possible embolus migration. Painful congestive hepatomegaly is not uncommon.

Clinical signs

The clinical diagnosis of tricuspid insufficiency is based on three signs; xiphoid systolic murmur, systolic expansion of the liver and systolic venous pulse. The characteristic TI murmur is holosystolic, with a soft tone and a low or moderate intensity. It is located in general in the xiphoid area or in the lower part of the left sternal border. In the case of substantial right ventricular dilation it may be audible as far away as the apex, where it may be confused with mitral regurgitation even though it does not radiate to the axilla. Its most informative characteristic is the Rivero-Carvallo sign, i.e. its appearance and/or frank increase in intensity during deep inspiration (1). The murmur of a major regurgitation is sometimes accompanied by a third right sound (53,54) followed by a brief diastolic murmur with a blowing tone, even in the absence of any associated stenosis (52,55). Although valuable for diagnostic purposes when present, this murmur is unfortunately not always present even in the case of a severe regurgitation (56); the frequency of its occurrence varies greatly from one series to another (45% in Lingamneni's angiographic series (50) and 97% in Salazar's clinical series (54)).

The systolic venous pulse should be searched with the patient in the semi-recumbent position, with the neck slightly bent and the head slightly rotated to the left. It appears as a wave motion in the upward direction following the path of the jugular veins, and may be suppressed, unlike arterial pulses, by gentle compression. Occasionally it is clearly marked and readily detectable even in varicose veins of the lower limbs (57). It is completely absent in other cases, even those with major regurgitation (54,56). It is, moreover, by no means a specific phenomenon, since it may also be observed, in the absence of any form of regurgitation, in patients with complete arrhythmia resulting from atrial fibrillation. Exceptionally, a venous systolic thrill and murmur may be present (58).

Systolic expansion of the liver is a major sign of tricuspid insufficiency. Rarely visible on inspection (causing a systolic rise in the anterior face of the right lobe below the costal margin), it is detectable by palpation, preferably during post-inspirational apnea, either by pressing the back of the closed fist on the lateral face of the right hypochrondrium or by palpation with both hands. This again is not a constant phenomenon and various assessments have been made of its frequency; 21% for Lingamneni in moderate to severe regurgitation, 76% for Muller and 91% for Salazar. Hepatomegaly is almost always present. It may be painful and may lead to hepato-jugular reflux in the case of right ventricular failure (59). It is often accompanied in the advanced stage of the disease by splenomegaly, even in the absence of any bacterial lesion (54). Characteristic changes appear on the face in the advanced forms, consisting of a combination of erythrocyanosis, pallor and subicterus (Shattuk facies), as well as changes in the patient's general state, involving asthenia and in particular cachexia due to the fall in cardiac output.

Clinical picture in other etiologies of organic tricuspid insufficiency

These etiologies normally involve isolated regurgitation. The functional symptoms are restricted in this case to effort dyspnea without orthopnea or any paroxysmal phenomena, hepatic pain and possibly, in the case of a major regurgitation, manifestations of right ventricular insufficiency. Some etiologies have specific clinical characteristics (in bacterial TI, for example, the clinical picture combines the normal signs of septicemia due to endocarditis with those of septic pulmonary migration; thoracic pain, cough, purulent sputum with radiologic evidence of diffuse pulmonary shading, frequently leading to abscess formation). The clinical signs of tricuspid insufficiency are not always clear. Sterilization of the lesions can in general be obtained by antibiotic therapy alone, but in some cases of Gram-negative or fungal endocarditis surgery is unavoidable. This applies to about 25% of cases (60,61).

In traumatic TI the functional tolerance depends on the extent of the lesions; a schematic distinction can be made between the rupture or tearing of a papillary muscle, which will usually lead to a rapid progression, and chordal ruptures, which may

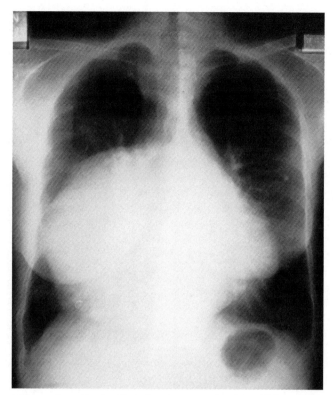

Figure 6.1-1: Chest X ray of a patient with isolated traumatic tricuspid insufficiency. Note the right atrial enlargement.

occasionally remain symptom-free over very long periods (32 years in one case reported by Morgan (62)). The clinical picture has no clearly marked characteristics apart from the frequent pericardial effusions noted during the initial period. There is however the possibility of a secondary cyanosis as a result of a right-left shunt in the event of a reopening of the patent foramen ovale or of an associated ASD (63,64).

Electrocardiography

The ECG is only exceptionally normal in tricuspid insufficiency. The readings are influenced by the associated heart condition and no specific abnormality can be identified. Atrial fibrillation has been noted in two thirds of cases by a number of authors (52-54,56). Where a sinus rhythm is present, the atrial ECG is virtually never normal, in most cases exhibiting an appearance of bi-atrial overload and clear evidence of right atrial hypertrophy in v1. The ventricular ECGs are also mainly abnormal, in most cases with evidence of right ventricular or bi-ventricular hypertrophy linked with the associated mitral disease. Numerous authors have stressed the frequent initial negative waves at $v3_R$ and v1 with q-R aspects attributable to the right atrial dilation opposite the parasternal electrodes. The frequency of intraventricular conduction disorders in traumatic tricuspid insufficiency is also worth emphasizing; a complete or incomplete

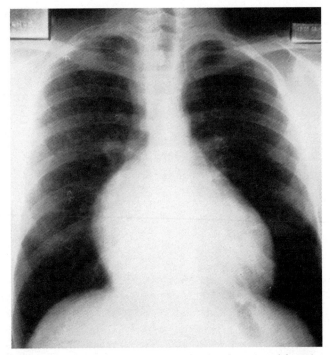

Figure 6.1-2: Chest X ray in a case of severe mitral valve disease and functional tricuspid insufficiency.

right bundle branch block has been found in more than 90% of all observations and is associated in half of the cases with left bundle branch hemiblock, more often anterior than posterior. These conduction disorders are probably of traumatic origin and may induce a paroxysmal atrioventricular block, necessitating a pacemaker (65).

Radiologic data

The right atrium is prominent. There is no strict correlation between the magnitude of the atrial dilation and the regurgitant volume (Fig. 6.1-1 and 6.1-2). The dilation of the right atrium is often masked by that of the right ventricle and the left atrium in the case of an associated cardiopathy. The systolic expansion of the right atrium is apparent in the radioscopic image in less than 10% of cases.

Phonocardiogram

This topic has been fully covered in Chapter 3.1 (66).

DOPPLER ECHOCARDIOGRAPHY

Doppler echocardiography is currently the reference complementary examination in tricuspid insufficiency, simultaneously enabling a definite and etiologic diagnosis to be arrived at and a semiquantitative assessment of the extent of the regurgitation to be made.

Definite diagnosis

Contribution of echocardiography

Two-dimensional echocardiography only provides indirect evidence of tricuspid insufficiency in the form of right ventricular volume overload, which is not very sensitive and not specific. Before the introduction of the Doppler technique, contrast echocardiography was used to diagnose TI by revealing a systolic reflux of particles from the right heart cavities into the inferior vena cava or the supra-hepatic veins. In experienced hands this technique provided a definite diagnosis in almost 100% of cases (67,68).

Contribution of the Doppler technique

Doppler echocardiography has become the method of choice for diagnosing TI. The sensitivity and specificity of the method are close to 100% irrespective of the mode (continuous- or pulsed-wave, or color)(69-76). With continuous-wave Doppler, the tricuspid insufficiency appears in the form of a glove finger curve which is unidirectional and recorded exclusively in the negative zone. With pulsed-wave Doppler, the characteristic feature of TI is the presence of a turbulent, retrograde flow from the right ventricle into the right atrium, producing a spectrum of rectangular appearances, equally distributed between positive and negative values as a result of an aliasing phenomenon. The diagnosis is easy with color Doppler; the tricuspid insufficiency appears in the form of a predominantly blue jet which originates at the leaflet coaptation and extends to a varying extent into the right atrium. Color Doppler is of particular value in the case of eccentric jets, where it greatly facilitates the diagnosis. In the difficult case of patients who are not very echogenic, this procedure can be improved by the simultaneous performance of a contrast test (77).

Physiologic regurgitation

A small, so-called physiologic tricuspid insufficiency has been found in 60% to 100% of all normal subjects, depending on the particular series. Three conditions must be met before the use of the term "physiologic tricuspid insufficiency" may be justified; (a) the absence of a tricuspid murmur during auscultation, (b) normal movements and texture of the leaflets under echocardiography and (c) the absence of dilation of the right heart cavities (78-81).

Etiologic diagnosis

In functional tricuspid insufficiency the leaflets have normal texture and kinetic properties. Measurement of the surface area of the tricuspid annulus by two-dimensional echocardiography is in practice extremely difficult (46). In rheumatic TI the leaflets are thickened, in particular at their free margin, and tricuspid stenosis is sometimes present simultaneously (82). In the case of regurgitation following endocarditis, the diagnosis is based on the presence of vegetation, sometimes associated with chordal rupture. The vegetation is visualized two-dimensionally in the form of echogenic masses, sessile or pediculate, attached to the leaflets but without restricting their movements (83,84). They may be extensive, diminishing in size or disappearing after septic pulmonary migration. Two-dimensional echocardiography is used for the diagnosis of tricuspid valve prolapse, which appears as a displacement of the coaptation line above the annular plane (80-82,84). Less frequently the tricuspid prolapse is secondary to chordal rupture, identified by the complete eversion of a leaflet into the right atrium. In tricuspid insufficiency due to carcinoid tumours, the leaflets take on a characteristic appearance; they are thickened, excessively echogenic, especially at their free end, retracted and not very mobile. Sometimes a loss of coaptation occurs during systole resulting in a massive TI (85-88). Traumatic injury of the thorax may cause chordal rupture (89). Usually it is difficult to image this by transthoracic echocardiography, which nevertheless reveals the inversion of the free margin of a leaflet into the right atrium. TI is frequently present in right ventricular necrosis, where akinesia of the free or diaphragmatic wall is noted, accompanied by dilation of the right ventricle, frequently with a paradox septal movement.

Transesophageal echocardiography may be of value, irrespective of the etiology, in patients who are insufficiently echogenic when examined by TTE.

Quantification of tricuspid insufficiency

The contribution of two-dimensional echocardiography

The degree of dilation of the right heart cavities or of the inferior vena cava is not a very specific parameter. Some authors have attempted to measure the diameter of the annulus in functional regurgitations in order to predict the need for annuloplasty (90,91). Chopra (90) found that 88% of her patients with tricuspid annulus dilation (diastolic diameter > 38 mm) benefited from tricuspid surgery accompanied by valve replacement in the left heart. Annuloplasty should also be envisaged in the case of a reduction in the percentage shortening of the tricuspid annulus (maximum diastolic diameter less minimum systolic diameter/maximum diastolic diameter) to below 25%.

The contribution of color Doppler

Color Doppler provides a means of measuring the extent of the regurgitation (75). Some authors (77,90) assess the tricuspid insufficiency as moderate where the maximum surface area is 4-8 cm^2 or where the ratio of the area of the regurgitant jet surface to that of the right atrium is less than 34%. The condition is considered to be serious, on the other hand, where the maximum surface area reaches 9 or 10 cm^2 and where the ratio of the surface areas exceeds 35% or 40%. This quantification of tricuspid insufficiency is in practice open to serious criticism, since the dimensions of the regurgitant jet are influenced by many factors other than the regurgitant volume, for example the equipment and settings used, the echogenicity of the patient, the hemodynamic conditions and the direction of the regurgitant jet.

Pulsed-wave Doppler

The laminar characteristics of the regurgitant flux are a clear criterion of severe tricuspid insufficiency; in the paper by Minagoe (92), 19 out of 21 patients with a laminar flow were suffering from severe TI. Unfortunately this criterion lacks sensitivity and its absence does not exclude the possibility of a major regurgitation. Analysis of the flow rate in the inferior vena cava, and in particular in the hepatic veins during expiratory apnea, appears to be a much more valuable criterion. In normal subjects (93) the recorded flow velocity curve consists of two negative waves (with the flow moving away from the sensor in the direction of the right atrium); a profound systolic wave, corresponding to atrial relaxation, and a diastolic wave of lesser amplitude, corresponding to the passive filling of the right ventricle. The ratio of the maximum systolic and diastolic flow velocities is greater than one.

Tricuspid insufficiency is accompanied by a reduced amplitude of the systolic wave, if not its complete inversion, as a result of the retrograde flow induced in the right atrium. Numerous authors have studied the maximum systolic velocity divided by the maximum diastolic velocity ratio as a means of quantifying TI (94-96). This ratio correlates well with the angiographic grading, although there is some overlapping in the values between the different gradings.

Continuous-wave Doppler

Continuous-wave Doppler is of no value for the quantification of tricuspid insufficiency. It does however enable the estimation of the systolic pulmonary arterial pressure on the basis of the maximum flow velocity in TI. Using the simplified Bernoulli equation, the systolic right atrioventricular gradient is found to be 4 V2 (97).

RADIONUCLIDE TECHNIQUES

Few papers have dealt with the value of radionuclide techniques for the diagnosis and quantification of tricuspid insufficiency. Lumia (98) correlated the extent of TI in 51 patients, revealed by the first passage of a radionuclide angiogram, with the results of the right ventricular angiogram. The sensitivity of the radionuclide technique was found to be 93%, its specificity 90% and the correlation between the quantification values obtained by the two methods was good. Handler (99) found a reduction in the regurgitation index (defined as the ratio of left heart to right heart output) and a very clearly marked increase in the hepatic expansion index (obtained by analyzing the variations in hepatic activity) in nine patients, all suffering from major TI. These results appear, however, to be rather incomplete, and further studies are needed in order to obtain an accurate assessment of the value and precise significance of these radionuclide techniques.

HEMODYNAMIC EXPLORATIONS

Cardiac catheterization, once the method of choice for the diagnosis and quantification of tricuspid insufficiency, based on analysis of the pressure curves and on right ventricular angiography, has become less favored since the advent of Doppler echocardiography.

Pressure curves

Analysis of the right atrial pressure curve enables us to distinguish three patterns which correspond theoretically to increasing degrees of regurgitation. In type I the normal morphology is retained, the X wave on the curve being more prominent than the Y. In type II the X wave tends to disappear, becoming shallower than the Y wave, with a parallel increase in the amplitude of the V wave. In type III, the X wave disappears completely, being replaced by a positive systolic wave, on occasion of considerable amplitude, enclosing the V wave and imparting a ventricular appearance to the atrial curve. It is to be noted that these are not fully reliable criteria, even when supported by a deep inspiration, which may render them more sensitive. Even a major tricuspid insufficiency may not be accompanied by any change in the morphology of the pressure curve provided that sinus rhythm is maintained (100). On the other hand, type II curves may be observed in the absence of any regurgitation in patients with atrial fibrillation (101).

The mean right atrial pressure is normally high in patients with tricuspid insufficiency (50). Where it exceeds 10 mmHg in the absence of an associated stenosis, this normally indicates an extensive TI. The pressure may still be normal even with major regurgitations, although this in no way excludes the diagnosis of tricuspid insufficiency. On the other hand, an increase during inspiration or at least a constant pressure (as opposed to a physiological drop in pressure) is regarded by Lingamneni (50) as a sensitive though not specific diagnostic factor. The right ventricular enddiastolic pressure may be normal or high, indicating in this case a right ventricular insufficiency. The pulmonary arterial pressure has long been used as a means of distinguishing organic and functional regurgitations, although this criterion appears to be very unreliable, since in several large series (13,50) no correlation was found between pulmonary arterial pressure, pulmonary arterial resistance, cardiac index and the extent of regurgitation.

Right ventricular angiography

This technique has long been criticized as a means of quantifying tricuspid insufficiency because of the frequent risk of regurgitation artefacts (30% according to Cairns (101)), resulting from interference with leaflet movement induced by the catheter or by ventricular extrasystoles during injection of the contrast medium. These difficulties have been surmounted by the use of pre-shaped (102) or balloon catheters (103). Assessment of the dimensions of the regurgitant jet is based on the rapidity, density, extent and shading of the atrial cavity, bearing in mind that allowance must be made for the dimensions of the right heart cavities, the right ventricular contractility and the type of regurgitation (since a narrow jet appears to have greater density than an area jet (104,105)). The organic or functional nature of TI may often be determined by this method (106); an area regurgitation, covering the whole surface of a dilated but otherwise normal annulus accompanied by closing of the leaflet in two movements indicates a functional origin, whereas a localized regurgitation in jet form, an annulus with normal size but irregular diameter and leaflet closure in a single movement argue in favor of organic TI. It must be emphasized in any case that this angiographic technique prolongs an already long hemodynamic exploration in subjects with multivalvular disease who are in some cases already very weak. Since the introduction of Doppler echocardiography, therefore, right ventricular angiography is only infrequently used.

The recording of intracardiac sound (107) and the study of dilution curves (108,109) have been completely abandoned.

POSTOPERATIVE OUTCOME

The outcome of tricuspid insufficiency, ignored during the surgical treatment of left sided valvular disease, has been the subject of considerable research, the results of which are sometimes contradictory. There are various reasons for the disparities between different patient series; an unequal distribution of the most serious heart conditions between the groups classified as good or bad results (110) in particular, and the variable criteria adopted for defining tricuspid insufficiency, assessing its organic or functional nature and its quantification. Intraoperative data and in particular a mere tactile approach are obviously insufficient and hardly reliable in this context (111-115).

Nevertheless, all authors regard the treatment of major tricuspid insufficiency as desirable to ensure the quality of long term results, since the secondary regression of a TI cannot be relied on and its persistence has been responsible for a number of late failures. The outcome of tricuspid regurgitation appears to depend on a wide range of factors:

- The quality of the repair of the left sided valvulopathy appears to be fundamental. Any incomplete or unsatisfactory repair, whether due to malfunction of a prosthesis, impaired systolic or diastolic left ventricular function or failure to treat the valve lesion, will result in persistence of TI as a consequence of the continuing pulmonary arterial hypertension.
- The preoperative cardiac status influences the outcome depending on the duration and extent of the TI, the degree of cardiomegaly and the deterioration of bi-ventricular systolic function. A major, long-standing TI in a patient with a highly dilated heart is very unlikely to regress (111,113).
- The organic or functional nature of the regurgitation also plays a part. Duran (112), on the basis of pre- and postoperative hemodynamic and angiographic studies, noted the invariable persistence of organic TI, while 50% of functional TIs could be expected to regress as a result of the decreasing pulmonary arterial resistance.
- The contractility of the right ventricle also exerts an influence by determining the percentage shortening of the annulus (44,45). This explains a number of unfavorable outcomes despite a satisfactory correction of left heart lesions.

Assessment of the effect of preoperative medical treatment on the existence and magnitude of the TI appears to be a simple and fairly sensitive means of predicting the postoperative outcome. In the absence of an organic lesion, the progress is usually favorable under medical treatment. The opposite is true for organic lesions (116). Details of the surgical treatment are given in Chapter 8.6.

References

1. Rivero-Carvallo JM. Signo para el diagnostico de las insufficiencas tricuspides. Arch Inst Cardiol Mex 1946;16:531-540
2. Silver MD, Lam JH, Ranganathan N et al. Morphology of the human tricuspid valve. Circulation 1971;43:333-348
3. Deloche A, Guerinon J, Fabiani JN et al. Etude anatomique des valvulopathies rhumatismales tricuspidiennes. Application a l'etude critique des differentes methodes d'annuloplastie. Arch Mal Coeur 1974;64:497-505
4. Waller BF, Moriarty AT, Eble JN, Davey DM, Hawley DA, Pless JE. Etiology of pure tricuspid regurgitation: based on annular circumference and leaflet area: analysis of 45 necropsy patients with clinical and morphologic evidence of pure tricuspid regurgitation. J Am Coll Cardiol 1986;7:1063-1074
5. Hauck AJ, Freeman DP, Ackermann DM, Danielson GK, Edwards W. Surgical pathology of the tricuspid valve: a study of 363 cases spanning 25 years. Mayo Clin Proc 1988;63:851-863
6. Dressler FA, Roberts WC. Infective endocarditis in opiate addicts. Analysis of 80 case studies at necropsy. Am J Cardiol 1989;63:1240-1257
7. Roberts WC, Buchbinder NA. Right sided valvular infective endocarditis: a clinico-pathologic study of twelve necropsy patients. Am J Med 1972;53:7-19
8. Stephenson LW, Mac Vaugh H, Kastor JA. Tricuspid valvular incompetence and rupture of the ventricular septum caused by nonpenetrating trauma. J Thorac Cardiovasc Surg 1979;77:768-772
9. Boisselier P, Lombaert M, Rey JL et al. Insuffisance tricuspidienne et anevrysme ventriculaire droit traumatique. A propos d'un cas. Arch Mal Coeur 1981;74:1465-1469
10. Eisenberg S, Suyemato J. Rupture of a papillary muscle of the tricuspid valve following acute myocardial infarction. Circulation 1964;30:588-591
11. Roberts WC, Sjoerdsma A. The cardiac disease associated with the carcinoid syndrome: carcinoid heart disease. Am J Med 1964;36:5-34
12. Morrison DA, Ouitt T, Hammermeister KE. Functional tricuspid regurgitation and right ventricular dysfunction in pulmonary hypertension. Am J Cardiol 1988;62:108-112
13. Dickerman SA, Rubler S. Mitral and tricuspid valve regurgitation in dilated cardiomyopathy. Am J Cardiol 1989;63:629-631
14. Daniels SJ, Mintz GS, Kotler MN. Rheumatic tricuspid valve disease: two dimensional echocardiographic hemodynamic and angiographic correlations. Am J Cardiol 1983;51:492-496
15. Aceves S, Carral R. The diagnosis of tricuspid valve disease. Am Heart J 1947;34:114-130
16. Ahn AJ, Segal BL. Isolated tricuspid insufficiency: clinical features, diagnosis and management. Prog Cardiovasc Dis 1966;9:166-193
17. Roger V, Carpentier A, Arie A, Vahanian A, Enriquez-Sarano M, Acar J. L'insuffisance tricuspidienne traumatique. A propos d'un cas traite par chirurgie conservatrice. Arch Mal Coeur 1987;80:677-681
18. Gayet C, Pierre B, Delahaye JP, Champsaur G, Andre-Fouet X, Rueff P. Traumatic tricuspid insufficiency. An underdiagnosed disease. Chest 1987;92:429-432
19. Gerry JL, Bulkley BH, Hutchins GM. Rupture of the papillary muscle of the tricuspid valve. A complication of cardiopulmonary resuscitation and a rare cause of tricuspid insufficiency. Am J Cardiol 1977;40:825-828
20. Chandraratna PAN, Lopez JM, Fernandez JJ et al. Echocardiographic detection of tricuspid valve prolapse. Circulation 1975;51:823-826
21. Weinreich DJ, Burke JF, Bharati S, Leu M. Isolated prolapse of the tricuspid valve. J Am Coll Cardiol 1985;6:475-481
22. Jackson D, Gibbs HR, Zee-Cheng CS. Isolated tricuspid valve prolapse diagonal by echocardiography. Am J Cardiol 1986;80:281-284
23. Chandraratna PAN, Littman BB, Wilson D. The association between atrial septal defect and prolapse of the tricuspid valve: an echocardiographic study. Chest 1978;73:839-842
24. Morganroth J, Jones RH. Chen CC et al. Two-dimensional echocardiography in mitral aortic and tricuspid valve prolapse. The clinical problem, cardiac nuclear imaging considerations and a proposed standard for diagnosis. Am J Cardiol 1980;46:1164-1177
25. Ogawa S, Hayashi J, Sasaki H. et al. Evaluation of combined valvular prolapse syndrome by two-dimensional echocardiography. Circulation 1982;65:174-180
26. Werner JA, Schiller NB, Prasquier R. Occurrence and significance of echocardiographically demonstrated tricuspid valve prolapse. Am Heart J 1978;96:180-186
27. Gooch AS, Maranhao V, Scampardonis G et al. Prolapse of both mitral and tricuspid leaflets in systolic murmur-click syndrome. N Engl J Med 1972;287:1218-1222
28. Maranhao V, Gooch AS, Yang SS et al. Prolapse of the tricuspid leaflets in the systolic murmur-click syndrome. Cathet Cardiovasc Diagn 1975;1:81-90
29. Rippe JM, Angoff G, Sloss LJ et al. Multiple floppy valves: an echocardiographic syndrome. Am J Med

1979;66:817-824

30. Chen CC, Morganroth J, Mardelli TJ et al. Tricuspid regurgitation in tricuspid valve prolapse demonstrated with contrast cross-sectional echocardiography. Am J Cardiol 1980;46:983-987

31. Descaves C, Daubert JC, Langella B et al. L'insuffisance tricuspidienne des infarctus du myocarde biventriculaire. Arch Mal Coeur 1985;78:1287-1295

32. Raabe DS, Chester AC. Right ventricular infarction. Chest 1978;73:96-99

33. Penther P, Boschat J, Blanc JJ, Etienne Y. L'insuffisance tricuspidienne dans les infarctus posterieurs par ischemie de l'artere coronaire droite. Etude anatomique. Arch Mal Coeur 1985;78:907-912

34. Mc Allister RG, Friessinger GC, Sinclair-Smith BC. Tricuspid regurgitation following inferior myocardial infarction. Arch Intern Med 1976;136:95-99

35. Zone DD, Botti RE. Right ventricular infarction with tricuspid insufficiency and chronic right heart failure. Am J Cardiol 1976;37:445-458

36. Acar J, Auriol M, Lainee R et al. Cardiopathie carcinoide et tumeur de l'ovaire; a propos d'un cas anatomoclinique. Ann Med Interne 1970;121:329-340

37. Herreman F, Vernant P, Cachera JP et al. Insuffisance tricuspidienne severe et tumeur carcinoide primitive de l'ovaire. Succes du remplacement valvulaire a long terme. A propos d'une observation. Arch Mal Coeur 1978;71:72-80

38. Pellika PA, Tajik AJ, Khanderia BK et al. Carcinoid heart disease. Clinical and echocardiographic spectrum in 74 patients. Circulation 1993;87:1188-1196

39. Harley JB, McIntosh CL, Kirklin JJ et al. Atrioventricular valve replacement in the idiopathic hypereosinophilic syndrome. Am J Med 1982;73:77-81

40. Lauper J, Frand M, Milo S. Valve replacement for severe tricuspid regurgitation caused by Libman-Sacks, endocarditis Br Heart J 1982;48:294-297

41. Gibbs KL, Peardon MJ, Strickman NE et al. Hemodynamic compromise (tricuspid stenosis and insufficiency) caused by unruptured aneurysm of the sinus of valsalva. J Am Coll Cardiol 1986;7:1177-1181

42. Bana DC, MacNeal PS, Lecompte PD et al. Cardiac murmurs and endocardial fibrosis associated with methysergide therapy. Am Heart J 1974;88:640-655

43. Limacher MC, Ware A, 0'Heara ME, Fernandez GC, Young JB. Tricuspid regurgitation during pregnancy, two-dimensional and pulsed Doppler echocardiographic observations. Am J Cardiol 1985;55:1059-1062

44. Simon R, Oelert H, Borst HG et al. Influence of mitral valve surgery on tricuspid incompetence concomitant with mitral valve disease. Circulation 1980;62(Suppl I):152-157

45. Ubago JL, Figueroa A, Ochoteco A et al. Analysis of the amount of tricuspid valve annular dilatation required to produce functional tricuspid regurgitation. Am J Cardiol 1983;52:155-158

46. Tei C, Pilgrim JP, Shah PM et al. The tricuspid valve annulus: study of size and motion in normal subjects and in patients with tricuspid regurgitation. Circulation 1982;66:665-671

47. Mikami T, Kudo T, Sakurai N et al. Mechanisms for development of functional tricuspid regurgitation determined by pulsed Doppler and two-dimensional echocardiography. Am J Cardiol 1984;53:160-163

48. Tsakiris AG, Mair DD, Seki S et al. Motion of the tricuspid valve annulus, in anesthetized intact dogs. Circ Res 1975;36:43-48

49. Come PC, Riley MF. Tricuspid annular dilatation and failure of tricuspid leaflet coaptation in tricuspid regurgitation. Am J Cardiol 1985;55:599-601

50. Lingamneni R, Cha SD, Maranhao V et al. Tricuspid regurgitation: clinical and angiographic assessment. Cathet Cardiovasc Diagn 1979;5:7-17

51. Louie EK, Bieniarz T, Moore AM, Levitsky S. Reduced atrial contribution to left ventricular filling in patients with severe tricuspid regurgitation after tricuspid valvulectomy. A Doppler echocardiographic study. J Am Coll Cardiol 1990;16:1617-1624

52. Himbert J, Joly J, Lenegre J. Etude clinique de 111 cas d'insuffisance tricuspidienne. Sem Hop Paris 1958;34:794-814

53. Muller O, Shillingfrod J. Tricuspid incompetence. Brit Heart J 1954;16:195-207

54. Salazar E, Levine HD. Rheumatic tricuspid regurgitation: the clinical spectrum. Am J Med 1962;33:111-129

55. Delzant JF, Forman J, Machado G et al. Insuffisance tricuspidienne fonctionnelle et organique (A propos de 60 cas etudies par catheterisme et phonocardiographie intracavitaire). Arch Mal Coeur 1968;61:305-332

56. Cha SD, Desai RS, Gooch AS et al. Diagnosis of severe tricuspid regurgitation. Chest 1982;82:726-731

57. Brickner PW, Scudder WT, Weinrib M. Pulsating varicose veins in functional tricuspid insufficiency. Circulation 1962;25:126-129

58. Amidi M, Irwin JM, Salerni R et al. Venous systolic thrill and murmur in the neck. A consequence of severe tricuspid insufficiency. J Am Coll Cardiol 1986;7:942-945

59. Maisel AS, Atwood JE, Goldberger AL. Hepatojugular reflux: useful in the bedside diagnosis of tricuspid regurgitation. Ann Intern Med 1984:101:781-782

60. Friedlander G, Bouvet E, Witchitz S et al. L'endocardite infectieuse chez les drogues. Nouv Presse Med 1981;10:3045-3048
61. Ginzton LE, Siegel RJ, Criley JM. Natural history of tricuspid valve endocarditis: a two dimensional echocardiographic study. Am J Cardiol 1982;49:1853-1859
62. Morgan JR, Forker AD. Isolated tricuspid insufficiency. Circulation 1971;43:559-564
63. Bardy GH, Talano JV, Meyers S et al. Acquired cyanosis heart disease secondary to traumatic tricuspid regurgitation: case report with a review of the literature. Am J Cardiol 1979;44:1401-1406
64. Bensaid J, Maurat JP, Cherrier F et al. Resultats du remplacement monovalvulaire tricuspidien par une bioprothese. A propos de 21 cas. Arch Mal Coeur 1980;73:1313-1317
65. Gougne G; Dessouter P, Fernandez F et al. Insuffisance tricuspide traumatique avec bloc auriculo-ventriculaire syncopal. Coeur Med Interne 1979;18:501-507
66. Scheck-Krejca H, Zilstra F, Roelandt J, Vletter-Mc Ghie J. Diagnosis of tricuspid regurgitation: comparison of jugular venous and liver pulse tracings with combined two-dimensional and Doppler-echocardiography. Eur Heart J 1986;7:937-938
67. Meltzer RS, Van Hoogenhuyze D, Serruys PW et al. Diagnosis of tricuspid regurgitation by contrast echocardiography. Circulation 1981;63:1093-1099
68. Lieppe W, Behar VS, Scallion R et al. Detection of tricuspid regurgitation with two-dimensional echocardiography and peripheral vein injections. Circulation 1978;57:128-132
69. Waggoner AD, Quinones MA, Young JB et al. Pulsed Doppler echocardiographic detections of right-sided valve regurgitation. Am J Cardiol 1981;47:279-286
70. Curtius JM, Thyssen M, Breuer HW, Loogen F. Doppler versus contrast echocardiography for diagnosis of tricuspid regurgitation. Am J Cardiol 1985;56:333-336
71. Miyakate K, Okamoto M, Kinoshita N et al. Evaluation of tricuspid regurgitation by pulsed Doppler and two-dimensional echocardiography. Circulation 1982;66:777-784
72. Lesbre JP, Genuyt L, Lalau JD, Kalisa A, Andrejak MT, Boey S. Apport du Doppler pulse au diagnostic d'insuffisance tricuspidienne. Arch Mal Coeur 1984;77:1481-1493
73. Garcia-Dorado D, Falzgraf S, Almazan A et al. Diagnosis of functional tricuspid insufficiency by pulsed-wave Doppler ultrasound. Circulation 1982;66:1315-1321
74. Veyrat C, Kalmanson D, Farjon M et al. Non-invasive diagnosis and assessment of tricuspid regurgitation and stenosis using one and two dimensional echo-pulsed Doppler, Br Heart J 1982;47:596-605
75. Suzuki Y, Kambaia H, Kadota K et al. Detection and evaluation of tricuspid regurgitation using a real time two-dimensional color coded Doppler flow imaging system: comparison with contrast two-dimensional echocardiography and right ventriculography. Am J Cardiol 1986;57:811-815
76. Berger M, Haimowitz A, Van Tosh A, Berdoff RL, Goldberg E. Quantitative assessment of pulmonary hypertension in patients with tricuspid regurgitation using continuous wave Doppler ultrasound. J Am Coll Cardiol 1985;6:359-365
77. Waggoner AD, Barzilai B, Perez JE, Saline contrast enhancement of tricuspid regurgitant jets detected by Doppler color flow imaging. Am J Cardiol 1990;65:1368-1371
78. Yoshida K, Yoshikawa I, Shakudo M. Color Doppler evaluation of valvular regurgitation in normal subjects. Circulation 1988;78:840-847
79. Berger M, Hecht SR, Van Tosh A, Lingamu U. Pulsed and continuous wave Doppler echocardiographic assessment of valvular regurgitation in normal subjects. J Am Coll Cardiol 1989;13:1540-1545
80. Choong CY, Abascal VM, Weyman J et al. Prevalence of valvular regurgitation by Doppler echocardiography in patients with structurally normal hearts by two-dimensional echocardiography. Am Heart J 1989;117:636-642
81. Klein AL, Burstow DJ, Tajik AJ et al. Age related prevalence of valvular regurgitation in normal subjects: a comparative color flow examination of 118 volunteers. J Am Soc Echo 1990;2:54-63
82. Cormier B, Dorent R, Dewilde J, Richaud C, Preud'homme G, Acar J. Etude du mecanisme etiologique des regurgitations valvulaires en echo-Doppler. Arch Mal Coeur 1990;83:805-814
83. Chandraratna PAN, Aronow WS. Spectrum of echocardiographic findings in tricuspid valve endocarditis. Br Heart J 1979;42:528-532
84. Berger M, Delfin LA, Jelveh M et al. Two-dimensional echocardiographic findings in right sided infective endocarditis. Circulation 1980;61:855-860
85. Howard RJ, Drobac M, Rider WD et al. Carcinoid heart disease: diagnosis by two dimensional echocardiography. Circulation 1982;66:1059-1065
86. Callahan JA, Wroblewski EM, Reeder GS, Edwards WD, Seward JB Tajik AJ. Echocardiographic features of carcinoid heart disease. Am J Cardiol 1982;30:762-770
87. Lundin L, Norheim I, Landelius J, Oberg K, Theodorsson-Norheim E, Carcinoid heart disease relationship of circulating vasoactive substances to ultrasound detectable cardiac abnormalities. Circulation 1988;77:264-269
88. Tribouilloy C, Slama MA, Rey JL, Marek A, Quiret JC, Lesbre JP. Demonstration par echo-Doppler d'une

atteinte polyvalvulaire au cours d'une cardiopathie carcinoide. Arch Mal Coeur 1989;82:109-114
89. Watanabe T, Katsume H, Matsukubo H et al. Ruptured chordae of the tricuspid valve due to non penetrating trauma: echocardiographic findings Chest 1981;80:751-753
90. Chopra HK, Nanda NC, Pan P et al. Can two-dimensional echocardiography and Doppler flow mapping identify the need for tricuspid valve repair? J Am Coll Cardiol 1989;14:1266-1274
91. Fischer EA, Goldman ME. Simple rapid method for quantification of tricuspid regurgitation by two-dimensional echocardiography. Am J Cardiol 1989;63:1375-1378
92. Minagoe S, Rahimtoola SH, Chandraratna PAN. Significance of laminar systolic regurgitant flow in patients with tricuspid regurgitation: a combined pulsed wave, continuous-wave Doppler and two-dimensional echocardiography. Am Heart J 1990;119:627-635
93. Appleton CP, Hattle LK, Popp RL. Superior vena cava and hepatic vein Doppler echocardiography in healthy subjects. J Am Coll Cardiol 1987;10:1032-1039
94. Diebold B, Touati R, Blanchard D, Peronneau P, Guermonprez JL, Maurice P. Quantitative assessment of tricuspid regurgitation by pulsed Doppler echocardiography. Br Heart J 1983;50:443-449
95. Pennestri F, Loperfido F, Salvatori MP et al. Assessment of tricuspid regurgitation by pulsed Doppler ultrasonography of the hepatic veins. Am J Cardiol 1984;54:363-368
96. Sakai K, Nakamura K, Satomi G, Kondo M, Hirosawa K. Evaluation of tricuspid regurgitation by blood flow pattern in the hepatic vein using pulsed Doppler technique. Am Heart J 1984;108:516-523
97. Yock PG, Popp RL. Non invasive estimation of right ventricular systolic pressure by Doppler ultrasound in patients with tricuspid regurgitation. Circulation 1984;70:657-662
98. Lumia FJ, Patil A, Germon PA et al. Tricuspid regurgitation by radionuclide angiography and contrast right ventriculography: a preliminary observation. J Nucl Med 1981;22:804-809
99. Handler B, Pavel DG, Pietras R et al. Equilibrium radionuclide gated angiography in patients with tricuspid regurgitation. Am J Cardiol 1983;51:305-310
100. Rubeiz GA, Nassar ME, Dagher IK. Study of the right atrial pressure pulse in functional tricuspid regurgitation and normal sinus rhythm. Circulation 1964;30:190-193
101. Cairns KB, Kloster FE, Bristow JD et al. Problems in the hemodynamic diagnosis of tricuspid insufficiency. Am Heart J 1968;75:173-179
102. Cha SD, Maranhao V, Lingamneni R et al. A new technique: right ventriculography using a preshaped catheter. Cathet Cardiovasc Diagn 1978;4:311-316
103. Ubago JL, Figueroa A, Colman T et al. Right ventriculography as a valid method for the diagnosis of tricuspid insufficiency. Cathet Cardiovasc Diagn 1981;7:433-441
104. Baron MG. Angiocardiographic evaluation of valvular insufficiency. Circulation 1971;43:599-605
105. Carlsson E, Gross R, Holt RG. The radiological diagnosis of cardiac valvular insufficiencies. Circulation 1977;55:921-933
106. Geschwind H, Tenaillon A, Samii K et al. Evaluation des lesions tricuspidiennes par la cineangiographie. Coeur 1975;6:687-701
107. Soulie P, Baculard P, Bouchard F et al. Catheterisme des cavites droites par le micromanometre dans les valvulites tricuspidiennes. Arch Mal Coeur 1961;54(Suppl I):131-146
108. Collins NP, Braunwald E, Morrow AG. Detection of pulmonic and tricuspid valvular regurgitation by means of indicator solutions. Circulation 1959;20:561-568
109. Hansing LE, Rowe GG. Tricuspid insufficiency: a study of hemodynamics and pathogenesis. Circulation 1972;45:793-799
110. Pluth JR, Ellis FH. Tricuspid insufficiency in patients undergoing mitral valve replacement: conservative management annuloplasty or replacement. J Thorac Cardiovasc Surg 1969;58:484-491
111. Carpentier A, Deloche A, Hanania G et al. Surgical management of acquired tricuspid valve disease. J Thorac Cardiovasc Surg 1974;67:53-65
112. Duran CMG, Pomar JL, Colman T et al. Is tricuspid valve repair necessary? J Thorac Cardiovasc Surg 1980;80:849-860
113. Fournier C, Gay J, Gerbaux A. Evolution a long terme des insuffisances tricuspides non operees apres correction chirurgicale des valvulopathies mitrales et mitro-aortiques. Arch Mal Coeur 1975;68:907-913
114. Fournier C, Gay J, Gerbaux A. Evolution a long terme des insuffisances tricuspides operees au cours de la correction chirurgicale des valvulopathies mitrales et mitro-aortiques. Arch Mal Coeur 1975;68:915-921
115. Braunwald E. Tricuspid regurgitation in Braunwald heart disease. A text book of cardiovascular Medicine (4th Ed); WB Saunders Philadelphia 1992;1055-1058
116. Colonna D, Duron F, Levy JP et al. Evaluation pre et per-operatoire de l'insuffisance tricuspidienne. Coeur 1975;6:661-670

Tricuspid Stenosis

Charles Starkman

Among the acquired valvular heart diseases, stenosis of the tricuspid valve (TS) is rare. Despite a net decline in the industrialized countries, the most frequent etiology remains post-rheumatic fibrosis. TS is therefore part of a multivalvular attack which nearly always includes mitral stenosis (MS) and often an aortic valve lesion as well. This difficult diagnosis, sometimes suspected on cardiovascular examination, is based on Doppler echocardiography and cardiac catheterization, possibly enhanced by pharmacodynamic tests. When the TS is tight, its correction, generally surgical, is required at the same time as that of the other valvular defects.

PATHOLOGY OF PRIMARY TRICUSPID VALVE STENOSIS

Post-rheumatic tricuspid stenosis

The history of the disease can be divided into three successive periods (1):

The anatomic/clinical period

This period extended from the start of the 18th century to 1950 (1-4). In 1704 Homberg attributed jugular venous dilatation and pulse to the result of right heart dilatation. In 1769, Morgagni demonstrated in an anatomical presentation that TS might be responsible for these venous signs. In 1806, Corvisart showed that stenosis of an atrioventricular valve can produce a precordial thrill. With the discovery of the stethoscope (Laennec 1819), Bertin in 1824 described the diastolic murmur and Duroziez in 1868 clarified the tricuspid diastolic murmur. In 1891, Shattuck observed that TS could occur in association with mitral stenosis in the event of peripheral venous stasis and distinguished the tricuspid from the mitral murmur.

With the commencement of the 20th century came the external recordings: in 1902, MacKenzie recorded the presystolic venous pulse accompanying the tricuspid murmur. In 1932, Zeisler linked the presystolic murmur in the tricuspid area to the great A wave of the jugular venous pulse. In 1946 in the case of incompetence, and in 1950 for stenosis, Rivero-Carvallo (5) showed the importance of maximum inspiration for eliciting tricuspid auscultatory signs.

The development of catheterization and surgery (4-9)

From 1951 Gorlin laid down the hemodynamic criteria for TS, i.e. the concept of pressure gradient and methods for estimating the valvular area. The construction of the micromanometer enabled the completion of the hemodynamic examination to include the recording of intracardiac sounds (10,11). In 1960, Perloff recorded the tricuspid presystolic murmur in the right ventricle (RV), where it is more intense than in the pericardial region, increases during inspiration and is accompanied by a mid-diastolic component which is inaudible in the precordium. In parallel, lesions were being discovered and clarified by contact with the tricuspid valve during the early commissurotomies on the closed heart in 1952 by Trace and Bailey (12).

The development of ultrasound methods

Joyner (13) published the first observations of TS by ultrasound in 1967. After anatomic scanning validation of the sections (14) obtained from two-dimensional (2D) echocardiography were published from 1982 onwards. The TS observations linking M-mode and 2D-echo showed not only the sensitivity of ultrasound in the diagnosis of organic tricuspid valve pathology but also its inability to demonstrate the degree of stenosis (15-22). At the same time, the application of the Doppler effect in the evaluation of intracardiac blood flow was developed. This was capable, in combination with the scan, of making a decisive contribution to the qualitative and quantitative diagnosis of TS (23-25).

PATHOMORPHOLOGY (1,3,26-34)

The normal tricuspid orifice

The normal tricuspid orifice is larger than the mitral orifice, and the valve has three leaflets inserted into a ring of 11.5 - 13.5 cm in circumference, resulting in an orifice area of approximately 8 cm^2. The leaflets are denoted as anterior which is the largest, septal and posterior, being separated by three commissures, the definition of which is more difficult than in the case of the mitral valve since the free edges of the anterior and septal leaflets have deep notches and the posterior leaflet is made up of two or three scallops separated by clefts. Commissures are in general defined by the variety of chordae known as "fan-shaped" chordae. Apart from the three commissural fan-shaped chordae, the tricuspid valve has, on average, 22 other chordae tendineae which are inserted into the ventricular side of the leaflets on the free edge as well as the rough part, the intermediate smooth area and into the base two millimeter from the ring. Intra-operatively, during tricuspid palpation, a normal orifice will permit the entry of three gloved fingers.

Post-rheumatic disease (32)

In predominant stenosis, there is nearly always an associated mild incompetence; the main lesion is a fusion of the three commissures. The leaflets are thickened and their free edges are slightly retracted. They retain, however, their flexibility over almost all their width. The chordae are only slightly involved. The annulus retains its normal dimensions. In the case of combined stenosis and a varying degree of incompetence, which is the most frequent case, the three commissures are fused to a variable degree. Fibrosis of the fused commissures is fairly dense and overlays the leaflets. The free edges of the leaflets are thick and rimmed. The chordae are in general thickened and retracted. The annulus is slightly dilated or remains normal. The damage is diffusely spread over the valvular tissue and chordae but there is no calcification.

PATHOPHYSIOLOGY (9,26)

The hemodynamic consequence of TS is a mean diastolic gradient between the right atrium (RA) and right ventricle (RV) of ≥ 2.0 mmHg at rest. The decreased cardiac output can be responsible for a borderline gradient in the resting state. The diagnosis can therefore be established by rapid i.v. infusion followed, if necessary, by an injection of atropine which causes the elevation of the mean diastolic gradient in the case of TS.

A mean diastolic gradient of 5.0 mmHg is sufficient to raise the mean right atrial pressure to a level sufficient to produce jugular venous distension, hepatomegaly, edema of the lower limbs or even ascites. TS also results in a fall in cardiac output at rest and a poor increase on effort, explaining the weakness and dyspnea in this state. The almost constant association of mitral stenosis with TS particularly decreases cardiac output, explaining the only modest elevation of the systolic pressure in the right ventricle, pulmonary artery and left atrium in double stenosis when compared with isolated mitral stenosis, and the relative protective effect of TS against the paroxysmal attacks of mitral stenosis.

OCCURRENCE

The prevalence of post-rheumatic disease of the tricuspid valve varies widely in different published series: high in postmortem series preceding the antibiotic era and in developing countries (30% to 67%) (28,35), lower in the early surgical series (20%, of which 5% was TS) (17,24,28,34). Post-rheumatic damage was estimated to occur in between 53% and 69% of pathology specimens of the resected tricuspid valve postoperatively since 1963 (33,34), with a net decline in those operated upon most recently; the series reported by Hauck found an incidence of 79% between 1963 and 1967, and 24% between 1983 and 1987. In the latter autopsy series of patients dying from valvular cardiopathy, the occurrence of TS was estimated at between 5% and 7% (32,34). So, post-rheumatic damage to the tricuspid valve induces, in general, a pure incompetence, less often a disease combining stenosis and marked incompetence and rarely a mainly predominant or pure stenosis (37).

A previous history of acute rheumatic fever is found in two out of three cases, in more than three cases out of four they are women between the age of 20 and 50 years (10,36,38,39). Multiple valve disease is nearly always present, inevitably consisting of a mitral stenosis and, in two thirds of cases, aortic disease (3,9,10,36,38-40). Very rare cases of isolated TS have been reported (41-45). A rheumatic etiology is probable in patients with a previous history of acute rheumatic fever, seen during surgery with slight mitral thickening (41) or with the post-surgical long term appearance of signs of moderate mitral stenosis (44). Congenital TS is possible in other cases (42,43,45) in the absence of a past history of acute rheumatic disease, in the presence of a cardiac murmur since infancy and in the absence of valvular or other associated anomalies on ultrasound and hemodynamic examination (45).

CLINICAL DATA

TS should be looked for in multivalvular patients. Careful analysis of functional signs, the results of clinical examination and phonomechanography affected by respiration, the ECG and chest x-ray establish the diagnosis of TS in three out of four cases prior to hemodynamic investigation (8-10,36,38,39), and currently echo Doppler is a valuable tool in the non-invasive diagnostic procedure.

Functional discomfort is dominated by weakness, effort dyspnoe and, as a result of systemic venous hypertension, liver tenderness, cervical discomfort caused by venous distension and pulse in the neck which is intensified on effort, or even peripheral edema and/or ascites. These signs contrast sharply with the rarity of the signs of pulmonary congestion even when mitral stenosis coexists.

Sinus rhythm is common. There is, in this case, a presystolic jugular and hepatic expansion on mechanogram recordings; the jugulogram registers a large and pointed A wave, a small V wave, a depression, and Y flattened with a very gradual descending slope, reflecting the absence of the right ventricular rapid filling phase. In the event of atrial fibrillation, the presystolic expansion disappears. The signs of systemic venous congestion are significant provided that they are not accompanied by signs of pulmonary arterial and capillary hypertension, i.e. palpation of a dilated right ventricle in the epigastric region and at the left sternal border, or a snapping of the second sound in the pulmonary region, or pulmonary alveolar rales. Palpation can detect a pulsatile thrust of the dilated right atrium at the right border of the sternum, a diastolic thrill in the lower part of the left sternal border, appearing or reinforced on inspiration.

Auscultatory signs are difficult to interpret due to the coexistence of mitral stenosis. One looks for a quieter zone between the apical site of mitral auscultation and the site of tricuspid auscultation situated in the mid and lower left sternal border. Inspiration and effort enhance the signs of TS whilst expiration and Valsalva maneuver reduce them. The diastolic murmur is more acute, earlier and shorter than that of a mitral origin. In sinus rhythm, it is mainly presystolic, climbing to a crescendo then waning to end before the first sound whilst the mitral murmur follows on up to the first sound.

In atrial fibrillation, it is limited to early diastole where it only appears during inspiration. The opening snap of the tricuspid valve has a poor diagnostic value. One can only be sure of its presence when the two opening snaps are heard, mitral at the apex, tricuspid at the lower part of the left border of the sternum. Their order varies with the degree of each stenosis (46); the more severe stenosis results in the earlier snap. The second sound is not split in the pulmonary area as on inspiration TS prevents the inspiratory increase of flow (10).

Investigations

On ECG (10,28,36,38,39), sinus rhythm is seen in more than 50% of cases despite an associated mitral stenosis. In this case the PR interval is often lengthened and can be shifted downwards as a result of the increase in the atrial T wave. There is the appearance of a right atrial overload contrasting with the absence of right ventricular overload; the P wave is more than 0.25 mV in II and III and aVF, and the P axis is greater than +70°. Right atrial dilatation can give rise to an interventricular septal rotation inducing a low QRS voltage in V1 with an initial q wave with a qr, qrs or qs appearance (3,26). Voltage increases from V2 (Fig. 6.1-3).

As a result of double stenosis, the electric appearance is often that of a bi-atrial

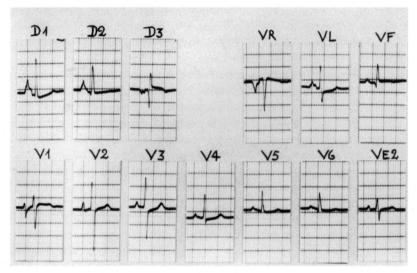

Figure 6.1-3: Electrocardiogramm: Tricuspid stenosis with mitral stenosis. Note the bi-atrial overload.

overload: pronounced and wide P waves in II-III-aVF and biphasic with an initial pronounced positivity followed by an increased negativity in V1.

On chest x-ray the cardiac silhouette is enlarged typically with a contrast between a dilated right atrium and the absence of signs of capillary and pulmonary arterial hypertension despite an associated mitral stenosis. In the frontal view, the right atrial dilatation gives a projection of the inferior right arch with a regular semi-circular edge extending to the dome of the right diaphragm below. The distance between the median line and the most external point of the inferior arch exceeds 50 mm (28,40). The dilatation of the superior vena cava upstream of the right atrium gives a vertical opacity to the right border of the trachea in which place one can note the superimposed opacity of the dilated azygos vein. On the opposite side, the trunk and branches of the pulmonary artery are not dilated and there is no pulmonary vascular overload. This topic is also discussed in Chapter 3.5.

Ultrasonic exploration (14-21,23-25,47-55) combines 2D- and M-mode echo-cardiography, and the study of trans-tricuspid blood flow using pulsed and continuous color flow Doppler. The difficulties in quantitative assessment with Doppler are due, on the one hand, to the presence or otherwise of atrial fibrillation, and on the other, to the tricuspid gradient variations during the respiratory cycle. Therefore, four to five cycles in sinus rhythm and nine to ten cycles in the presence of atrial fibrillation must be averaged by studying the gradient over one respiratory cycle during sinus rhythm and over two respiratory cycles in the case of atrial fibrillation. One can attempt to standardize the recording by collecting data during apnea following normal inspiration (51).

Echocardiographic imaging (14) is completed through the parasternal long axis window visualizing the anterior and posterior leaflets, and the parasternal short axis and the apical four-chamber windows visualizing the septal leaflet. If the transthoracic image is of poor quality, transesophageal echocardiography can complete the investigation.

M-mode guided by 2D-echo can measure the thickness of the tricuspid leaflets, the maximum opening of the anterior leaflet and its closing slope, as well as record the reduced and/or paradoxical motion of the septal and posterior leaflets. The thickening of the leaflets and their paradoxical motion are signs of organic valve damage, the reduction in the closing slope, even below 30mm/sec has no value as it is also influenced by right side cavity compliance, cardiac output, pulmonary pressure and the state of the pericardium. On the other hand, a maximum opening amplitude of the anterior leaflet of less than 10 mm would suggest a stenosis (47).

On 2D-echo, contrary to the mitral orifice, no section allows planimetry of the tricuspid orifice. Showing evidence of post-rheumatic damage, the thickening of the three leaflets and their reduced opening ability create the appearance of a diastolic dome where the distance separating the extremities of the valves at the summit of the dome is clearly less than the distance separating their base of insertion on the same section. There is also a "one time" valve closure. However, this diastolic dome appearance, even if it involves the three leaflets, is not specific to stenosis; in a consecutive series of 42 patients with this appearance on ultrasound, Ribeiro only recorded a mean diastolic gradient equal to or greater than 2 mmHg at catheterization at rest or during exercise in 22 patients. Echocardiography is therefore a sensitive method for detecting rheumatic damage in the tricuspid valve, but not for specifying the degree of stenosis.

Doppler echocardiography has therefore been decisive in enabling the calculation of the tricuspid diastolic gradient, using the simplified Bernoulli equation, in the estimation of associated tricuspid incompetence, and, to a certain degree, in the estimation of the functional valvular area. For further details see Chapter 3.2.

Normally (52,54,55), the anterograde diastolic trans-tricuspid flow consists of two elements, i.e., E wave, corresponding to early diastolic filling which rapidly declines, and the a wave, corresponding to the flow related to right atrial contraction. The maximum speed of the E wave is between 0.30 and 0.65 m/s, that of the a wave between 0.20 and 0.45 m/s. The E/a ratio is between 1.2 and 1.3. The half-time of the fall in the diastolic gradient (PHT) is between 30 and 50 ms. The velocity time integral (VTI) measured at the level of the tricuspid annulus by an apical four-chamber view is 8.7 ± 1.9 cm, with a range of 5.3 to 15.9 cm.

In TS, the maximum early diastolic speed of the E wave is equal to or higher than 1.0 m/s. The PHT is slowed down and a gradient is still present in late diastole both in sinus rhythm and in atrial fibrillation. However, this gradient can be increased by numerous factors: associated tricuspid incompetence, the inspiratory phase in the respiratory cycle, tachycardia and other factors increasing the cardiac output. Estimation of the effective valvular orifice should therefore be related to the calculation of the mean diastolic gradient. Two methods are proposed:

- the calculation of a constant ratio to the PHT. The constant is either that proposed by Hatle for the calculation of the mitral surface, i.e. 220, or that proposed by Fawzy, extracted from the ratio of constants used for the hemodynamic estimation of mitral and tricuspid orifice areas, i.e. 190. The effective tricuspid orifice calculated by this method is therefore 220/PHT or 190/PHT, the latter correlating better with the orifice area estimated from catheterization by Fawzy (50), whilst a good correlation was obtained with the 220 constant by Denning (55).
- the continuity equation (54) can be applied to the aortic or pulmonary orifice as a reference on the condition that the TS is pure and the reference orifice is normal.

One can therefore state that

effective tricuspid orifice = subaortic surface x subaortic VTI/tricuspid VTI
or
effective tricuspid orifice = PA trunk surface x PA trunk VTI/tricuspid VTI

Hemodynamic exploration consists of pressure and cardiac output recordings. The recording of intracardiac sounds and cineangiography can complete this examination. Low cardiac output, a slight RA-RV gradient and the usual association of tricuspid incompetence complicate the hemodynamic calculation of the tricuspid valvular area (9,28,38). The main hemodynamic appearance of TS is therefore the presence of a ≥ 2.0 mmHg mean diastolic gradient. A recording of excellent quality is necessary for the simultaneous measurement of RA-RV pressures, and is best achieved with a double lumen catheter and by curve standardization and eliminating artifacts.

The right atrial pressure curve in sinus rhythm has a large a wave which can reach the value of the right ventricular systolic pressure (26,40). Its descent is progressive, terminated by a notch coincidental with valve opening. The right atrial mean pressure is raised. The right ventricular pressure curve is unaltered. In sinus rhythm, the gradient is therefore at its peak during right atrial contraction. In atrial fibrillation, the gradient is at its peak in early diastole.

In deep inspiration the gradient increases due to physiologic inspiratory depression in the right ventricular diastolic pressure, whilst the right atrial pressure is hardly changed (4,9,10). As a result of the low cardiac output, the mean diastolic gradient can be less than 2.0 mmHg. An approach aimed at increasing the cardiac output should therefore complete the examination under continuous monitoring of clinical tolerance and capillary pulmonary pressure. That proposed by Ribeiro (51) consists of the rapid infusion of physiologic saline resulting in the mean right atrial pressure rising to 12 mmHg. The mean diastolic gradient is then recalculated. If it is still lower than 2.0 mmHg and if the heart rate is less than 85 beats/min, an intravenous injection of 0.6 mg of atropine is given with the further measurement of the gradient.

In a prospective series of 33 cases evaluated by Ribeiro with echocardiographic evidence of TS, 11 patients had a mean basal diastolic gradient of ≥ 2.0 mmHg. Of the remaining 22 cases, the gradient increased to more than 2.0 mmHg in four patients with the above mentioned procedures. Thirteen of these 33 patients underwent perioperative evaluation of the tricuspid orifice, estimated at between 1.0 and 2.0 cm^2 in cases with a spontaneous or induced gradient of ≥ 2.0 mmHg, versus more than 3.0 cm^2 in cases where the gradient remained below 2.0 mmHg.

Moreover, in comparison with isolated mitral stenosis, mitral and tricuspid stenosis in combination result in lower cardiac output, pulmonary arterial and capillary pressures (8,9,26).

Intracardiac sound and simultaneous pressure reading (3,4,10,11,38) is useful in recording the opening tricuspid snap and the diastolic murmur in the right ventricle and their exact timing (4).

Cineangiography is carried out with contrast injection into the RA and the RV in 30° right anterior oblique position (26,42,43,56). Atrial injection reveals a dilated RA with thickened walls, emptying progressively into the RV by a narrow jet and reduced tricuspid valve leaflet motion, forming the appearance of an atrial concave dome in diastole. Right ventricular injection gives the appearance of a diastolic ring due to stagnation of the contrast media between the tricuspid annulus and the base of the valve leaflets which have reduced opening and closing motion. It also facilitates the observation of any associated tricuspid incompetence.

TREATMENT

In multivalvular patients, the existence of a hemodynamically significant TS with a valvular surface of less than 2.0 cm^2 and a mean diastolic gradient in general of more than 5.0 mmHg will require correction (26).

Surgery

The first closed tricuspid commissurotomies from 1952 onwards gave satisfactory results, especially in the case of pure or predominant stenosis and by being restricted to an incomplete tricuspid commissurotomy to avoid the creation of a significant incompetence (28,36,38).

This technique was abandoned in favor of open heart surgery with a good assessment the lesions and selection of the appropriate correction which will, where possible, be conservative. Of 150 tricuspid operations, 26 of which had significant tricuspid stenosis, conservative intervention was carried out in 96% of cases at the Broussais Hospital between 1968 and 1972 (37). This commissurotomy, performed under direct vision, comprised the opening of the three commissures, or, if the valve was badly affected, an opening limited to two commissures was undertaken whilst leaving the fusion between the anterior and posterior leaflets intact to avoid creating a serious incompetence (26,37). The correction of this orifice is concluded by a Carpentier annuloplasty reducing the annular dilatation and the often associated incompetence (30).

Where conservative action is impossible, or if the plasty is deemed to be unsatisfactory, replacement of the tricuspid valve should be performed. Preference should then be given to bioprostheses, that is mounted aortic homografts (58,59) or heterografts (26,60-66). Numerous complications have been described with mechanical prostheses in the tricuspid position:

- with ball prostheses, poor accommodation of the cage in the right ventricle, embedding of the the cage into the wall of the RV subsequent to the postoperative reduction in its size, thrombosis and fibrin deposits around the orifice and on the bars impeding the motion of the ball, are all stenosing features of this type of prosthesis (26,67-71);
- with tilting disc prostheses, there is a better hemodynamic function but a significant risk of thrombosis (72,73);
- there is a non-negligible risk of thrombosis with bileaflet prostheses.

The implantation of a bioprosthesis in the tricuspid position reduces the incidence of these complications, gives good hemodynamic results and satisfactory durability (26,60,61,66).

The surgical results of TS corrections are difficult to assess for two reasons; on the one hand because multiple valvular surgery is undertaken, and on the other hand because surgical techniques have changed during the last thirty years of valvular surgery. Early mortality, which used to be greater than 20% during double and triple mechanical valve replacement, has been reduced significantly by conservative surgery (37) or by the implantation of a biologic prosthesis if necessary (59,61,62,64), and by early indication of surgery in multiple valvular disease. Long term results depend on the satisfactory correction of the left sided valvulopathies and on the absence of right ventricular dysfunction. In the case of multiple valve disease with tricuspid biologic prostheses, actuarial survival was 86% for Mikaeloff at five years and 75% at nine years (59,62). Guerra and McGrath suggested a lower long term survival of 20%-25% at 14 to 15 years and a high early mortality of 15%-30% for tricuspid replacements of any cause (65,66). More than two out of three survivors were in functional class I or II.

Whether the tricuspid intervention is a commissurotomy/annuloplasty or a bioprosthesis implantation, hemodynamic, and recently ultrasonic investigations demonstrate the persistence of a postoperative trans-tricuspid diastolic gradient, generally below 4.0 mmHg, and a residual tricuspid incompetence following conservative surgery.

Percutaneous tricuspid valvulotomy

Fifteen cases have been published since the first dilatation by Khalilullah in 1987 (74), 13 of which were post rheumatic TS; one case of isolated TS with normal mitral valve on ultrasound (45) and one case of TS occurring in carcinoid syndrome (97). The first six cases (74-77) were isolated tricuspid dilatations for tight tricuspid stenosis associated with a moderate mitral stenosis. The seventh case (78) was a tight TS associated with a mitral re-stenosis where the tricuspid stenosis alone was dilated. The next five cases involved multiple valvulotomies, four mitral and tricuspid and one case of a triple tricuspid, aortic and mitral valvulotomy (81). These 12 patients were older than 50 years of age whilst the thirteenth patient was a woman of 74 years with moderate mitral disease and severe tricuspid stenosis (83).

The immediate results were satisfactory, with a fall in the mean diastolic gradient of 5-9 mmHg to two or less, and an increase in the orifice area by catheter data from 0.7-1.3cm^2 to 1.6-2.7cm^2. Correlations with the effective orifice estimated by Doppler using the Hatle formula were satisfactory.

Follow up was between two months and three years for the four cases of Ribeiro (82), with clinical, orifice area and gradient stability. For further details see Chapter 7.2.

A few cases of stenotic percutaneous porcine or pericardial bioprosthetic valvulotomies in the tricuspid position should be mentioned (84-86). Generally these only result in a temporary improvement and can only therefore be indicated as palliative treatment when the risk of re-intervention is judged to be too great.

TS IN NON-RHEUMATIC ENDOCARDIAL DISEASE

Cardiac involvement in carcinoid syndrome (26,87-98)

The first description of valvular damage to the right heart in the presence of a carcinoid tumour was made by Milman in 1943. The carcinoid syndrome is due to the excessive production of serotonin or 5-hydroxytryptamine and also bradykinin, substance P, dopamin, histamine, kallikrein and prostaglandins by the tumor or by its metastases. The primary tumor is usually gastrointestinal, particularly in the small intestine and appendix (26,88,89). The secretion from the tumor therefore reaches the liver via the portal circulation, where it is inactivated. It is the tumor secretion from hepatic metastases released in an active form into the hepatic veins which reach the right side of the heart via the inferior vena cava. Other locations, especially ovarian, are responsible for tumor secretions reaching the heart directly via the inferior vena cava without hepatic transfer. Cardiac damage occurs in two out of three cases of carcinoid syndrome but only one in four present with a clinical and hemodynamic picture.

Pathomorphology

Lesions of the left heart are in general minor, perhaps due to inactivation of tumour secretion coming from the right side of the heart during its passage through the lungs. More severe left heart damage is possibly induced by a patent foramen ovale with a right to left shunt, or if the carcinoid tumour is bronchial, as in this case the tumour secretion directly enters the pulmonary veins. The lesions are mainly located in the right side of the heart: sclerotic retraction is present in the pulmonary and tricuspid valves, greatly diminishing their mobility, rendering them stenotic (especially the pulmonary valve) and incompetent (mainly the tricuspid valve). The sclerosis extends to the chordae tendineae and papillary muscles of the tricuspid valve, to the right ventricular and atrial endocardia, the inferior vena cava, and also to the coronary sinus and the pulmonary artery. There is no associated intra-cavity thrombosis.

The histologic appearance is that of superficial plaques consisting of a slightly cellular endocardial fibrosis made up mainly of smooth muscle fibres embedded in a stroma rich in mucopolysaccharides and collagen fibres, whilst elastic fibres are almost absent. These fibrotic plaques are secondary to endocardial damage from tumor secretions, but the precise mechanism is unknown.

Diagnosis

Cardiac involvement should be systematically investigated in carcinoid syndrome as it can be insidious. It must be distinguished from hyperkinetic states without valvular damage linked to the hypersecretion of kinins (87,88). 2D-echo appears to be an accurate method of establishing the diagnosis (89,93); the leaflets of the tricuspid valve are thickened and almost immobile in a semi-open position during the entire cardiac cycle, following the movements of the annular ring. This appearance is quite different from the diastolic dome of post-rheumatic tricuspid stenosis. The pulmonary valve is thickened and the right heart cavities are dilated. Doppler confirms and quantifies the generally predominant incompetence of the tricuspid valve and the mainly stenotic pulmonary valve. The degree of change in the diastolic function of the right ventricle following the development of ventricular plaques is difficult to quantify taking into account the associated valvular pathology.

Treatment

Valvular damage due to the carcinoid syndrome is progressive and represents, at the hemodynamic stage, a prognostic factor of mortality. However, carcinoid tumors, even at the stage of hepatic metastases, often have a fairly long history of more than five years.

This slow progression of the tumor makes cardiac surgery justified when valvular damage is severe and symptomatic with signs of congestion. The tricuspid valve is replaced. If the carcinoid tumor can be removed in a satisfactory way in the absence of metastases, then a tricuspid bioprosthesis can be inserted. If the carcinoid tumor or metastases remain, then the insertion of a mechanical prosthesis should be recommended as recurrence of carcinoid plaques on a bioprosthesis is possible (33,95,96). In the case of a mechanical prosthesis, vitamin K antagonists are usually well tolerated.

A commissurotomy should first be performed on the stenosed pulmonary valve (88,94). Ablation of the pulmonary valve without replacement (valvectomy) is nowadays recommended in the absence of cardiac pathology on the left side of the heart (33,95,96), as it only induces a moderate and well tolerated pulmonary incompetence. Percutaneous tricuspid valvulotomy for tight stenosis with a moderate tricuspid incompetence has been described in the case of carcinoid syndrome in a patient of 77 years with progressive signs of congestion and hepatic metastases (97,98). The orifice area increased from 0.9 to 1.4 cm^2 with a partial improvement of the signs of congestion during a follow up of over one month. The absence of commissural fusion in this type of pathology, the persistence of a tight TS after the procedure and the presence of a moderate to severe incompetence makes this only a palliative procedure for patients judged to be inoperable.

Miscellaneous forms of tricuspid stenosis

Hypereosinophilic syndrome (Löffler's endocarditis) generally affects the endocardium; very rarely cases with mitral and tricuspid stenotic lesions have been described(99). Endocarditis arising from *acute disseminated lupus erythematosus* very rarely leads to TS (39,100). *Bacterial endocarditis* of the tricuspid valve is accompanied by bulky vegetations which can give the appearance of tricuspid stenosis.

INDIRECT STENOSIS DUE TO COMPRESSION OR OBSTRUCTION OF THE VALVE

Intracavital tumors

Myxomas account for more than half of primary cardiac tumors in the adult (101,102). Twenty-five percent of myxomas are situated in the right heart. These are pedunculated tumors arising from the atrial septum and moving into the tricuspid orifice during diastole. Their discovery is related to valvular obstruction: asthenia, dyspnea on effort, postural malaise, peripheral congestive signs, or to pulmonary embolism. Echocardiography is of diagnostic value.

Muscular tumors can develop in lower or upper part of the inferior vena cava extending to the right atrium and protruding into the tricuspid orifice, either as a benign operable leiomyoma (103), which sometimes requires a second intervention to remove the venous part of the tumor distant from the heart (104), or a malignant leiomyosarcoma, which is generally inoperable (103).

Parietal tumors

These are in general due to metastases; post mortem studies on malignancies have shown cardiac metastases in up to 20% of the cases (105). Numerous cancers can be implicated, especially melanomas. The picture is dominated by pericardial damage; endocardial damage is generally silent. Melanomatous nodular metastases (105) or undifferentiated cancers bulging outwards into the right atrium or surroundings of the tricuspid valve can create the appearance of TS.

Hydatid cysts in the wall of the right atrium (108) or of the upper part of the interventricular septum (107) can also create TS symptoms.

Extracardiac tumors

Neighbouring tumors invading the right atrium producing obstruction of the tricuspid valve have been described, sometimes arising from malignant pleural mesotheliomas (109) or malignant thymomas (110).

Pericardial effusion and constriction

Acute: The picture of acute TS has been described concomitant with tense focal sero-fibrinous or blood stained pericardial effusions situated in contact mainly with the right heart at the level of the tricuspid annulus (111,112),

-   at the time of recurrence of an acute pericarditis, the first episode of which was drained a month earlier (113);
- after open heart surgery, blood stained isolated effusion with the picture of a delayed TS has been described on the fifth and also the 20th day after surgery (115); - after rupture of a myocardial infarct into a partially isolated compartment of pericardial adhesions in a patient who had undergone a double bypass procedure five years earlier (116);
- following thoracic trauma (117).

Chronic: A diastolic murmur in the tricuspid region increasing during inspiration has been seen in constrictive pericarditis with the presence of a diastolic gradient across the orifice at catheterization. The valve being normal, the proposed mechanism was the effect of constriction at the level of the right atrioventricular annulus (112,118,119).

Iatrogenic causes linked to prolonged catheterization of the right heart

A case of extensive thrombosis extending from the superior vena cava into the right atrium and obstructing the tricuspid orifice, induced by the presence of an intravenous feeding catheter (120) has been reported, as well as a case of a pacemaker probe forming a loop under the valve, resulting in a secondary fibrosis of the sub-valvular apparatus immobilizing the tricuspid leaflets in the closed position, with a clinical picture of TS 14 years after the insertion of the pacemaker (121).

The external compression of the right ventricle by a non-ruptured aneurysm of the non-coronary sinus of Valsalva was reported as presenting the clinical picture of TS in a 28-year-old man (122).

References

1. Acar J. Cardiopathies Valvulaires Acquises. Flammarion Medecine Science Paris 1985; 386-399
2. Sinclair-Smith BC, Newman EV. Tricuspid valve disease. An historical and physiological perspective. Trans Am Clin Climatol Assoc 1969;81:143-159
3. Colonna D, Meilhac B, Levy JP. Lesions tricuspidiennes. Encycl Med Chir Paris Coeur-Vaisseaux 2. 1979;11014 A 10
4. Wooley CF, Fontana ME, Kilman JW et al. Tricuspid stenosis, atrial systolic murmur, tricuspid opening snap and right atrial pressure pulse. Am J Med 1985;78:375-384
5. Rivero-Carvallo JM. El diagnostica de la estenosis tricuspides. Arch Inst Cardiol Mexico 1950;20:1
6. Gorlin R, Gorlin SG. Hydraulic formula for calculation of the area of the stenotic mitral valve, other cardiac valves, and central circulatory shunt. Am Heart J 1951;41:1-29
7. Ferrer MI, Harvey RM, Kuschner M et al. Hemodynamic studies in tricuspid stenosis of rheumatic origin. Circ Res 1953;1:49
8. Yu PN, Harken DE, Lovejoy FW et al. Clinical and hemodynamic studies of tricuspid stenosis. Circulation 1956;13:680-691
9. Killip T, Lukas DS. Tricuspid stenosis: physiologic criteria for diagnosis and hemodynamic abnormalities. Circulation 1957;16:3-13
10. Perloff JK, Harvey WP. Clinical recognition of tricuspid stenosis. Circulation 1960;22:346-364
11. Soulie P, Colonna D, Forman J et al. Le retrecissement tricuspidien. Etude hemodynamique et phonocardiographique intracardiaque. Arch Mal Coeur 1965;58:1273-1295
12. Trace HD, Bailey CP, Wendkos MH. Tricuspid valve commissurotomy with a one year follow-up. Am Heart J 1954;47:613
13. Joyner CR, Hey EB, Johnson J. Reflected ultrasound in the diagnosis of tricuspid stenosis. Am J Cardiol 1967;19:66-73
14. Tajik AJ, Seward JB, Hagler DJ et al. Two-dimensional real time ultrasonic imaging of the heart and great vessels: technique, image orientation, structure, identification and validation. Mayo Clin Proc 1978;53:271
15. Escojido N, Salomon M, Bousquet JP et al. Apport de l'echocardiographie au diagnostic des valvulopathies tricuspidiennes. A propos de 103 cas. Arch Mal Coeur 1978;71:1083-1088
16. Grimberg D, Kechrid R, Halphen C et al. Approche echocardiographique des valvulopathies tricuspidiennes. Actualites cardio-vasculaires medico-chirurgicales Masson Paris 1980;3-14
17. Grimberg D, Starkman C, Rachoin R et al. Diagnosis of acquired organic tricuspid valvular disease and tricuspid regurgitation by echocardiography. IX World Congress of Cardiology Moscou 1982;0696
18. Guyer D, Gillam L, Dinsmore R et al. Detection of tricuspid stenosis by two dimensional echocardiography. Am J Cardiol 1982;49:104
19. Guyer DE, Gillam LD, Foale RA et al. Comparison of the echocardiographic and haemodynamic diagnosis of rheumatic tricuspid stenosis. J Am Coll Card 1984;3:1135-1144
20. Daniels SJ, Mintz GS, Holter MN. Rheumatic tricuspid valve disease. Two dimensional echocardiographic hemodynamic and angiographic correlations. Am J Cardiol 1983;51:492-496
21. Morin D, Lardoux H, Bruchner I et al. Apport de l'echocardiographie TM au diagnostic du retrecissement tricuspide. Arch Mal Coeur 1983;76:323-332
22. Nanna M, Chandraratna PA, Reid C et al. Value of two dimensional echocardiography in detecting tricuspid stenosis Circulation 1983;67:221-224
23. Kalmanson D, Veyrat C. Nouvelle technique d'exploration mitrale et tricuspidienne. La velocimetrie scanner-Doppler pulse. Nouv Presse Med 1980;9:638
24. Veyrat C, Kalmanson D, Farjon M et al. Non invasive diagnosis and assessment of tricuspid regurgitation and stenosis using one and two dimensional echo-pulsed Doppler. Br Heart J 1982;47:596
25. Diebold B, Touati R, Blanchard D et al. Non invasive evaluation of tricuspid stenosis using Doppler echocardiography. Circulation 1983;68(Suppl III):920
26. Braunwald E. Heart Disease. A textbook of cardiovascular medicine. 4th Edition. WB Saunders Company Philadelphia 1992;1053-1055
27. Jallut H. Le retrecissement tricuspidien acquis. Etude etiologique anatomique clinique et hemodynamique basee sur 17 observations. These Paris 1955
28. Kitchin A, Turner R. Diagnosis and treatment of tricuspid stenosis. Br Heart J 1964;26:354-379
29. Silver MD, Lam JHC, Ranganathan N et al. Morphology of the human tricuspid valve. Circulation 1971;43:338-348
30. Deloche A, Guerinon J, Fabiani JN et al. Etude anatomique des valvulopathies rhumatismales tricuspidiennes. Application a l'etude critique des differentes methodes d'annuloplastie. Arch Mal Coeur 1974;67:497-506
31. Roberts WC, Sullivan MF. Combined mitral valve stenosis and tricuspid valve stenosis. Morphologic observations after mitral and tricuspid valve replacement or mitral replacement and tricuspid valve commissurotomy. Am J Cardiol 1986;58:850-852

32. Penther P, Boschat J, Etienne Y et al. Les atteintes rhumatismales de la valve tricuspide. Etude des types anatomiques et des possibilites de dilatation. Arch Mal Coeur 1988;81:1079-1083
33. Hauck AJ, Freeman DP, Ackermann DM et al. Surgical pathology of the tricuspid valve: a study of 363 cases spanning 25 years Mayo Clin Proc 1988;63:851-863
34. Eways EA, Roberts WC. Clinical and anatomic observations in patients having mitral valve replacement for mitral stenosis and simultaneous tricuspid valve replacement. Am J Cardiol 1991;68:1367-1371
35. Libman E. Characterization of various forms of endocarditis. J Am Med Ass 1923;80:813-818
36. Coblence B, Daumet P, Daussy M et al. Etude de 13 cas de retrecissement tricuspide; criteres diagnostiques chirurgicaux, resultats. Arch Mal Coeur 1967;60:1593-1614
37. Carpentier A, Deloche A, Hanania G et al. Surgical management of acquired tricuspid valve disease. J Thorac Cardiovasc Surg 1974;67:53-65
38. Colonna D, Maurat JP, Acar J et al. Indications et resultats de la commissurotomie tricuspide Coeur Med lnterne 1969;8:209-220
39. Gibson R, Wood P. The diagnosis of tricuspid stenosis. Br Heart J 1955;17:552-562
40. Goodwin JF, Rab SM, Sinha AK et al. Rheumatic tricuspid stenosis. Br Med J 1957;5058:1383-1389
41. Finnegan P, Abrams LD. Isolated tricuspid stenosis. Br Heart J 1973;35:1207-1210
42. Gueron M, Hirsch M, Borman J et al. Isolated tricuspid valvular stenosis. The pathology and merits of surgical treatment. J Thorac Cardiovasc Surg 1971;63:760-764
43. Keefe JF, Wolk MJ, Levine HJ. Isolated tricuspid valvular stenosis. Am J Cardiol 1970;25:252-257
44. Morgan JR, Forker AD, Gates JR et al. Isolated tricuspid stenosis. Circulation 1971;44:729-732
45. Robalino BB, Whitlow PL, Marwick T et al. Percutaneous balloon valvotomy for the treatment of isolated tricuspid stenosis. Chest 1991;100:867-869
46. Lisa CP, Tavel ME. Tricuspid stenosis: graphic features which help in its diagnosis. Chest 1972;61:291-293
47. Shimada R, Takeshita A, Nakamura M et al. Diagnosis of tricuspid stenosis by M-Mode and two-dimensional echocardiography. Am J Cardiol 1984;53:164-168
48. Perez JE, Ludbrook PA, Ahumada GG. Usefulness of Doppler echocardiography in detecting tricuspid valve stenosis. Am J Cardiol 1985;55:601-603
49. Parris TM, Panidis IP, Ross J et al. Doppler echocardiographic findings in rheumatic tricuspid stenosis. Am J Cardiol 1987;60:1414-1416
50. Fawzy ME, Mercer EN, Dunn B et al. Doppler echocardiography in the evaluation of tricuspid stenosis. Eur Heart J 1989;10:985-990
51. Ribeiro PA, Al Zaibag M, Sawyer W. A prospective study comparing the haemodynamic with the cross sectional echocardiographic diagnosis of rheumatic tricuspid stenosis. Eur Heart J 1989;10:120-126
52. Berman GO, Reichek N, Browson D et al. Effects of sample volume location, imaging view, heart rate and age on tricuspid velocimetry in normal subjects. Am J Cardiol 1990;65:1026-1030
53. Pearlman AS. Role of echocardiography in the diagnosis and evaluation of severity of mitral and tricuspid stenosis. Circulation 1991;84(Suppl I):193-197
54. Lesbre JP, Tribouilloy C. Echograhie Doppler des cardiopathies valvulaires acquises. Flammarion Medecine Sciences Paris 1992;121-135
55. Dennig K, Henneke KH, Rudolph W. Assessment of tricuspid stenosis by Doppler echocardiography J Am Coll Card 1987;9:237
56. Geschwind H, Tenaillon A, Samll K et al. Evaluation des lesions tricuspidiennes par la cineangiographie Coeur 1975;687-703
57. Ribeiro PA, Al Zaibag M, Al Kasab S et al. Provocation and amplification of the transvalvular pressure gradient in rheumatic tricuspid stenosis. Am J Cardiol 1988;61:1307-1310
58. Mikaeloff P, Fleurette J, Transy MJ et al. Indications, resultats des remplacemenst tricuspidiens par homogreffe valvulaire aortique. Coeur 1975 VI No. Special;559-571
59. Mikaeloff P, Convert G, Fleurette J et al. Remplacement de la valve tricuspide par homogreffe valvulaire aortique. Resultats cliniques et hemodynamiques a plus de 5 ans. Nouv Prese Med 1981;10:1131-1134
60. Carpentier A. Heterogreffes et bioprotheses valvulaires. 1965-1975. Coeur 1975;6:587-600
61. Delahaye JP, Rondepierre D, Gaspard P et al. Le remplacement valvulaire tricuspidien par la prothese de Hancock. Arch Mal Coeur 1981;74:281-288
62. Mikaeloff P, Delahaye JP, Convert G et al. Resultats precoces et tardifs des triples remplacements valvulaires. Utilisation d'une bioprothese en position tricuspidienne. Arch Mal Coeur 1981;74:719-726
63. Kratz JM, Crawford FA, Stroud MR et al. Trends and results in tricuspid valve surgery. Chest 1985;88:837-840
64. Chaouch H, Kafsi N, Ben Ismail M. Indications et resultats de la chirurgie des atteintes organiques de la valve tricuspide. Arch Mal Coeur 1989;82:879-884
65. Mcgrath LB, Gonzalez-Lavin L, Bailey BM et al. Tricuspid valve operations in 530 patients. 25 year assessment of early and late phase events. J Thorac Cardiovasc Surg 1990;99:124-133
66. Guerra F, Bortolotti U, Thiene G et al. Long term performance of the Hancock porcine bioprosthesis in the

tricuspid position. A review of 45 patients with fourteen-year follow-up. J Thorac Cardiovasc Surg 1990;99:838-845

67. Ben Ismail M, Abid F, Sirinelle A et al. Thromboses tardives sur protheses en position tricuspide. Arch Mal Coeur 1981;74:289-296

68. Ben Ismail M, Curran Y, Bousnina A. Devenir au long cours des protheses en position tricuspide. Arch Mal Coeur 1981;74:1035-1044

69. McGoon DC, Sanfelippo PM. Remplacements polyvalvulaires en particulier de la valve tricuspide. Coeur 1975;VI No. Special 643-648

70. Piekarski A, Dewide J, Dumoulin P et al. Les triples remplacements valvulaires. Arch Mal Coeur 1979;72:1196-1202

71. Kurnik PB, Saffitz JE, Ahumada GG et al. 19-year longevity of isolated tricuspid valve replacement. Am Heart J 1985;109:904-905

72. Bowen TE, Tri TB, Wortham DL. Thrombosis of a St Jude Medical tricuspid prosthesis. J Thorac Cardiovasc Surg 1981;82:257-262

73. Thorburn CW, Morgan JJ, Shanahan MX et al. Long term results of tricuspid valve replacement and the problem of prosthetic valve thrombosis. Am J Cardiol 1983;51:1128-1132

74. Khalilullah M, Tyagi S, Yadav BS et al. Double-balloon valvuloplasty of tricuspid stenosis. Am Heart J 1987;114:1232-1233

75. Al Zaibag M, Ribeiro P, Al Kasab S. Percutaneous balloon valvotomy in tricuspid stenosis. Br Heart J 1987 VI No. Special;57:51-53

76. Ribeiro PA, Al Zaibag M, Al Kasab S et al. Percutaneous double balloon valvotomy for rheumatic tricuspid stenosis. Am J Cardiol 1988;61:660-662

77. Goldenberg IF, Pedersen W, Olson J et al. Percutaneous double balloon valvuloplasty for severe tricuspid stenosis. Am Heart J 1989;118:417-418

78. Bourdillon PDV, Hookman LD, Morris SN et al. Percutaneous balloon valvuloplasty for tricuspid stenosis: hemodynamic and pathological findings. Am Heart J 1989;117:492-494

79. Berland J, Rocha P, Mechmeche R et al. Valvulotomie percutanee dans l'association stenose mitrale-stenose tricuspide. A propos de trois observations. Arch Mal Coeur 1990;83:1585-1589

80. Bethencourt A, Medina A, Hernandez E et al. Combined percutaneous balloon valvuloplasty of mitral and tricuspid valves. Am Heart J 1990;119:416-418

81. Konugres GS, Lau FYK, Ruiz CE. Successive percutaneous double-balloon mitral, aortic and tricuspid valvotomy in rheumatic trivalvular stenoses. Am Heart J 1990;119:663-666

82. Ribeiro PA, Al Zaibag M, Idris MT. Percutaneous double balloon tricuspid valvotomy for severe tricuspid stenosis: 3-year follow-up study. Eur Heart J 1990;11:1109-1112

83. Shaw TRD. The Inoue balloon for dilatation of the tricuspid valve: a modified over-the-wire approach. Br Heart J 1992;67:263-265

84. Feit F, Stecy PJ, Nachamie MS. Percutaneous balloon valvuloplasty for stenosis of a porcine bioprosthesis in the tricuspid valve position. Am J Cardiol 1986;58:363-364

85. Wren C, Hunter S. Balloon dilation of stenosis bioprosthesis in tricuspid valve position. Br Heart J 1989;61:65-67

86. Chow WH, Cheung KL, Tai YT et al. Successful percutaneous balloon valvuloplasty of a stenotic tricuspid bioprosthesis. Am Heart J 1990;119:666-668

87. Acar J, Auriol M, Lainee R et al. Cardiopathie carcinoide et tumeur de l'ovaire. A propos d'un cas anatomo-clinique. Ann Med Interne 1970;121:329-340

88. Bletry O, Godeau P. Cardiopathie carcinoide. Encycl Med Chir Paris. Coeur 1977;11014 C-10

89. Callahan JA, Wroblewski EM, Reeder GS et al. Echocardiographic features of carcinoid heart disease. Am J Cardiol 1982;50:762-768

90. Ferrans VS, Roberts WC. The carcinoid endocardial plaque. An ultrastructural study. Hum Pathol 1976;7:387-409

91. Lundin L, Norheim I, Landelius J et al. Carcinoid heart disease: relationship of circulatory vasoactive substances to ultrasound detectable cardiac abnormalities. Circulation 1988;77:264

92. Menzies DG, Campbell IW, Starkey IR. Infective endocarditis complicating tricuspid valve disease in the carcinoid syndrome. Brit Med J 1988;296:682

93. Taber M, Askenazi J, Ribner H et al. The tricuspid valve in carcinoid syndrome. An echocardiographic study. Arch Intern Med 1983;143:1033-1034

94. Hendel N, Leckie B, Richards J. Carcinoid heart disease: eight year survival following tricuspid valve replacement and pulmonary valvotomy. Ann Thorac Surg 1980;30:391-395

95. Disesa VJ, Mills RM, Collins JJ. Surgical management of carcinoid heart disease. Chest 1985;88:789-791

96. Lundin L, Hansson HE, Landelius J et al. Surgical treatment of carcinoid heart disease. J Thorac Cardiovasc Surg 1990;100:552-561

97. Mullins PA, Hall JA, Shapiro LM. Balloon dilatation of tricuspid stenosis caused by carcinoid heart

disease. Br Heart J 1990;63:249-250

98. Dalvi B. Balloon dilatation of tricuspid stenosis caused by carcinoid heart disease. Letter to the editor. Br Heart J 1991;65:113

99. Weyman AE, Rankin R, King H. Loffler's endocarditis presenting as mitral and tricuspid stenosis. Am J Cardiol 1977;40:438-444

100. Ames DE. Systemic lupus erythematous complicated by tricuspid stenosis and regurgitation; successful treatment by valve transplantation. Ann Rheum Dis 1992;51:120-122

101. Nasser WK, Davis RH, Dillon JC et al. Atrial myxoma: I- Clinical and pathologic features in nine cases. Am Heart J 1972;83:694-704. II - Phonocardiographic, echocardiographic and angiographic features in nine cases. Am Heart J 1972;83:810

102. Soulie P, Acar J. Les myxomes de l'oreillette droite. Arch Mal Coeur 1961;54:241-273

103. Mandelbaum J, Pauletto FJ, Nasser WK. Resection of a leiomyoma of the interior vena cava that produced tricuspid valvular obstruction. J Thorac Cardiovasc Surg 1974;67:561-567

104. Gonzalez-Lavin L, Lee RH, Falk L et al. Tricuspid valve obstruction due to intravenous leiomyomatosis. Am Heart J 1984;108:1544-1545

105. Thomas JH, Panoussopoulos DG, Jewell WR et al. Tricuspid stenosis secondary to metastatic melanoma. Cancer 1977;39:1732-1737

106. De Cock KM, Gikonyo DK, Lucas SB et al. Metastatic tumour of right atrium mimicking constrictive pericarditis and tricuspid stenosis. Br Med J 1982;285:1314

107. Erol C, Candan I, Akalin H et al. Cardiac hydatid cyst simulating tricuspid stenosis. Am J Cardiol 1985;56:833-834

108. Mancuso L, Bondi F, Marchi S et al. Cardiac hydatid disease with clinical features resembling tricuspid stenosis. Am Heart J 1987;113:1234-1236

109. Walters LL, Taxi JB. Malignant mesothelioma of the pleura with extensive cardiac invasion and tricuspid orifice occlusion. Cancer 1983;52:1736-1768

110. Gunn J, Walker DR, Boyle RM. Malignant thymoma causing tricuspid valve obstruction. Eur Heart J 1990;11:854-856

111. Beaver WL, Dillon JC, Jolly W. Pseudo-tricuspid stenosis, a rare entity. Chest 1977;71:772-774

112. Cintron GB, Snow JA, Fletcher RD et al. Pericarditis mimicking tricuspid valvular disease. Chest 1977;71:770-772

113. Baruchin MA, Hecht SR, Berger M. Reversible tricuspid stenosis. Demonstration with two-dimensional echocardiography and continuous wave Doppler. Chest 1991;100:852-853

114. Young SG, Gregoratos G, Swain JA et al. Delayed postoperative cardiac tamponade mimicking severe tricuspid valve stenosis. Chest 1984;85:824-826

115. Zahler R, Breisblatt W, Hashim S et al. Isolated right atrial tamponade by serous fluid simulating tricuspid stenosis. Am J Med 1985;79:531-534

116. Silver MA, Hilgard JH, Murabit I et al. Right atrial tamponade simulating tricuspid stenosis following acute myocardial infarction. Am Heart J 1986;111:984-986

117. Wray TM, Prochaska J, Fisher RD et al. Traumatic pericardial hematoma simulating tricuspid valve obstruction. John Hopkins Med J 1975;137:147-150

118. McGinn JS, Zipes DP. Constrictive pericarditis causing tricuspid stenosis. Arch Intern Med 1972;129:487-490

119. Schrire V, Gotsman MS, Beck W. Unusual diastolic murmurs in constrictive pericarditis and constrictive endocarditis. Am Heart J 1968;76:4-12

120. Chakravarthy A, Edwards WD, Fleming CR. Fatal tricuspid valve obstruction due to a large infected thrombus attached to a Hickman catheter. J Am Coll Card 1987;257:801-803

121. Old WD, Paulsen W, Lewis SA et al. Pacemaker lead-induced tricuspid stenosis: diagnosis by Doppler echocardiography. Am Heart J 1989;117:1165-1166

122. Gibbs KL, Reardon MJ, Strickman NE et al. Hemodynamic compromise (tricuspid stenosis and insufficiency) caused by an unruptured aneurysm of the sinus of Valsalva. J Am Coll Card 1986;7:1177-1181

Chapter 6.2

Multivalvular Disease

Guy Hanania, Jean-Pierre Maroni, Marc Terdjman

The incidence of multivalvular disease primarily of rheumatic origin has sharply decreased over the past twenty years, at least in developed countries, in parallel with the decline in rheumatic fever (1).

The clinical profiles and evolution of these entities depend, for the most part, upon the type of involvement, regurgitation or stenosis, the extent of each of them and the association of the different valves affected. Pathophysiologically, a proximal (upstream) stenosis can protect against the repercussions of a distal (downstream) valvulopathy, when the cardiac chambers are located between the two lesions. In contrast, a downstream stenosis may aggravate the consequences of an organic regurgitation upstream. The extent of each of these valvular defects produces highly variable clinical and evolutive profiles for which any systematization includes an arbitrary element. The co-existence of two or even three lesions can lead to a minimization of the clinical expression of one of them or to a modification of the natural evolution of the disease.

Thus clinical diagnosis of multivalvular disease has certain blind spots that phonocardiography, radiology and electrocardiography can help to illuminate. Nevertheless, before the advent of echocardiographic and Doppler techniques, recourse to hemodynamic and angiographic studies was essential. At present, preoperative catheterization remains highly desirable in the context of multivalvular involvement, in order to confirm the type and extent before deciding on the approach regarding each orifice, even if these hemodynamic and angiographic findings often serve only to further support the echocardiographic diagnosis (2,3).

The progress made over the years in the field of cardiac surgery has led to very significant improvement in results, despite the progressive aging of the populations treated. This improvement has been particularly clear for patients with mitral plus aortic involvement whose double organic lesions do not necessarily aggravate the prognosis if surgery is performed sufficiently early. However, this progress is less evident in patients with mitral plus tricuspid lesions that more often correspond to mitral valvulopathies allowed to evolve naturally for too long than to double organic pathologies that continue to suffer heavy surgical mortality.

This chapter addresses only mitral-aortic involvement and trivalvular lesions; mitral-tricuspid disease is treated in detail elsewhere in this volume.

FREQUENCY

The incidence of multivalvular disease compared to that of monovalvular lesions has been estimated in old autopsy studies and more or less recent surgical investigations. In an old autopsy study (1940), Clawson (4) found 323 multiple lesions among 779 autopsies of patients with a known valvulopathy, i.e. 41.5%. In a more recent post mortem study (1960-1980) of 1,010 cases, Roberts (5) observed a similar percentage (39%), but the morphologic multivalvular lesions with significant impairment corresponded to only 27% of them.

Surgical investigations, which only counted the orifices operated on, yielded smaller percentages, ranging from 11.5% for Duvoisin et al. (6) to 14% for Teply et al. (7) and Dubost et al. (8) and up to 27% for Pellegrini et al. (9) and 28% for Pinzaki et al (10). Only the surgical series of Isom et al. (11) presented a percentage similar to that found in the old autopsy studies. i.e. 40%.

In a French co-operative study (12) comparing the valvulopathies treated surgically in 1973 to those in 1983, the indications for multivalvular interventions decreased from 25% in 1973 to 18% in 1983.

In the context of multivalvular disease, mitral-aortic involvement is by far the most common. Most of the studies, both post mortem and surgical, estimated that these lesions represent 57% to 69% of the multiple pathologies (4-6,8). Pellegrini et al. (9), in a series of patients operated on between 1963 and 1973, observed only 48% mitral-aortic involvement among their population of multivalvulopathies. In contrast, Teply et al. (7) reported a rate of 86% mitral-aortic lesions in 2,135 patients with multivalvular disease who underwent surgery between 1961 and 1981. For a series of patients that underwent surgery between 1983 and 1986, Pinzani et al. (10) found that about 87% had mitral-aortic involvement. The percentage of mitral-aortic lesions ranged from 58% to 69.5% in the French co-operative study (12) cited above. This progressive rise in the percentage of mitral-aortic pathologies among multivalvular diseases should be considered in the light of the rarity of indications for tricuspid surgery as a consequence of earlier surgical intervention. Indeed, compared to the entire population operated on for valvular disease, the percentage of mitral-aortic lesions did not vary significantly, only decreasing from 14.5% to 12.4%.

Organic mitral-tricuspid involvement is rare, evaluated to be 2% to 4% in the autopsy series. Isolated tricuspid stenosis is very unusual and, in most cases, is observed in association with a tight mitral stenosis.

In the French study comparing surgical indications for valve surgery in 1973 versus 1983 (12), the proportion of mitral-tricuspid lesions in which both valves were operated on decreased significantly from 7.1% to 4.7% for the reasons cited above.

Trivalvular disease, which represents 7% (4) to 10% (5) of the cases in post mortem studies, only corresponds to 1% to 3% of the surgical series (6,9). In the French study (12), the percentage of interventions on the three orifices decreased from 3.4% in 1973 to 1% in 1983.

Quadrivalvular disease is extremely rare and has generally been an isolated and old observation (13,14).

ETIOLOGIES AND ANATOMIC-ECHOCARDIOGRAPHIC FINDINGS

Each of the etiologies of multivalvular disease exhibits corresponding anatomic and pathologic changes clearly demonstrated by two-dimensional echocardiographic imaging. These alterations are not different from those seen in monovalvular disease. On the other hand, Doppler velocimetry, which reflects hemodynamic status, reveals the particularities of each association.

Therefore, in this chapter, we will describe each of the principal etiologies, its frequency, its anatomic particularities and its echocardiographic presentations, reserving Doppler findings for the characterization of each of the principal valvular diseases.

Rheumatic heart disease

Rheumatic fever is the predominant etiology of multivalvular lesions. Although its frequency in developed countries has diminished sharply, it remains the most common cause of multivalvular involvement, in contrast to isolated valvular lesions, for which a degenerative pathology is primarily responsible (1,12).

The very high prevalence of rheumatic fever in developing nations explains the frequency of multivalvular disease in these countries. For Roberts and Sullivan (15), in an autopsy series, the most common association was that of double mitral-aortic stenoses (15%), three times more frequent than the association of mitral stenosis with aortic regurgitation (6%). Braunwald (16) found aortic regurgitation to be associated with mitral stenosis very frequently (two-thirds of cases) but significant lesions were present in only 10% of them. For Delahaye et al. (17), 27.7% of the mitral stenoses operated on were associated with aortic regurgitation, whereas the coexistence of aortic stenosis or mixed disease was noted in only 8% of patients. Aortic and mitral interventions were performed in only 7.1% of the 202 patients who underwent surgery.

Double regurgitations of rheumatic origin are less frequent, representing only 4% for Roberts and Sullivan (15). The combination of aortic stenosis and organic mitral regurgitation is even rarer in the context of this etiology. The anatomic lesions of each of the valves implicated do not differ from those observed in monovalvular disease of the same origin. These pathologies are clearly visualized by echocardiography.

Mitral involvement affects the valve leaflets and the subvalvular apparatus in the form of valvular thickening, predominantly at the extremities of the leaflets, valve retraction, commissural fusion, calcification, and thickening-fusion-calcification of the subvalvular apparatus. These different modifications can lead to an isolated stenosis of the mitral valve, mitral disease or, more rarely, rheumatic mitral insufficiency, isolated and pure because of the absence of a commissural fusion and associated with retraction essentially of the posterior leaflet, which is immobile in the intermediate open position. Thus, the anterior leaflet, whose movement is normal during diastole, exhibits excessive movement towards the left atrium during systole, above the plane of the mitral annulus, because of the now insufficient area support normally provided by the posterior leaflet.

In aortic involvement, as for the mitral valve, one or more of the cusps are thickened, the centripetal evolution of the commissural fusions ends at a fibrous diaphragm, and the cusps have calcification of various sizes. Thus, depending upon the extent of these alterations and according to their association, semilunar valve movement restriction can give rise to either aortic valve stenosis or regurgitation, or mixed valvular disease combining both these elements equally.

In tricuspid involvement, as above, the leaflets are thickened, particularly at their extremities, and are retracted with a more or less important loss of mobility. These lesions most often lead to mixed tricuspid disease and only rarely to pure stenosis or regurgitation.

Infective endocarditis

These vegetations are responsible for 6% to 7% of multivalvular diseases (1,12) and are the second most common cause of these lesions. The most common pathology is double mitral-aortic regurgitations (occurring in 13% of the cases of endocarditis for Witchitz et al. (18)). Endocarditic trivalvular pathologies are very rare (18). The anatomic lesions are classical: rupture of the chordae tendineae, vegetations, valvular perforations, and intracardiac abscess. Transthoracic (TTE) and transesophageal echocardiography (TEE) clearly visualize these elements at both the valvular and paravalvular levels (19).

Valve involvement presents as vegetations that vary in size and are characterized by their hyperechogenicity and their mobility. At the level of the aortic valves, the vegetations are located on the ventricular face, on mitral leaflets they are situated on the atrial side. Their identification is better with TEE, the sensitivity of which is 100% versus 63% for TTE, while the specificities of the two modes are comparable, at about 98% (20). These vegetations are sometimes difficult to recognize because they arise on altered valves (as seen in rheumatic fever) or because of myxomatous degeneration of the valves or floppy valve syndrome. Furthermore, they are associated with destructive lesions: rupture and tearing of the aortic or mitral valves result during diastole in an eversion of a cusp into the ejection chamber of the left ventricle or during systole in an eversion of the free end of the mitral leaflet into the left atrium.

When valvular pathologies are present, paravalvular lesions must also be sought, particularly by TEE: an abscess at the level of the anterior portion of the aortic root or the fibrous aortic-mitral trigone yields a dense structure when it is pus-filled or a cystic one when it is fistulated. These lesions can be complicated by fistulation with the surrounding cavities creating communications between the aorta and the right atrium, the left ventricle, or the left atrium.

Dystrophic and degenerative valvulopathies

These pathologies can be responsible for double mitral and aortic regurgitations with the anatomic lesions typical of the latter and require surgical intervention (21).

At the level of the aorta, the following entities may or may not coexist: dilatation of the aortic root in its ascending segment, dilatation of the aortic annulus itself, and/or prolapse of one or several cusps, the texture of which may be myxomatous.

At the level of the mitral annulus, two types of degenerative lesions are observed: myxomatous degeneration with floppy valve syndrome accompanied by elongation of the chordae tendineae and sometimes their rupture, and fibroelastic degeneration (frequently seen in the elderly) with thin (pellucid) valves and fragile chordae tendineae often complicated by rupture clearly visible on TEE images.

In addition to double regurgitation, the degenerative pathology can also be responsible in the aged individual for stenosis of the calcified aorta and organic mitral insufficiency attributable to calcification of the mitral apparatus.

Rare multivalvular diseases

The other more uncommon etiologies of valvular heart disease can affect two orifices.

Carcinoid tumors of the small intestine metastasized to the liver and those of the ovary can also be responsible for double involvement, this time affecting the tricuspid and pulmonary valves (22). Fibrous plaques develop in the mural and valvular endocardia leading to the formation of regurgitant and stenotic lesions (23). *Löffler's fibroplastic* endocarditis *and endomyocardial fibrosis of tropical regions give rise to mitral and* tricuspid involvement resulting in regurgitant lesions, ventricular compliance disorders and mural thrombi. Double mitral-tricuspid valve replacements associated with endocardial resection have been performed in these forms of fibrous endocarditis (24). *Rheumatoid arthritis* affects the aortic and mitral orifices and may cause leakage of these valves. *Libman-Sacks (syndrome)* lupus endocarditis consists of verrucous endocarditic lesions that usually develop on the ventricular face of the mitral leaflets, the opening of which is diminished as a consequence. More rarely, an association of mitral and aortic involvement has been described that gives rise to both regurgitant and stenotic pathologies at the levels of the two respective orifices (25,26). *Mitral-aortic calcification,* sometimes causing valvular stenosis, have been found in hemodialysis patients.

MITRAL-AORTIC VALVULOPATHIES

The following associations are treated successively: double mitral and aortic stenoses, mitral stenosis and aortic regurgitation, and double mitral and aortic regurgitations. The rarest combination of lesions, aortic stenosis-organic mitral regurgitation, is reviewed in detail in Chapter 5.1 in Volume I.

Mitral and aortic stenoses

Almost always of rheumatic origin, this double pathology now poses less of a problem in terms of positive diagnosis since the advent of Doppler echocardiography, than in terms of precise and respective evaluation of the two valvular lesions, because the therapeutic indications for each orifice are defined by this evaluation.

The presence of two successive stenoses, proximal and distal to the left ventricle, protect the latter from the deleterious effects of the aortic stenosis, or at least reduce its clinical expression and hemodynamic consequences (27,28). These latter are, however, marked by a larger decrease in cardiac output than in the case of an isolated aortic stenosis.

In terms of symptoms, this double pathology is characterized by the dominance of the upstream mitral stenosis which is responsible for the classical pulmonary edema manifestations (effort-induced or paroxysmal dyspnea, hemoptysis), but also the possible thromboembolic consequences associated with left atrial dilatation and stasis (palpitations, systemic emboli).

On auscultation, the mitral stenosis usually predominates while the systolic ejection murmur of the aortic stenosis may be of low intensity (29). Verification of the latter in the aortic area with cervical radiation and diminution of the second heart sound serves to orient the clinician towards this association.

More rarely, the aortic stenosis is loud. The perception of an accentuated second heart sound in the pulmonary area, an opening snap at the apex and a diastolic rumbling murmur, which must be distinguished from a possible diastolic murmur accompanying

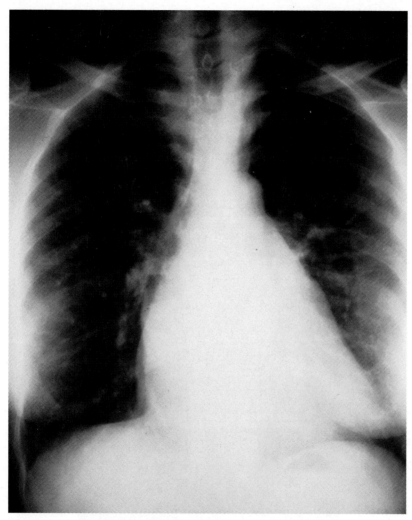

Figure 6.2-1: Typical triangular mitral silhouette with convex left middle arc, an over-extended right border, double outline, with no radiologic argument supporting an aortic valvulopathy in a patient with double mitral-aortic stenoses, both tight.

the aortic stenosis, leads the physician to envisage a double valvulopathy.

Before the development of echocardiographic and Doppler techniques, phonocardiography and pharmacodynamic tests were needed to determine the precise origins of the murmurs and their antero- or retrograde character (30). Amylnitrite reinforced the intensity of the anterograde diastolic rumbling murmur of a mitral stenosis but reduced that of the retrograde murmur of aortic insufficiency. On the other hand, vasoxine hydrochloride diminished the intensity of the systolic murmur of an aortic stenosis but enhanced that of the retrograde holosystolic murmur of a mitral insufficiency.

Radiologically, signs of mitral stenosis are generally clearer than those of aortic valve stenosis, with dilatation of the left atrium visible on the middle arc of the left border and

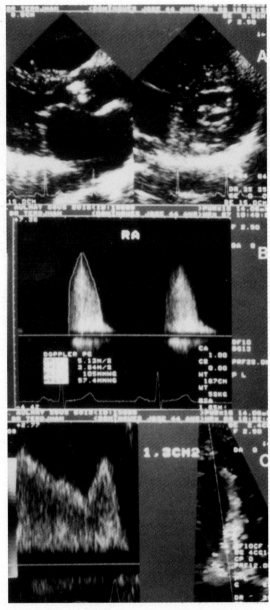

Figure 6.2-2: Echocardiographic and Doppler cardiac images of a patient with aortic and mitral stenoses. A. Echocardiography: longitudinal section through the parasternal window (left) and transverse transmitral section (right). Thickening and hypokinesis of the aortic cusps and the mitral leaflets, respectively, during systole and diastole; bicommissural fusion and planimetry of the mitral orifice open during diastole (1.4cm^2). B. Continuous wave Doppler echocardiography at the level of the right parasternal window. The mean left ventricle-aorta (LV-Ao) gradient was 57 mmHg, the aortic area was calculated to be 0.6 cm^2 using the continuity method. C. Continuous wave Doppler through the apical window. Tight mitral stenosis (area calculated to be 1.3 cm^2 using the HPT method).

at the level of the over-extended right border, possibly with a double silhouette, whereas the left ventricular hypertrophy associated with aortic valve stenosis can be invisible or discrete (Fig. 6.2-1). The presence of valvular calcification in both mitral and aortic sites during fluoroscopy examination is a good argument for double stenotic lesions, but sometimes one appearing late in the evolution of the disease.

The electrocardiogram (ECG) also provides indirect evidence supporting a double valvulopathy, such as unusual atrial fibrillation for an isolated aortic stenosis or unexplained left ventricular hypertrophy for an isolated mitral stenosis.

Echocardiographic and Doppler cardiac examination (Fig. 6.2-2) enable, in the majority of cases, the presence of two stenoses to be confirmed, together with the evaluation of the respective importance of each one and cardiopulmonary repercussions. The left ventricle remains small in size; its walls are hypertrophied sometimes moderately. Quantification of an aortic stenosis has become easy since the arrival of Doppler echocardiography (continuity method at both ends of the aortic orifice).

The degree of mitral valve stenosis can be adequately evaluated by planimetry of the orifice by cardiac imaging when it is possible to clearly delineate the internal outline. The continuity method, in the absence of an associated regurgitation at the level of the two orifices, will enable the mitral area to be calculated. As far as the half-pressure time (HPT) method described by Hatle et al. (31) is concerned, it becomes unreliable when left ventricular compliance is sharply decreased. Indeed, in this latter case, the HPT is abnormally decreased and thereby overestimates the mitral area (32).

Finally, as in all the other valvulopathies, the effects of these double stenoses on pulmonary pressure can be evaluated by Doppler examination, particularly in the case of an associated tricuspid insufficiency.

Hemodynamic assessment remains necessary despite these echocardiographic and Doppler findings, even though it usually merely confirms the information obtained with the Doppler technique in the context of double stenoses. Doppler transvalvular gradient estimates measured at either the level of the mitral orifice or that of the aortic orifice do not always adequately evaluate the severity of the stenoses because of the typical decrease in cardiac output in this double valvulopathy.

Calculation of the areas according to the method of Gorlin and Gorlin (33), in the absence of regurgitation in the pathology envisaged, confirms the degree of each of the valvular defects.

Hemodynamic assessment, as for all isolated or associated mitral valvulopathies, provides information on the pulmonary pressures and, in particular, on the existence of pulmonary precapillary arterial hypertension and functional tricuspid insufficiency.

Angiographic evaluation is not contributive in the case of double stenoses and left ventriculography is not recommended in the case of tight aortic stenosis. Dye injection into the coronary circulation only provides a relevant contribution in the case of clinical angina, rare in this association, and in patients over the age of 50 years (34).

The therapeutic indications determined by these tests are based on the degree of functional disability, the extent of each of the two stenoses and the changes in the mitral apparatus. In the case of a negligible aortic stenosis and when the mitral apparatus will tolerate it, a percutaneous transvenous mitral commissurotomy can be envisaged. However, the risks inherent in using this procedure if the extent of the aortic stenosis is underestimated must be emphasized. In the case of extensive and poorly tolerated double stenoses, the most commonly prescribed treatment is double replacement of the valves with mechanical prostheses or with an aortic prosthesis associated with surgical mitral commissurotomy. To avoid anticoagulant therapy, particular situations can be corrected by associating open-heart mitral commissurotomy and an aortic bioprosthesis or double mitral and aortic bioprostheses.

Mitral stenosis and aortic regurgitation

The association of discrete aortic incompetence and tight mitral stenosis occurs frequently (16). More rarely, the two valvulopathies are significant. It is of the utmost importance that the preoperative evaluation quantifies these two lesions precisely, since the clinical and paraclinical expressions of aortic regurgitation can be minimized by a tight mitral stenosis.

Most often, mitral stenosis is evident and the nature of the diastolic sound perceived at the left border of the sternum is explored, with the following findings: 1) a simple radiating of the stenotic rumbling murmur whose timber can become muffled in this auscultation area; 2) an aortic regurgitation associated with a holodiastolic murmur that is initially protodiastolic phonocardiographically and that is reinforced by vasoxine hydrochloride; 3) much more rarely, a pulmonary insufficiency murmur (Graham Steells' murmur) is heard in the context of pulmonary artery hypertension, a stage that in principle is usually rarely attained during the natural evolution of mitral stenosis. The coexistence of a significant mitral stenosis and a negligible aortic insufficiency is a situation observed in 60% of pure and tight mitral stenoses (16) and reparation of the discrete aortic leak is not necessary. The latter will be just slightly louder after the removal of the mitral obstacle but will not have any hemodynamic consequences.

This is not the case in the rarer situation (10%) in which a tight mitral stenosis and aortic regurgitation of a larger volume lead the physician to recommend double valve correction. Usually, cardiac auscultation in these cases enables recognition without difficulty of the coexistence of the two pathologies with diastolic rumbling murmur of good intensity at the apex and a holodiastolic murmur characteristic of aortic regurgitation in the aortic area and at the left edge of the sternum. These findings are further supported, on the one hand, by typical signs of aortic insufficiency, both clinical (widening of the differential arterial pressure) and paraclinical (left ventricular dilatation seen radiographically and echocardiographically, left ventricular hypertrophy seen on the ECG and, on the other hand, the manifestations indicating mitral stenosis (left atrial dilatation seen radiologically and atrial fibrillation seen on the ECG).

More rarely, the aortic regurgitation dominates the clinical picture, with frank peripheral signs, the perception of a diastolic rumbling murmur at the apex orienting the cardiologist towards a hypothesis of Flint's murmur in the light of the importance of the aortic incompetence. The presence of other stethoscopically heard sounds of "Duroziez' rhythm" (snap of the first heart sound, opening snap of the mitral valve) evokes an associated mitral stenosis, usually moderate, that can be confirmed by echocardiographic and Doppler examinations.

Once confirmed, the respective importance of the two valvulopathies has to be determined

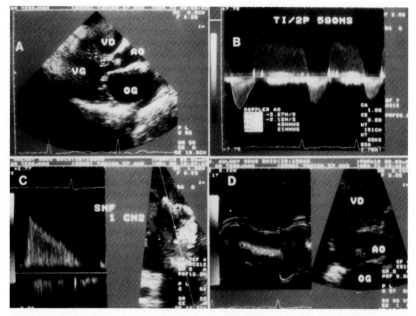

Figure 6.2-3: Echocardiography and Doppler examination of a patient with mitral stenosis and aortic involvement. A. Echocardiography: longitudinal section through the parasternal window during diastole showing the limited mitral opening, thickening of the two mitral leaflets and the aortic cusps. B, C and D. Doppler echocardiography: The aortic disease is of moderate importance: mean systolic LV-Ao gradient was 21 mmHg, the aortic area was calculated to be 1.2 cm² using the continuity method. B. The diameter of the aortic regurgitant jet at its origin was five millimeter during telediastole by color Doppler flow (D) and an HPT of 590 ms on the decreasing maximal velocities of the aortic insufficiency by continuous wave Doppler echocardiography (B). The diameter of the mitral stenosis was calculated to be 1 cm² using the HPT method (C). The extent of the mitral stenosis can be underestimated because of the associated aortic regurgitation.

and a decision made whether or not to repair them both simultaneously. Information provided by Doppler echocardiography is less specific in this association than in the case of double stenosis (Fig. 6.2-3). The left ventricle is dilated by a diastolic overload, which is usually moderate. In the case of significant aortic regurgitation, the mitral area cannot be calculated using the HPT method because of its tendency to overestimate, thereby demonstrating the contribution of mitral planimetry in cardiac imaging. Sometimes, when the pulmonary annulus is easily discerned, the continuity method can be applied at the level of the mitral and pulmonary orifices in the absence of regurgitation at either or both of these sites.

The aortic regurgitation can be quantified using continuous wave Doppler (HPT) to study the decreased velocity during diastole in the left ventricular ejection chamber, but here also, the level of the left ventricular telediastolic pressure, aortic and left ventricular compliance and the amount of aortic resistance can frustrate this method. The flow can be further analyzed by means of pulsed Doppler in the isthmic region, mapping of the regurgitant jet of aortic insufficiency into the left ventricular ejection chamber and the dimensions of the jet at its origin. The multiple methods used show the difficulty encountered in quantifying the aortic regurgitation.

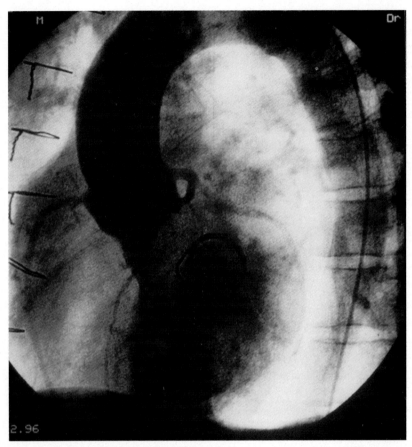

Figure 6.2-4: Aortic cineangiography with a left anterior oblique of 60°. Demonstration of a voluminous aortic regurgitation in a patient who had undergone mitral valve replacement for mitral stenosis several years earlier.

As in all multivalvular diseases and particularly when the problem of quantifying the regurgitation arises, hemodynamic and angiographic analyses (Fig. 6.2-4) are essential to determine the true extent of the aortic insufficiency evaluated during injection into the aortic root (35). Underestimation of the reflux will lead to the treatment of only the mitral valvulopathy, a factor aggravating the long term prognosis. For Delahaye et al. (17), leaving a grade I aortic insufficiency intact did not change the long term prognosis for the surgical treatment of mitral stenosis (72.7% survival at 20 years), whereas failure to treat grade II or higher aortic regurgitation significantly altered survival at the same endpoint (49.7%).

In the final analysis, perioperative examination, either at the beginning or the end of cardiopulmonary bypass, can be used to revise a possible minimization of the aortic leak, especially when it interferes with mitral surgery.

The interventions recommended depend upon the respective importance of the two valvulopathies.

When the mitral stenosis is tight and the aortic regurgitation is discrete, the latter is left untouched and the mitral stenosis is treated, whenever possible, by percutaneous transvenous mitral commissurotomy.

When the mitral stenosis is tight and the aortic insufficiency is moderate, a range of therapeutic possibilities is available depending upon the results of the presurgical evaluation; in certain cases, isolated percutaneous transvenous mitral commissurotomy can be performed leaving the aortic regurgitation intact, though the repercussions must be subjected to regular monitoring afterwards. Most commonly, dual repair is necessary, combining aortic and mitral valve replacements or aortic valve replacement and open mitral commissurotomy. Finally, when the aortic regurgitation is extensive, it must be corrected. The approach to the mitral valve depends upon the extent of the stenosis and the type of lesion, varying from no surgery, open-heart mitral commissurotomy or mitral valve replacement.

Aortic and mitral insufficiency

In contrast to mitral-aortic involvement including mitral stenosis, always of rheumatic origin, the association of the two regurgitations reflects more diverse etiologies. This situation may be of rheumatic origin, but sometimes the lesions are of the degenerative myxomatous type with valve prolapse, in the context, or not, of Marfan's syndrome, with elongation and rupture of the chordae tendineae. More rarely, it results from a dual infection of infective endocarditis with a particularly severe evolution (29,36). In this association, the aortic regurgitation is usually predominant, masking the clinical expression of the mitral insufficiency. Especially in the latter case, it is not always easy to differentiate between an organic and a functional origin by simple dilatation of the annulus.

These double regurgitations are often poorly tolerated with extensive dilatation of the left ventricle induced during diastole by both the aortic regurgitation and the increased left atrioventricular flow. Upon auscultation, in addition to the holosystolic regurgitation murmur of mitral insufficiency and holodiastolic aortic incompetence, a protodiastolic gallop rhythm is often heard. Phonocardiography and pharmacodynamic tests confirm the retrograde origin of the two murmurs with parallel enhancement with vasoxine hydrochloride and concomitant diminution with amylnitrite. The ECG usually indicates a clear enlargement of the left atrium or atrial fibrillation and left ventricular hypertrophy of the diastolic type, except in the case of acute double regurgitations. Fluoroscopy reveals left atrioventricular dilatation, except in the case of acute bacterial regurgitations, but it reveals this condition in all cases with highly increased overall cardiac kinetics associating oscillation of the cardio-aortic shadow and expansion of the left atrium and the pulmonary veins with pulmonary vascular overload.

Echocardiographic and Doppler cardiac examinations further define the organic mitral involvement and the effect on the left-side chambers, and quantify the regurgitant jets. Left ventricular diastolic overload is marked. Regurgitations are easily identified by color Doppler flow echocardiography with limited interaction between the two refluxes. Furthermore, their quantification remains easy with this technique when they are extensive. Such regurgitations give rise to broadly elongated jets, either into the left ventricle in the case of aortic insufficiency or into the left atrium in the case of mitral incompetence. In contrast, quantification becomes less accurate for intermediate pathologies (37). In the latter case, aortic and left ventricular angiographies are needed to quantify the two regurgitations and to evaluate the left atrial and ventricular dilatation and ventricular kinetics (35).

Hemodynamic study usually confirms the poor tolerance with frank elevation of the telediastolic left ventricular pressure, the pulmonary capillary pressure with v wave of mitral regurgitation and increased pulmonary pressures.

The aortic lesion is always repaired surgically with prosthetic or homograft valve replacement. Repair of the mitral defect also consists of valve replacement in most cases. When the anatomic lesions are amenable, reconstructive mitral valvuloplasty complemented by the insertion of an annuloplasty ring can be envisaged (38).

Aortic stenosis and mitral insufficiency

Fortunately, the association of these two lesions is rare. Its functional tolerance is poor, with rapid onset of pulmonary repercussions, which are responsible for its seriousness. This pathology is treated in detail in another chapter in this volume.

TRIPLE VALVULOPATHIES

Triple valvular involvement is rare, representing no more than 1% to 3% of surgical series. Most often, they are the association of a functional tricuspid insufficiency and a mitral-aortic valvulopathy. More rarely, triple organic lesions occur.

Triple aortic-mitral-tricuspid regurgitations can be observed in the context of diffuse dystrophic lesions of the three orifices (39). More unusually, the three valves can be affected with bacterial endocarditis. Symptomatologic specificity relies on the existence of predominant right-sided heart signs with exertion-induced and spontaneous hepatalgia and attenuations of signs of left ventricular insufficiency. During the clinical examination, a holodiastolic aortic regurgitation murmur coexists with a holosystolic reflux murmur in the apex-axillary and xiphoid areas, where the inspiratory increase is not always evident. Signs of congestive heart failure attest to the right-sided lesion with painful systolic hepatomegaly, hepatojugular reflux and distended jugular, all associated with edema of the lower limbs.

Radiographs show frank cardiomegaly with heightened kinetics and overall dilatation affecting the four chambers. The EGG can demonstrate bi-atrial hypertrophy but the sinus rhythm is often replaced by atrial fibrillation. Bi-ventricular enlargement is not always seen and a normal ventriculogram can contradict the radiologic image of cardiomegaly. Echocardiography provides etiologic indications with images of valvular prolapse, elongated or ruptured chordae tendineae, dilatation of the annuli and information concerning the size and the kinetics of the heart chambers. Doppler remains limited in the quantification of regurgitations but, in contrast, provides information on pulmonary pressures.

Hemodynamic and angiographic assessments are essential for the specific determination of the respective involvement of each of the three valves and the necessity for triple valvular surgery. To repair the aortic insufficiency, a replacement valve is required in association with double mitral and tricuspid repair when the latter is anatomically possible. When the latter is not feasible, the mitral and tricuspid valves are replaced.

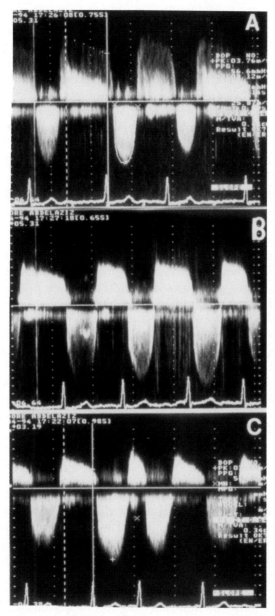

Figure 6.2-5: Quantitative continuous wave Doppler study of a triple valvulopathy of rheumatic origin. A. Aortic disease: mean systolic LV-Ao gradient of 43 mmHg, the aortic area was calculated to be 0.7 cm² using the continuity method, HPT of the aortic regurgitation jet was 543 ms. B. Mitral disease: mean diastolic left atrium-left ventricle gradient of 20 mmHg, mitral area was calculated to be 1.1 cm² using the HPT method on the mitral diastolic flow. C. Tricuspid disease: mean diastolic right atrium-right ventricle gradient of 8 mmHg, tricuspid area was calculated to be 1.2 cm² using the HPT method. The maximal systolic velocity of the tricuspid regurgitation enabled the systolic pressure in the pulmonary artery to be estimated at 64 mmHg.

Triple mixed aortic-mitral-tricuspid disease, more common than triple stenoses (40-42), are of rheumatic origin. Their symptomatology depends upon the respective part played by each of the three lesions, with the possibility of congestive heart failure dominated by right-heart signs. Sometimes, the clinical picture recalls that described for mitral-aortic valvulopathies, where the predominant manifestations reflect the mitral pathology, that is to say, dyspneic pulmonary symptoms.

Auscultation is burdened with sounds associating diastolic and systolic murmurs in all classical areas, with the particularity of inspiratory enhancement of systolic-diastolic xiphoid auscultation which should, in principle, be sought. Chest x-ray almost always shows overall cardiomegaly with images of pulmonary vascular overload and possible mitral and/or aortic valvular calcification. The ECG shows atrial fibrillation with signs sometimes dissociated with bi-ventricular hypertrophy. Echocardiography and Doppler, in addition to providing anatomic information (43), enables evaluation of the pulmonary repercussions. Quantification of the valvular defects in this situation, as in the others, is frustrated by the association of regurgitation and stenosis (Fig. 6.2-5). Catheterization prior to recommending surgical reparation of the lesions is more essential in this case than in the others. Hemodynamic assessment provides information concerning the left and right ventricular telediastolic pressures, and pulmonary pressures in the search for pulmonary pre-, post- or mixed-capillary arterial hypertension.

The surgical intervention usually consists of double mitral-aortic valve replacement associated with tricuspid valvuloplasty or, more rarely, with a the insertion of a tricuspid bioprosthesis.

ACQUIRED PULMONARY VALVULOPATHIES

Finally, in the context of acquired multivalvular disease, pulmonary involvement is extremely unusual. Such lesions were previously described during the course of major and long-standing rheumatic valvulopathies (13,14) and, more recently, in the context of tricuspid-pulmonary right-heart involvement during the progression of carcinoid disease, especially of primary ovarian origin (22).

The clinical picture is that of right-sided heart failure without autonomous pulmonary involvement (no thromboembolic disease or chronic bronchopathy) and without left-heart involvement, in particular, without mitral and/or aortic valvulopathy.

The etiologic diagnosis is supported by the search for a primary tumor by abdominal echocardiography or the measurement of serotonin derivatives, the choice of analyses being oriented by the clinical particularities expressed (abdominal pain, flush syndrome).

Echocardiography confirms the anatomic involvement of the tricuspid and pulmonary valves, identifies an infiltration, assesses its extent, and evaluates valvular hypokinesis (44). This valvular involvement gives rise to stenotic and regurgitant forms recognized by Doppler examination (45).

In the absence of hepatic metastases, some of these patients can benefit from surgical treatment (46,47).

Pulmonary insufficiency, mentioned above as an element for a possible differential diagnosis in the context of mitral-aortic involvement, is actually seen more rarely because it corresponds to an advanced stage of mitral valve disease that is rarely attained in the populations consulting cardiology departments in developed nations.

The diagnostic profile of acquired pulmonary valve disease includes very severe pulmonary arterial hypertension associated with the clinical signs of causal mitral valvulopathy (usually stenosis), functional tricuspid insufficiency, pulmonary arterial hypertension with a loud second heart sound in the pulmonary area, and a holodiastolic Graham Steell's murmur of pulmonary insufficiency.

At this stage, the ECG very often shows atrial fibrillation with signs of right ventricular hypertrophy. The chest x-ray shows a middle arc, convex at its superior part, and right ventricular enlargement with a supradiaphragmatic apex. Pulmonary transparency is usually enhanced at this stage. Echocardiographic and Doppler examinations confirm the pulmonary origin of the murmur and, because of the existence of tricuspid insufficiency, enable the calculation of the systolic pulmonary arterial pressure, which is generally very high. At this stage, the prognosis is poor.

SURGICAL TREATMENT OF MULTIVALVULAR DISEASE

Surgery is usually recommended for patients with symptomatic multivalvular disease. Nonetheless, in asymptomatic or minimally symptomatic patients, certain parameters indicating myocardial repercussions of the multiple valvular pathologies can prompt the physician to propose surgery (7,48). Thus, significant cardiomegaly, low cardiac output and modification of the ejection fraction of the left ventricle are factors to be considered in the decision to operate or not (49,50).

Modalities

Each valvulopathy responsible for significant deleterious effects should be corrected; minor involvement of a valvular orifice can be neglected keeping in mind the risk represented by a subsequent re-intervention (51). Associated involvement, particularly coronary or aortic, should be treated at the same time (42,52).

Aortic valve disease is corrected by valve replacement (mechanical prosthesis or, in certain cases, a bioprosthesis or homograft). The long term efficacy of conservative reconstructive surgery to repair acquired pathologies of this orifice has not yet been proven.

Mitral valvulopathy can be treated by valve repair or replacement with a mechanical valve or bioprosthesis (53). Percutaneous transvenous mitral commissurotomy is only justifiable when the aortic involvement can be neglected or in the case of mitral-tricuspid lesions, when the latter can either be left intact or repaired using the same method. Thus, Berland et al. (54) reported on three cases of double percutaneous transvenous commissurotomies in patients suffering from mitral-tricuspid stenoses of rheumatic origin.

The choice of prosthesis to replace mitral and aortic valves, when necessary, depends upon the typical criteria used in this situation, such as the patient's age, socio-economic class and aptitude to comply with anticoagulant therapy, and the possibility of a later re-intervention without too high a risk (53,55).

When both left heart valves have to be replaced, it is logical to recommend either two mechanical prostheses or two bioprostheses. It would indeed be unreasonable to add the risk of anticoagulant therapy for a mechanical prosthesis to that of early deterioration and thus re-intervention faced with a bioprosthesis (16).

Tricuspid correction depends upon the type of lesion (56- 61). Organic tricuspid disease benefits from repair or, if it is impossible, replacement with a bioprosthesis (42,59,62-65). Because of the high rate of thrombosis that occurs on mechanical prostheses in the tricuspid position, they are no longer used.

The extent of functional regurgitation due to dilatation of the annulus can be examined perioperatively (58), to determine the need for repair, which in turn can be effected with one of the various repair techniques available (56).

Organic pulmonary involvement in acquired valvular cardiopathies is usually attributable to carcinoid heart disease (66,67). It can take the form of pulmonary stenosis or mixed pulmonary disease and is associated with organic tricuspid regurgitation. Pulmonary endocarditis is extremely rare (66), as are significant lesions due to rheumatic fever. Surgical treatment consists of valve excision; only in certain cases is the valve replaced with a prosthesis.

Functional pulmonary insufficiency can develop as a consequence of pulmonary artery hypertension during valve disease of the left heart. No intervention is necessary in this type of lesion because it usually regresses in parallel with the decrease of pulmonary artery hypertension after reparation of the diseased valves of the left heart.

Results

Mortality attributable to multivalvular replacements, both early (during the first month following the intervention) and delayed (two months or more post surgery), has regressed markedly. This improvement is linked to several factors, especially to progress made in myocardial protection, which is even more important in these interventions because the cardiopulmonary bypass is much longer than that required for monovalvular replacement (68,69). In the report by Gersh et al. (70) describing 91 triple valve replacements performed between 1961 and 1984, the perioperative mortality rate was 7% for patients undergoing surgery during the last eight years versus 24% overall mortality for the series.

Other factors contributing to this prognostic improvement are the choice of prostheses and their improved performance and, above all, the functional status of patients at the time of surgery (16,41). The tendency over the last few years has been to operate on older patients but at an earlier stage in their valvular disease, which improves the long term prognosis; thus Coll-Mazzei et al. (71) reported that 85% of the deaths of the patients who underwent triple valve replacement had New York Heart Association (NYHA) grade IV valvular heart disease preoperatively.

For double mitral-aortic replacements, the perioperative mortality rate in more recent series was less than 10%. Actuarial survival at 10 years varies according to the series but remains around 50% (7,57,62,65,68,72)(Table 6.2-I).

For double mitral-tricuspid replacements, the patient series are smaller and heterogeneous. Indeed, mechanical prostheses were initially used in the tricuspid position but no longer are, as in the case of triple valve replacements, bioprostheses are now recommended. Nonetheless, early mortality still exceeds 10% (59,65,73). Long term actuarial survival depends upon the type of prosthesis implanted (53).

For triple valve replacements, reported perioperative mortality varies from 5% to 37% (48,61,70,71,74,75). The disparity reflects the age and heterogeneity of the studies. The beneficial role of new techniques of cardioplegia and the less advanced character of the

Table 6.2-I. Early mortality and long term survival of patients with mitral-aortic replacements.

Author (ref)	Study period	Patients (n)	Prosthesis type	Perioperative mortality (%)	Long term survival
Teply et al. (7)	1960-80	253	Starr	18	45% at 10 yrs 27% at 15 yrs
Cohn et al. (65)	1972-77	58	Hancock	3.40	75% at 6 yrs
Tandon et al. (62)	1971-80	54	Ionescu	10	94.7% at 3.5 yrs
Duran et al. (57)	1974-79	102	Hancock	13.70	78% at 6 yrs
Stephensonet al. (68)	1973-83	150	diverse	6	35% at 8 yrs
Mikaeloffet al. (72)	1970-85	322	diverse mechanical	5.90	70% at 10 yrs

cardiopathy at the time of the intervention are factors contributing to the better immediate prognosis.

Actuarial survival at 10 years varies between 40% and 60% (7,42,52,70,71,74-76) (Table 6.2-II). Studies of surviving patients have noted constant functional improvement (71,75). Thus, among the 29 survivors in the series of Gersh et al. (70), 79% are NYHA class I and II, as are 70% of the survivors in the population described by Bourezak et al. (74). This favorable clinical evolution is correlated with a regression of cardiomegaly (75) and a return towards normal hemodynamic parameters (16).

Intermediate and long term complications of surgery are mainly accidents associated with the presence of prostheses and the necessity for anticoagulant therapy. Multiple mechanical prostheses expose the patient to the risk of a thromboembolic accident (about 10 events per 100 patient-years (70,75)), for which the clinical picture varies widely depending upon whether it is a prosthetic thrombosis whose evolution can rapidly become dramatic or a systemic embolic accident. On the other hand, hemorrhagic accidents are the consequence of the anticoagulant therapy and are mostly attributable to excessive dosage. Bioprostheses, regardless of their position, expose the patient to the risk of primary valve failure, responsible for regurgitation or sometimes valvular stenosis, and necessitate a new intervention. Finally, regardless of the type of prosthesis, evolution after surgery can be complicated by aggravation of a pre-existing myocardial dysfunction, the development of endocarditis, or a periprosthetic leak.

Table 6.2-II. Early mortality and long term survival of patients with triple valve replacements.

Author (ref)	Study period	Patients (n)	Perioperative mortality (%)	Long term survival
Piekarski et al. (61)	1966-77	34	14	66% at 5 yrs
Bourezak et al. (74)	1967-79	90	37	40% at 10 yrs
Gersh et al. (70)	1961-84	91	24	40% at 10 yrs 25% at 15 yrs
Michel et al. (75)	1968-84	22	13.6	61% at 6 yrs
Coll-Mazzei et al. (71)	1970-84	37	5.40	58% at 10 yrs

In these patients, the use of tricuspid mechanical prostheses darken the prognosis because of their poor hemodynamic performance in this position and their tendency towards thromboembolic complications (52,59). This latter risk is even greater when a disc prosthesis is used compared to a ball prosthesis. The specific risk associated with a ball prosthesis corresponds to the encasement of the struts of the cage in the right ventricular endocardium, thereby decreasing the size of the chamber (61) when pulmonary artery hypertension regresses. The movement of the ball is thus limited and thrombosis occurs more frequently.

In contrast, tricuspid bioprostheses have a much better hemodynamic profile (62,65,75,77) that is even further improved by using aortic homografts in this position (78). The problem, as in positions in the left heart, is the risk of primary valve failure of these substitutes, although this is lower.

Conservative tricuspid surgery is indicated in trivalvular or mitral-tricuspid disease when a functional tricuspid insufficiency exists. The long term prognosis is based on the underlying right ventricular function, which is difficult to evaluate. Indeed, correction of left-heart hemodynamic anomalies and thus the diminution of pulmonary circulation pressures decreases the volume of the tricuspid regurgitation, even when it has not been corrected. However, in the latter case, half the patients have persistent regurgitation, which is a factor of poor long term prognosis, and thus favors surgical repair when the tricuspid insufficiency is considered to be significant in pre- and perioperative examinations (41,79).

Late mortality in patients who underwent double valve replacements with conservative tricuspid surgery is comparable to that of triple replacements (48,56,60) and the intervention is characterized by clear-cut functional improvement.

CONCLUSION

Multivalvular disease has occurred less frequently in recent years because of the lower incidence of rheumatic disease but nevertheless remains an important chapter in the discussion of valve pathologies. These entities are marked by their particularly wide variability in terms of the clinical picture observed, which reflects the diversity of associations possible, with various degrees of regurgitation and stenosis at each of the orifices affected. For these reasons, the clinical and evolutionary profiles are very diverse and render more difficult the exact quantification of the role played by each of the lesions.

Echocardiography and especially Doppler echocardiography have greatly facilitated the diagnosis and evaluation of multivalvular diseases. Nevertheless, the typical complexity of the findings renders hemodynamic and angiographic assessments necessary in almost all cases before the therapeutic indications can be defined.

Multivalvular pathologies have also benefited greatly from the advances made in cardiac surgery, the techniques protecting the myocardium and in postoperative intensive care. The perioperative mortality and morbidity observed in these patients is coming closer and closer to that seen in patients with single valve replacement, provided that the surgical indications are pursued sufficiently early in the natural evolution of these pathologies.

Reference
1. Acar J, Michel PL, Dorent R et al. Evolution des etiologies des valvulopathies operees en France sur une periode de 20 ans. Arch Mal Coeur 1992;85:411-415

2.	Acar J, Luxereau P. Indications operatoires et valvulopathies acquises. Arch Mal Coeur 1981;74:249-253
3.	Delahaye JP. Les examens invasifs dans les valvulopathies acquises de l'adulte. Arch Mal Coeur 1985;78:993-997
4.	Clawson BJ. Rheumatic heart disease. Am Heart J 1940;20:454-474
5.	Roberts WC. Morphologic features of the normal and abnormal mitral valves. Am J Cardiol 1983;51:1005-1027
6.	Duvoisin GE, Wallace RB, Henry Ellis Jr F, et al. Late results of cardiac valve replacement. Circulation 1968; 38(Suppl II):75- 85
7.	Teply JF, Grunkemeier GL, d'Arcy Sutherland H, et al. The ultimate prognosis after valve replacement: an assessment at twenty years. Ann Thorac Surg 1981;32:111-117
8.	Dubost Ch, D'Allaines C, Blondeau P. La chirurgie des cardiopathies tricuspidiennes dans le cadre des lesions polyvalvulaires. Ann Chir Thorac Cardiovasc 1968;7:557-564
9.	Pellegrini A, Peronace B, Marcazzan E. Resultats a distance de 1 190 cas de remplacement valvulaire par une prothese artificielle. Ann Chir Thorac Cardiovasc 1975;14:121-130
10.	Pinzani A, de Gevigney G, Pinzani V, et al. L'insuffisance cardiaque droite pre- et postoperatoire des mitraux et mitro-aortiques. Arch Mal Coeur 1993;86:27-34
11.	Isom OW, Spencer FC, Glassman E. Long term results in 1375 patients undergoing valve replacement with the Starr-Edwards cloth- covered steel ball prosthesis. Ann Thorac Surg 1977;186:310-322
12.	Hanania G, Champeau B, Collin P, et al. Evolution en 10 ans des valvulopathies acquises operees en France. Etude multicentrique. Arch Mal Coeur 1986;79:1402-1410
13.	Ayres SM, Arditi LI, Lanbrew CT, Lukas DS. Quadrivalvular rheumatic heart disease: report of a case with marked stenosis of all valves. Am J Med 1962;32:467
14.	Vela JE, Contreras R, Sosa FR. Rheumatic pulmonary valve disease. Am J Cardiol 1969;23:12-18
15.	Roberts WC, Sullivan MF. Combined mitral valve stenosis and tricuspid valve stenosis: morphologic observations after mitral and tricuspid valve replacements or mitral replacement and tricuspid valve commissurotomy. Am J Cardiol 1986;58:850-852
16.	Braunwald E. Valvular heart disease. In Braunwald E (ed). Heart disease. Saunders, Philadelphia 1991;1007-1077
17.	Delahaye F, Delaye J, Ecochard R, et al. Influence of associated valvular lesions on long term prognosis of mitral stenosis. A 20-year follow up of 202 patients. Eur Heart J 1991;12(Suppl B):77-80
18.	Witchitz S, Gibert C, Witchitz J, et al. Les indications chirurgicales dans l'endocardite infectieuse. A propos de 320 malades dont 114 operes. Arch Mal Coeur 1981;74:735-745
19.	Karalis DG, Ross JJ, Brown BM, Chandrasekaran K. Transesophageal echocardiography in valvular heart disease. In: Frankl WS, Brest AN. (eds). Valvular heart disease: comprehensive evaluation and treatment. 2nd Ed. Cardiovascular Clinics. FA Davis, Philadelphia 1993:105-123
20.	Erbel R, Rohmann S, Drexler M, et al. Improved diagnostic value of echocardiography in patients with infective endocarditis by transesophageal approach. A prospective study. Eur Heart J 1988;9:43- 53
21.	Nelson RM, Vaughan CC. Double valve replacement in Marfan's syndrome. J Thorac Cardiovasc Surg 1969;57:732-737
22.	Wynne J, Braunwald E. The cardiomyopathies and myocardities: toxic, chemical and physical damage to thc heart. In: Braunwald E (ed). Heart disease. Saunders, Philadelphia 1991:1394- 1450
23.	Lundin J, Landelius J, Andren B, Oberg K. Transesophageal echocardiography improves the diagnostic value of cardiac ultrasound in patients with carcinoid heart disease. Br Heart J 1990;64:190-194
24.	Dubost Ch, Maurice P, Gerbaux A. The surgical treatment of constrictive fibrosis endocarditis. Ann Surg 1976;184:303-307
25.	Mossard JM, Walter P, Brcchenmacher C. Atteinte cardiaque au cours d'un syndrome lupique. Etude cliniquc et morphologique a propos d'un cas ayant necessite un double remplacement valvulaire. Arch Mal Coeur 1977;70:1203-1208
26.	Rawsthorne L, Ptacin MJ, Choi H. Lupus valvulitis necessitating double valve replacement. Arthritis Rheum. 1981;24:561- 564
27.	Honey M. Clinical and hemodynamic observations on combined mitral and aortic stenosis. Br Heart J 1961;23:545-555
28.	Urrichio JF, Goldberg H, Sinah KP, et al. Combined mitral and aortic stenosis: clinical and physiological features and results of surgery. Am J Cardiol 1959;4:479-491
29.	Terzaki AK, Cokkinos DV, Leachman RD, et al. Combined mitral and aortic valve disease. Am J Cardiol 1970;25:588-601
30.	Baragan J, Fernandez F, Thiron JM. Les lesions associees. In: Bailliere (ed). Phonocardiologie dynamique. Paris 1976:194-243
31.	Hatle L, Brubakk A, Tromsdal A, Angelsen B. Non-invasive assessment of pressure drop in mitral stenosis by Doppler ultrasound. Br Heart J 1978;40:131-140
32.	Loyd D, Eng D, Ask P, Wranne B. Pressure half-time does not always predict mitral valve area correctly.

J Am Soc Echo 1988;1:313- 321

33. Gorlin R, Gorlin NG. Hydraulic formula for the calculation of the area of the stenotic mitral valve, other cardiac valves, and central circulatory shunts. Am Heart J 1951;41:1-29
34. Danchin N, Khalife K, Neimann JL, et al. Etude retrospective du role de la coronarographie systematique chez les patients valvulaires. Arch Mal Coeur 1984;77:1026-1032
35. Roberts WC. Reasons for cardiac catheterization before cardiac valve replacement. N Engl J Med 1982;306:1291-1293
36. Shine KI, De Sancis RW, Sanders CA. Combined aortic and mitral incompetence: clinical features and surgical management. Am Heart J 1968;76:728-735
37. Lesbre JP, Tribouilloy C. Echographie Doppler des cardiopathies valvulaires acquises. Flammarion Medecine-Sciences, Paris 1993:1-215
38. Carpentier A. Chirurgie reconstructrice de la valve mitrale. In: Acar J (ed). Cardiopathies valvulaires acquises. Flammarion Medecine-Sciences, Paris 1985:554-561
39. Jeresaty RM. Mitral valve prolapse. Raven Press, New York 1979
40. Mikaeloff Ph, Delahaye JP, Convert G, et al. Resultats precoces et tardifs des triples remplacements valvulaires. Utilisation d'une bioprothese en position tricuspidienne. Arch Mal Coeur 1981;74:719-726
41. Piekarski A, Dewilde J. Les polyvalvulopathies. In: Acar J (ed). Cardiopathies valvulaires acquises. Flammarion Medecine-Sciences, Paris 1985:416-441
42. Stephenson LW, Kouchoukos NT, Kirklin JW. Triple valve analysis replacement: an analysis of eight years' experience. Ann Thorac Surg 1977;23:237-242
43. Daniels SI, Mintz GS, Kotler MN. Rheumatic tricuspid valve disease: two-dimensional echocardiographic, hemodynamic and angiographic correlations. Am J Cardiol 1983;51:492-496
44. Tribouilloy C, Slama MA, Rey JL, et al. Demonstration par l'echo-Doppler d'une atteinte polyvalvulaire au cours d'une cardiopathie carcinoide. Arch Mal Coeur 1989;82:109-114
45. Pellikka PA, Tajik AJ, Khandheria BK, et al. Carcinoid heart disease. Clinical and echocardiographic spectrum in 74 patients. Circulation 1993;87:1188-1196
46. Giuttierez FR, McKnight RC, Jaffe AS. Double porcine valve replacement in carcinoid heart disease. Chest 1982;81:101-103
47. Hendel N, Leckie B, Richards J. Carcinoid heart disease: 8 years' survival following tricuspid valve replacement and pulmonary valvotomy. Ann Thorac Surg 1980;30:391-395
48. Livi U, Bortolotti U, Rizzoli G, et al. Surgical treatment of patients with triple heart valve disease. Results and analysis of factors affecting the surgical outcome. Thorac Cardiovasc Surg 1982;30:288-291
49. Acar J, Vahanian A, Michel PL, et al. Faut-il operer les valvulopathies mitrales a- ou paucisymptomatiques? Arch Mal Coeur 1992;85:1837-1843
50. Delahaye JP, Machuron C, Heinen I, de Gevigney G. Faut-il operer un aortique asymptomatique? Arch Mal Coeur 1992;85:1845-1849
51. Rossiter SJ, Craig-Miller D, Stinson EB. Aortic and mitral prosthetic valve reoperations. Early and late results. Arch Surg 1979;114:1279-1283
52. San Felippo PM, Giuliani ER, Danielson GK, et al. Tricuspid valve prosthetic replacement: early and late results with the Starr Edwards prosthesis J Thorac Cardiovasc Surg 1976;71:441-445
53. Perier P, Deloche A, Chauvaud S. Comparative evaluation of mitral valve repair and replacement with Starr, Bjork, and porcine valve prosthesis. Circulation 1984;70(Suppl I):187-192
54. Berland J, Rocha P, Mechemeche R, et al. Valvulotomie percutanee dans l'association stenose mitrale-stenose tricuspide. Arch Mal Coeur 1990;83:1585-1589
55. Bonchek LI. Current status of cardiac valve replacement: selection of a prosthesis and indications for operations. Am Heart J 1981;101:96-105
56. Carpentier A, Deloche A, Hanania G, et al. Surgical management of acquired tricuspid valve disease. J Thorac Cardiovasc Surg 1974;67:53-65
57. Duran CMG, Pomar JL, Comman Th, et al. Is tricuspid valve repair necessary? J Thorac Cardiovasc Surg 1980;80:849-860
58. Iwa T, Watanabe Y, Tsuchiya K, et al. Improved surgical treatment of tricuspid insufficiency in combined valvular diseases. J Cardiovasc Surg 1980;21:604-613
59. Judgutt BI, Fraser RJ, Lee SJK, et al. Long term survival after tricuspid valve replacement. J Thorac Cardiovasc Surg 1977;74:20- 27
60. Peterffy A, Jonasson R, Bjork VO. Ten years' experience of surgical management of triple valve disease. Scand J Thorac Cardiovasc Surg 1979;13:191-198
61. Piekarski A, Dewilde J, Dumoulin P, et al. Les triples remplacements valvulaires. Arch Mal Coeur 1979;72:1196-1202
62. Tandon AP, Whitaker W, Ionescu MI. Multiple valve replacement with pericardial xenograft. Clinical and hemodynamic study. Br Heart J 1980;44:534-540
63. Guerra F, Bortolotti U, Thiene G, et al. Long term performance of the Hancock porcine bioprosthesis in

the tricuspid position. A review of forty-five patients with fourteen-year follow up. J Thorac Cardiovasc Surg 1990;99:838-845

64. Donzeau-Gouge P, Villard A, Olivier M, et al. Reintervention tricuspidienne dans la chirurgie des valvulopathies rhumatismales. A propos de 24 cas. Arch Mal Coeur 1984;77:255-261

65. Cohn LH, Koster JK, Mee RBB, Collins JJ. Long term follow up of the Hancock bioprosthetic heart valve. Circulation 1979;60(Suppl I):87-92

66. Altrichter PM, Olson LJ, Edwards WD, et al. Surgical pathology of the pulmonary valve: a study of 116 cases spanning 15 years. Mayo Clin Proc 1989;64:1352-1360

67. Disesa VJ, Mills Jr RM, Collins Jr JJ. Surgical management of carcinoid heart disease. Chest 1985;88:789-791

68. Stephenson LW, Edie RN, Harken AH, Edmunds Jr LH. Combined aortic and mitral valve replacement: changes in practice and prognosis. Circulation 1984;69:640-644

69. Nitter-Hauge S, Horstkotte D. Management of multivalvular heart disease. Eur Heart J 1987;8:643-646

70. Gersh BJ, Schaff HV, Vatterott PJ, et al. Results of triple valve replacement in 91 patients: perioperative mortality and long term follow up. Circulation 1985;72:130-137

71. Coll-Mazzei JV, Jegaden O, Janody P, et al. Results of triple valve replacement: perioperative mortality and long term results. J Cardiovasc Surg 1987;28:369-373

72. Mikaeloff Ph, Jegaden O, Rumolo A, Bonnefoy JY. Le double remplacement valvulaire mitro-aortique: 322 cas operes entre 1970 et 1985. Arch Mal Coeur 1988;81:71-79

73. King RM, Schaff HV, Danielson GK. Surgery for tricuspid regurgitation late after mitral valve replacement. Circulation 1984;70(Suppl I):193-197

74. Bourezak SE, Chauvaud S, Romano M, et al. Triple remplacement valvulaire. Bilan de 90 operes. Arch Mal Coeur 1984;77:724- 729

75. Michel PL, Houdart E, Ghanem G, et al. Combined aortic, mitral and tricuspid surgery: results in 78 patients. Eur Heart J 1987;8:457-463

76. McManus R, Grunkemeier G, Starr A. Late results of triple valve replacement: a 14-year review. Ann Thorac Surg 1978;25:402-409

77. Mikaeloff Ph, Delahaye JP, Convert G, et al. Resultats precoces et tardifs des triples remplacements valvulaires. Utilisation d'une bioprothese en position tricuspidienne. Arch Mal Coeur 1981;74:719-726

78. Mikaeloff Ph, Convert G, Fleurette J, et al. Remplacement de la valve tricuspide par homogreffe valvulaire aortique. Resultats cliniques et hemodynamiques a plus de 5 ans. Nouv Presse Med 1981;10:1131-1134

79. Delaye J, Gaillarde B, Delahaye JP. L'insuffisance tricuspidienne apres correction chirurgicale des valvulopathies mitro- aortiques: causes de sa persistance et de sa recidivre. Arch Mal Coeur 1975;68:899-907

Chapter 6.3

Endocarditis

Dieter Horstkotte and Cornelia Piper

HISTORICAL SURVEY

The first description of a pancarditis in the course of an acute rheumatic fever, the recognition of endocardial involvement in the inflammation process and the logical designation of this syndrome as "endocarditis", are attributable to the nineteenth century Parisian cardiologist Buoillaud (1), after the vegetation typical of many forms of endocarditis had already been described by Riviere in 1646 and infective endocardial lesions by Lancisi in 1706 and Morgagni in 1761.

In his Gulstonian Lectures in 1885, William Osler distinguished between acute, prognostically unfavorable endocarditis and a chronic, prognostically distinctly more favorable form (2), without being able to explain the reason for these differences in the course of the disease.

No etiologic differentiation between the forms of endocarditis was made until the beginning of this century. Hugo Schottmüller was the first to distinguish between bacterial and rheumatic endocarditis in 1910 (3). It remained for Rudolf Virchow to detect bacteria in the cardiovalvular vegetation and thus to show the involvement of micro-organisms in the development of certain forms of endocarditis (4).

Although the increase in medical knowledge up to the middle of the 20th century with regard to the pathogenesis, clinical signs and symptoms, and the natural course of the disease was impressive, with few exceptions the prognosis remained hopeless even after the introduction of sulfonamides. A prognostically more decisive step in the therapy was achieved with the use of penicillin.

In October 1940, Henry Dawson, in New York, carried out the first low-dosed, parenteral treatment with penicillin on a patient with sub-acute bacterial endocarditis (5). The infection, and a re-infection three years later, could be controlled by means of medication. By 1947, six authors had reported on 69 patients who had been treated with low total daily doses of 0.06-0.34 million units of penicillin for 10 to 103 days. The infection could be controlled in 50 (72.5%) of these patients (6).

The prognosis of patients with sub-acute bacterial endocarditis further improved at the beginning of the fifties after Tom Hunter had demonstrated, in vitro, the bactericidal synergism of penicillin and streptomycin against streptococci (7). At the same time, it became known that antibiotics in bactericidal dosages are essential for the treatment of endocarditis. The high percentage of therapeutic failures in the case of treatment with bacteriostatically effective tetracyclines and chloramphenicol, respectively, substantiated this effectively (8,9).

Apart from the development of further groups of successfully applied antibiotics, the improvement of diagnostic possibilities, up to and including non-invasive echocardiographic detection of endocardial vegetation in 1973 (10,11), as well as microbiologic testing methods to demonstrate the pathogenic agent and to test the bactericidal qualities of antibiotics and combinations of antibiotics in vitro, surgical intervention during acute endocarditis has made a substantial contribution to improving the prognosis.

The first successful surgical treatment of a native valve endocarditis was carried out in 1960 by Kay (12). He removed the tricuspid valve, which was infected by a fungal endocarditis, from a patient on whom he operated because of an acquired ventricular septal defect. The aortic and mitral valves were replaced in 1965 and 1967, respectively (13,14), because of florid endocarditis. Since then, acute surgical intervention has had a firm place in the treatment of otherwise uncontrollable endocarditis.

Recommendations for the prevention of bacterial endocarditis, which were considerably modified in 1977 on the basis of animal experiments (15), have existed since 1955 (16).

ANATOMY AND DEFINITIONS

The endocardium lines the myocardial areas facing the cavities of the heart (parietal endocardium), forms the cover of the semilunar valves, which is supported by hard fibrous lamina (valvular endocardium), and is an essential component of the tendinous fibers of the atrioventricular valve apparatus (chordal endocardium). The endocardial cover of the cardiac valves is thicker on the proximal circulation side and, in the case of the atrioventricular valves, is composed of three layers, namely the endothelium, stratum subendothelial and stratum myoelasticum, which also contain non-striated muscle cells. The semilunar valves are always muscle-free. On the distal side (remote from the bloodstream) all cardiac valves are composed of two layers, namely the endothelium and stratum subendothelial. The atrial endocardium is thicker than the ventricular. Branched, corresponding, non-striated muscle cells give the ventricular endocardium elastic properties and thus allow active regulation of passive resistance upon diastolic dilation. The endocardium itself, and normal human semilunar valves, contains no vessels.

From a functional point of view, the endocardial endothelium serves as the structural and metabolic barrier between the intracardiac blood and thrombogenic subendothelial structures (17). The normal endocardium does not activate plasmatic coagulation and does not make it possible for thrombocytes and other cellular blood constituents to adhere. Thus it fulfils, to a high degree, the requirements of a thromboresistant surface, which is based on the considerable synthesis capacity of the endothelium, including the development of the von Willebrandt factor (18).

Inflammations of the valvular and the parietal endocardium, as well as of the endothelium of the large vessels close to the heart, in the case of which, strictly speaking, an endarteritis is concerned, are collectively referred to as endocarditis. Some forms of endocarditis, such as endocardial fibroelastosis and endomyocardial fibroses, chiefly affect the valvular endocardium. In the case of the latter, differentiation must be made between microbial and non-microbial causes. Endocarditis caused by micro-organisms is, in imitation of Anglo-American linguistic usage, imprecisely also referred to as "infective endocarditis", in order to convey that the infections can be caused by bacteria,

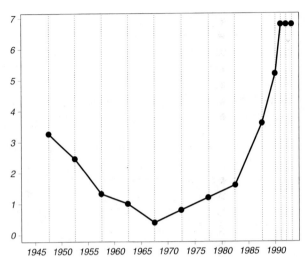

Figure 6.3-1: Changing incidence of infective endocarditis per 100,000 inhabitants in the catchment area of the University of Düsseldorf.

fungi and, possibly, also by viruses. Of the non-bacterial inflammations of the valvular endocardium, rheumatic endocarditis (cf. below (Rheumatic endocarditis)), which is usually a part of a pancarditis, non-bacterial thrombotic endocarditis (cf. below (Non-bacterial thrombotic endocarditis)) and Libman-Sacks endocarditis, which complicates systemic lupus erythematosus (cf. below (Endocardial involvement in the case of SLE)), as well as Löffler's endocarditis (cf. below), are clinically significant.

INFECTIVE ENDOCARDITIS (IE)

INCIDENCE

The precise morbidity rate of the disease, which is not notifiable in any country of the world, is unknown. Based on the voluntary notification system in France (French Registry) the incidence of clinically diagnosed endocarditis is 0.0024% per year, with men (0.0032%) more frequently affected than women (0.0016%) (19). Since more than half of the endocarditis established by autopsy up to the beginning of the nineties remained undiagnosed during the lifetime of the persons affected, and in some cases have continued to do so even after imaging methods, such as transesophageal echocardiography, became available, due to the non-utilization of these methods of diagnosis, there are probably still a considerable number of unknown cases. With an increase in degenerative heart valve defects (calcific aortic stenosis, degenerative mitral insufficiency), predisposing to endocarditis, as well as patients with palliatively operated, congenital and acquired cardiac defects, including patients with prosthetic implant materials, a higher incidence is to be expected (17).

Clinical observations of the case material in the own admission area, defined in relation to the population figure, as well as reported incidences from other closed population collectives, allow to conclude that the number of treated cases of endocarditis is, at present, still higher (0.0068%) (20) and continues to increase. Due to a lack of field studies, it is not clear to what this increase in incidence since the beginning of the seventies is to be attributed and why, in the late eighties, the incidence of endocarditis rose above that at the end of the Second World War (Fig. 1). The probable causes are:

- the increase in degenerative heart valve defects (calcific aortic stenosis, congenital mitral insufficiency), predisposing to endocarditis, as well as the increase in patients with palliatively operated (congenital and acquired) cardiac defects, which have led to an identifiable increase in incidence (21);

- the introduction of echocardiography and, more recently, also transesophageal echocardiography, so that a method is available which allows the involvement of the endocardium in obscure cases of septicemia to be demonstrated and endocarditis diagnosed in otherwise undefined cases.

Etiology and microbiology

The prerequisite for the development of an infective endocarditis (IE) is the colonization of the endocardium, in the train of exogenic or endogenic bacteremias, by micro-organisms capable of reproduction. Exogenic bacteremias of short duration normally occur during diagnostic or therapeutic intervention. Arterial and venous accesses, indwelling catheters, respirator treatment, and infections (pyelonephritis, bronchitis, meningitis, skin infections) can cause persisting endogenic bacteremias.

Although, under appropriate conditions almost all micro-organisms can cause an IE, gram-positive cocci constitute approximately 90% of endocarditis pathogens. The broad application of antibiotics, the increase in the general life expectancy (increase in skin and urinary tract infections and malignant growths), the considerably improved prognosis, as a result of surgical intervention, with respect to patients with congenital and acquired cardiac defects, as well as the extension of invasive examinations have resulted in

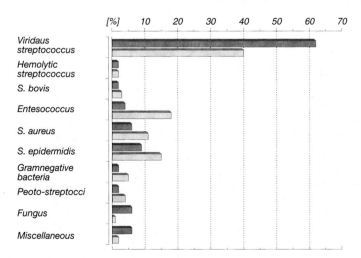

Figure 6.3-2: Prevalence of native valve endocarditis pathogens during 1968-1982 (n = 107) (dark bars) vs. 1983-1992 (n = 192). Note the decreased incidence of infections caused by viridans streptococcus and the increased staphylococcus and enterococcus proportions.

Table 6.3-I: Microbiology of infective endocarditis, taking into account the susceptibility of micro-organisms which are important for the pathogenesis of IE.

Penicillin-sensitive cocci (MIC$_{PEN}$ < 0,1 µg/ml)
- *Viridans streptococci*
  S. sanguis I (gordonii), S. mitior (mitis), S. sanguis II, S. mutans, S. milleri, S. salivarius, S. lactis, nutrionally variant streptococci (NVS)

- *D. streptococci*
  S. bovis

- *β-hemolytic streptococci*
  group A (S. pyogenes), group B (S. agalactiae), group C (S. equisimilis), group F and group G

- Pneumococci

Enterococci and resistant staphylococci (MIC$_{PEN}$≥> 0,1 µg/ml)
- *Enterococci*
  E. faecalis, E. faecium

Staphylococci and micrococci
- *Coagulase-positive staphylococci*
  S. aureus
- *Coagulase-negative staphylococci*
  S. epidermidis, S. hominis, S. hemolyticus
- *Micrococcus spp*

Gram-positive bacilli
- *Corynebacteria*
  C. xerosis, C. pseudodiphtheriticum, C. jeikeium
- *Lactobacillus spp*
- *Erysipelothrix rhusiopathiae*
- *Listeria monocytogenes*
- *Nocardia asteroides*

Gram-negative bacilli
- *Enterobacteria*
  E. coli, Salmonella spp, Serratia marcescens
- *Pseudomonas*
  P. aeruginosa
- *Other gram-negative bacilli*
  Hemophilus parainfluenza[1], H. aprophilus[1]; Actinobacillus actinomycetem-comitans[1]; Brucella melitensis; Cardiobacterium hominis[1], Eikenella corrodens[1]; Kingella kingae[1], Acinetobacter calcoaceticus; Legionella pneumophilia

Gram-negative cocci
- *Neisseria*
  N. meningitides and other species with the exception of N. gonorrhoeae

Mycobacteria (especially rapidly growing mycobacteria)
M. chelonae, M. fortuitum

Rickettsia and chlamydia
Coxiella burnetii (Q-fever)
Chlamydia trachomatis, Chlamydia psittaci

Anaerobic germs
- *Peptostreptococci*
- *Bacteroides spp*

Funghi
- *Candida spp*

---

[1] have been summarized as HACEK-group

---

distinct shifts in the pathogenic spectrum of infective endocarditis (Fig. 2) (22). A classification of the endocarditis pathogens which takes into account the sensitivity of the pathogen to antibiotics is useful for the clinician (Table 6.3-I).

Penicillin-sensitive streptococci

Nearly all viridans streptococci (α-hemolysis), hemolytic (β-hemolysis) and non-hemolytic streptococci, as well as Landsfield Group D streptococci, which are now classified as the genus "enterococcus", are sensitive to penicillin ($MIC_{pen} < 0.1$ µg/ml).

Streptococci sensitive to penicillin have a special adhesion mechanism which allows them to adhere to the projecting non-bacterial, thrombotic vegetation (see below). Hydrophobic interactions, or specific coupling enzymes between endogenous collagenous substances and the fibrillar polysaccharides of the bacterial capsule (glycocalix), which allow the bacteria, even with a high flow velocity, to firmly adhere to the non-bacterial thrombotic vegetation (23-25), serve this purpose.

Viridans streptococci, approximately one percent of which have a relatively high resistance to penicillin ($MIC_{pen} \geq 0.1$ µg/ml), are often responsible for a subacute, prognostically favorable course of the disease. Their pathogenetic significance lies in the fact that they are part of the flora of the parodontium and oropharynx and can very easily infect a previously damaged endocardium due to their adhesion mechanisms.

The chief representative of Lansfield Group D streptococci, which are sensitive to penicillin, is streptococcus bovis, which causes an infective endocarditis with a sub-acute or chronic course. Dental treatments, chronic inflammatory intestinal diseases or malignant gastrointestinal growths are to be found in the infection anamneses of these patients (28). In a number of studies, streptococcus bovis, biotype I has been found significantly often in the blood cultures of patients with gastro-intestinal tumours, usually malignant colorectal growths, or chronic inflammatory intestinal diseases.

S. pyogenes and S. pneumoniae are significant as pathogens in drug-addicts or immunocompromised patients (29).

Enterococci and moderately penicillin-sensitive streptococci

The species streptococcus faecalis and streptococcus faecium, formerly referred to as enterococci, have been classified as belonging to the genus enterococcus since 1984 (30). Serologically, they can be assigned to the Lansfield Group, but they differ from the streptococcus species, inter alia, due to a positive pyrolidonyl-acrylamidase reaction (31). To date, about 12 enterococci species have been discovered, most of which have been isolated in humans (32).

The two most important species of enterococci, as far as infective endocarditis is concerned (E. faecalis and E. faecium), decompose mannitol and hydrolyse arginine; they do not decompose sorbose and sorbitol is only decomposed by E. faecalis. Enterococci dispose of a couple of adherence and virulence factors, as well as an aggregation substance, which are particularly important for the pathogenesis of endocarditis (33-38). For the diagnosis of E. faecalis endocarditis an ELISA can be applied (39).

The percentage of enterococci in the pathogenic spectrum of bacterial endocarditis has risen constantly over the past few years (Fig. 2). In this context, E. faecalis accounts for up to 90% and E. faecium for up to 10% of clinically isolated enterococci, while the other species have only been observed in individual cases. Enterococci are involved to the same degree in ambulatorily and clinically acquired infections. A primary infection (urinary tract infection, intraabdominal and intrapelvic infections, soft-tissue infections, including infections of burn wounds, decubital ulcers, diabetic gangrene) frequently precedes an enterococcal endocarditis (34,40,41). Enterococci were demonstrated in 5%-13% of positive blood cultures from endocarditis patients (42,43,44), where E. faecalis also dominated (Fig. 2).

Of particular interest is the age and sex distribution of the incidence of enterococcal endocarditis; it occurs most frequently in men, chiefly after the age of 50 and in connection with complicated urinary tract infections, while women are mostly affected at an age at which they are capable of gestating. In some reports, instrumental manipulations in the urogenital area have been seen to be responsible for bacteremia of this type in up to 50% of cases (44). Other routes of entry are decubital ulcers, intravenous catheters, or infected injection sites in the case of drug-addicted patients. Another route, which has been given little attention in the past, is endodontitis, in which enterococci are often involved (45).

Approximately one percent of viridans streptococci are only moderately sensitive to penicillin (MIC$_{pen}$ ≥ 0.1 μg/ml), including vitamin B6 (pyridoxine)-dependent streptococci, the hemocultural evidence of which always arouses a suspicion that an infective endocarditis is present.

Staphylococci

Staphylococci comprise approximately 30 species, of which only a few are of definite pathogenic significance as far as humans are concerned. The currently common division into coagulase-negative and coagulase-positive types can neither be molecular-genetically corroborated nor does it allow an evaluation of the pathogenicity. However, it is adhered to for practical bacteriologic diagnostic reasons.

Staphylococcus aureus grows easily in conventional media (sheep-blood agar), produces cell wall-bonded coagulase (fibrinogen receptor) and also releases coagulase. In addition, it forms numerous other enzymes and toxins which allow bacterial persistency and spreading into the infected tissue. The determination of antibodies against teichoic acid is diagnostically useful (46).

S. aureus endocarditis exhibits an acute or hyperacute course, and is frequently complicated by intracardial abscesses, the formation of fistulae, sinus Valsalva aneurysms and perforations (47). A sanitation without operation is only rarely successful and, even with early surgical intervention, a mortality rate of more than 20% must be expected. Endocarditis is often the result of a primary infection (skin injuries, primary local inflammations of the skin, pneumonia, otitis media, osteomyelitis, empyema, septicemia in the case of infected indwelling catheters, and following implantation of joint or vascular prostheses), whereby renal insufficiency, diabetes mellitus and alcoholism, in particular, promote its development. If such infections sustain bacteremias, which occurs in 30%-65% of cases, a secondary endocarditis must be expected. In addition S. aureus endocarditis occurs after cardiac surgical interventions and in the case of intravenous drug abuse. Predisposing cardiac defects are frequently missing. Multiple septic embolism is typical (Fig. 3).

The most significant species in the S. epidermidis group are S. epidermidis and the often multi-resistant S. hemolyticus. S. epidermidis is the most common cause of endocarditis in prosthetic cardiac valves, although perioperative prosthetic infections are rare nowadays. In the case of prosthetic endocarditis, the special interaction between the staphylococci and the implanted polymer material takes effect. What is decisive is the ability, above all, of the coagulase-negative staphylococci to irreversibly adhere to the polymer surfaces and to develop into multiple cell layers in which, parallel to surface growth, they produce an extracellular mucosal substance in which the cell layers become embedded (Fig. 4).

Gram-positive rod-shaped bacilli

Endocarditis as a result of gram-positive rod-shaped bacilli (Table 6.3-I) is rare; its diagnosis is made more difficult by its slow growth in bloodcultures. A variety of corynebacteria (in particular, the multi-resistant taxon JK) have caused suppurating endocarditis in patients with congenital cardiac defects or heart valve prostheses (48-50).

Lactobacilli chiefly cause subacute endocarditis following dental surgery, usually in patients with predisposing cardiac defects (51). Erysipeloid endocarditis (erysipelothrix rhusiopathia) cannot affect a previously undamaged endocardium, takes an acute course and is prognostically unfavorable. Normally, the native aortic valve is affected, while prosthetic endocarditis with this pathogen has not, as yet, been reported (52). Listeriosis endocarditis is chiefly encountered in males above the age of 50 and in dialysis patients (53,54). They have a tendency towards septo-embolic complications.

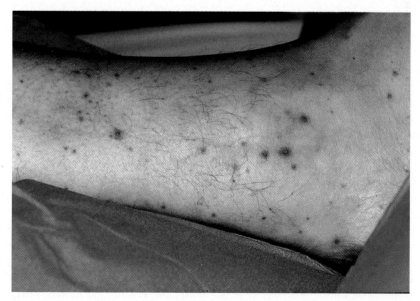

Figure 6.3-3: Multiple septic emboli in a 56-year-old male patient with acute staphylococcus aureus endocarditis.

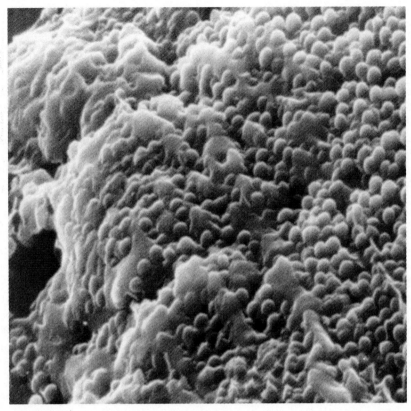

Figure 6.3-4: Surface interaction between staphylococci and synthetic material. Coagulase-negative staphylococci are particularly capable of adhering irreversibly to such surfaces and to produce an extracellular matrix which totally embeds the bacteria. (Courtesy of G. Peters, Münstes.)

Persons with artificial valves and patients without predisposing cardiac defects also frequently contract the disease. Infective endocarditis caused by Legionella pneumophila, actinomycetes (nocardia) and spore-producing bacilli (bacillus cereus, B. subtilis, clostridium perfringens) is limited to individual cases, chiefly to patients with immunosuppression and/or prosthetic cardiac valves (52,55,56).

Gram-negative rod-shaped bacilli

Without any essential change in the incidence, gram-negative rod-shaped bacilli have accounted for approximately 5% of all reported cases of endocarditis in the last 20 years (see above). The pathogens develop aerobically and, due to the length of their generation cycle, growth limits and other requirements with respect to the quality of microbiologic diagnostics, differentiation is made between a non-fastidious group (escherichia coli, serratia marcenscens, salmonella, pseudomonas aerogenosa and cepacia, actinobacter calcoaceticus) and a fastidious group (cardiobacterium hominis, actinobacillus actinomycetemomitans, hemophilus parainfluenzae and aprophilus, kingella kingae, eikenella corrodens, campylobacter fetus, and brucella). In the case of the latter, demonstration of the pathogenic agent is difficult and requires accurate microbial diagnosis (58-60). Except in the case of campylobacter and brucella, bacteremia demonstrated as a result of fastidious gram-negative rod-shaped bacilli always indicate, to a high degree, the presence of an endocarditis, so that these bacteria have been placed together in an independent group (HACEK group: hemophilus, actinobacillus actinomycetem-comitans, cardiobacterium hominis, eikenella corrodens, kingella kingae). Enterobacteria and non-fermenting, gram-negative rod-shaped bacilli belong to the non-fastidious group.

E. coli endocarditis is rare. In approximately 50% of patients, the endocarditis is preceded by urinary tract infections or urologic instrumentation. The mitral valve is the predominant site of infection. Valvular destruction is rare, but large vegetations are frequent, and with a reported mortality rate of up to 60%, the prognosis is poor (59,61).

Salmonella infections have been considerably more frequently diagnosed in the last few years (62-64). When antibiotic therapy is uncompromisingly applied, the endocarditis is conservatively controllable, otherwise, the mortality is high (63).

The left cardiac valves are predominantly affected in the case of acute or subacute serratia endocarditis. Long term hospitalization, alcohol and drug abuse, the implantation of vascular prostheses, urinary and respiratory tract infections (possibly caused by respirator treatment), predispose to serratia endocarditis, which is frequently complicated by the development of large vegetations, embolisms and valvular destruction, and has a high mortality rate (65,66). Other enterobacteria (Table 6.3-I) only rarely cause an endocarditis, following, as a rule, infections or therapeutic or diagnostic intervention in the urogenital tract (67,68).

Particular significance is attached to fastidious gram-negative rod-shaped bacilli in the case of suspected endocarditis if it has not been possible to demonstrate the pathogen on the basis of blood cultures (culture-negative endocarditis), if a target-specific search for HACEK-group pathogens is necessary (see below), or if, in the case of patients where endocarditis is not suspected, these pathogens are found in hemocultures (high probability of endocarditis, exclusion or confirmation of an endocarditis by means of all appropriate diagnostic means). The course is often decidedly chronic.

Gram-negative cocci

Gram-negative cocci were often endocarditis pathogens in the pre-antibiotic era; today, they are rare. Infective endocarditis, which has been caused over the last few years by N. gonorrhoeae, usually took an acute course and affected young adults without predetermined cardiac defects (69). N. meningitidis usually caused acute endocarditis on native valves, frequently following a preceding meningitis (70).

Mycobacteria

Infective endocarditis caused by mycobacteria (M. fortuitum, M. cheloneae) is extremely rare and has only appeared, up to now, in particular circumstances (sternum osteomyelitis, dialysis patients with mechanical heart valve prostheses) (71). These mycobacteria are a rapidly-growing species. With slow-growing species, a large portion of cases affected possibly remain undiagnosed.

Rickettsia and chlamydia

Since Q-fever endocarditis can only be diagnosed serologically, via complement fixation titers of counterphase I and II antigens, or histologically, it has probably been underdiagnosed in the past. Extremely chronic courses (one to two years after contraction of the primary disease) have been recorded, so that, to a high degree, secondary complications (glomerulonephritis, hepatic dysfunction, etc.) first led to diagnosis (72,73). Due to the intracellular persistence of the pathogen, a definitive cure is difficult, and long term therapy over at least one year is necessary (74).

Chlamydia endocarditis is, at least in central Europe, rare. It usually affects the aortic valve and is often accompanied by pericarditis. Anamnestic evidence of contact with birds (Ch. psittaci) or a sojourn in endemic regions (Ch. trachomatis) (75) is diagnostically significant.

Anaerob bacteria

The rare anaerobic endocarditis is usually subacute, occasionally acute, and achieves its importance due to the fact that some anaerobic organisms are part of the flora of the oral and pharyngeal cavities, so that, for example, following dental intervention, they can normally be found in blood cultures (peptostreptococci, bacteroides) (59,76).

Fungi

About 2% of all reported cases of infective endocarditis (4% of prosthetic valve endocarditis) are caused by fungi, a quarter of them in drug-dependent patients. Apart from drug abuse, other immunodeficit states (malignant growths, immunosuppressive therapy, diabetes mellitus) play a role as far as these opportunistic infections are concerned. More than 90% of fungal endocarditis is caused by three genera of fungi; candida types (77-79) account for about two thirds (in 50% of these, candida albicans), aspergillus for 17% (80,81) and histoplasma capsulatum, which is insignificant in central Europe, for approximately 7%. The course is subacute or chronic. Typically, there are large vegetations, which seldom remain unrecognized with echocardiography. Hemocultural demonstration is unsuccessful in at least 20% of cases, so that serologic diagnosis (antibodies, galactomannae) is useful (82).

Pathogenesis

Since the endocardium and normal human semilunar valves have neither vessels nor lymph tracts, potential micro-organisms must reach the site of the infection from the intracardiac blood. Since previously undamaged endocardium is resistant to colonization by micro-organisms, platelet/fibrin deposits are the prerequisite for the development of an infection (Fig. 5). Non-bacterial thrombotic vegetation (ATV) normally develops where there is rheumatic or traumatic damage of the endocardial endothelium as a result of bacterial toxins (staphylococci-α toxin, streptolysin-O) or complement activation. Flow-related changes at the closure edges of the valvular endocardium, which result in increased regeneration and loss of antithrombogenicity of the endothelial cells, are detectable even with a low degree of flow-disturbance (e.g. turbulent flow).

The quite low degree of cardiovascular dysfunction, which can be caused by endothelial damage, explains why, in a portion of the patients with IE, no so-called predisposing cardiac defects are determinable. Two thirds of the patients, however, exhibit congenital, rheumatic, post-infective, or degenerative valvular changes. The preferred locations are distributed in an exemplary way: where there are obstructions, they are post-stenotically localized; with incompetent atrioventricular valves, they are on the atrial side; with semilunar valves, on the ventricular side. Jet-type flows can also cause endocardial damage remote from the lesion (e.g. McCallum patch in the case of mitral insufficiency, or on the pulmonary artery wall opposite a patient ductus) (83-85).

An infection of the ATV requires that an adequate number of pathogens reach it and remain adhered (Fig. 6). The prerequisite for this is a failure of macrophag activation or of humoral defence against infections as a result of the infective power of the pathogen (virulence), inadequate complement activation (serum bactericidia) or elimination capacity of the reticulo-histiocyte system with respect to the infective agent (clearance). Diseases with complement consumption, reduced cellular immunoreactivity and immunosuppressive serum factors (immunodeficiency syndrome, terminal renal

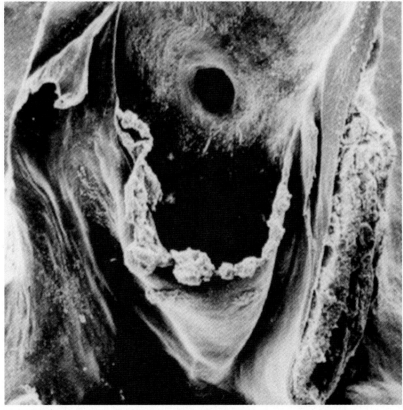

Figure 6.3-5: Rat experiment. Abacterial thrombotic vegetation on the free edge of an aortic cusp, subsequent to endocardial damage caused by an indwelling catheter. Reproduced with permission from Horstkotte D, Bodnar E (eds). Infective Endocarditis. 1st Edition; 1992, ICR Publishers, London.

insufficiency, alcoholism, drug abuse) are accompanied by reduced serum bactericidal effect and clearance (53,86-90).

The ability of potential endocarditis pathogens to adhere to the ATV is determined by their adhesive power and the nature of the vegetation. An adhesion occurs more easily on fresh thrombi, rich in platelets while, in the case of thrombocytopenia, the growth of the vegetation is slowed down (91,92). Diseases which promote the development of an ATV (leukemia, cirrhosis of the liver, various carcinomas, colitis ulcerosa, systematic lupus erythematodes) are, therefore, associated with an increased incidence of IE (93,94). From the point of view of the bacteria, the factors which promote adhesion are linked to the ability of the pathogen to produce glucoproteins such as fibronectin and thus allow the build up of a polysaccharide lawn on the outer cell wall membrane (glycocalix) (95-98) (Fig. 6).

After infection of the vegetation, the bacteria can easily multiply, since humoral defence mechanisms can hardly be effective due to the lack of vascularization of the endocardium and the fact that the fibrin deposits constitute an effective barrier against phagocytes. As a result of multiplication of the pathogens, the accumulation of cell detritus, as well as the accumulation of platelets and fibrin, the vegetation grows until the diffusion of nutrients from the intracardiac blood becomes the limiting factor. The metabolism of the endocarditis pathogens is then restricted, and they multiply only slowly. The reduced reduplication rate explains why, occasionally, even with very long treatment with bactericidal antibiotics, sterilization of the vegetation is not achieved.

Numerous phenomena associated with IE are the expression of a distinct immunologic response. These include the polyclonal (IgG, IgM, IgA) and pathogen-specific activation of immunoglobulin synthesis, as well as the activation of

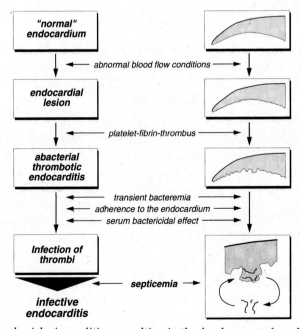

Figure 6.3-6: Pathophysiologic conditions resulting in the development of an abacterial thrombotic vegetation and its subsequent infection by circulating micro-organisms.

Table 6.3-II: Infections, diagnostic and therapeutic interventions likely responsible for bacteremia within four weeks prior to the manifestation of infective endocaridits (University of Düsseldorf 1975-1993, n=237).

	n	%
dental procedures	35	21,3
purulent bronchitis, pneumonia	13	7,9
oropharyngeal and respiratory tract interventions	10	6,1
sinusitis	5	3,0
urgent abdominal surgery	12	7,3
chronic inflammatory bowl disease	7	4,3
cholangitis, cholecystitis	5	3,0
elective abdominal surgery	5	3,0
invasive gastrointestinale diagnostics[1]	4	2,4
acute gastroenteritis	3	1,8
urologic procedures	14	8,5
urosepsis	8	4,9
spontaneous discharge of ureter stones	7	4,3
gynaecologic procedures	3	1,8
adnexitis	2	1,2
septic delivery	1	0,6
indwelling catheters, intensive care	8	4,9
intravenous drug abuse	4	2,4
chronic hemodialysis	4	2,4
wound infections, trauma	14	8,5
	164	69,2
no source identified	73	30,8

[1] coloscopy n=2, sigmoidoscopy n=1, barium enema n=1

immunoglobulin synthesis against auto-antibodies (93,99-102). The presence of circulating immune complexes can be diagnostically significant, and is responsible for numerous complications (arthritis, vasculitis, glomerulonephritis, Janeway lesion) (103-109). In addition, an activation of the complement system occurs with consumption of C3, C4 and CH50, as well as immunologic epiphenomena (positive rheumatoid factors, cryoglobulins). Stimulated phagocytosis is the cause of monocytosis and splenomegaly.

Predisposition

Predisposing factors of a general medical nature (diabetes mellitus, terminal renal insufficiency, cirrhosis of the liver, viral hepatitis, alcohol abuse, immunosuppressive therapy, radiation, congenital and acquired immunodeficiencies, malignant growths) (53,93,110,111) have to be differentiated from cardiac predisposition (already existing endocardial damage). In addition, the increased incidence of bacteremia also plays a role in the case of patients where terminal renal insufficiency (dialysis), diabetes mellitus (skin lesions), drug abuse (intravenous injections), burns, or polytrauma are involved, as well as during intensive medical treatment (53,112,113).

A humoral defence deficiency also exists in patients with chronic inflammatory intestinal diseases, so that the increased incidence of endocarditis in this group of patients is explainable (27). On the other hand, the disturbed cellular immune response in HIV-positive patients or patients manifestly suffering from AIDS, is not, apparently, accompanied by a dramatic increase in the incidence of endocarditis. The possible reason for this is that, in the mainly young, previously undamaged patients, there is no cardiac predisposition. If there is cardiac manifestation in AIDS patients, this is usually quiescent, so that the precise degree of prevalence is unknown. At autopsy, cardiac involvement is found in 28%-73% of cases, most frequently non-bacterial ("marantic"), thrombotic vegetation with consecutive pulmonary or systematic embolisms.

Referred to the total population, no increased risk of endocarditis can be determined with respect to mitral valve prolapse without accompanying mitral insufficiency and secundum type atrial septal defect. As far as all other congenital and acquired cardiac defects are concerned, there is a more or less increased risk of endocarditis (cf. Table 6.3-IX).

Causes of predisposing bacteremia

Knowledge of the causes of bacteremia which precede an IE is of decisive importance as far as their primary prophylaxis is concerned (114-116). In the immediate anamnesis of endocarditis patients, dental surgery, infections of the respiratory tract and surgical intervention involving the oropharynx or respiratory tract, can be determined in approximately 25% of cases (Table 6.3-II). The bacteremia in the case of these surgical interventions, are chiefly caused by penicillin-sensitive streptococci, staphylococcus epidermidis or peptostreptococci.

An abdominal operation, diseases, or diagnostic intervention in the gastrointestinal tract have been found to have preceded a contraction of endocarditis in approximately 15% of cases. The predominant pathogens are enterococci and gram-negative rod-shaped bacilli, as well as coagulase-negative and positive staphylococci. Patients with chronic inflammatory intestinal diseases contract an endocarditis significantly more frequently (usually S. faecalis, S. mitis, S. bovi, S. aureus, or peptostreptococci) than the general population.

Urologic interventions, an urosepsis, or the spontaneous discharge of calculus in the ureter are to be found in the past history of 13% of patients in whom endocarditis is later established. The pathogens are chiefly enterococci but occasionally gram-negative rod-shaped bacilli. Endocarditis as a result of wound infections, skin injuries or indwelling catheters is, in most cases, caused by staphylococci. With the increasing range of diagnostic and interventional techniques in cardiology, particularly in the case of considerably predisposed patients (heart valve defects) and operations of long duration (e.g. valvuloplasty), there are increasing reports of subsequent endocarditis (117-119), so that endocarditis prophylaxis must be applied with particular care in these cases.

Pathology

The classification of endocarditis into acute, subacute and chronic forms originates from the pre-antibiotic-antibiotic era when, without causal therapy, diseases were classified into those which led to death within six weeks and those with a longer course. Subacute IE usually results from infection by less virulent or facultative pathogens (viridans streptococci, S. epidermidis, some gram-negative rod-shaped bacilli, fungi). Enterococcal endocarditis frequently takes a course midway between acute and sub-acute. Acute courses are, as a rule, caused by obligatory pathogenic agents (S. aureus, β-hemolytic streptococci, some gram-negative rod-shaped bacilli). Acute endocarditis can also occur as a complication of other primary infections. While subacute IE usually affects patients with already existing heart valve defects, while in the case of acute endocarditis, previously slightly damaged valves are also frequently affected.

The clinically significant pathologic aspects of IE are its activity, localization and complications. The high percentage (86%) of endocarditis of the native left-sided cardiac valves and prosthetic endocarditis, makes it clear that the valvular endocardium, including the tendinous fibers of the atrioventricular valve and the suture ring of prosthetic cardiac valves, are the most significant preferred locations as far as the development of an endocarditis is concerned (83,84,120,121). The incidence ratio of left to right-side endocarditis has, as a result of the increase in degenerative cardiovascular defects predominantly affecting the aortic valves over the last few years, shifted further in favor of the left cardiac valve (Table 6.3-III). Among left-side infections, aortic valve endocarditis dominates.

Table 6.3-III: Topography of infective endocarditis based on 420 consecutive patients (University of Düsseldorf, 1970-92).

	n	%	Σ
Endocarditis, valvular endocardium involved			
- native left sided heart valves			
- aortic valve	142	33,8	
- mitral valve	71	16,9	
- aortic plus mitral valve	40	9,5	60,2
- native right sided heart valves			
- pulmonary valve	2	0,5	
- tricuspid valve[1]	9	2,1	2,6
- aortic valve endocarditis in non valvular			
obstructions of the left ventricular outflow tract	3	0,7	0,7
Endocarditis, valvular plus mural endocardium involved			
- congenitals with intracardiac shunts	12	2,9	2,9
- persistent ductus apertus	1	0,2	
- aortic coarctation	3	0,7	
- systemic to pulmonary shunts	11	2,6	3,6
Endocarditis parietalis, no shunt lesion	2	0,5	0,5
Prosthetic valve endocarditis			
- aortic prostheses	64	15,2	
- mitral prostheses	43	10,2	
- aortic plus mitral prostheses	17	4,0	29,5

[1] in four cases later involvement also of the left sided heart valves

In 90% of cases, the clinical picture of left ventricular endocarditis is that of a systematic infection or a septicemia (121,122). Predisposing cardiovascular defects frequently exist. The most frequent causes of death are myocardial insufficiency, following acute valvular destruction, and uncontrolled septicemia (123). Compared to this, endocarditis of native, right cardiac valves tends to manifest itself more as pneumonia (septic thromboembolisms) than as systematic infections (124-127). Cardiac symptoms are, as a rule, rare; frequently, there is no cardiac murmur and, in almost all cases, predisposing factors can be determined (intravenous drug abuse, alcohol abuse, indwelling venous catheters), while predisposing cardiovascular defects are rare. The most common cause of death is respiratory insufficiency following septic pulmonary infarctions. A left ventricular endocarditis develops during the course of about half the cases of primary right ventricular endocarditis.

Endocarditis with non-valvular obstruction of the left ventricular outflow tract (e.g. HOCM, or subvalvular membranous aortic stenosis) predominantly affects the aortic valve, the endocardium of which is damaged on the ventricular side as a result of the jet-type and turbulent blood flow (128). With HOCM, less frequently, the mitral valve, which in the case of advanced HOCM is often secondarily insufficient, can also be affected. Even with increasing destruction of the aortic valve, in the majority of cases no serious aortic insufficiency results since the muscular obstruction of the left ventricular outflow tract prevents serious regurgitation.

Of the lesions with intracardiac shunts, both patients who had and those who did not have tetralogy of Fallot repair, as well as those who underwent palliative surgery (e.g. systemic-pulmonary shunts), are particularly predisposed (129). Patients with ventricular septal defect and concomitant aortic insufficiency, in case of which normally the prolapsing aortic valve is infected, also carry a high risk of endocarditis. Isolated septum defects can also lead to an endocardial lesion and, secondarily, to a tricuspid valve endocarditis or to a parietal endocarditis of the right ventricular wall. Formerly, a persisting duct was considered to carry a high risk of endocarditis and, even with hemodynamically insignificant shunt volumes, operation was recommended. Actually, however, the risk of endocarditis appears to be lower than, for example, in cases with palliative systemic-pulmonary shunts.

All cases of microbiologically cured endocarditis exhibit cardiac defects, more than 50% of which are hemodynamically significant. Residual morphologic defects following atrioventricular endocarditis are ruptured chordae (valvular prolapse), perforation of the cusps, substance defects, and frequently fusion of the commissures. Cured aortic valve endocarditis frequently exhibits perforations or other substance defects of the semilunar valves, and/or periannular aneurysms or fistulas following drained ring abscesses. Even minor valvular changes are accompanied by changed flow conditions and can become hemodynamically significant after decades.

Case history and clinical picture

Case history

The general anamnesis helps to estimate the duration of the signs and symptoms of the infection (fever, pallor, indisposition, decrease in vitality, arthralgia, etc.) and to make the general medical factors predisposing to endocarditis evident (see above). The specific anamnesis serves to ascertain previously determined cardiac murmurs and cardiac defects, as well as circumstances which could have caused endocarditis (Table 6.3-II).

Symptoms and clinical findings

The declining number of cases of streptococcal endocarditis, with an increase in staphylococci and enterococci as endocarditis pathogens, has essentially contributed to the increase in the percentage of acute, and in some cases fulminant courses of the disease, so that a certain "structural change" has occurred in the clinical picture of endocarditis (Table 6.3-IV). A general malaise (fatigue, languor, recurrent outbreaks of sweating, a sudden drop in efficiency) and, in almost all cases, continuous or remittent fever, exists in

Table 6.3-IV: Clinical symptoms and findings at hospital admission and prognosis of patients with native valve infective endocarditis.

symptoms/prognosis	1986/1992[1] %	1971/1980[2] %
fever	95	92-98
lack of appetite, nausea	73	68-82
outbreaks of sweat	61	42-73
dyspnoe	56	8-55
paleness	42	56-87
shivering attack	41	15-64
athralgias, myalgias	41	25-51
palpitations	37	16-29
non-focal neurologic symptoms	29	14-33
tendency to hemorrhages	25	3-9
angina pectoris	12	1-7
pathologic murmurs	91	86-100
- of these, first appearance of murmurs	65[3]	-
lung edema	46	-
cutaneous manifestations, typical for endocarditis	32	7-9
RBBB/LBBB	24	12-44
conduction disturbances in the ECG	19	8-31
splenomegaly	16	29-52
ventricular arrhythmias	9	0-6
vasculitis	9	0-12
drumstick finger	1	3-58
increased BSR	94	88-100
leucocytosis	71	34-87
erythrocyturia/hematuria	44	33-89
proteinuria	51	17-63
anemia	42	43-89

[1] Number of consecutive patients (Department of Medicine, University Düsseldorf 1986-1992)

[2] Indications according to pooled statistics published between 1972 and 1981

[3] Re-examined patients with available patient files for comparison

approximately 90% of patients. It may not exist in the case of older patients with subacute forms, patients with terminal renal insufficiency, cerebral hemorrhages or medication-induced endocarditis (antipyretica, antibiotics). A newly developing regurgitant murmur is looked upon as evidence of an endocarditis. In the case of suspected atrioventricular valvular insufficiency, it should be remembered, from a differential diagnosis point of view, that systolic murmurs are frequent in patients with acute (increased cardiac output) or chronic infections (anemia). Patients with acute endocarditis often have no cardiac murmur in the initial clinical examination, but in the majority of cases this develops under antibiotic therapy. There are also frequently no cardiac murmurs in the case of tricuspid valve endocarditis. In case of tachycardia, the unexperienced often fails to recognize the diastolic cardiac murmur indicative of an aortic insufficiency.

The most common cardiac complication of IE is valvular insufficiency, which is found very much more frequently in the case of infections of the aortic valve than in the case of mitral valve endocarditis (21,130). Following left-side valvular insufficiency, there is an acute volume overload and dilation of the left chamber, which only the stiffness of the pericardium counteracts mechanically. With the exception of less severe cases, in which the acute decrease of the effective stroke volume can be compensated for by an increase in heart rate, a cardiac pump failure occur relatively quickly (113).

A regionally confined myocarditis, which occurs in approximately 30% of cases, can be the result of circulating immunity complexes, bacterial toxins or a vasculitis (131,132).

Myocardial infarction can be the result of septic thromboembolism, mycotic aneurysms, or inflammations of the coronary arteries (coronary artery thromboses). The intracardiac fistulae and abscesses detectable in up to 80% of IE cases predominantly occur with S. aureus or enterococcal endocarditis, and chiefly affect the annulus of the aortic valve (133). The rupture of a mycotic aneurysm can lead to a pyohemopericardium, pericardial tamponade, atrial and ventricular septum defects, or aortopulmonary windows. Most frequently, there are perforations of a sinus Valsalva in the left or right ventricle or in the right atrium. Left-ventricular to right-atrial shunts (acquired Gerbode defect), which peregrinate the root of the aorta, are rare in the case of aortic valve endocarditis.

The majority of extracardiac endocarditis complications consist of arterial embolisms, which can be infective or non-infective (130,134-137). The incidence of clinically diagnosed arterial embolisms is 15%-35%. A much higher percentage can be recorded in series of autopsies, in which the kidney and the central nervous system are affected in particular.

Focal embolic glomerulonephritis or renal infarctions are less frequent in the course of an IE than diffuse complex-mediated nephritis, which can manifest itself as interstitial nephritis or acute or chronic proliferative glomerulonephritis (106,107,138-144). With increasing serum concentration, complex-mediated nephritis is becoming more frequent, is accompanied by bacteriuria and hematuria, and histologically, often comprises a focal, subacute glomerulonephritis (Löhlein focal nephritis) with immunity complex deposits on the basal membranes of the glomeruli. A proteinuria of more than 150 mg/day must be considered as prognostically unfavorable (138,140,145). An antimicrobial therapy, in particular, with a combination of potential nephrotoxic antibiotics, can be a contributory cause of an acute renal failure (146-148).

A diffuse vasculitis as a result of the accumulation of circulating immunity complexes

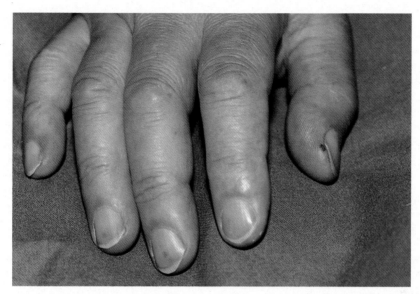

Figure 6.3-7: Osler nodes on the right thumb of a 52-year-old male patient with native valve endocarditis caused by viridans streptococci.

on the vascular endothelium, with consecutive activation of the complement system, can, besides the myocardium and the renal glomerula, affect the central nervous system (aseptic meningoencephalitis) and the skin (104,108,149). Complex-mediated vasculitis or embolisms can be at the root of the changes in the skin, which can be typically observed following endocarditis. So-called mycotic aneurysms have been reported in 2%-15% of cases and chiefly occur in the later course of an endocarditis. Predominantly, the cerebral vessels (24.1%), the limbs (13.8%), the coronary arteries (10.3%), the thoracic aorta including the sinus Valsalva, the abdominal aorta and its branches (27.6%), and predominantly the splenic or other mesenteric arteries are affected (Table 6.3-V) (150-154). Viridans streptococci and other less virulent bacteria cause mycotic aneurysms more frequently than, for example, staphylococci (147).

An anemia-related pallor occurs in approximately a quarter of patients with chronic forms of IE. A lupus-like, butterfly-shaped facial erythema is extant. Septic skin or cerebral thromboembolisms are observed in approximately 20% of patients. As an indication of the decreasing number of chronic forms, splenomegaly has become rarer.

Typical skin and eye manifestations are:

- Osler nodes: Pin-head to pea-sized, bluish-red tumefactions, usually on the finger or toe pads, which are tender on pressure. These are the result of embolisms, possibly with consecutive vasculitis (Fig. 7) (155-159). In contrast to a pyodermia, Osler nodes disappear without suppuration a few days after the infective endocarditis is medically controlled. Parallel to the decrease of "lenta" cases, the frequency of Osler nodes has decreased from 70% to 10%-15% (160).

- Janeway efflorescences: Painless, maculous, 1-5 mm, irregularly defined, hemorrhagic efflorescences on the palmar and plantar surfaces of the feet, more rarely, also on the

Table 6.3-V: Mycotic aneurysms complicating infective endocarditis. Pooled data from Cates et al. (153) and Horstkotte (154).

Incidence:		29/798 (3,6%)
Localization:	Thoracic aorta[1]	n=7 (24.1%)
	Cerebral arteries	n=7 (24.1%)
	Mesenteric arteries	n=5 (17.2%)
	Limb arteries	n=4 (13.8%)
	Coronary arteries	n=3 (10.3%)
	Abdominal aorta	n=1 (3.4%)
	Other sites	n=2(6.9%)

[1] including the sinus of Valsalva

arms and legs, which become pale under pressure (103,161).

- Subungual hemorrhages (splinter hemorrhages) are frequently observed in infections of differing origin and are not specific as far as an IE is concerned (162,163) (Fig. 7).

- Petechia are the result of sepsis-related thrombocytopenia, which are often localized on the trunk or the oral and pharyngeal mucosa. Complex-mediated vasculitis possibly contributes towards their development (164).

- Roth spots in the retina appear as cotton wool foci, the perivasal lymphocytic aggregates of which are attributable to edema and hemorrhages (165-167).

Due to a concomitant infective involvement a progressive but reversible splenomegaly as a consequence of a follicular hyperplasia is observed more often the longer the endocarditis is active. With the decrease in lenta cases and an increase in more acute courses, the percentage of patients presenting with splenomegaly has significantly decreased (Table 6.3-IV). In autopsy series, splenic abscesses have been found in approximately 10% of cases (160-162). Due to a lack of awareness, splenic abscesses are not suspected in most cases until autopsy (169). Routine abdominal sonography or scintigraphy, therefore, should be considered in all patients with infective endocarditis, especially in those who have signs or symptoms referable to the left upper quadrant, or with persistent sepsis for more than 72 hours despite adequate antibiotic treatment.

Severe, prognostic significant complications of IE are cardiac or aortic root abscesses, aneurysms and fistulas. Micro-abscesses are found in nearly all cases of aortic valve endocarditis and most cases with mitral valve endocarditis if special attention is paid to them intra-operatively. Depending on the causative organism, micro-organisms tend to increase in size (see above). If an annular abscess is drained to one side, for example into the ascending aorta, an aneurysm results. Perforation and drainage of two sides results in an intracardiac or peri-annular fistula which is often accompanied by significant regurgitation. Clinically, the drainage of an abscess is frequently accompanied by a septic reaction or a pyodermia in patients with a so far controlled infection. The clinical deterioration is transient and recovery usually manifests within 24 hours.

Peri-annular spreading of the infection can be found intra-operatively in approximately 25% of cases with endocarditis involving the mitral or the tricuspid valve, while in the aortic position a percentage of 40%-50% is reported (170,171). The diagnosis of even small annular abscesses is easily possible with echocardiography, especially with transesophageal echocardiography (see below). In cases where the endocarditis is complicated by a pericarditis, a pericardial effusion or an AV-block, abscesses should be suspected and transesophageal echocardiography performed.

In approximately one third of all native valve endocarditis cases, the clinical course is accompanied by neurologic complications (172-175). The mortality of uncomplicated versus neurologically complicated cases of infective endocarditis is 15% versus 41% (172). The majority of neurologic complications are consequences of septic or aseptic embolisms. They may be divided into:

- cerebral vascular occluding embolisms

- intracerebral hemorrhage complicating (mycotic) aneurysms

- brain abscesses, and

- meningitis or meningoencephalitis.

The latter may be divided into septic and aseptic forms. The frequency of cerebral embolic complications varies significantly between 15% and more than 80% (176). According to large surveys, cerebral embolic complications are most frequent (approximately 58%) while meningitis (25%), intracerebral hemorrhagic (15%) and brain abscesses (10%) have been found less frequently (172). Focal neurologic symptoms (e.g. hemiplegia, hemianopsia) are the reason for hospital admission in 3%-5% of patients with later proven bacterial endocarditis. If non-focal neurologic symptoms are also regarded, 52% to 58% of patients with endocarditis demonstrate neurologic symptoms when they are admitted to hospital. Staphylococcus aureus (isolated on multiple brain abscesses, meningitis), streptococcus viridans (cerebral thromboembolic events, lympho-monocytere meningitis) and S. pneumonea (purulent meningitis) are frequently associated with neurologic complications.

Laboratory tests

A sometimes distinctly increased BSR is the most common laboratory finding in patients with IE. While with a normal BSR, a bacterial endocarditis is improbable, due to the numerous possible causes, an increased BSR is only of minor significance from a differential diagnosis point of view. Repeated determination of the BSR is useful for therapy control. After an endocarditis has been cleaned up, an increased BSR occasionally continues for some months.

A leukocytosis exists in more than 60% of all patients with IE. In the case of acute endocarditis, it is practically always present, usually with leukocyte counts of 25,000-50,000/mm^3. With sub-acute courses of the disease, often not more than 8,000 mm^3 are found. Leukopenia can be caused by gram-negative pathogens or the antibiotic therapy.

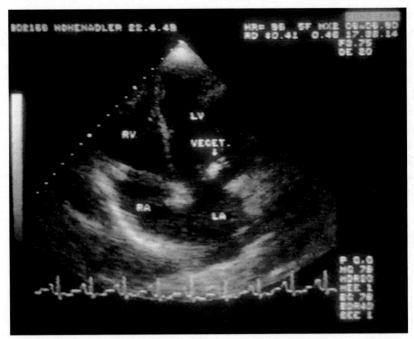

Figure 6.3-8: Staphylococcus epidermidis vegetation on the mitral valve diagnosed by TTE.

A normochromic, normocyte anemia occurs in 50%-80% of cases. Stimulation of the reticulo-histiocyte system leads, particularly in the case of subacute forms, to an increase in plasma cells in the bone marrow. In 15%-25% of cases, macrophages are detectable in the capillary blood.

A renal involvement usually manifests itself primarily as proteinuria (approximately 50% of patients with IE). The degree of loss of renal protein is jointly responsible for the reduction of the albumin and total protein in the serum. In the electrophoresis, there is, in addition, an increase in the α_1, α_2 and γ-globulins. A (micro-) hematuria is observed in half of the patients with proteinuria. In over 90% of cases, circulating immune complexes (CIC) can be detected. The development of immunoglobulins can, *inter alia*, lead to complement consumption and to the determination of positive rheumatoid factors, antinuclear antibodies, antibodies against myocardial structures non-striated musculature and skeletal musculature, cryoglobulins, and macroglobulins. The serum complement consumption manifests itself in an increase in the C-reactive protein which, in the case of patients with IE, is normally increased to over 5 mg% and, in 20% of patients, to over 30 mg%. CIC's are jointly responsible for numerous secondary complications of IE, such as nephritis, vasculitis and pericarditis.

Except for the recognition of septic pulmonary embolisms, radiologic examinations are of no diagnostic value in the case of right ventricular endocarditis, but they are useful for controlling the course (heart size, pulmonary vascular obstruction, pneumonia).

Electrocardiographically, AV blocks have been reported in approximately 20% of cases (177), which may indicate intracardiac abscesses or fistulas, or an accompanying myocarditis. Less frequently, intraventricular conduction disorders or bundle-branch

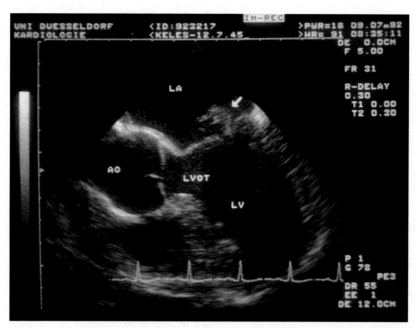

Figure 6.3-9: Same patient as in Fig. 8. The vegetation is larger when viewed by TEE which also demonstrates micro-abscesses not seen by TTE.

blocks are reported. In our own experience, conduction disorders have been found more frequently within 100 days after manifestation of the initial endocarditis symptoms, while in the later course their incidence is less frequent. However, it is of clinical importance that 2.1% of AV blocks grade I and II and 0.9% of a total AV blocks occur later than 100 days after the initial manifestation of endocarditis (Table 6.3-VI). Ventricular tachycardia, ventricular fibrillation or sudden death have been observed in 0.6% of our patients within 100 days although these patients were hospitalized or had frequent out-patient controls. Later than 100 days after the initial symptoms of endocarditis, another eight patients (2.4%) presented with ventricular arrhythmia or died suddenly (Table 6.3-VI).

Echocardiography: Transthoracic echocardiography is indispensable for detection of vegetation and, thus, for confirmation of the diagnosis (10,11). In two-thirds (according to the literature, 35%-85%) of cases, it furnishes evidence corroborating the tentative diagnosis of the later established case of endocarditis. Proof of vegetation with a diameter of <2 mm can frequently not be reliably furnished as a function of previously existing valvular changes. Moreover, fresh vegetation from an endocarditis which has been cured cannot always be reliably distinguished from rheumatic or degenerative valvular abnormalities, although, normally, there are differing reflex characteristics (178,179). Abscesses larger than 10 mm (180,181), valve perforation (182) or mitral valve aneurysms (183) can also be reliably demonstrated in the majority of patients with two-dimensional echocardiography.

In the case of indefinite transthoracic echocardiographic findings, and to detect smaller vegetations, transesophageal echocardiography (TEE) is the examination

Table 6.3-VI: Conduction disturbances and ventricular arrhythmias complicating the late (> 30 days) course of infective endocarditis (154).

	30-100 days	> 100 days
AV-block I°/II°	21/356 (5.9%)	7/337 (2.1%)
AV-block III°	5/356 (1.4%)	3/337 (0.9%)
VT,VF, sudden death[2]	2/356 (0.6%)	8/337(2.4%)

[1] within 100-365 days; events which occur later than 365 days were not considered to be due to endocarditis;
[2] ventricular tachycardia/fibrillation

technique of choice (Figs. 8 and 9). The diagnosis of abscess cavitations smaller than 5 mm, which regularly fail to show up on transthoracic echocardiography, is frequently achieved with this technique. Apart from confirmation of the diagnosis, repeated echocardiographic examinations also serve to observe the growth development and nature of endocarditic vegetations, morphologic changes in the valve and the left ventricular diameter and contractions (184-195). The role of transthoracic as well as transesophageal echocardiography of the detection management of vegetations with or without thromboembolic complications is further outlined below.

Isotope imaging: Of the nuclear medical examinations, scintigraphy with gallium-76-citrate is employed as a non-specific search method for larger cardiac and secondary foci of inflammation. An accumulation can be achieved in florid vegetations with indium-111-oxine-marked leukocytes or granulocyte fractions (200,201). Studies are being carried out on the application of monoclonal antibodies in the nuclear medical diagnosis of endocarditis (207).

Microbiologic diagnosis

Apart from demonstration of the pathogen in at least two independently extracted blood cultures (BC), standard micro-biologic diagnosis includes an antibiogram and a quantative serial tube dilution test, with determination of the minimum inhibitory concentration (MIC) and the minimum effective bactericidal concentration (MBC) of antibiotics or combinations of antibiotics.

The extraction of the BC under the most stringent sterile conditions, proper transportation, and the provision of the information to the laboratory that the BC has been extracted under suspicion of an IE, are obvious requirements. It is not practical to only extract BC's during fervescence since, with florid endocarditis, a continuous bacteremia usually exists. Four sets of two (two aerobic or one aerobic and one anaerobic) venous BC's per 24 hours are usually sufficient for demonstration of the pathogenic agent if 5-10 ml of blood are taken, in each case, in nine times the volume of a rich bouillon. However, the bacterial count in the peripheral blood can vary considerably, and is frequently below 100 bacteria/ml blood, so that the extraction of more than eight BCs/24 hours or the extraction of larger quantities of blood can be useful.

Should it not be possible to demonstrate the pathogenic agent in patients with florid

ENDOCARDITIS 621

endocarditis without antibiotic therapy, in spite of the BC being properly extracted and processed, thought must be given to atypical bacteria (e.g. micro-aerophilic, nutritionally variant, pyridoxin-dependent streptococci), which need culture media with specific growth factors or vitamins, rather than to rare pathogens. On the other hand, pathogens can be present which adhere relatively tightly to the tissue or pass through the capillary system only with difficulty (e.g. yeasts) and, therefore, are only to be found in low counts in the peripheral blood. However, it has not proven useful to extract arterial BC's in the latter case, either (43,202,203). The attempt to demonstrate the pathogenic agent on the basis of bone marrow cultures or on the basis of peripheral septic embolism foci (204) is more promising. Even in these cases, however, two BC's extracted independently of each other must provide a uniform demonstration of the pathogenic agent.

The incidence of so-called culture-negative endocarditis (see below), is given in the literature as 3%-41%. This wide variation is proof of the differing quality standards in the micro-biologic diagnosis of endocarditis. The quality of the hemoculture technique can, *inter alia*, be judged on how frequently bacteremia as a result of hemophili, or pyridoxin-dependent streptococci, are diagnosed in the respective laboratory, since both pathogens are only demonstrable in the case of a faultless technique.

Delayed demonstration of the pathogenic agent due to non-specific antibiotic treatment considerably worsens the prognosis of endocarditis patients, so that, in the case of suspected endocarditis, provided no vital risk is involved, the administration of antibiotics must be avoided until there is hemoculture demonstration of the pathogenic agent. Demonstration of the pathogenic agent also requires more time in the case of bacteria with a long generation period or slow growth. This applies, for example, to fastidious gram-negative rod-shaped bacilli, neisseria, anaerobia, pyridoxin-dependent streptococci, some gram-positive rod-shaped bacilli, fungi, mycobacteria, and rickettsia burnettii. Tricuspid valve endocarditis, which takes a chronic course, is also more difficult to diagnose on the basis of hemocultures.

Should surgical intervention be necessary, the excised valvular tissue should always be conserved for microbiologic analyses.

Due to the antigen properties of enterococci, candida, cryptococci, histoplasma, brucella, chlamydia, rickettsia burnetti, salmonella, aspergillus and mycoplasma, demonstration of specific antibodies is possible in the case of infection with these pathogens (205).

Culture-negative endocarditis: In published series, the incidence of culture-negative endocarditis (CNE) varies between 3% and more than 41%. This striking difference in itself shows that deficiencies in the extraction of blood samples, as well as in microbiologic diagnosis, are the essential reasons for the, at present, high percentage of CNE in clinically established cases of endocarditis (e.g. transesophageal echocardiography). In a number of patients, preceding antibiotic therapy must, apparently, take the blame for the absence of positive blood cultures. The persistent negative influence of a non-specifically commenced antibiotic therapy on the demonstration of the pathogenic agent is made clear by examinations in which, with unselected patients with established IE, a demonstration of the pathogenic agent was achieved within 48 hours in 97% of cases, provided no antibiotic therapy had been commenced.

Sixty-eight percent of the patients in whom antibiotics had been employed during the course of the disease, but more or less discontinued long before admission to hospital, demonstration of the pathogenic agent was achieved within 48 hours, dropping to 27% in patients who were still undergoing antibiotic treatment at the time of admission. In these patients, demonstration of the pathogenic agent was also delayed in the further course of the disease and the number of cases of culture-negative endocarditis was higher.

Completely suppressive phases following antibiotic therapy last for up to six days. In addition, it could be shown in experiments that, in the presence of antibiotics, the positivity of the blood culture is dependent on the ratio of concentrations of antibiotics in the hemoculture medium to the MIC of the respective micro-organisms; 161 of 162 cultures were positive, with a ratio of < 1:10, 52 of 108 (48%) with a ratio of 1:10 to 1:1, and 0 of 54, with a ratio of > 1:1 (206). Generally, antibiotics are inactivated as a result of neutralization (e.g. aminoglycosides by liquid) or dilution of the blood in the media (approximately 1:10). An additional elimination of the antibiotic effect can be achieved by employing a lysis centrifugation system (e.g. "isolator") or a radiometric system with exchange resins (Bactec) (207), although the effect of the resins, even those of the non-radioactive variety (Bactec 26 plus), has been questioned (208). The addition of penicillinase carries with it the risk of contamination and should remain limited to one bottle (209).

An indicator as far as the quality of the microbiologic laboratory is concerned is the isolation of hemophili, of which the species H. influencae and H. parainfluencae only grow on rich media. This is verified by an analysis of reported series of cases of endocarditis, in which the percentage of CNE was 23.3% when hemophilus was not identified, while in 14 series with demonstration of hemophilus it was only 16.2% (p < 0.001) (210). Apart from hemophilus, metabolically defective streptococci and anaerobia

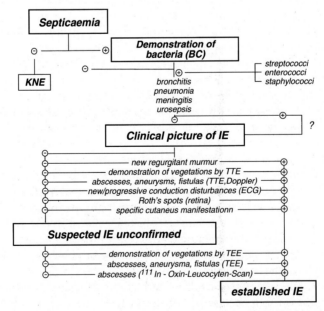

Figure 6.3-10: Flow chart of the tentative diagnosis of endocarditis. BC: blood culture; TTE: transthoracic echocardiography; TEE: transesophageal echocardiography.

Table 6.3-VII: Micro-organisms and reasons for culture-negative endocarditis (after 214).

Micro-organism	Reason	Remedy	Literature
Anaerobic germs	lack of anaerobic subcultures from normal blood cultures	anaerobic subcultures [a]	215,216
- Peptostreptococcus anaerobius	SPS[b] - susceptibility	blood cultures without SPS or addition of gelatine (1,2%)[a]	217
Brucella sp.	slow growing	incubation for three weeks[a]	218,219
Campylobacter sp.	suboptimal environment for growing	Septi-Chek (BCB, Roche) BACTEC, Isolator	220,221
Chlamydia sp.	lack of growing	serology (KBR, MIF)	222
Corynebacterium sp. (especially C.jeikeium)	slow growing	incubation for three weeks[c]	215,223
Coxiella burnetii	no growing	serology (Phase I and II-antibodies)	224
Fungi	poor growing	longer incubation periods, BACTEC, BCB-Lysis, Isolator; Serology?[d]	225,226,227
Gardnerella vaginalis[e]	SPS-susceptibility	BK without SPS or addition of gelatine (1,2%)	228
HACEK[f]	slow growing	incubation for two weeks subcultures of the anaerobic bottle	215, 229, 230, 231
Legionella sp.	poor growing	subcultures of BCYE[g] Agar	232
Mycobacterium sps.	no or poor growing	BACTEC, Isolator[a]	233,234
Mycoplasma hominis	no or poor growing	no SPS of addition of gelatine (1,2%), BACTEC	235, 236
Neisseria gonorrhoeae	SPS-susceptibility	no SPS or addition of gelatine (1,2%), Isolator	237, 238, 239
Nocardia sp.	slow growing	long incubation period, BACTEC[a], Isolator[a] excision of (cutaneous) manifestation	240, 241
Streptobacillus moniliformis	SPS-susceptibility	no SPS or addition of gelatine (1,2%)	242
Streptococcus defectivus S. adjacens (NVS)[h]	poor growing	subcultures on chocolate medium, Amme	243

[a] so far no experience with blood cultures in patients with proven endocarditis
[b] SPS = Liquoid
[c] the vast majority became positive within seven days of incubation
[d] hyphomycetes are growing rarely in blood cultures
[e] has not been reported as causative organism for endocarditis so far
[f] Hemophilus-Actinobacillus-Cardiobacterium-Eikenella-Kingella
[g] buffered Charcoal-Yeast Extract

are "index micro-organisms" which also provide information on the quality of the microbiologic diagnosis (211,212).

When CNE is suspected, consultation between the clinician and the microbiologist, is of by far the greatest importance. When employing special techniques or media, the following steps are recommended:

- Additional blood cultures must be drawn; no consensus has yet been reached on the number. The literature contains no information on a possible better yield from hemocultures which are extracted during fervescence. Arterial hemocultures are not superior (43). No corresponding data are available on bone marrow cultures in the case of endocarditis, although these would appear to be practical (204).

- In the case of negative blood cultures during antibiotic therapy, discontinuation of the antibiotic and extraction of cultures from the third day onwards (43).

- Consideration, on the part of the clinician, as to whether, on the basis of the anamnesis of the course of the disease and (typical) complications which may have occurred, one of the micro-organisms specified in Table 6.3-VIA could be involved.

- Reconsideration of the hemoculture technique and the possible employment of other methods (Table 6.3-VII).

Due to the widely differing causes of a culture-negative endocarditis, a uniform scheme of therapy cannot be specified. If, in the case of patients who have not been antimicrobially treated, hemocultures remain negative after other diagnostic strategies have been exhausted (Table 6.3-VII), that pathogen should first be treated which is most frequently encountered in the group of endocarditis patients to which the affected person belongs (213) (see below). As far as endocarditis in drug-dependent patients is concerned, these are S. aureus, streptococci, enterococci, candida spp. and gram-negative rod-shaped bacilli. In the case of nosocomial (not associated with artificial valves) endocarditis, consideration must be given, in particular, to S. aureus, coagulase-negative staphylococci and enterococci (214). In patients over 60 years of age, S. aureus, enterococci and S. bovis endocarditis should be considered first. In the case of early prosthetic endocarditis, thought should first be given to coagulase-negative staphylococci and, in addition, to gram-negative rod-shaped bacilli, S. aureus, fungi, and corynebacteria. With delayed postoperative endocarditis, coagulase-negative staphylococci and viridans streptococci are the most frequent.

The mortality of CNE is distinctly higher than in the case of early demonstration of the pathogenic agent and target-specific treatment. Prompt defervescence is, without a doubt, a prognostically effective parameter.

Differential diagnosis

As far as deliberations in terms of differential diagnosis in the case of undiagnosed endocarditis are concerned, differentiation must be made between two situations (Fig. 10):

(a) The febrile condition not clarified in the differential diagnosis requires the careful exclusion of an inflammatory local finding and a system disease or a tumour, which could explain the fever. Where there is evidence of septicemia, its most frequent causes must first be clarified (bronchitis, pneumonia, urosepsis, cholecystitis, meningitis). In the case of septicemia as a result of streptococci, enterococci or staphylococci, a primary IE, or a secondary IE which has developed following other infections, must also be taken into consideration at an early stage of differential diagnosis. Then an echocardiographic examination (TEE) is indicated. The probability that an IE is the cause of a fever of unknown origin (FUO) would, assuming an appropriate diagnostic investigation and consideration of the definition of an FUO, be below 5%.

(b) Confusing clinical pictures are frequently encountered in differential diagnosis when complications of a previously undiagnosed IE are responsible for the initial clinical signs and symptoms. If these complications primarily manifest themselves with cardiac symptoms (e.g. valvular insufficiency, arrhythmia, AV blocks), the, today usual, clarification by means of differential diagnosis - which always includes echocardiographic examinations - leads, in the majority of cases, to an early detection of endocardial vegetation. On the other hand, in the case of non-cardiac manifestation, clarification by means of differential diagnosis can be difficult. Therefore, an IE should be excluded by means of differential diagnosis whenever thromboembolism, glomerulonephritis, vasculitis, and (non-bacterial) meningoencephalitis of unknown origin occur.

Suspected but unconfirmed endocarditis

This exists if, in the case of a septicemia with hemoculturally demonstrated pathogenic agents, the clinical picture is that of an IE, but an endocardial involvement in the infective process cannot be demonstrated (no or little change in the cardiac murmur; no positive evidence of vegetation is furnished via transthoracic echocardiography (TTE); the ECG reveals no (progressive) conduction disorders indicative of myocardial involvement; skin and retina manifestations typical of an IE). Regarding cardiac murmurs, it must be remembered that, in patients where bacterial endocarditis has been established, a cardiac murmur develops in almost all cases, since isolated involvement of the parietal endocardium is rare and the infection of the valvular endocardium results in valvular damage. In the case of acute endocarditis, however, an increasing percentage of patients have been observed in the last few years who had no cardiac murmurs in the initial clinical examination and in whom a murmur first developed later, usually under antibiotic therapy (244). This applies, in particular, to acute, isolated tricuspid valve endocarditis (245). Therefore, the initial absence of a cardiac murmur does not exclude the existence of an endocarditis.

On the other hand, it must be taken into account that systolic murmurs can frequently be auscultated under highly feverish or septic conditions, or in the case of anemia, due to the increased cardiac output. Therefore, only distinct valvular insufficiency murmurs which, upon comparison with previous findings, are really new or (evaluating the given hemodynamic situation) have become more severe, are usable.

Where there is unconfirmed suspected endocarditis, transesophageal echocardiography (TEE) is now the examination technique of choice. While in two thirds (according to the literature, 34%-84%) of later established cases of endocarditis TTE furnishes a finding which corroborates the tentative diagnosis (180,246,247), TEE, with at least a sensitivity of 93%, a specificity of 95% and a positive prognostic value of 93%, is, in high measure, the appropriate method of demonstrating an existing endocardial involvement (smaller degrees of vegetation, abscesses) (180,248-250).

TEE can trigger off a bacteremia. The probability of positive hemocultures under a TEE, and the consequences thereof, are, at present, the subject of controversy, since the studies published show deficiencies in terms of methodics (251-254). Although the majority of authors do not consider an antibiotic prophylaxis necessary when conducting a TEE, this should be applied where there is an unconfirmed suspicion of endocarditis (not, however, in the case of culture-negative endocarditis), since:

(a) contrary to CNE, the pathogen causing the infection is already known, and

(b) if an infective endocarditis actually exists as a result of a recent bacteremia, the patient carries a certain risk of contracting a secondary infection, so that an even more unfavorable prognosis may result.

In the case of suspected intracardiac abscesses, but without pathologic TEE findings, scintigraphy with gallium-76-citrate can be used as a non-specific search method and to detect secondary foci of inflammation (255). Accumulations have been achieved in florid vegetations with indium-111-oxine-marked granulocyte fractions (256); the method cannot, however, be considered to have been validated.

Intracardiac catheter diagnosis to confirm a previously unconfirmed, suspected endocarditis is obsolete, since - as is the case with auscultation and Doppler echocardiography - only valvular stenosis or insufficiency can be diagnosed, but an endocarditis can neither be confirmed nor excluded. Particularly in the case of aortic valve endocarditis, a transvalvular intracardiac catheter examination is associated with a high percentage of thromboembolic complications. Examinations in which the catheter does not pass through the aortic valve (coronary angiography, aortography) are also associated with a high risk of thromboembolic complications, so that an accurate technique is also imperative in these situations.

Using a mathematical model, after prospective analysis of the course of the disease, findings and complications typical, but not demonstrative, of endocarditis were analysed in 108 consecutive patients with later confirmed IE (15 of these were patients with unconfirmed suspected endocarditis) to determine their value for confirmation of the diagnosis. Based on this analysis, the individual parameters were weighted, with respect to their diagnostically informative value, with one to four points within the framework of a point-score system. The model employed resulted in a classification of the diagnosis as retrospectively correct as far as the 93 patients with initially confirmed endocarditis, as well as the 15 patients with initially unconfirmed suspected endocarditis were concerned, when nine or ten score points were attained. Upon prospective testing on the following 129 consecutive patients, in 121 (93.8%) cases, the score system proved to be valid for predicting the later established diagnosis, so that the score system can be alternatively applied in the case of an undiagnosed suspected endocarditis (Table 6.3-VIII).

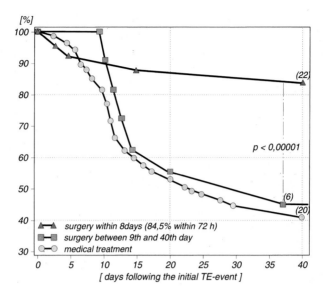

Figure 6.3-11: Survival after cerebral embolism complicating native valve endocarditis.

Course and prognosis

In the pre-antibiotic era, almost all patients with IE died as a result of the uncontrollable infection. Since effective antibiotics have become available, the prognosis has become distinctly more favorable. As far as the following complications of endocarditis are concerned, the prognosis is persistently worse, so that urgent surgical intervention must be considered (see below).

Vegetation and thromboembolic complications

Carefully considering the operative risk taken during active infective endocarditis and the preventive benefit of such an urgent surgical intervention, transesophageal echocardiography contributes significantly to the decision making:

(a) Generally, the risk of thromboembolic complications is higher in mitral than in isolated aortic valve endocarditis (257).

(b) With respect to sound reflection characteristics, the experienced examiner may differentiate between acute ("fresh") vegetations and more dense vegetations which already show a tendency to organize themselves. The latter are accompanied by a much lower incidence of embolic complications (258,259).

(c) Mobile vegetations are generally diagnosed earlier and more frequently than abnormal masses which are fixed to the leaflets. Mobile vegetations and larger vegetations have a higher incidence of thromboembolic complications than fixed vegetations and those of smaller diameters. This holds especially true for vegetations attached to the highly mobile parts of the mitral leaflets, which are exposed to

Table 6.3-VIII: Criteria for the diagnosis of unproven native valve endocarditis.

Criteria	Score
Cardiac predisposition present, high risk group (previous endocarditis,	1
artificial material)	2
General predisposition	
- elevated	1
- high risk group	2
Regurgitant murmur	
- existent	1
- proven new murmur	4
Positive blood culture	
- streptococci	3
- enterococci	2
- staphylococci	1
- HACEK and other micro-organisms typical for endocarditis	4
Thromboembolic complications	4
Manifestation of conduction disturbances	3
Vegetation	
- Uncertain dignity	2
- floating	4
Intracardial abscesses or fistulas suspected	4
Cutaneous or retinal manifestation	
- uncertain	1
- typical	4
All cases appropriately grouped retrospectively if more than	9 points
Prospective evaluation of the Scoresystem	121/129 (93,8%)

extreme accelerations during the heart cycle (260). According to our own experience, as well as the experience of other centers, vegetations more than 10mm in diameter which are attached to the mobile segments of the mitral leaflets represents an independent indication for surgical intervention, as the risk of thromboembolic complications is 27% within 10 days after demonstration of vegetation and 76% within 30 days (113,261).

(d) The risk of recurrent episodes after first manifestation of a thromboembolic complication is high if vegetations are still demonstrated by transesophageal echocardiography after first manifestation of the thromboembolic event

(257,260,262). In more than 50% of cases recurrence of a thromboembolic event manifests within 30 days after the initial episode (113,263). Our experience suggests that a surgical intervention within 72 hours is suggested in the case of cerebral manifestation of the embolism. The progressive manifestation of the brain barrier disturbance after the expiry of this period worsens prognosis and, later than eight days after the event, compared to conservatively treated patients, no longer results in an improvement in the prognosis (257) (Fig. 11). Other authors have observed a favorable prognosis even with longer intervals if no hemorrhagic cerebral infarction has occurred, which in these cases have to be excluded by cranial tomography (264).

(e) Spontaneous echo-contrasts which occur during acute bacterial endocarditis appear, particularly in the case of staphylococcal endocarditis, to indicate a thrombotic condition and thus a high risk of thromboembolic complications (194,265).

(f) Kissing vegetations involving the anterior mitral leaflet as a complication of primary aortic valve endocarditis results in secondary mitral valve endocarditis in a high percentage of patients. There is also a significant risk of secondary destruction of the mitral valve. If a surgical intervention is performed early, in the majority of cases the mitral valve can be repaired and mitral valve replacement can be avoided. In these cases early surgical intervention is therefore useful and should be performed as soon as a mitral regurgitation is present, the mitral kissing vegetation increases in size despite antibiotic therapy or if the endocarditis is not definitely controlled by antibiotic therapy (266).

Persisting septicemia in spite of antibiotic treatment

A septicemia persisting for more than 48 hours in spite of target-specific (i.e. directed towards the pathogen isolated from hemocultures) antibiotic therapy, has a persistent negative influence on the prognosis of an infective endocarditis if β-hemolytic streptococci, enterococci or staphylococci, but not if viridans streptococci, are the causal pathogens (263). The surgical removal of the source of the septicemia leads to a statistical improvement in the prognosis (262).

Acute renal failure

Apart from embolic events and a diffuse glomerulonephritis, an acute renal failure during the course of an infective endocarditis can also be pre-renally or toxically (co-factor: antibiotic therapy) induced. Continuous hemofiltration is then indicated. Hemodialysis treatment does not constitute an adequate alternative either, due to the cardiac situation. Irrespective of the genesis, acute renal failure is indicative of such a drastic deterioration in the prognosis that early surgical intervention is wise.

Acute valvular regurgitation and myocardial failure

If cardiac insufficiency occurs following an aortic valve endocarditis, the prognosis is particularly bad since the myocardium has not adapted to the acute, increased volume loading and, contrary to the case with mitral insufficiency, there is no possibility of unloading of the increased enddiastolic volume against a low degree of resistance. Therefore, an operation is urgently indicated for patients with a severe acute aortic insufficiency and pulmonary edema which cannot be quickly cleared up conservatively. In a few, less difficult cases, a recompensation can be attempted. With a heart rate of 120 per minute, the diastolic duration, decisive with respect to the regurgitation fraction, is optimally shortened. If applicable, pace-maker therapy is indicated in the case of patients where the course is complicated by the occurrence of an AV block.

The occurrence of a pulmonary edema following an acute, infection-related mitral insufficiency, must be evaluated differently in terms of the prognosis. Even a slight to medium degree of mitral insufficiency, which has developed acutely, can result in a pulmonary edema (267). This is not a manifestation of a left ventricular myocardial insufficiency, but the consequence of the left atrial pressure, increased during systole as a result of the higher left ventricular enddiastolic pressure, and increased during diastole as a result of the regurgitation volume. Since, in these cases, there is no significant myocardial contractility dysfunction, recompensation is often successful, particularly if left ventricular impedance is favorably influenced by the use of vasodilators. More caution should, therefore, be shown in diagnosing an urgent valve replacement than in the case of acute aortic regurgitation (267).

Treatment of infective endocarditis

The successful treatment of an IE is essentially determined by quick confirmation of the diagnosis, to which the timely and correct microbiologic examination contributes to differing degrees (see above). With an equal degree of frequency, diagnostic, as well as therapeutic, errors bring catastrophic consequences in their wake.

General conservative treatment and observation of the course

General conservative treatment measures include comparison of the liquid and electrolyte balances, taking into consideration fever-related liquid losses on the one hand and the degree of cardiac insufficiency on the other, as well as, if applicable, symptomatic therapy, lowering of the fever by physical and medical means and the recompensation of a cardiac insufficiency. If possible, indwelling catheters should be avoided. Where there are difficult venous conditions, a peripheral venous access, by means of a thin-calibre, flexible, indwelling cannula, is justifiable if this is changed at least once a week and carefully taken care of. Specific sanitation of a source of infection causal of the IE (pathogen conformity) should be aimed at during antibiotic treatment. A non-specific elimination of possible sources of infection is pointless.

Anticoagulants and corticosteroids are relatively contra-indicated in the case of patients with IE. Anticoagulants have no proven influence on the development of the degree of endocarditic vegetation or the incidence of septic embolic complications (see below). Based on both clinical and animal experiments, treatment with coumarin derivates is, as far as IE is concerned, associated with an increased percentage of, in some cases serious, hemorrhagic complications. Except in the case of patients with an uncomplicated course of a prosthetic endocarditis, when the IE is florid, coumarin derivatives should be dispensed with and, if necessary, heparin used.

Observation of the course of patients with IE includes, apart from regular measurement of the blood pressure and pulse, checking of the cardiac and pulmonary auscultation findings, control of the BSR, the red and white cell count, platelet count, the coagulation situation, the urinalysis, and the substances usually eliminated in the urine. Even with courses which appear uncomplicated, an ECG should be taken twice a week to record impulse transmission and conduction disturbances (AV block, bundle-branch blocks) and repolarisation disorders in good time. If changes are registered in the ECG, a daily ECG is required. In the case of a more severe conduction disorders and ventricular arrhythmias, there must be monitor-control. Echocardiographic observations of development serve to evaluate endocardial vegetation, as well as to control the cardiac diameter and the cardiac function. With a clinically uncomplicated course, they should be repeated at least once per week.

Adjuvant treatment: While a more favorable effect has been demonstrated when glycocorticoids were administered in large doses in the case of septicemia/septic shock in animal experiments, a prognostic benefit of this treatment has not been substantiated in clinical studies (268). In the case of confirmed endocarditis, the use of glycocorticoids should be approached very critically.

In approximately 15% of patients with acute infective endocarditis who develop a thrombopathy, there is disseminated intravascular coagulation; in 35% of cases there is a hepatic synthesis dysfunction with a consecutive decrease in the vitamin K-dependent coagulation factors and, in approximately 50% of cases, an isolated platelet dysfunction as the result of direct damage to platelets by bacteria, toxins and immunity complexes. Only where there is a disturbance of plasmatic hemostasis to the disadvantage of the anticoagulant potential is AT III substitution indicated. The damage to the endothelial cells caused by α-toxin, with a consecutive disturbance in the vascular permeability ("capillary leak syndrome"), observed in endocarditis caused by S. aureus cannot be influenced by modulation of the coagulation system, but it can be possible to achieve some affect with C1 esterase inhibitors.

To date, there are no established findings on the probable but unsubstantiated value of the early use of polyvalent immunoglobins (Ig-GAM) in the individual case to prevent the toxic effect of bacterial exotoxins (e.g. streptolysin O-producing streptococci, S. aureus, pseudomonas). On the other hand, established immunoglobulin conditions indicate the treatment of septic patients with Ig-GAM concentrations (296). The rapid inactivation of bacterial toxins and, thus, favorable influencing of the course of the septicemia, as a result of treatment with specific immunoglobins (e.g. pseudomonas immunoglobin) is also substantiated.

Specific monoclonal antibodies, which can recognize and bind the lipid A portion of the exotoxin, have been developed to neutralize exotoxic gram-negative bacteria (270). Their value is debated, since, as they must be used at a very early stage, their too hasty use prior to confirmation of a gram-negative septicemia appears to worsen the prognosis. In the majority of EU countries, licensing of Centoxin® has at, present, been suspended.

The almost refractory vasodilation and "capillary leak syndrome" seen in the case of fulminant endocarditis are the result of the uncontrolled contact activation of the complement system. The C1 inhibitor plays a major role in the regulation of the complement, as does the bradykinin-kinin system. After their activation, both systems release vasoactive peptides (*inter alia*, bradykinin, anaphylatoxin). Treatment with C1-inhibitor concentrations also results, in the individual case, in a drastic improvement in those clinical pictures which, on the basis of empirical experience, hardly appear to be promising (271). The diagnostic framework and the optimum point for treatment have not as yet been clarified. The presently recommended dosage (6000 IE initially, 3000 IE after 12 hours, 2000 IE after 24 hours, and 1000 IE after 36 hours) has not yet been validated.

Differential diagnosis of shock in the case of IE: When shock symptoms appear following an IE, hemodynamic monitoring is indicated in order to clarify the cause of the shock and to control treatment. The essential differential diagnosis is that between a septic circulatory situation and a primary myocardial cause, usually due to acute volume loading in the case of acute valvular insufficiency, to which the myocardium has not adapted (263). Occasionally, inflammatory myocardial involvement in the infection process or a myocardial distensibility disturbance ("septic shock myocardium"), clinically and hemodynamically reminiscent of "pericardial tamponade" caused by toxins and mediators, is (jointly) responsible for a cardiogenic shock. Mixed forms (septic and cardiogenic shock) frequently occur, with a differing formation of the subcomponents. The prognosis for these is particularly unfavorable. With acute myocardial decompensation, a dilation of the heart is rather unusual, since the stiffness of the pericardium counteracts this. Therefore, a normal cardiac silhouette in the X-ray picture of the thorax does not exclude acute myocardial decompensation.

Specific antimicrobial treatment

IE differs from other infections due to the embedding of the pathogens in vegetation comprising cellular detritus, fibrin and platelets, which partially protect against cellular and humoral immunologic response. Due to the lack of vascularization of the endocardium, antibiotics can only enter the vegetation via diffusion from the intracardiac blood (see above). Both factors complicate specific antimicrobial treatment and require observation of the following therapeutic principles.

To overcome exposure protection, high diffusion gradients of the antibiotic must be achieved. After testing the MIC and MBC of the antibiotic and combinations of antibiotics, a large-dose, bactericidally effective therapy is imperative. Testing of the antimicrobial sensitivity in the agar diffusion test is inadequate as far as therapeutic decisions are concerned. The exposure protection of the pathogen carries the risk of relapses in the case of an insufficiently long therapy, so that, even in the case of uncomplicated endocarditis, therapy over a period of four weeks is recommended. Therapeutic regimens, with ambulant medication or medication only once per day, have also been successfully tested with respect to uncomplicated cases of endocarditis caused by viridans streptococci (272,273). These ambulant schemes of therapy, shortened in terms of time or reduced with regard to the antibiotics used, have regularly failed in the case of endocarditis not caused by viridans streptococci (274).

Special recommendations apply with respect to combinations of antibiotics and some infections which are difficult to clean up (e.g. those caused by enterococci, staphylococci, some gram-negative bacteria, and fungi). In order to reliably achieve the required serum level and to prevent the unreliable taking of tablets and uncertain gastrointestinal

Table 6.3-IX: *Pharmacokinetic data and drug monitoring for antibiotics often used in endocarditis therapy (263).*

antibiotics	passing of urine %	Clearance (ml x min^{-1} x kg^{-1})	half-life period/h	therapy control[1,2] minimal level	peak levels[1]
Gentamicin	> 90	0.73$_{CREAT}$ ± 0.06	2-3	< 2 µg/ml	3-10 µg/ml[4]
Mezlocillin	8-22	1.44$_{CREAT}$ ± 0.23	1.3 ± 0.4	-	-
Oxacilling	46 ± 4	6.1 ± 1.7	0.4 ± 9.7	-	-
Penicillin G	> 80	~ 5.0	0.5 ± 0.2	-	-
Streptomycin	39 ± 12	~ 0.4	5.3 ± 2.2	< 5 µg/ml	20 µg/ml
Tobramycin	90	0.7$_{CREAT}$	2.2 ± 0.1	< 5 µg/ml	< 10 µg/ml
Vancomycin	> 90	1.09 ± 0.07	5.6 ± 1.8[3]	< 5 µg/ml (< 10 µg/ml)[5]	< 25 µg/ml (< 45 µg/ml)[5]

[1] Serum level determinations are not indicated in betalactam-antibiotics because of the wide therapeutic range

[2] Not generally necessary for therapy control

[3] Under hemodialysis approx. 180 h

[4] Minimal peak level in enterococcal endocarditis

[5] In strict indications, the higher serum levels are acceptable to treat active endocarditis (275,276)

adsorption, a parenteral therapy should be given preference as a matter of principle. The specific treatment of endocarditis pathogens according to their MIC and MBC constitutes the optimum antibiotic treatment. It cannot be improved by the administration of additional antibiotics because of an unjustified need to be cautious. Non-specific treatment, i.e. treatment which is commenced without knowing of the endocarditis pathogen and/or its antimicrobial sensitivity, is paid for with a worsening of the prognosis, and is only justified, after proper conservation of the appropriate materials for microbiologic examination, if the septic clinical picture does not allow commencement of the treatment to be postponed.

In the case of bacterial endocarditis, the renal and hepatic excretion mechanisms of pharmaceutics are normally disturbed, so that drug monitoring is necessary (263). Determination of the serum antibiotic level is an indispensable component part of endocarditis therapy, since, on the one hand, high rates of diffusion are decisive as far as the result of the treatment is concerned and, on the other hand, changes in the renal function, the cardiac output (septicemia, valvular insufficiency) or pharmacologic interactions can have a lasting influence on the serum level. Antibiotics with a potential nephro- and ototoxic effect (audiogram prior to the commencement of therapy) require particularly careful monitoring of the treatment, particularly if they are employed in a combined form (e.g. vancomycin plus aminoglycosides). The minimum serum level (serum level concentration prior to the administration of sequential medication) suffices for routine monitoring of treatment (Table 6.3-IX).

High-dosage antibiotic treatment, such as is employed in the treatment of IE, is frequently accompanied by secondary effects, even with optimum treatment monitoring:

- thrombopenia or platelet dysfunctions, which are caused, in particular, by some β-lactam antibiotics.
- pseudomembranous colitis (or "antibiotic-associated colitis"), which, with appropriate host disposition, is caused by toxins of chlostridia (above all, chlostridium difficile), if the growth conditions for these gram-positive anaerobia are improved by lincomycin, clindamycin, cephalosporins, penicillins and, with the exception of vancomycin and metronidazol, almost all other antibiotics (277,278).

Irrespective of the dosage, this complication occurs in some cases only weeks after the commencement of therapy or even after conclusion of therapy and, when unrecognized or untreated, is fatal. The most frequent clinical symptoms are hemorrhagic diarrhoea, severe abdominal pain and fever. Standard therapy consists of an immediate interruption of treatment with the causal, or probably causal, antibiotics and oral treatment with 125-500 mg vancomycin every six hours for seven to ten days or with metronidazol (3 x 500 mg/day) (279,280). Antidiarrhea agents, or substances which inhibit the peristaltics, prolong the symptoms and negatively affect the prognosis.

- A rare complication after too rapid infusion of vancomycin is the "red man syndrome", which is accompanied by a maculo-papular erythema, primarily on the upper half of the body, coupled with anaphylactoid reactions, such as pruritus, dyspnea, possible hypotension, and other, general histamine-mediated symptoms, up to and including shock (281,282). With slower infusion and avoidance of serum concentrations > 25 µg/ml, the serum concentrations of the components of the glycopeptide mix, which are responsible for the anaphylactoid reaction, are also kept so low that this secondary effect does not occur. For quite some time, in the majority of EU countries, only batches of purified vancomycin (chromatographically purified vancomycin, vancomycin CP), in which, with a high degree of probability, those components which are responsible for the red man syndrome have been eliminated, have been supplied. Nevertheless, the recommendation to still infuse vancomycin CP slowly, over at least 45 to 60 minutes, should be adhered to for the time being.

- Depending on the dosage, vancomycin and aminoglycoside damage the nervous vestibulo-cochlearia (N. VIII) and the kidneys. Symptoms of the damage are vertigo, tinnitus, reversible and irreversible hearing defects up to and including loss of hearing. Ototoxicity is generally observed in the case of excessively increased serum concentrations and, for example, very rarely occurs with vancomycin concentrations of less than 30 µg/ml. The ototoxic effect of vancomycin is promoted when aminolycosides, certain diuretics such as ethacrynic acid in large doses, or furosemide are administered. An acute renal failure is also usually only observed in the case of very high vancomycin serum levels. Nephrotoxicity, which was formerly very frequent, is, today, rare if the upper limit of the vancomycin level is observed and the vancomycin dosage is adapted to the renal function (275). In addition, when aminoglycosides and vancomycin are administered simultaneously, an interstitial nephritis occasionally occurs, so that, because of the oto- and nephrotoxicity, particularly careful drug monitoring is required (282). With antibiotic combinations using aminoglycosides, the toxicity of the treatment may be reduced by administering the aminoglycoside once per day.

Table 6.3-X: Therapy recommendations during infective endocarditis after identification of pathogens.

pathogen	other conditions	antibiotics antimycotic	dosage	length of therapy
penicillin-sensible streptococci (MHK_{Pen} < 0.1 μg/ml)	no penicillin	Penicillin G[1,2] plus Gentamicin[4,5]	4-6 x 5 Mio U/d 3 x 1 mg/kg/d[6]F[6]	at least 4 weeks[3] 2 weeks
	penicillin	Vancomycin plus[7,8] Gentamicin[4,5]	4 x 7.5 mg/kg/d[9] 3 x 1 mg/kg/d[6]	4 weeks 2 weeks
enterococci and less penicillin-sensible streptococci (MHK_{Pen} > 0.1μg/ml)	penicillin-sensibility	Mezlozillin[10] plus Gentamicin[4,5,13]	3 x 5 g/d 3 x 1 mg/kg/d[6]	4(-6) weeks 4(-6) weeks[11,12]
	penicillin	Vancomycin plus[7,8,14,15] Gentamicin[4,5,13]	4 x 7.5 mg/kg/d[9] 3 x 1 mg/kg/d[6]	4(-6) weeks[11,12] 4(-6) weeks[11,12]
staphylococci	PSSA; penicillin-sensible strains (MHK_{Pen} ≤ 0.125 μg/ml)	Penicillin G plus Gentamicin[4,19]	4-6 x 5 MioU/d 3 x 1 mg/kg/d[6]	4(-6) weeks 3(-5) days
	MSSA; penicillin-resistant methicillin-sensible strains	(Dicl-, Flucl)-Oxacillin[1,17,18] plus Gentamicin[4,19]	4-6 x 2g/d 3 x 1 mg/kg/d[6]	4(-6) weeks 3(-5) days
	($MHK_{Oxâ}$ ≤ 1μg/ml) MRSA; methicillin-resistant strains ($MHK_{Oxâ}$ > 1μg/ml)[20]	Vancomycin[7,9] plus Gentamicin[4,19]	4 x 7.5 mg/kg/d[9] 3 x 1 mg/kg/d[6]	4(-6) weeks 5-14 days
Pseudomonas aeruginosa	in vitro sensibility testing mandatory	Azlocillin plus[1,21] Tobramycin[4]	4 x 5g/d 3 x 1.5mg/kg/d[22]	6 weeks and more 6 weeks and more
E. coli, Klebsiellae, Serratia, Proteus		Cefotaxim plus[1] Gentamicin[4]	4 x 2g/d 3 x 1.5 mg/kg/d[22]	4(-6) weeks 4(-6) weeks

Hemophilus, Actino-bacillus, Cardiobac-terium hominis, Eikenella, Kingella (HACEK)	Mezlocillin plus[23] Gentamicin[4]	4 x 5 g/d 3 x 1.5 mg/kg/d[22]	4(-6) weeks 4(-6) weeks
Candida and other fungi	Amphotericin B[24] Flucytosin[24]	up to 0.6 mg/kg/d[24] 3-4 x 50 mg/kg/d	6 weeks and more 6 weeks and more

[1] infusion for 30 minutes

[2] with uncomplicated clinical courses and highly susceptable germs Penicillin monotherapy for at least four weeks (6 x 5 Mio. U/d) should be preferred, if the risk for aminoglykosid side effects is high (pre-existent renal failure, damage of N. VIII, age > 65 years).

[3] with uncomplicated cases lasting for less than three months the duration of therapy may be reduced to two weeks if the patients are < 35 years.

[4] infusion for 30 minutes after application of a β-Lactam-antibiotic

[5] With sensitive germs Streptomycin (2 x 0.5 g/d) may be an alternative in micro-organisms sensitive to Streptomycin

[6] Controll of serum levels (see. Table 6.3-IX) necessary. Maximum dosage for Gentamicin 240 mg/day

[7] infusion for at least 60 minutes

[8] Cefazolin (3 x 1-2 g/d) combined with Gentamicin (4 weeks) may be an alternative

[9] With a serum level < 25 μg/ml, dosage can be increased; maximum dosage 2g/day

[10] Mezlozillin in vitro and in animal experiments more effective than Ampicillin or Vancomycin

[11] Identical length of therapy for the components of a combined antibiotic therapy, because only the combination of antibiotics has a bactericidal effect.

[12] with complicated courses, large vegetations (> 5mm) proven by echocardiography and a duration illness > two months therapy should not be less than six weeks.

[13] Up to 80% of enterococci demonstrate high-level-resistances against streptomycin

[14] Imipenem (3-4 x 1 g/d), 50 mg/kg/d or ca. 4 g/d may be an alternative

[15] Animal experiments and preliminary clinical results show Teicoplanin to be also effective

[16] In uncomplicated courses therapy for four weeks may be sufficient

[17] Up to 50% of coagulase-negative staphylococci may be oxacillin-resistant

[18] With staphylococci susceptible to penicillin (MHK$_{Pen}$ < 0.125 μg/ml) therapy as with penicillin-sensible streptococci

[19] With coagulase-negative staphylococci and well directed indication (abscesses, intracardial fistulas, implantation of prothetic material) 3 x 300 mg Rifampin is added

[20] Vancomycin-susceptable (MIC$_{Vanp}$ < 1.6 mg/ml) staphylococci

[21] Piperacillin (4 x 5 g/d) or Ceftazidin (4 x 2 g) may be an alternative

[22] With high dosages of aminoglycosides daily serum level controls are mandatory (see Table 6.3-IX). Maximal dosages for Gentamicin 240 mg/day

[23] Ampicillin (4 x 5 g/d) or Cefotaxim (4 x 2 g/d) may be an alternative

[24] Special therapeutic guidelines for therapy (see text)

Penicillin-sensitive streptococci: Penicillin-sensitive streptococci (*inter alia*, viridans streptococci, microaerophilic streptococci, S. bovis) are growth-inhibited by penicillin concentrations < 0.1 µg/ml (MIC_{Pen} < 0.1 µg/ml). Since some species are penicillin-tolerant (low MIC_{Pen}, high MBC_{Pen}), complete in vitro sensitivity testing by means of the qualitative serial tube dilution test (283-286), is recommended. Above all, β-lactam antibiotics and aminoglycosides are potentially bactericidal. Standard treatment consists of the combination of penicillin G and an aminoglycoside because, in almost half the cases, a synergetic effect is also achieved if the pathogen is only slightly sensitive to aminoglycosides alone (287-289). Animal experiments also substantiate a more rapid pathogen elimination from the endocarditic vegetation when combinations are used for treatment (290).

Taking into consideration therapeutically desirable diffusion gradients on the one hand, and the risk of a dosage-dependent cytotoxic reaction (so-called penicillin allergy) on the other, individual doses of penicillin of 5 million units and total daily doses of 20-25 million units, have proven beneficial. Application is by means of short-term infusion over 30 minutes. Of the aminoglycosides, gentamicin and streptomycin have been tested for combination therapies. However, approximately 1% to 2% of viridans streptococci exhibit a high level resistance (HLR; MIC ≥ 2000 µg/ml) to streptomycin, so that only gentamicin can be used. The aminoglycoside must be administered after the β-lactam antibiotic. Differing from the daily dosages stated in Table 6.3-X, in the case of potentially fatal infections, up to three doses of 1 µg/kg body weight can be administered for the first two to three days of treatment. For practical purposes, the aminoglycoside is infused within 30 minutes via the same entry.

The dosages stated (Table 6.3-X) must be controlled by means of serum-level determination and, particularly in the case of patients with renal insufficiency, adapted. With a combination of β-lactam antibiotics and aminoglycosides, due to the pharmacokinetics, a single application of the usual total daily dosage, via a 60 minute infusion every 24 hours, has been considered advantageous, particularly in the case of patients with previously existing renal dysfunction or of advanced age (291,292). This therapy, however, has not been proven effective in endocarditic patients. A penicillin monotherapy with six doses of 5 Mill IU/day can only be beneficial in the case of an uncomplicated endocarditis and highly sensitive pathogens if there is a high risk of aminoglycosid toxicity, for example in the case of existing renal dysfunction or previous damage of the Ist or VIIIth cranial nerve. The duration of the treatment is usually four weeks for penicillin G and two weeks for aminoglycoside. In the case of young patients with uncomplicated endocarditis and an infection anamnesis of less than three months, a penicillin therapy shortened to two weeks is justifiable (285).

If there is penicillin intolerance, the combination of vancomycin or cephacolin with gentamicin is recommended (Table 6.3-X).

With a MBC_{linco} < 45 µg/ml, endocarditis caused by viridans streptococci or S. bovis can also be alternatively treated with three doses 3g lincomycin hydrochloride daily over a period of four weeks (293), provided the infusions are administered slowly (< 50 mg/kg/hour). Infusion rates of approximately 30 mg/kg/hour are recommended (293). The high lincomycin sensitivity of the S. bovis species constitutes a unique exception among the otherwise lincomycin-insensitive streptococci of the serologic group.

Enterococci and moderately penicillin-sensitive streptococci: Enterococci are resistant to β-lactam antibiotics and vancomycin in concentrations which otherwise inhibit the cell wall synthesis of gram-positive bacteria or are only bacteriostatic. In these cases, the MIC and MBC usually differ by several titer stages. In the case of penicillin concentrations above an optimally effective concentration in vitro, the bactericidal effect is diminished (paradox bactericidal effect, "eagle" effect). Resistance and eagle effect are most pronounced in the case of E. faecium. The reason for the resistance lies in the low degree of bonding of the penicillins or the low affinity of penicillin-bonded proteins as far as the enterococci are concerned. Besides this, many species of enterococci exhibit a β-lactamase with respect to penicillin and ampicillin; their resistance to these antibiotics has, however, not essentially increased (294). This enzyme can be inactivated by β-lactamase inhibitors such as clavulanic acid or sulbactam.

It is to be assumed that the tolerance of some species of enterococci towards cell wall-active antibiotics, such as penicillin, ampicillin and vancomycin, has been acquired over the course of the last ten to fifteen years (294).

The monotherapy of enterococcal endocarditis, already attempted in 1946, regularly fails. On the other hand, the combination of penicillin plus streptomycin, empirically used even before 1954, is largely successful (295,296) because, by this means, a higher degree of absorption of amino-glycoside antibiotics into the bacterial cell is achieved (297). Consequently, the synergically effective combination with an aminoglycoside is, due to the normally resulting bactericidal effect, indispensable.

Since the end of the seventies, high level resistance (HLR) to streptomycin (HLR$_{strepto}$ > 2000 μg/ml) has been observed in numerous enterococci isolates. This resistance, caused by ednylising enzymes, renders the combination of penicillin and streptomycin useless. However, in the case of E. faecalis with a HLR to streptomycin, combinations of penicillin with canamycin, tobramycin, amicacin, gentamicin, or netilmicin are effective (297), whereas combinations of this type in the case of E. faecium species highly resistant to streptomycin are not successful, because their chromosomally coded aminoglycoside acetylase also inactivates these antibiotics (297,298).

In the case of both species, a plasma-coded 3' phosphotransferase can lead to resistance to canamycin and its derivates (297). An antagonism between penicillin and amicacin has also been observed (299). Of the enzymes mentioned, gentamicin is the least attacked and, except for a few species in the case of which gentamicin is only absorbed by the bacterium to an inadequate degree, is the most suitable as a combination partner. The synergistic effectiveness of different aminoglycosides should be tested in each case.

In principle, penicillin, vancomycin or ampicillin derivates can be used in combination with gentamicin. In the case of enterococcal endocarditis, a combination therapy of 20-30 million units of penicillin or 12 g ampicillin plus three doses of 2 mg/kg gentamicin, is recommended, whereby peak levels of 3 μg/ml should be attained. In animal experiments and in vitro, the ampicillin derivate mezlocillin exhibits the most favorable activity, so that, subject to an appropriate microbiologic sensitivity test, a four-week combination of mezlocillin and gentamicin is considered to be the therapy of choice. Streptomycin (2 x 7.5 mg/kg) can also be used instead of gentamicin, in which case the peak serum level should be approximately 20 μg/ml (300,301). In the case of a complicated course, therapy over a period of six weeks is recommended. Instead of mezlocillin, the use of vancomycin or, in the case of a MBC$_{linco}$ < 4 μg/ml, lincomycin has been clinically tested and the use of teicoplanin, tested in animal experiments, for patients with a penicillin intolerance (Table 6.3-X) can be recommended.

Since 1979, with increasing frequency, both E. faecalis and E. faecium species which exhibit a high resistance to gentamicin (MIC > 2000 µg/ml), have been isolated (297,302-304). Combination of penicillin and aminoglycoside in these cases has little effect. A continuous infusion of ampicillin is under discussion as an alternative. A simultaneously existing β-lactamase can be inactivated by means of a combination with clavulanic acid or sulbactam (305). In the case of enterococci strains with a pronounced resistance, early surgical intervention should be considered, since the infection is otherwise barely controllable (300).

Staphylococci: As far as the treatment of staphylococcal endocarditis is concerned, a distinction must be made between native and prosthetic endocarditis. In the case of native-valve endocarditis caused by staphylococci, due to the embedding of the bacteria in a vegetation comprising fibrin, detritus and corpuscular blood elements, considerable exposure protection exists.

With the present resistance situation, it must be assumed that more than 90% of all S. aureus strains from clinical material produce a penicillinase, which rapidly inactivates penicillin as a result of hydrolytic cleavage of the β-lactam ring. In those rare cases in which the staphylococcus is not able to produce a penicillinase, the administration of penicillin G is the remedy of choice, because isoxazolyl penicillins exhibit a high degree of secondary effects (interstitial nephritis, neutropenia, hepatotoxicity) (287,306-309) and, above all, because the auto-activity of penicillin G *vis a vis* sensitive S. aureus strains is greater, by about the factor 10, than that of penicillinase-resistant penicillins. Therefore, the greatest possible bactericidal effect is to be expected with strains of this type. The daily dose should be 10-30 million units (for patients with a body weight above 100 kg, up to 40 million units) and is normally divided into four to six individual doses in the form of short term infusions (Table 6.3-X). The duration of the therapy ranges between four and six weeks. In addition, an aminoglycoside, preferably gentamicin, is administered in daily dosages of 3 µg/kg (divided into three individual doses) for three to five days. Similarly to streptomycin, a synergism with β-lactam antibiotics has also been demonstrated with respect to gentamicin, both in vitro and in animal experiments (310,311). This synergism could also be confirmed in clinical studies. The basic molecular mechanism is a massively increased penetration of the aminoglycoside into the staphylococci cells after the β-lactam antibiotic has taken effect.

The administration of a penicillinase-resistant isoxazolyl penicillin is imperative in the case of penicillinase-producing streptococci. Oxacillin, dicloxacillin and flucloxacillin are available for this purpose, whereby dicloxacillin and flucloxacillin offer pharmacokinetic advantages, without a therapeutic superiority having, as yet, been clinically demonstrated. A daily dosage of 8-12g, divided into three to four individual doses, and combination with gentamicin, are required in order to achieve adequate efficacy levels and rates of diffusion in the vegetation. In animal experiments and, with non-drug dependent patients, also clinically, combination with an aminoglycoside resulted in a rapid sterilization of the vegetation. In view of the high percentage of S. aureus endocarditis which, when pathogen elimination is delayed, require operation during the florid infection stage, and the still high mortality rate, a combination therapy should always be given priority.

When a methicillin-resistant staphylococcus strain (incidence generally < 5%) is demonstrated, in the case of corresponding sensitivity (MIC_{vanco} - 1.6 μgml), the administration of 2 g/day vancomycin, divided into three to four individual doses, is the therapy of choice (312). At the same time, care must be taken that short term infusion is effected over a period of at least 45 minutes, because, otherwise, vancomycin-typical secondary effects (red man syndrome) can occur (see above).

Due to the usually slow sterilization of the vegetation and, consequently, a prolonged bacteremia, a six-week therapy is normally required (313). A synergism between vancomycin and gentamicin (or fosfomycin) appears probable, although, to date, contrary to the combination with β-lactam antibiotics, only a few animal experiments or clinical studies exist. The addition of the aminoglycoside should continue beyond the, otherwise recommended, period of three to five days (Table 6.3-X) and, as a rule, should cover a period of 5-14 days. In a certain percentage of cases, staphylococci are gentamicin-resistant; in such cases, the MIC determined in vitro is the factor which decides whether, nevertheless, a combination is practical. In the case of high-level resistance (MIC > 1000 μg/ml), it is not wise. A possible alternative in these cases is netilmicin, since the resistance mechanism with respect to aminoglycoside-modified enzymes fails in this instance. Gentamicin-resistant strains can, therefore, be netilmicin-sensitive.

Although, in principle, rifampin acts antagonistically in combination with isoxazolyl penicillin, after appropriate in vitro microbiologic tests, the additional administration of rifampin should be considered when abscesses, intracardiac fistulas or prosthetic valve endocarditis are demonstrated, since rifampin is also effective against phagocyted staphylococci and, in vitro, accelerates the sterilization of abscesses (314-316).

Right ventricular endocarditis constitutes a special case as far as parenteral drug abuse is concerned (317,318). In these cases, not only is a high percentage to be expected with S. epidermidis as the pathogen, but also other coagulase-negative staphylococci of the S. epidermidis group, such as S. hominis and S. hemolyticus. With respect to the pathogenic clarification of this situation, attention is drawn, on the one hand, to the fact that parenterally applied narcotics contain micro-crystals and, on the other hand, to the theory that due to the unhygienic conditions, the injection of large numbers of staphylococcoccal organisms from the normal skin flora, which overtax the humoral and cellular immune response and can, thus, adhere to the preformed vegetation, is possible. However, there is no experimental evidence to support this hypothesis. Clinically, right ventricular endocarditis as a consequence of recurrent dissemination in the lungs often appears as pneumonia. It can occur recurrently and, prognostically, is astonishingly benign. Therapy is, as a rule, the same as for other types of staphylococcal endocarditis (Table 6.3-X). However, the therapy can usually be of very much shorter duration (two to three weeks). There are also reports of successful oral therapies.

Gram-negative pathogens: Endocarditis as a result of gram-negative bacteria is rare and the pathogens multifarious (Table 6.3-I). Standardized recommendations regarding antibiotic treatment are pointless. Since sensitivity to the antibiotics can differ greatly, the therapy is dependent on the in vitro sensitivity test. On the basis of animal experiments and limited clinical experience, the following can be stated as a guide.

Pseudomonas endocarditis can be treated by means of a combination of azlocillin and piperacillin (five doses of 4g per day) with gentamicin, tobramycin (three doses of 1-1.5

mg/kg per day) or netilimicin. The duration of therapy is at least six weeks. With aortic and/or mitral valve endocarditis as a result of pseudomonas aeruginosa, an early valve replacement and, subsequently, a six-week, large-dose antibiotic therapy are usually required. Inadequate experience is available with regard to monotherapy with ciprofloxacin, which is accompanied by considerably less toxic side effects, so that an attempted therapy is only justified in well-founded, exceptional cases (319-321).

As far as IE as a result of enterobacteria (E. coli, klebsiella, serratia, proteus) is concerned, therapeutic experience with the combination of a β-lactam antibiotic, e.g. cefotaxim (4 x 2 g/day) plus gentamicin, is available (322-324). As a rule, therapy over a period of at least six weeks is required.

In the case of endocarditis as a result of hemophilus, cardio-bacterium hominis, actinobacillus, eikenella, and kingella, mezlocillin or ampicillin (4 x 5 g/day) are the antibiotics of choice (Table 6.3-X) (234,325-332). Combination with an aminoglycoside (eg. 3-5 mg/kg/day gentamicin) is, in the case of complicated courses or echocardiographic detection of vegetation, definitely recommended.

Fungi: Without surgical intervention, fungal endocarditis can be cured only in exception cases. In the case of endocarditis caused by species of candida, antimycotic treatment is the therapy of choice, in the synergistically effective combination of amphotericin B and 5-flucytosin (333,334). After using small initial doses and gradually increasing these, amphotericin B is administered in doses of up to 1 mg/kg/day, with simultaneous administration of high volumes and NaCl to reduce nephrotoxicity. The maximum total dose should not exceed 3.0 g. Monitoring of the hematopoesis and renal function is necessary during the therapy. A distinct increase in the body temperature, as well as hypotensive responses of the circulatory system, which should not be confused with septic reactions, often occur, particularly at the beginning of therapy. When antimycotica are applied over several hours, there are usually fewer side effects. When amphothericin B, emulgated in lipid solutions, is applied, or when amphothericin B, embedded in liposomes (Ambisome®), is used, there are much fewer secondary effects (335,336). In the case of fungal endocarditis not caused by candida (e.g. aspergillus), after an appropriate sensitivity test, the combination with 5-flucytosin can, occasionally, be dispensed with.

Culture-negative endocarditis: Therapy is effected taking into account the clinical signs and symptoms and, particularly, on the basis of patient-related factors, such as drug abuse, artificial valve implantation, age, etc. (see above). Where there is an acute clinical course, a triple combination of isoxazolyl penicillin, penicillin G and an aminoglycoside (preferably gentamicin) is recommended. Where the onset is sub-acute, treatment is chiefly directed towards penicillin-sensitive streptococci (Table 6.3-IX). In the case of penicillin intolerance, a combination therapy with vancomycin and gentamicin is recommended.

Surgical therapy

Retrospective analysis of the course of the disease in patients with endocarditis supplies numerous arguments in favor of surgical intervention immediately typical complications occur (21,263,266,337-349). In addition, several factors can also come together which, although each in itself is not an indication for surgery, in combination, on the basis of available empirical experience, indicate a valve replacement for prognostic reasons (Table 6.3-XI).

It is undisputed that urgent surgical intervention is indicated in the case of patients with IE and a severe or progressive myocardial insufficiency as a consequence of an acute valvular regurgitation or obstruction. About 80% of fatalities in the case of IE, which occur in spite of effective antibiotic therapy, are attributable to this complication. Early surgical intervention is also accepted when there is an uncontrollable infection (see above). In some of these cases it must be assumed that the antibiotic therapy is ineffective. In the case of persistent septicemia in spite of suitable and appropriately dosed antibiotic treatment following a sensitivity test of the original pathogen, consideration must, on the other hand, first be given to the existence of an abscess.

In the case of endocarditis, indication for an operation should, in general, not be made dependent on the causative pathogen alone. An exception is endocarditis caused by fungi, gram-negative bacteria and highly resistant enterococci or staphylococci, since conservative therapy normally fails in these cases.

Surgery may be performed in the acute state of infective endocarditis, early after the first manifestation of symptoms, or late.

Early surgical intervention is reserved for those patients in whom the prognosis is

Table 6.3-XI: Indication for a surgical intervention in active infective endocarditis of native (N-IE) and prosthetic heart valves (P-IE). If more than five points are achieved, a valve replacement (N-IE) or a prosthetic valve exchange (P-IE) is indicated. Due to the favorable prognosis of endocarditis involving right sided valves, this is listed with -2 points.

findings	scores	
	N-IE	P-IE
heart failure - manifest,therapeutic refractory or progressive	5	-
- manifest, but satisfactorily conservative recompensationable	3	-
- latent	1	2
fungal endocarditis	5	5
persistant sepsis (< 48 h, despite adequate antibiotic therapy)	5	5
other pathogens than viridans streptococci	1	2
first septic thromboembolic event	3	3
recurrent thromboembolic events	5	5
echocardiographic detection of vegetations	1	1
endocarditis involving right sided valves only	-2	0
rupture of the papillary muscle or of chordae tendineae	3	-
ruptured sinus-valsalvae-aneurysm, ventricular septum defect	4	4
AV-block, progressive conduction disturbances or intracardial abscesses	4	4
small paravalvular dehiscence	-	2
large paravalvular dehiscence, marked tilting of the prosthetic valve	-	5
early prosthetic valve endocarditis (< 60 days)	-	2
mitral kissing vegetations in aortic valve endocarditis	4	4
isolated endocarditis of the aortic or of more than one valve	2	2
isolated mitral valve endocarditis	1	1

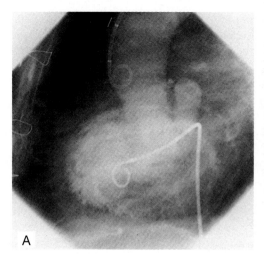

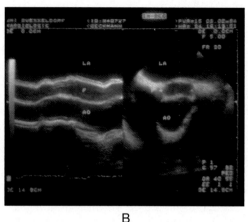

Figure 6.3-12: Paravalvular fistula after a medically cured prosthetic endocarditis on a St. Jude
Medical valve. Reoperation was later indicated because of the hemodynamically significant
regurgitation. A. Angiogram showing the left ventricle, ascending aorta and the paraprosthetic
fistula. B. Corresponding transesophageal echocardiographic findings: M-mode (left) and 2-D
(right). LA: left atrium; F: fistula; AO: ascending aorta.

otherwise very unfavorable, or in whom manifestation of complications are likely. Early
surgical intervention should generally be considered after two to four weeks of
antibiotic treatment for patients in whom the endocarditis has caused a significant
valvular defect with or without compensated heart failure. Indications for late surgical
interventions are the same as for non-infective acquired valvular lesions.

Cardiac failure due to extreme aortic regurgitation following endocarditis has a very poor
prognosis since the myocardium is not adapted to the acute volume overload and cannot
eject blood (as opposed to acute mitral regurgitation) against lower resistance. These patients
are protected only for a short time by the competent mitral valve against a progressive and
conservatively practically untreatable lung edema. For patients with severe acute aortic
insufficiency and progressive lung edema, therefore, there is no alternative to an urgent
surgical intervention. With diuretics or chronic veno-venous filtration, vasodilator therapy,
eventually increasing of the heart rate to shorten diastole and, thus, the regurgitation time, a
partial recompensation may be possible. These patients should be operated early, which
means that in case of a non-progressive aortic regurgitation there is often time for a two to
three week antibiotic treatment to sterilize the local situation (113).

Manifestation of a lung edema complicating an acute mitral insufficiency due to an
endocarditis has a different prognostic significance. Even mild to moderate acute mitral
regurgitations may result in a lung edema which is not a consequence of a left
ventricular myocardial failure but of the increasing left atrial pressures due to the
regurgitation volume. In these cases, myocardial contractility may not be significantly
compromised and recompensation is often possible, especially if vasodilators are used
to favorably influence the left ventricular impedance (113).

In cases with pre-existent severe aortic regurgitation or stenosis with or without
associated mitral regurgitation, early surgery within the first three weeks after starting

the antibiotic therapy is advisable because it prevents secondary complications and sudden occurrence of acute cardiac failure requiring emergency procedures (see above).

The impact of large and/or mobile vegetations on the indication for surgical intervention has been discussed elsewhere in this chapter.

Therapeutic procedure when thromboembolic complications occur is a moot point. Although a higher mortality rate has been proven with respect to these patients, there are diverging statements regarding the point at which a relapse is to be expected following a single thromboembolic complication. Reports are increasing that, with the exception of IE as a result of streptococcus viridans, the prognosis of the patients is improved if an operation is performed following the first septic embolism (see above). Where the indication for an operation is doubtful, the echocardiographic demonstration of massive vegetation is an additional argument in favor of an early operation (Fig. 7).

In addition, the occurrence of an acute renal failure is an indication for an operation because, irrespective of the genesis of the acute renal failure, the prognosis of these patients is significantly more unfavorable without an operation than with surgical intervention (see above).

The choice of valve substitute to be used in valve replacement during acute infective endocarditis remains controversial. As long as there are no abnormal cardiac morphologies and no persistent sepsis the standard techniques and the standard devices can be used. If annular or subannular myocardial abscesses are found intraoperatively, most experienced centers recommend the use of a free-hand homograft which can be individually fashioned and sutured to cover the infected area. In all other cases, differential use of biologic versus mechanical heart valves should follow those indications set up for other etiologies.

PROSTHETIC VALVE ENDOCARDITIS

Apart from acute mechanical dysfunctions, infections of artificial cardiac valves are subject to the highest mortality rate of prosthesis-related complications (20,21,263).

Incidence

Differentiation must be made between so-called early and late prosthetic valve endocarditis; with improvements in surgical management, the low degree of contamination during the cardiopulmonary bypass and perioperative antibiotic prophylaxis, early prosthetic endocarditis (defined as within 60 days postoperatively) is rare (350). Its incidence has decreased from over 4% prior to 1970 to far below 1%. Even with tight control of the patients, the incidence of late prosthetic endocarditis must be assumed to be approximately 0.3%/year of follow up. There is a constant hazard rate. The incidence with respect to mechanical prostheses is somewhat lower than for patients with bioprostheses (350).

Etiology and microbiology

The etiology of prosthetic endocarditis does not fundamentally differ from that of native-valve endocarditis, whereas, as far as the microbiology is concerned, there are distinct differences. Streptococci and enterococci are found more frequently in the case of native-valve endocarditis, and fungi, staphylococci and mixed infections more frequently with respect to prosthetic endocarditis (350-355) . Methicillin-sensitive S. epidermidis, in particular, has a high affinity to implanted or passage-applied foreign bodies, above all, if they are plastic coated. It is the typical pathogen of a prosthetic endocarditis (356,357).

Pathogenesis and pathology

Heart valve prostheses manufactured from plastic materials allow potential endocarditis pathogens no adhesion provided they are free of thrombi. Therefore, infections in mechanical prostheses usually emanate from the suture ring or thrombi which have developed in the vicinity of the suture ring, i.e. in areas where the blood is recirculated (358). On the other hand, an infection of a bioprosthesis can remain limited to the cusps, initiate their secondary degeneration and exhibit only a slight tendency to involve the suture ring or to suppurate (359-361).

The subdivision into early endocarditis, with the appearance of symptoms of the infection in the first 60 days after implantation of the prosthesis, and late endocarditis, which only manifests itself for the first time subsequent to this period, is of historical significance; in the sixties and seventies, early endocarditis was subject to a distinctly higher mortality rate. The time limit of 60 postoperative days was chosen arbitrarily. The subdivision still has a certain significance due to the fact that the spectrum of pathogens for early and late endocarditis differs; in the first postoperative weeks, the non-endothelialized suture ring of the prosthesis makes it easier for circulating bacteria to adhere. The interaction between staphylococci and the implanted polymer material is of considerable pathognomic significance as far as prosthetic endocarditis is concerned. What is perhaps most significant is the ability of coagulase-negative staphylococci to irreversibly adhere to the polymer surfaces, growing into multiple cell layers and forming a matrix of extracellular mucosal substance and host proteins. On the basis of these pathogenic findings, the question as to whether a staphylococcal prosthetic endocarditis, with involvement of the artificial surfaces in the infection, can be cleaned up at all with conservative medication and whether or not a reoperation is necessary in each case, are the subjects of debate at present.

Clinical picture and diagnosis

A prosthetic endocarditis is confirmed when, apart from septicemia, involvement of the implant in the infection process is demonstrated. When the tentative diagnosis is unconfirmed, the microbiologically isolated pathogen can be significant (Table 6.3-XIV).

Involvement of the prosthesis can manifest itself in a periprosthetic dehiscence or interference of the prosthetic occluder by thromboendocarditic vegetation (349). In addition to newly occurring stenotic or insufficiency murmurs, echocardiographically documented vegetation or intracardiac abscesses, abnormal movement of the base of the prosthesis or the prosthetic occluder in the fluoroscopic examination, as well as conduction disorders which are manifest for the first time, indicate a prosthetic endocarditis (362-368). Periprosthetic regurgitation can be localized by means of color

Doppler echocardiography, with transesophageal echocardiography providing considerably more informative results (255,369-373) (Fig. 12). The diagnosis is frequently made only after the appearance of typical complications (pulmonary congestion, periprosthetic dehiscence, chronic intravascular hemolysis, thromboembolism).

If there is no evidence of a typical constellation of a septicemia, with positive hemocultures and a prosthetic dysfunction, or of vegetation or intracardiac abscesses, demonstration of a prosthetic endocarditis is difficult. The probability that a prosthetic endocarditis nevertheless exists, can be checked in these cases by means of a retrospective point-scoring system (Table 6.3-XII).

Differential diagnosis

From the point of view of differential diagnosis, when endocarditis is suspected within the first few months after artificial valve replacement, non-infective dehiscence and excessive endothelial growth (tissue ingrowth) in the area of the suture ring, in particular, must be taken into consideration. When endocarditis is suspected later in the course, and the excursion of the prosthetic occluder is inhibited, prosthetic valvular thrombosis and fibrous tissue ingrowth must be considered.

Course and prognosis

Possible complications of a prosthetic endocarditis are, in principle, similar to those of a native-valve endocarditis. The by far most frequent complication is infection-mediated periprosthetic dehiscence.

Valvular insufficiency, septic embolisms and a persistent septicemia are, proportionally, more frequently observed than in the case of native valve endocarditis. The prognosis of patients with prosthetic endocarditis has distinctly improved over the last few years; while in the Sixties, more than 80% of all patients died, the mortality rate today is probably less than 15%. Apart from advances in the field of diagnostics and conservative treatment, this improvement in the prognosis is primarily attributable to earlier surgical intervention.

Treatment and prophylaxis

The treatment of prosthetic endocarditis does not fundamentally differ from that of native endocarditis; sanitation by means of drug therapy is, however, more difficult than in the case of native valve endocarditis, so that, as far as the alternative treatments stated in Table 6.3-X are concerned, the most highly dosed therapy, combination therapy and the therapy of longest duration must always be chosen. In addition, the diagnosis with respect to surgical re-intervention must be made in good time. This applies, in particular, when a hemodynamically significant perivalvular dehiscence occurs. No binding recommendations can be made with regard to the decision as to whether, in the case of a florid prosthetic endocarditis, conservative treatment should be continued or there should be a surgical intervention. With certain courses of the disease, available results provide evidence of a superiority of combined surgical and drug therapy as opposed to conservative treatment alone (Table 6.3-XI).

Prosthetic endocarditis caused by staphylococci, which are often of nosocomial origin

Table 6.3-XII: Retrospectively drawn-up and prospectively proven score-system in unproven tentative diagnosis of prosthetic valve endocarditis.

	endocarditis after valve implantation	
	within one year	later than one year
septicemia and blutcultural demonstration of the infective agent of:		
- streptococci	1	3
- enterococci	1	3
- staphylococci	3	3
- gram-negative bacteria	3	2
- mixed infections	2	3
- funghi	2	1
- other germs	1	1
clinical signs of an endocarditis	2	3
emboli	1	1
first manifestation of conduction disturbances	1	2
echocardiographic demonstration of:		
- vegetations (without earlier findings available)	2	2
- vegetations (with earlier findings available for comparison)	4	4
- ring abscesses, intracardial abscesses	4	4
new insufficiency or stenotic murmur	2	2
demonstration of a prosthestic malfunction	2	4
all cases (n=61) are correctly diagnosed retrospectively with more than	8 scores	10 scores
prospective confirmation of the score-system by a prospective testing	6/7 (85.7%)	9/31 (93.5%)

and exhibit multi-resistance, poses a particular problem. Contrary to the case with native valve endocarditis, almost without exception, penicillinase-producing strains of S. aureus and S. epidermidis are involved. In addition, over 50% of coagulase-negative staphylococci strains isolated in the case of endocarditis patients are not only penicillinase-producers, but are also methicillin-resistant.

Based on these preconditions, the therapy regimen for treating prosthetic endocarditis as a result of staphylococci must be considerably more aggressive. If a penicillinase-producing, but methicillin-sensitive, strain is demonstrated, treatment consists of a combination therapy with isoxazolyl penicillin, gentamicin and rifampin. Contrary to the case with native valve endocarditis, the daily dosage of gentamicin should be gradually increased to up to 5 mg/kg body weight and administered over a period of two weeks. The additional application of rifampin (900 mg/day in three individual oral doses) is, according to studies available to date, superior to the combination of isoxazolyl penicillin and gentamicin. The isoxazolyl penicillin and rifampin therapy should continue for at least six weeks; in individual cases, particularly when coagulase-negative staphylococci are involved, therapy of longer duration may be required; in extreme cases, where a prosthetic endocarditis caused by coagulase-negative staphylococci is concerned and a reoperation can definitely not be performed, treatment can be necessary over a period of one year.

In the case of methicillin-resistant strains, or if there is a penicillin allergy, isoxazolyl penicillin must be replaced by vancomycin. In the combination therapy with an isoxazolyl penicillin and gentamicin, an alternative concept provides for the parenteral application of fosfomycin instead of rifampin. In this context, the daily dosage is 15g-20g, divided into three to four individual doses. Attention must be paid to the comparatively high administration of sodium.

When effectiveness is demonstrated in vitro (absolutely necessary in the case of coagulase-negative staphylococci), the possibility of using the new glycopeptide antibiotic, teicoplanin, which can be applied once per day, on average, also exists. Only as result of this is the possibility of an ambulant therapy available.

Hemodynamically significant suture dehiscence is particularly feared after reoperation during florid prosthetic endocarditis. Suture dehiscence, which requires renewed surgical intervention, occurs in approximately 20% of patients. However, mortality is not higher than in the case of valvular reoperation generally.

RHEUMATIC ENDOCARDITIS

Rheumatic endocarditis, which in the acute stage, is part of a pancarditis, will be discussed here.

Incidence and pathogenesis

An acute rheumatic fever is now only rarely observed in central Europe. However, apart from degenerative heart valve defects, chronic valvular lesions following rheumatic endocarditis still constitute the largest nosologic group of acquired valvular diseases; approximately 50% of mitral stenoses requiring operation today, and approximately 30% of mitral insufficiencies, are attributable to rheumatic fever or equivalent rheumatic processes. The percentage of degenerative, ischemia-related, and so-called "relative" mitral insufficiencies, is, however, distinctly increasing. In the case of aortic stenoses requiring operation, the percentage is lower, namely 39% with respect to the primary bicuspid aortic valve and 49% with respect to the tricuspid aortic valve, because a constantly increasing percentage of older patients exhibit a degenerative, calcifying aortic stenosis (374,375).

The pathogenesis of acute rheumatic fever has not been conclusively clarified. The role of the M protein in the β-hemolysing streptococci of serologic Group A, which acts as an antigen and possibly triggers off an autoimmune reaction, is undisputed (376,377). The antibodies formed exhibit cross-reactions with, on the one hand, streptococcal substances and, on the other, with proteins in a variety of tissues, and appear to have a sensitizing effect, so that, in the case of a renewed streptococcal infection, typical rheumatic fever reactions are triggered off in the myocardial sarcolemma (rheumatic myocarditis), the endocardium (rheumatic endocarditis), the pericardium (rheumatic pericarditis), the synovia (acute rheumatic fever), the main arteries (erythema annular), the renal glomerula (diffuse glomerulonephritis), and the pleura (pleurittis) (378-380). This pathogenesis also explains why the relapse of a rheumatic fever is of such great significance as far as the development of a manifest valvular defect is concerned.

The development of a rheumatic fever has a prerequisite, i.e. the existence of a streptococcal infection, in general, for 10 or more days, usually involving an infection of the upper respiratory tract, a scarlet fever or a tonsillitis (375,381,382). Initial cardiac involvement within the framework of the new, acute attack of rheumatic fever is co-determining as far as the later development of rheumatic valvular changes are concerned. Patients in whom no cardiac murmur (mitral insufficiency, aortic insufficiency) is present during the acute rheumatic fever and in whom the ECG has revealed no changes later develop a rheumatic heart valve defect only in exceptional cases (383). In comparison to this, up to two thirds of the patients with cardiac insufficiency during rheumatic carditis exhibit considerable morphologic changes in the mitral valve, and these, usually, develop valvular heart disease within 10 years after the acute illness.

On the other hand, with effective prophylaxis over a period of decades, no rheumatic valvular defect occurs in the majority of patients, whereas a hemodynamically significant valve defect develops within a few years in about half of the patients in whom cardiac consequences of the initial illness (cardiac murmur, cardiac insufficiency) are still present at the time of a relapse (384).

Thus rheumatic relapses determine the prognosis of patients more than the initial cardiac involvement in the case of single episodes of rheumatic fever.

What is significant in terms of the pathogenesis is that the interval between an anamnestically confirmed rheumatic fever with carditis and symptoms of a secondary valvular defect can be between one and 35 years. On average, symptoms of a mitral valve defect appear more than 16 years later, and those of an aortic valve defect more than 23 years later.

In southern Europe, North Africa and Third World countries, the latent period can be considerably shorter and, not infrequently, a valve disease requiring operation can occur even before the age of 20. More frequent and more serious carditis relapses are blamed as being the cause.

Clinical picture and diagnosis of rheumatic carditis

The criteria designated by Ducket Jones for the diagnosis of an acute rheumatic fever have been frequently improved and supplemented by more recent findings (385). With the aid of these, an acute rheumatic fever can be diagnosed with a high degree of reliability. A rheumatic carditis occurs less frequently in adults than in children. The pericardium, myocardium and endocardium, are often simultaneously affected (rheumatic pancarditis). The existence of a carditis can be deemed to be established if, within the framework of a rheumatic fever, a cardiomegaly, with or without cardiac insufficiency, develops and/or cardiac murmurs occur for the first time. Diagnosis is simplified if, in addition, a pericarditis (pericardial friction rub, serofibrinous fluid from the pericardial space) or changes in the ECG are detectable. A cardiomegaly requires an echocardiographic examination.

Apart from flow murmurs due to the increased cardiac output in the case of fever and anemia, relative valvular insufficiencies are frequent with acute rheumatic carditis due to cardiomegaly caused by myocarditis or acute valvulitis. In addition, rheumatic myocarditis causes early electrocardiographic changes, most frequently prolonged AV time, up to and including a total AV block, and S-T changes, chiefly in the left precordial chest leads, as well as extension of the Q-T interval. Less frequently, bundle-branch blocks, as well as atrial and ventricular arrhythmias, are observed.

Treatment and prophylaxis

In the acute stage of rheumatic fever, due to the carditis, normally detectable in children and less frequently established in adults, bed rest is, in particular, recommended if a cardiac involvement is established on the basis of a newly occurring cardiac murmur, a cardiomegaly, or ECG changes are established. To eliminate the causal streptococcal infection, treatment with penicillin must be initiated without delay and continued for at least 10 days. A postponement of the commencement of treatment for up to a maximum of 24 hours is considered justifiable in order to demonstrate the streptococci, since the clinical picture of rheumatic fever generally permits no doubt with respect to the diagnosis. As a rule, 1-2 million IU/day are adequate as an oral dose of penicillin for adults; higher doses of penicillin have no affect on secondary cardiac manifestations (386).

In the case of symptomatically severe courses, additional steroids should be administered after establishment of the diagnosis. The dosage must be orientated towards the therapeutic effect, and is usually 60-100 mg/day prednisolon or equivalent doses of another corticosteroid. After therapy for three to six days, the dose is gradually reduced. In the case of less severe courses, treatment with salicylic acid derivates in large doses is recommended. The initial treatment with four doses of 1.5-2.5g acetylsalicylic acid per day for adults is halved after a few days and maintained for a few weeks. The use of steroids and salicylic acid derivates constitutes only a symptomatic therapy. There are no indications that they have an influence either on the duration of the rheumatic fever or on the development of a later heart valve defect. If, in the case of florid carditis, there are signs and symptoms of a cardiac insufficiency, a therapy with ACE inhibitors, diuretic treatment and, after exclusion of stimulus conduction dysfunctions, a digitalization, are indicated.

Of decisive importance as far as the development of a manifest rheumatic heart valve defect is concerned are the incidence and severity of rheumatic fever relapses, their interval from the initial attack and the age of the patients at this point in time. The occurrence of relapses can be reliably obviated by means of a long term penicillin therapy in terms of a secondary prophylaxis (388). Penicillin therapies which are initiated following the renewed occurrence of symptoms of an infection of the upper respiratory tract cannot reliably prevent relapses, so that only long term prophylaxis over many years promises success.

OTHER PRIMARY FORMS OF ENDOCARDITIS

NON-BACTERIAL THROMBOTIC ENDOCARDITIS

Non-bacterial thrombotic vegetation (ATV) plays a major role in the pathogenesis of endocarditis (see above). Apart from the case of endocardial damage, it is also to be found in the case of hypercoagulability following neoplasms, circulating immune complexes, or a septicemia (389-391). Where there are malignant growths, particularly adenocarcinoma, ATV is seen in autopsies, e.g. five times more frequently than in patients without neoplasms. In the case of disseminated intravascular coagulation (DIC) following a staphylococcal septicemia, ATV, which is also observed following viral infections, for example caused by the Coxsackie-B4 virus, is also found, with a disproportionately high frequency, in autopsies. Where there are circulating immune complexes, both direct damage to the endocardial endothelial cells and a hypercoagulability are significant as far as the development of ATV is concerned. Libman-Sacks endocarditis, complicating systematic lupus erythematosus, is an example for immunity complex-related ATV. Endocarditis verrucosa simplex, observed in marantic patients of advanced age, also belongs to this morphologic circle.

Endocardial fibroelastosis

Endocardial fibroelastosis (EFE) is pathomorphologically characterized by fibrous thickening of the left ventricular, less frequently, also of the left atrial endocardium, and occurs, to an increasing degree, familially (392). Etiologically, acquired forms are, in addition, suspected following prenatal subendocardial hypoxia or perinatal endocardial infections (393,394). Differentiation is made between a primary, dilatative form, with involvement of the endocardium of the left ventricle and the left cardiac valves, and secondary EFE, which is usually accompanied by a thickening of the mural endocardium and consecutive obliteration of the left ventricular cavity. It is chiefly found in patients with a pressure-loaded left ventricle and consecutive myocardial hypertrophy since birth (aortic stenosis, coarectation critical aortic stenosis in early infancy, with and without hypoplastic left heart syndrome (394).

Primary endomyocardial fibroelastosis in patients without accompanying congenital cardiac defects, apart from the left ventricle, also affects the mitral and aortic valves, and is usually associated with small degrees of non-bacterial thrombotic vegetation. In about half the cases, there is a mitral insufficiency since the subvalvular apparatus can be included in the process. The patients usually become noticeable in the first year of life, as a result of tachycardia, gallop rhythm, as well as indirect indications of a cardiac insufficiency (somnolence, deficient suction, dyspnea, coughing, pallor), and normally exhibit negative T-waves in the left precordial ECG leads, as well as an increased arteriovenous oxygen difference (395). From the point of view of therapy, the early application of, and long term treatment with, digital glycosides is indicated. In a few cases, heart transplantation has been performed, with moderate prognostic success (396).

Endomyocardial fibrosis

The endomyocardial fibrosis (EMF), chiefly encountered in the tropical rain forest belt, is the chronic, more rare endocarditis parietalis fibroplastica Löffler, the acute form of the same disease which is understood today to be part of the hypereosinophilia syndrome (397-402). Functionally, endomyocardial fibrosis results in a restrictive cardiomyopathy (403).

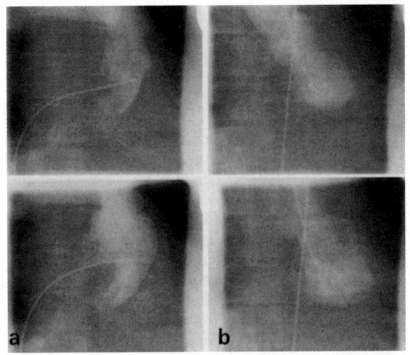

Figure 6.3-13: Angiocardiogram in Löffler's endocarditis complicating hypereosinophylic syndrome.
a. Obliteration of the apical segment of the right ventricle and filiform contrasts of the
intratrabecular spaces during diastole. b. Apical contrast defect of the left ventricle.

Tropical EMF is usually encountered in young patients, with no preference as to sex, without indications of a system disease being found (404). Due to its geo-epidemiologic propagation, a connection with parasitic diseases must be assumed (405). In 75% of cases, both, the right and left ventricular endocardium are affected; in 20% of cases, only that of the right ventricle (406). A pronounced eosinophilia, thromboembolic complications and atrioventricular valvular defects are rarely encountered, atrial fibrillation, on the other hand, frequently.

Idiopathic mural endocarditis (Becker's endocarditis), described in 1953, is probably the early manifestation of an EMF (407).

Löffler's endocarditis

Definition and incidence: In 1968, pronounced eosinophilia with, in some cases, a considerable degree of leukocytosis, was classified as the hypereosinophilia syndrome (HES) (408). Later, HES was more precisely defined as being an eosinophilia of the blood and bone marrow, persisting for more than six months (absolute eosinophile count > 1500/μl) with secondary organic manifestation (409).

Endocarditis parietalis fibroplastica (399), which takes a more acute and progressive course than tropical EMF, is the cardiac manifestation of the hypereosinophilia syndrome, in which, apart from the lungs, bone barrow and cerebrum and, more rarely, the kidneys, the gastrointestinal tract, the liver and the skin can be affected. Löffler's endocarditis is characterized by a thickening of the apical and subvalvular endocardium of both ventricles of the heart, normally accompanied by eosinophilia and, frequently, by thromboembolisms, eosinophilic infiltrates in the myocardium and, usually, widely disseminated parietal thrombi. To date, approximately 350 confirmed cases of the, probably too rarely diagnosed, disease, have been reported.

Etiology and pathogenesis: An eosinophilia of unclarified cause exists in approximately half the patients with Löffler's endocarditis. As far as the others are concerned, an eosinophilic leukemia (disputed as being an independent clinical picture) (approximately 25%) or, in the case of panarteritis nodosa, bronchial asthma, parasitosis and, less frequently, in the case of Hodgkin disease, carcinoma, malignant diseases of the reticulohistiocytary system, as well as where there is remedial drug intolerance, a relative eosinophilia is found (410).

The damage to the endocardium and myocardium (and also to other organic systems), is probably the result of eosinophilic infiltrates, with toxic cell damage due to eosinophilic peroxidase (EPO) and basic proteins. The major basic protein, which forms more than 50% of the protein content of the eosinophilic granula, activates inflammatory cells and, in high concentrations, has a cytotoxic effect. In addition, it is a potential stimulator of hemocyte aggregation (411) and is responsible, together with the cationic proteins which primarily affect the plasmatic coagulation system, for thrombotic and thromboembolic complications following the disease (401,412,413). The degree of stimulation of the eosinophiles, for example following type I immune reactions, parasitosis or remedial drug intolerance, is genetically controlled; its persistence is co-determined by the colony stimulating factor (CSF), which inhibits the chemotactic mobility of the eosinophiles. Secondly, non-specific thickening of the myocardium and endocardium, together with thrombotic vegetation, then develops in the heart and, ultimately, severe endomyocardial fibrosis.

Pathology: From a histopathologic point of view, an obliterative endoarteritis, as well as a periarteritis of the intramural coronary arteries, is found with respect to the endomyocardial infiltrations and necroses, chiefly comprising eosinophilic granulocytes, which exist with Löffler's endocarditis. The epicardial coronary arteries are not affected. At a later stage, a fibrosis, chiefly of the apical and subvalvular, less frequently, also of the valvular endocardium (mitral and tricuspid valves) of both ventricles develops, combined with widely disseminated parietal thrombi (Fig. 13). The endomyocardial fibrosis which ultimately develops leads to a pronounced diastolic dysfunction in terms of a restrictive cardiomyopathy (414,415).

Clinical picture and diagnosis: Cardiac involvement in the case of HES is frequent, and can be determined in 60% to 80% of cases when there is early diagnosis (416,417). Males between 20 and 50 years of age are predominantly affected (9:1). The peak age is in the 4th decade.

Apart from general symptoms of the infection, cardiomegaly, with or without indications of a right or left ventricular insufficiency, indications of a restrictive cardiomyopathy, dyspnea, thromboembolic complications, mitral insufficiency murmurs, and a third heart sound are typical cardial symptoms/findings. Non-specific ECG changes, with depression of the S-T segment and negative T-waves, are frequently encountered; conduction disturbances rarely.

In the terminal stage of HES, there may be little evidence of the obligatory eosinophilia in chemical laboratory tests. There are often non-specific changes in the immunologic system, such as an increase in the IgE, a reduced number of T-lymphocytes or an increase in circulating immune complexes. While bone marrow eosinophiles exhibit no morphologic irregularities, the peripherally circulating eosinophiles exhibit, to a higher degree, degranulation and vacuolation. This is held to be an indication of an increased release of cationic proteins and peroxidases (418,419).

In the early phases of Löffler's endocarditis, endomyocardial biopsy from the apex of the right ventricle is considered to be the diagnostic method of choice. At this point in time, the clinical findings may be discreetly pronounced and, except for the persisting hypereosinophilia, there may be no cardinal pathologic changes (420,421). The bioptic findings allow, in addition, the sometimes difficult differentiation between constrictive pericarditis (422). However, where there is widely disseminated thromboses, it can be difficult to acquire portions of the endomyocardium in an adequate quantity. Furthermore, it must be borne in mind that the fibrotic material in the, frequently obliterated, cavity allows biopsy only with difficulty (423). Activated eosinophiles and their liberated granular proteins can, particularly in the early necrotic phase, be detected both in the endomyocardium and in the mural thrombi by means of immunocytochemical methods (424,425).

In the advanced stage, 2D echocardiography provides a guide (Fig. 14). In this context, distinct thickening of the posterior mitral cusp is often exhibited, which can, occasionally, simulate vegetations (426). An apical obliteration of one or both ventricular cavities, caused by thrombotic material, and a distinctly increased echogenity of the endocardium, are typical (Fig. 12). On the other hand, the basal wall segments, usually free of this, often evidence hyperdynamic contractions (427-429). In advanced cases, the restricted diastolic filling can be confirmed by means of Doppler echocardiography. Moderate or even significant insufficiencies of the atrioventricular valves are frequent.

Hemodynamically, pressure curves, characteristic of a biventricular distensibility disorder, with early diastolic DIP and subsequent plateau formation, similar to that of a constrictive pericarditis, are to be found (430).

Angiocardiographically, there is an apical rounding of the right and/or left ventricles, with a lack of definition of the papillary muscles. A mitral insufficiency is frequent. In order to prevent dissolution of the thrombi, a right ventricular angiography, with laevocardiogram, or transseptal puncture of the left atrium is to be given preference over left ventricular catheteriztation. Since the biventricular findings are typical of Löffler's endocarditis, a right ventricular myocardial biopsy presents itself for confirmation of the diagnosis.

Differential diagnosis: Differentiation between an IE and a rheumatic valvular disease, particularly of the mitral valve, as well as a constrictive pericarditis or the different forms of restrictive cardiomyopathy, can only be made in the early stages of a Löffler's endocarditis on the basis of the differential blood chemistry, with demonstration of a pronounced hypereosinophilia, if applicable, by means of endomyocardial biopsy. In rare cases of initial manifestation in early infancy, an endocardial fibroelastosis must be excluded by means of differential diagnosis. Churg-Strauss granulomatous eosinophilic vasculitis (431,432), which can, likewise, also affect small and medium-sized coronary arteries and veins, can, on the basis of the usually typical extra-cardiac manifestations in

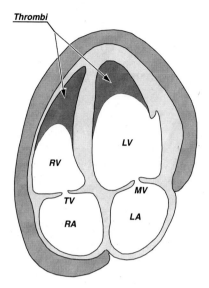

Figure 6.3-14: Schematic diagram of bi-ventricular filling defects in Löffler's endocarditis. RV: right ventricle; LV: left ventricle; RA: right atrium; LA: left atrium, TV: tricuspid valve; MV: mitral valve.

the area of the lungs and oropharynx, as well as of the histologic findings, be distinguished, without difficulty, from a necrotizing vasculitis. Cardiac thesaurismoses, cardiac amyloidosis and endocarditis involving a metastasising carcinoid, must be taken into account in differential diagnostic considerations.

Course and prognosis: In the majority of cases, the course progresses rapidly and usually leads, within two years, to a left ventricular (75%) or right ventricular (50%) insufficiency, as well as to hemodynamically significant mitral insufficiencies (40%) and/or tricuspid insufficiencies (15%). Thromboembolic complications occur in 20% of those affected, and are to blame for the majority of central and renal complications. Without operative intervention (thrombi removal and endocardial resections), the patients die as a result of the therapy-insensitive cardiac insufficiency.

Treatment: In the acute necrosis stage, the reduction of the eosinophilic granulocyte count and the elimination of the cardiotoxic cationic proteins of the eosinophiles take priority. Due to the irreversible myocardial changes in the terminal phase and the negative prognosis for untreated cases, with a mortality rate of 80% to 95% within three years (409,433,434), an early therapeutic attempt must be made to interrupt the disease process by the application of immunosuppressants and chemotherapeutics. In a relatively low number of cases, favorable results have been reported following the use of glucocorticoids, if applicable, combined with hydroxycarbamite or with alkaloids. In the case of therapeutic failure (435,436), a combination of chemotherapy with cytarabin and 6-thioguanine is recommended (435,436). Treatment with recombinant α-interferon constitutes a very promising therapeutic approach (437).

Anticoagulation with coumarin derivatives is always indicated in order to prevent thromboembolic complications. Where success is inadequate, a combination with platelet inhibitors should also be considered, regardless of the complications of hemorrhage.

In the fibrosis stage, a symptomatic therapy with ACE inhibitors and diuretics can be applied. In the case of atrial fibrillation, digitalization is indicated. In conservative, non-controllable cases of a consecutive cardiac insufficiency, endocardial resection, the high perioperative mortality rate of which is 20% to 30%, is indicated (438). In the case of hemodynamically significant atrio-ventricular valve insufficiency, due to the high thromboembolic risk, a bioprosthetic valve replacement is recommended (438,439,440). In late stages, resection of the fibrotic tissue and reconstruction of the atrioventricular valves has been described (441).

ENDOCARDITIS IN THE CASE OF DIFFERENT PRIMARY DISEASES

The pathogenesis of endocarditis, with the development of thrombotic vegetation in the case of structural damage to the endocardium, hypercoagulability and other factors, explains why numerous diseases can be accompanied by endocardial involvement. These include, *inter alia*, systemic lupus erythematosus (SLE), metastasising carcinoids, rheumatic arthritis, and spondylitis ankylopoetica (M. Bechterew).

Endocardial involvement in the case of SLE

Definition and incidence

Systemic lupus erythematosus is an acute or chronic disease of the vascular connective tissue, which often progresses intermittently, with the pathomorphologic picture of a diffuse micro-vasculitis and possible involvement of almost all organic systems (442). Cardiac involvement, in the form of a myocarditis or pericarditis, is stated to be 20% to 70% (443,444), but it has been detected in more than 90% of those affected at autopsy (444). In approximately one third of the clinically diagnosed cases of SLE (445), and approximately 50% of the post mortem cases, the disease is accompanied by an non-bacterial verrucosal endocarditis of the valvular and parietal endocardium (Libman-Sacks endocarditis) (446).

In Europe, the prevalence of systematic lupus erythematosus is, as a function of geographical and ethnic factors, approximately 0.07% (447).

Etiology and pathogenesis

Where there is a genetically determined susceptibility, an immunologic imbalance occurs between B and T lymphocytes as a result of a polyclonal hyperactivity of B lymphocytes, caused by a multiplicity of factors, with consecutive formation of antibodies, as well as increased immune response to microbial, pharmacologic and numerous other antigens (448,449). In over 90% of cases, ss-DNS antibodies, in 20%-40%, RF antibodies, in 60%-70%, ds-ss DNS antibodies, in 30%-40%, Sm antibodies, in 30%-40%, SS-A/Ro antibodies, and in 10%-15%, 22-B/La antibodies are detectable in the case of SLE. The inhibition of the immune reaction by male hormones explains the prevalence of the female sex, whereby women of an age at which they are capable of gestating are predominantly affected. The deposition of circulating immune complexes and complement factors in the endothelial cells of the endocardium initiate the local release of enzymes comprising polymorphonuclear leukocytes damaging to the endothelium. The endothelial damage results in the development of Libman-Sacks vegetation and also the destruction of deeper layers, particularly those of the valvular endocardium, so that a typical valvulitis develops (450).

Pathology

The small degree of vegetation, chiefly comprising detritus, fibrin, platelets and hematoxylin corpuscles, which exists in the case of SLE, corresponds to an atypical verrucosal endocarditis. The vegetation is predominantly found in the recesses formed by the ventricular walls and the cusps of the atrioventricular valves, more rarely on the ventricular surfaces of the atrioventricular valves, the subvalvular apparatus and the parietal ventricular and atrial endocardium, and only occasionally on the edges of the valve closure (451). The semilunar valves are sometimes also affected. Except for individual cases of perforated aortic semilunar valves, hemodynamically significant aortic valve defects as a result of an SLE has, to date, not been described. The valve function is only impaired in exceptional cases (452). Individual cases of acute mitral insufficiency due to rupture of the groups of tendinous fibers, are, however, known. Chronic, progressive mitral insufficiencies can occur as a result of the shortening of the tendinous fibers due to shrinkage of the cusp, or adhesion of the atrioventricular cusp to the ventricular endocardium.

Clinical picture and diagnosis of Libman-Sacks endocarditis

The cardinal clinical findings are an inconstant mitral insufficiency murmur, and, less frequently, that of a tricuspid or aortic insufficiency and, in exceptional cases, that of a mitral stenosis. Pulmonary venous congestion following a mitral insufficiency is rare in the case of SLE and, as a rule, can be conservatively controlled. With progressive dyspnea, or other indications of a cardiac insufficiency, hemodynamically significant pericardial effusion and a myocarditis, must, above all, be taken into consideration by means of differential diagnosis. Both are usually also the cause of the other cardiac symptoms and findings - such as conduction or repolarisation disturbances in the ECG, tachycardia, atrial fibrillation, ventricular arrhythmia, dry pericarditis, thoracodynia, gallop rhythm, or cardiomegaly (453). Transesophogeal echocardiography is the examination method of choice to determine specific morphologic valvular changes (445,454).

The lupus-associated vegetation differs from microbial vegetation due to its localization, manifestation and mobility, since it is located near the base of the cusps or leaflets oganicity, exhibits heteregenous echogenity with increased central reflexes as correlative of connective tissue or calcifying structures, and moves parallel to the affected valve. Contrary to this, microbial vegetation is usually localized on the edges of the cusps or leaflets with low echogenicity, and exhibits floating motions, i.e. disguising valve excursions.

In the case of contraction of SLE during pregnancy, the neonate can have a lupus-type clinical picture, including cardiac manifestations (in particular, congenital, total AV block, pericarditis) due to the transplacental passage of antibodies and circulating immune complexes. However, a termination of pregnancy on the basis of the filial diagnosis is not indicated. Attention must be paid to fetal bradycardia. On the other hand, a pronounced cardiac lupus manifestation on the part of the mother is adequate indication for a termination of pregnancy if an interruption of the immunosuppressive therapy appears not to be justifiable for the pregnancy period (455).

Course and prognosis

Contrary to acute rheumatic fever, in the case of acute SLE, there are only rarely hemodynamically significant valvular dysfunctions. Slight mitral and tricuspid valve insufficiencies are, on the other hand, frequently found. Chronic systemic lupus erythematosus, which occasionally leads to progressive valvular changes, up to and including a severe mitral and tricuspid insufficiency, is responsible for less than 0.2% of the mitral insufficiencies requiring operation (375). In rare cases, an acute mitral insufficiency can develop as a result of rupture of the chordae tendineae. Diagnosis of a valve replacement must then be made in the case of acute mitral insufficiency of another genesis. The involvement of the endocardium in the case of systemic lupus erythematosus is not, as a rule, the prognostically limiting factor (454,456).

Treatment

Anticoagulation, and therapy with corticosteroids, also in combination with azathioprine and/or cyclophosphamide has, in the case of systematic lupus erythematosus, only a negligible influence on the development of a Libmann-Sacks endocarditis or on the incidence and severity of a consecutive heart valve defect (457).

Endocarditis in the case of the carcinoid syndrome

Definition, etiology and pathology

Carcinoids, which develop from enterochromaffin cells, secrete endocrine-active substances such as serotonin, histamine, kinin, prostaglandins and, rarely, ACTH, gastrin, catecholamins, insulin, somatotropin, or calcitonin. The majority of tumours are found in the appendix and in the ileum, as well as in other segments of the gastrointestinal tract, in the pancreas, the bronchi, and the ovaries (458,459). Upon passage through the liver, lungs and brain, the endocrine-active substances are metabolized. If more than 2.5 mg of the 5-hydroxyindoleacetic acid from the serotonin metabolites are excreted in the urine per 24 hours, diagnosis of the carcinoid syndrome is confirmed (460).

A carcinoid syndrome exists if the endocrine-active substances - usually following metastatic spread to the liver from a small intestine carcinoid - can become systemically effective, due to the suspension of hepatic inactivation, and can reach the right ventricle. In the case of a carcinoid of the ovaries, the endocrine-active substances are drained directly into the vena cavae. A left ventricular involvement following pulmonary metastatic spread is observed in about one third of the patients (461). A metastatic spread occurs in approximately 25%-50% of patients, whereby carcinoids with a diameter of more than 2 cm frequently metastasise; smaller ones rarely.

The clinical symptoms of the carcinoid syndrome are serotonin-induced diarrhoea and abdominal cramps. In addition, bronchial spasms and a flush-type erythema of the skin, induced by kinin, occur. The attacks usually last a few minutes, but can last for hours. They vary in intensity and frequency, usually occur spontaneously, occasionally after excitement, greasy meals, consumption of alcoholic beverages, the taking of medication, and pressure on the tumour tissue. The cardinal symptoms, "flush" and "diarrhoea", are observed in practically all patients with the carcinoid syndrome, while a cardiac involvement can be determined in about two thirds of the patients, and bronchial spasms in one third (461,462).

It is assumed that the substances secreting in tumours damage the endocardial endothelium and cause a proliferation of myocytes and myofibroblasts, with an excessive formation of collagen fibrils and sour mucopolysaccharides (463). The thickening of areas of the endocardium, which develops at the same time, is predominantly localized to the sides of the tricuspid and pulmonary valves remote from the bloodstream, the atrial portions of the vena cavae, in the right atrium, including the coronary sinus, in the right ventricle and in the pulmonary trunk (464). Extremely rarely, changes are found in the left ventricle, chiefly to the mitral valve, but only when there is a right-left shunt or a bronchial carcinoid.

Clinical picture, diagnosis and treatment

Apart from the typical cardinal symptoms and findings of the metastasising carcinoid, in the case of cardiac manifestation, the auscultatory findings usually indicate a tricuspid valve insufficiency and/or pulmonary stenosis. Combined tricuspid disease is infrequent; combined pulmonary disease is rare (459,465). The clinical symptoms, as well as the phonocardiographic, radiologic, echocardiographic, hemodynamic, and angiocardiographic findings correspond to the extent of the valvular lesion.

In addition, endocardial thickening and hemodynamically increased cardiac outputs, can frequently be documented (461,462,466,467).

Apart from primary surgical treatment of the basic disease, carcinoids usually react well to cytostatic therapy, particularly with 5-fluorouracil, in addition, cyclophosphamide and adiamycin, are used, either alone or in combination, with a response rate of 20%-30%. Initial studies also show an effectiveness of human leukocyte interferons on carcinoids (408). Carcinoids are relatively resistant to a radiotherapy (409). Apart from symptomatic treatment with sandostatin (3 x 50-500 mg/day s.c.), cyproheptadin (8-32 mg/day), methysergid, antihistamines, and corticosteroids, digitalization and saluretic therapy are necessary in the case of patients with symptoms of a consecutive cardiac insufficiency. Methysergid has a certain intrinsic activity and can, thus, intensify endocardial fibrosis (470).

A valve replacement or pulmonary commissurotomy may be necessary, in rare cases, where right ventricular insufficiencies cannot be conservatively controlled (471).

Endocardial involvement in the case of rheumatoid arthritis

When the course of rheumatoid arthritis is florid, cardiac involvement can be determined in 10%-15% of cases at autopsy, whereas it is only clinically diagnosed in 1%-6% of patients (472). The rheumatoid granuloma consist of a central, fibrinoid necrosis and a wall of histiocytes, which is surrounded by the connective tissue (473).

The most frequent cardiac involvement is acute fibrinous pericarditis; less frequently, there is myocarditis with lymphocyte infiltrates, a coronaritis, an aortitis, or an endocardial involvement, in the case of which, the rheumatic granuloma can permeate the valvular endocardium and the parietal endocardium in the vicinity of the valves (474-476).

Typically, the central portions of the valves and the annuli are particularly affected. Only rarely does a hemodynamically significant valvular insufficiency result, usually when numerous granuloma become confluent and destroy the valve base, as well as the cusp and/or pockets. In individual cases, as a result of the rapid progression of this process, acute valvular insufficiencies can occur (477). As is the case with rheumatic fever, the mitral valve is far more frequently affected than the aortic valve. Apart from granulomatous endocardial infiltrations, non-specific, fibrotic and sclerosing endocardial changes are also observed (478). The clinical course and the prognosis of a rheumatoid arthritis are, except for the few cases of an acutely developing valvular insufficiency, not determined by the cardiac involvement.

Endocardial involvement in the case of ankylosing spondylitis

The percentage of patients with ankylosing spondylitis (Bechterew's disease) who exhibit a cardiovascular manifestation, is rising, with increasing duration of the disease, by approximately 0.3% per year of illness. In the case of ankylosing spondylitis, part of the endocardium of the left ventricular outflow tract, the aortic valves and the endothelium of the sinus Valsalva are affected in terms of a local inflammation and focal degeneration of the elastic and muscular fibers of the aortic media. Occasionally, the process can continue on the basis of the anterior mitral cusp and the membraneous ventricular septum.

The pathologic result is a dilation of the sinus Valsalva and the aortic anulus. Thickening of the connective tissue and loss of the coaptation of the aortic semilunar valves, resulting in an aortic or mitral insufficiency, are very rare. If the membraneous ventricular septum is also affected, the atrioventricular bundle or proximal portions of the three fascicles can be damaged.

Endocardial involvement in the case of sclerodermita

There can be endocardial involvement in rare cases following a sclerodermitis. The degenerative changes in the mitral and aortic endocardium then observed are slight. Hemodynamically significant valvular defects only occur in exceptional cases. The primary cardiac manifestation of sclerodermitis is that on the small coronary arteries, with consecutive ischemia, maculate cicatrisation and fibrosation, so that, following renal insufficiency as the second most frequent limiting organic manifestation, a myocardial pump failure develops.

Endocardial involvement in the case of Takayashu aortitis

In the case of the aortic arch syndrome (usually Type III), the degenerative infiltrative process of as yet unclarified etiology can also spread to the endocardium of the aortic valves and lead to an aortic insufficiency.

Endocarditis following radiation

In three quarters of the patients with radiation, in which the heart lies in the irradiation field and more than 3500 rad (35 Gy) are applied, an endomyocardial fibrosis, predominantly of the right ventricle, can be determined at autopsy. Apart from the endocardial fibrosis, papillary muscle dysfunctions, which can lead consecutively to a mitral and/or tricuspid valve insufficiency, have also been described. Aortic valve insufficiencies develop as a result of thickened semilunar valves (478-480). The clinical picture of endocarditis following radiation usually corresponds to a restrictive cardiomyopathy (482-484). If a cardiac murmur develops following radiation, frequent controls over a period of 12 months are required in order to evaluate progress (485).

References

1. Bouillaud JP. Quoted from: Flint A. Diseases of the Heart. VIII. Inflammatory affections of the heart. Endocarditis, myocarditis. Blanchara and Lea, Philadelphia 1859
2. Osler W. The Gulstonian Lectures on malignant endocarditis. Br Med J 1885;1:467-470,522-526,577-579
3. Schottmuller H. Endocarditis lenta. Munch Med Wschr 1910;57:617-619
4. Virchow, Winge, Hiberg. Quoted from Major RH. Notes on the history of endocarditis. Bull Hist Med 1945;17:351-359
5. Dawson MH, Hobby GL, Meyer K, Chaffee E. Penicillin as a chemotherapeutic agent. J Clin Invest 1941;20:434-436
6. Durack DT. Review of early experience in treatment of bacterial endocarditis, 1940-1955. In: Bisno AL (ed). Treatment of infective endocarditis, Grune & Stratton, New York 1981;1-14
7. Hunter TH. Speculations on the mechanism of cure of bacterial endocarditis. JAMA 1950;144:542-544
8. Kane LW, Finn JJ. The treatment of subacute bacterial endocarditis with aureomycin and chloromycetin. New Engl J Med 1951;244:623-626
9. Kerr A. Subacute bacterial endocarditis. Pullen FL (ed.) American lecture series, monograph of bannerstone division of American lectures in internal medicine. Charles C Thomas, Springfield 1955;274:343
10. Dillon JC, Feigenbaum H, Konecke LL, Davis RH, Chang S. Echocardiographic manifestations of valvular vegetations. Am Heart J 1973;86:698-704
11. Spangler RD, Johnson ML, Holmes JH, Blount SG. Echocardiographic demonstrations of bacterial vegetations in active infective endocarditis. J Clin Ultrasound 1973;1:126-128
12. Kay JD, Bernstein S, Feinstein D, Biddle M. Surgical cure of candida albicans endocarditis with open-heart surgery. N Engl J Med 1961;264:907-910
13. Wallace AG, Young WG, Osterhout S. Treatment of acute bacterial endocarditis by valve excision and replacement. Circulation 1965;31:450-453
14. Robicsek F, Payne RB, Daughtery HK, Sanger PWW. Bacterial endocarditis of the mitral valve treated by excision and replacement. Coll Works Cardiopulm Dis 1967;13:36-41
15. American Heart Association. Committee report on prevention of bacterial endocarditis. Circulation 1977;56:139-143
16. American Heart Association. Committee report on prevention of rheumatic fever and bacterial endocarditis through control of streptococcal infections. Circulation 1955;11:317-320
17. Thorgeirsson G, Robertson AL. The vascular endothelium - pathobiologic significance. A review. Am J Pathol 1978;93:803-848
18. Davis PF. Biology of disease. Vascular cell interaction with special reference to the pathogenesis of atherosclerosis. Lab Invest 1986;35:5-24
19. Delahaye F, Goulet V, Lacassin F, Ecochard R, Selton-Suty C, Hoen B, Briancon S, Etienne J, Leport C. Incidence, caracteristiques demographiques, cliniques, microbiologiques, et evolutives de l'endocardite infectieuse en France en 1990-1991. Med Mal Infect 1992;22:975-986
20. Horstkotte D. Microbiell Verursachte Endocarditis. Steinkopff, Darmstadt 1995
21. Horstkotte D, Bircks W, Loogen F. Infective endocarditis of native and prosthetic valves - the case for prompt surgical intervention? Z Kardiol 1986;75(Suppl II):168-192
22. McKinsey DS, Rutts TE, Bisno AL. Underlying cardiac lesions in adults with infective endocarditis. The changing spectrum. Am J Med 1987;82:681-687
23. Scheld M, Valine JA, Sande M. Bacterial adherence in the pathogenesis of endocarditis. J Clin Invest 1978;61:1304-1404
24. Absolom DR. The role of bacterial hydrophobicity in infection: bacterial adhesion and phagocytic

ingestion. Can J Microbiol 1988;34:287-298

25. Yamada KM, Ahimyama SH, Hasegawa E, Humphries MJ, Kennedy DW, Nagata K, Urushihara H, Olden K, Chen WT. Recent advances in research on fibrin and other cell attachment proteins. J Cell Biochem 1985;28:79-97
26. Brown EJ. The role of extracellular matrix proteins in the control of phagocytosis. J Leukocyte Biol 1986;39:579-591
27. Kreuzpaintner G, Horstkotte D, Losse B, Strohmeyer G. Increased risk of bacterial endocarditis in neoplastic and chronic inflammatory lesions of the gastrointestinal tract. Horstkotte D, Bodnar E (eds) Infective Endocarditis, ICR Publishers 1991;171-197
28. Ruoff KL, Miller SI, Garner CV, Ferraro MJ, Calderwood SB. Bacteremia with streptococcus bovis and streptococcus salivarius: clinical correlates of more accurate identification of isolates. J Clin Microbiol 1989;27:305-384
29. Finley JC, Davidson M, Parkinson AJ, Sullivan RW. Pneumococcal endocarditis in Alaska natives. A population based experience, 1978 through 1990. Arch Intern Med 1992;152:1641-1645
30. Schleifer KH, Klipper-Balz R. Transfer of streptococcus faecalis and streptococcus faecium to the genus enterococcus nom. rev. as enterococcus faecalis comb. nov. and enterococcus faecium comb. nov. Inst J Syst Bacteriol 1984;34:31-34
31. Facklam RR, Wahington II JA. Streptococcus and related catalase-negative gram-positive cocci. Balows A (ed): Manual of Clinical Microbiology, 5th edition. Am Soc for Microbiol, Washington 1991;238-257
32. Facklam RR, Collins MD. Identification of enterococcus species isolated from human infections by a conventional test scheme. J Clin Microbiol 1989;27:731-734
33. Straube E. Mikrobiologie und Antibiotikatherapie der Enterokokken-Endokarditis. Horstkotte D (ed) Bakterielle Endokarditis. SMV, Grafelfing 1992;130-141
34. Rouslathi E. Fibonectin and its receptors. Ann Rev Biochem 1988;57:357-413
35. Galli D, Lottspeich F, Wirth R. Sequence analysis of enterococcus faecalis aggregation substance encoded by the sex pheromone plasmid pADI. Molecular microbiol 1990;4:895-904
36. Guzmann CA, Pruzzo C, Lipira G, Calegari L. Role of adherence in pathogenesis of enterococcus faecalis urinary tract infection and endocarditis. Infection and immunity 1989;57:1834-1838
37. Lambert PA, Schorrock PJ, Aitchison EJ, Domingue PAG, Power ME, Costerton JW. Effect of in vitro growth conditions upon expression of surface protein antigens in enterococcus faecalis. FEMS microbiol immunol 1990;64:51-54
38. Ike Y, Hashimoto H, Clewell DB. Hemolysin of streptococcus faecalis subspecies zymogenes contributes to virulence in mice. Infection and immunity 1984;45:528-530
39. Burnie JP, Clark I. Diagnosing endocarditis with the cloned 112 kDa antigen of enterococcus faecalis. J Immunologic methods 1989;123:217-225
40. Centers for disease control: Nosocomial infections surveillance. Morbidity and mortality weekly report 1984-1986;35:1755-2255
41. Gross PA, Harkavy LM, Barden GE, Flower MF. The epidemiology of nosocomial enterococcal urinary tract infection. Am J Med Sci 1976;272:75-84
42. Hoge CW, Adams J, Buchanan B, Sears SD. Enterococcal bacterimia: To treat or not to treat, a reappraisal. Rev Infect Dis 1991;13:600-605
43. Wiemer M, Horstkotte D, Thomas L, Hadding U, Strauer BE. Bieten arteriell entnommene Blutkulturen Vorteile gegenüber Kulturen aus venösem Blut? Intensivmed 1993;30:225
44. Lewis CM, Zervos MJ. Clinical manifestations of enterococcae infection. Eur J Clin Microbiol infect Dis 1990;9:111-117
45. Glockmann E, Gunther E. Untersuchungen zur Beteiligung von Streptokokken an der Infektion des Wurzelkanals. Z gesamte Hygiene K 1988;34:594-595
46. Wheat J, Kohler RB, White A, Garten M, Wilkinson BJ. IgM and IgG antibody response to teichoic acid in infections due to staphylococcus aureus. J Infect Dis 1983;147:1101
47. Chambers HF, Korzeniowski OM, Sande MH. The National Collaborative Endocarditis Study Group. Staphylococcus aureus endocarditis: Clinical manifestations in addicts and non addicts. Medicine, Baltimore 1983;62:170-177
48. Lipsky BA, Goldberger AC, Tompkins LS, Plorde JJ. Infections caused by nondiphtheria corynebacteria. Rev Infect Dis 1982;4:1220-1235
49. Murray BE, Karchmer AW, Moellering RC. Diphtheroid prosthetic valve endocarditis. A study of clinical features and infecting organisms. Am J Med 1980;69:838-848
50. Van Scoy RE, Cohen SN, Geraci JE, Washington II JA. Coryneform bacterial endocarditis. Difficulties in diagnosis and treatment, presentation of three cases and review of literature. Mayo Clin Proc 1977;52:216-219
51. Meier B, Fischer E, Luthy R, Von Graevenitz A, Siegenthaler W. Endokarditis durch lactobacillus casei nach Aortenklappenersatz. Schweiz med Wschr 1981;111:601-603

52. Freland C. Les infections a erysipelothrix rhusiopathiae. Revue generale a propos de 31 cas de septicemies avec endocardite releves dans la litterature. Pathol Biol 1977;25:345-352
53. Leonard A, Raij L, Shapiro FL. Bacterial endocarditis in regularly dialyzed patients. Kidney Int 1973;4:407-422
54. Nieman RE, Lorber B. Listeriosis in adults: a changing pattern. Report of eight cases and review of the literature, 1968-1978. Rev infect Dis 1980;2:207-227
55. Lowry PW, Tompkins LS. Nosocomial legionellosis: a review of pulmonary and extrapulmonary syndroms. Am J Infect Control 1993;21:21-27
56. Vlachakin ND, Gazes PC, Hairston P. Nocardial endocarditis following mitral valve replacement. Chest 1975;63:276-279
57. Steen MK, Bruno-Murtha LA, Chaux G, Lazar H, Bernard S, Sulius C. Bacillus cereus endocarditis: report of a case and review. Clin Infect Dis 1992;14:945-946
58. Von Graevenitz A. Mikrobiologie der Endokarditis. Maisch B (Hrsg) Infektiöse Endokarditis. Perimed, Erlangen 1987;18-31
59. Cohen PS, Maguire JH, Weinstein L. Infective endocarditis caused by gram-negative bacteria: a review of the literature, 1945-1977. Prog cardiovasc Dis 1980;12:205-242
60. Ellner JJ, Rosenthal MS, Lerner PI, McHenry MC. Infective endocarditis caused by slow-growing, fastidious gram-negative bacteria. Medicine 1979;58:145-158
61. Carruthers MM. Endocarditis due to enteric bacilli other than Salmonellae: case reports and literature review. Am J Med Sci 1977;273:203-211
62. Schneider PJ, Nernoff III J, Gold JA. Acute Salmonella endocarditis. Archs Intern Med 1967;120:478-482
63. Hufnagel B, Saul F, Rosin H, Polonius MJ, Losse B. Mitralklappenendokarditis durch Salmonella enteritides. Z Kardiol 1993;82:654-657
64. Buff DD, Patel AD, Neches RB. Salmonella cholerasuis bacteremia and endocarditis in a patient with acquired immunodeficiency syndrome. NY State J Med 1993;93:147-149
65. Cooper R, Mills J. Serratia endocarditis. A follow up report. Archs Intern Med 1980;140:199-202
66. Von Graevenitz A. Endocarditis due to serratia marcescens. Von Graevenitz A, Rubin SJ (eds) The Genus Serratia, CRC Press, Boca Raton. 1980;170-172
67. Jerondi MO, Halim MA, Harder EJ. Brucella endocarditis. Brit Heart 1987;58:279-285
68. Reyes MP, Lerner AM. Current problems in the treatment of infective endocarditis due to pseudomonas aeruginosa. Rev infect Dis 1983;5:314-320
69. Felten-Papaiconomou A, Ruf C, Baudouy YP, Riou JY, Perol Y. Endocardite a gonocoque avec rupture d'aneurysme cerebral. Med Mal Infect 1982;13:189-193
70. Weetman AP, Matthews N, O'Hara SP, Amos N, Williams BD, Thomas JP. Menigococcal endocarditis with profound acquired hypocomplementemia. J Infect 1985;10:51-56
71. Wallace RJ, Swenson JM, Silcox VA, Good RC, Tschen JA, Stone MS. Spectrum of disease due to rapidly growing mycobacteria. Rev Infect Dis 1983;5:657-679
72. Tobin MJ, Cahill N, Gearty G, Maurer B, Blake S, Daly K, Hone R. Q-fever endocarditis. Am J Med 1982;72:396-400
73. Brouqui P, Dupont HT, Drancourt M, Berland Y, Etienne J. Chronic Q-fever. 92 cases from France, including 27 cases without endocarditis. Arch Intern Med 1993;153:642-648
74. Yeaman MR, Roman MJ, Baca OG. Antibiotic susceptibilities of two Coxiella burnetii isolates implicated in distinct clinical syndromes. Antimicrob Agents Chemother 1989;33:1052-1057
75. Jones RB, Priest JB, Kuo C. Subacute chlamydial endocarditis. J Am Med Ass 1982;247:655-658
76. Wilson WR. Treatment of infections caused by anaerobes. J Chemother 1991;3(Suppl II):7-11
77. Drutz D. The spectrum of fungal endocarditis. Calif Med 1971;115:34-40
78. Reisberg BE. Infective endocarditis in the narcotic addict. Prog Cardiovasc Dis 1979;22:193-204
79. Rubinstein E, Noriega ER, Simberkoff MS, Holzmann R, Rahal JJ. Fungal endocarditis: analysis of 24 cases and review of the literature. Medicine 1975;54:331-344
80. Kammer RB, Utz JP. Aspergillus species endocarditis. The new face of a not so rare disease. Am J Med 1974;56:506-521
81. Rinaldi MG. Invasive aspergillosis. Rev Infect Dis 1983;5:1061-1077
82. De Repentigny L, Reiss E. Current trends in immunodiagnosis of candidiasis and aspergillosis. Rev Infect Dis 1984;6:301-312
83. Rodbard S. Blood velocity and endocarditis. Circulation 1963;27:18-21
84. Lepeschkin E. On the relation between the site of valvular involvment in endocarditis and the blood pressure resting on the valve. Am J Med Sci 1952;224:318-322
85. Allen AC. Mechanism of localization of vegetations of bacterial endocarditis. Arch Pathol 1989;27:399-402
86. Durack DT, Beeson PB. Pathogenesis of infective endocarditis. Rahimtoola SH (ed) infective endocarditis. Grune & Stratton. New York, San Francisco, London 1978;1-28
87. Freedman LR, Valone J. Experimental infective endocarditis. Prog Cardiovasc Dis 1979;22:169-180

88. Niebel J. Infective endocarditis in immune-compromised patients. Horstkotte D, Bodnar E (eds) Infective Endocarditis. ICR Publishers, London 1991;154-162
89. Maisch B. Autoreactive mechanisms in infective endocarditis. Springer Semin Immunopathol 1989;11:439-456
90. De Castro S, Miglian G, Silvestri A, D'Amati G, Giannantoni P. Heart involvment in AIDS: a prospective study during various stages of the disease. Eur Heart J 1992;13:1452-1439
91. Sullam PM, Frank U, Yeaman MR, Tauber MG, Bayer AS, Chambers HF. Effect of thrombocytopenin on the early cause of streptococcal endocarditis. J Infect Dis 1993;168:910-914
92. Ford I, Douglas CW, Preston FE, Lowless A, Hampton KK. Mechanisms of platelet aggregation by streptococcus sanguis, a causative organisms in infective endocarditis. Br J Haematol 1993;84:95-100
93. Rosen P, Armstrong D. Infective endocarditis in patients treated for malignant neoplastic diseases. A postmortem study. Am J Clin Pathol 1973;59:241-246
94. Bulkley BH, Roberts WC. The heart in systemic lupus erythematosus and the changes induced in it by corticosteroid therapy. Am J Med 1979;58:243-248
95. Johnson CM. Staphyolococcus aureus binding to cardiac endothelial cells is partly mediated by a 130 kilodalton glycoprotein. J Lab Clin Med 1993;121:675-682
96. Lee JC, Takeda S, Livolsi PJ, Paoletti LC. Effects of in vitro and in vivo growth conditions on expression of type eight capsular polysaccharid by staphylococcus aureus. Infect Immun 1993;61:1853-1858
97. Tart RC, Van de Rijn I. Analysis of adherence of streptococcus defectivus and endocarditis-associated streptococci to extracellular matrix. Infect Immun 1991;59:857-862
98. Vercellott TGM, Lussenkop D, Peterson PK, Furcht LT, McCarthy JB, Jacob HS, Moldow CF. Bacterial adherence to fibrinonectin and endothelial cells: a possible mechanism for bacterial tissue tropism. J Lab Clin Med 1984;103:34-43
99. Maisch B, Eichstadt H, Kochsiek K. Immune reactions in infective endocarditis, part I: Clinical data and diagnosis relevance of antimyocardial antibodies. Am Heart J 1983;106:329-337
100. Nagai T, Tamura T, Kawai C. Clinical significance of titered circulating microbial antibody in bacteremia. Am J Clin Path 1982;77:430-435
101. Phair JP, Clarke J. Immunologie de l'endocardite infectieuse. Acquis Nouv Pathol Cardio-vasc 1980;22:267-284
102. Scheld WM, Calderone RA, Brodeur JP, Sande MA. Influence of preformed antibody on the pathogenesis of experimental candida albicans endocarditis. Infect Immmun 1983;40:950-955
103. Godeau P, Leport C, Rosenthal P. Traitement medical des endocardites infectieuses. Sem Hop Paris 1982;58:2291-2295
104. Burton-Kee J, Morgan-Capner P, Mowbray JF. Nature of circulating immune complexes in infective endocarditis. J Clin Path 1980;33:653-659
105. Carson DA, Bayer AS, Eisenberg RA, Lawrance S, Theofilopoulos A. IgG rheumatoid factor in subacute bacterial endocarditis - relationship to IgM rheumatoid factor and circulating immune complexes. Clin exp Immunol 1978;100-103
106. Neugarten J, Baldwin DS. Glomerulonephritis in bacterial endocarditis. Am J Med 1984;77:297-304
107. Nonnast-Daniel B, Ehrich JH, Eisenbach GM, Daniel WG, Kuehn DW, Lichtlen PR, Koch KM. Is renal involvement a prognostic parameter in patients with infective endocarditis? Eur Heart J 1984;5(Suppl C):93-96
108. Petersdorf RG. Immune complexes in infective endocarditis. New Engl J Med 1976;295:1534-1535
109. Schned ES, Inman RD, Parris TM, Kimberly RP, Redecha PB, Christian CL. Serial circulating immune complexes and mononuclear phagocyte system function in infective endocarditis. J Lab Clin Med 1983;102:947-959
110. Cooper G. Staphylococcus aureus bacteremia in diabetic patients. Endocarditis and mortality. Am J Med 1982;3:658-662
111. Cross AS, Steigbigel RT. Infective endocarditis and access site infections in patients on hemodialysis. Medicine 1976;55:453-466
112. Hubbel G, Cheitlin MD, Rapaport E. Presentation, management and follow up evaluation of infective endocarditis in drug addicts. Am Heart J 1981;102:85-94
113. Horstkotte D, Strauer BE. Intensivmedizinische Probleme in Diagnostik und Therapie der infektiösen Endokarditis. Intensiv Notfallmed 1992;17:6-17
114. Everett ED, Hirschmann JV. Transient bacteremia and endocarditis prophylaxis. A review. Medicine (Baltimore) 1977;56:61-77
115. Sipes JN, Thompson RL, Hook EW. Prophylaxis of infective endocarditis. A re-evaluation. Ann Rev Med 1977;28:371-391
116. Rechmann P, Seewald M, Thomas L, Horstkotte D. Untersuchungen zur Bakteriämie bei zahnärztlichen Eingriffen. Dtsch Zahnarzt Z 1986;41:996-999
117. Chirillo F, Cavarzerani A, Totis O, Bruni A, Giommi L, Marton F, Cuzzato V. Aortic endocarditis after

percutaneous balloon valvuloplasty. The role of transesophagal echocardiography in early detection and follow up. Am Heart J 1992;124:223-225

118. Kulkarni SM, Loya YS, Sharma S. Infective endocarditis following balloon dilation of mitral valve. Int J Cardiol 1992;34:103-105

119. Mermel LA, McCormick RD, Springman SR, Maki DG. The pathogenesis and epidemiology of catheter-related infection with pulmonary artery Swan-Ganz catheters. A prospective study utilizing molecular subtyping. Am J Med 1991;(Suppl 3B):5197-5205

120. Lopez JA, Ross RS, Fishbein MC, Siegel RJ. Non-bacterial thrombotic endocarditis. A review. Am Heart J 1987;113:773-784

121. Weinstein L, Schlesinger JJ. Pathoanatomic, pathophysiologic and clinical correlations in endocarditis. N Engl J Med 1974;291:1122-1126

122. Graves MK, Soto L. Left sided endocarditis in parenteral drug abusers: recent experience at a large community hospital. South Med J 1992;85:378-380

123. Varma MPS, McCluskey DR, Kahn MM, Cleland J, O'Kane HO, Adgey AA. Heart failure associated with infective endocarditis. A review of 40 cases. Br Heart J 1986;55:191-197

124. Bahl VK, Vasan RS, Jain P, Shrivastava S. Spectrum of right-sided infective endocarditis. An Indian experience. Int J Cardiol 1992;35:187-193

125. Calleja F, Eguaras MG, Chacon A, Vivancos R, Montero A, Concha M. Pulmonary valve endocarditis during puerperal sepsis. J Cardiovasc Surg (Torino) 1992;33:292-294

126. Grover A, Anand IS, Varma J, Choudhury R, Khattri HN, Sopru RP, Bidwai PS, Wahi PC. Profile of right-sided endocarditis. An Indian experience. Int J Cardiol 1991;33:83-88

127. Hecht SR, Berger M. Right-sided endocarditis in intravenous drug users. Prognostic features in 102 episodes. Ann Intern Med 1992;117:560-566

128. Roberts WC, Kishel JC, McIntosh CL, Cannon RO, Maron BJ. Severe mitral and aortic valve regurgitation, or both, requiring valve replacement for infective endocarditis complicating hypertrophic cardiomyopathy. J Am Coll Cardiol 1992;19:365-371

129. Horstkotte D, Paselk CH, Bircks W, Loogen F. Klinische Langzeitergebnisse nach Korrekturoperation einer Fallotschen Tetralogie. Z Kardiol 1993;82:552-562

130. Mills J, Utlay J, Abbott J. Heart failure in infective endocarditis: predisposing factors, course and treatment. Chest 1974;66:151-159

131. Pankey GA. Subacute bacterial endocarditis at the University of Minnesota Hospital 1939-1959. Ann Intern Med 1961;55:550-558

132. Kim HS, Weilbacher DG, Lie JT, Titus JL. Myocardial abscesses. Am J Clin Pathol 1978;70:18-21

133. Kan MN, Chen YT, Lee AYS. Comparison of transesophageal to transthoracic color Doppler echocardiography in the identification of intracardiac mycotic aneurysms in infective endocarditis. Echocardiography 1991;8:643-648

134. Jones HR, Seikert RG, Geraci JE. Neurologic manifestation of bacterial endocarditis. Ann Intern Med 1969;71:21-28

135. Kitts D, Bongard FS, Klein SR. Septic embolism complicating infective endocarditis. J Vasc Surg 1991;14:480-487

136. Ninet J, Gayet I, Etienne J, Bonvoisin B, Vignon E, Barthou JD, Delahaye JP, Pasquier J, Delaye J, Normand J. Bacterial endocarditis presenting as acute vertebral osteomyelitis: 14 cases. Eur Heart J 1984;5(Suppl C):101-105

137. Salgado AV. Central nervous system complications of infective endocarditis. Stroke 1991;22:1461-1462

138. Elliott JP, Smith RF. Peripheral embolization. Magilligan DJ, Quinn EL (eds) Endocarditis. Medical and Surgical Management. M Dekker, New York and Basle 1986;165-176

139. Glassock RJ, Cohen AG. Secondary glomerular disease. Brenner BM, Rector FC (eds) The Kidney. Saunders, Philadelphia-London-Toronto 1981;1536-1537

140. Löhlein M. Über hämorrhagische Nierenaffektionen bei chronischer ulceroser Endokarditis (embolische nicht eitrige Herdnephritis). Med Klin 1910;6:375-377

141. Heptinstall R. Focal glomerulonephritis. Pathology of the Kidney. Little Brown, Boston 1974;438-446

142. Morel-Maroger LJD, Herreman G, Godeau P. Kidney in subaccute endocarditis: pathological and immunofluorescence findings. Arch Pathol 1972;94:205-213

143. Neugarten J, Gallo GR, Baldwin DS. Glomerulonephritis in bacterial endocarditis. Am J Kidney Dis 1984;3:371-379

144. Pelletier LL, Petersdorf RG. Infective endocarditis: a review of 125 cases from the University of Washington Hospitals, 1963-1972. Medicine (Baltimore) 1977;56:287-313

145. Gutman RA, Striker GE, Gillifond BC, Cutler RE. The immune complex glomerulonephritis of bacterial endocarditis. Medicine 1978;51:1-6

146. Bennett WM, Muther RS, Parker RA, Feig P, Morrison G, Golper TA, Singer I. Drug therapy in renal failure: dosing guidelines for adults. Part I. Antimicrobial Agents, analgesics. Ann Intern Med

1980;93(Part I):62-89

147. Cobbs CG, Livingston WK. Special problems in the management of infective endocarditis. Bisno AL (ed) Treatment of infective endocarditis. Grune & Stratton, New York-London-San Francisco 1981;147-166

148. Moore RD, Smith CR, Lipsky JJ, Mellits ED, Lietman PS. Risk factors for nephrotoxicity in patients treated with aminoglycosides. Ann Intern Med 1984;100:352-357

149. Pruitt AA, Rubin RH, Karchmer AW, Duncan GW. Neurologic complications of bacterial endocarditis. Medicine 1978;57:329-343

150. Roach MR, Drake CG. Ruptured cerebral aneurysms caused by microorganisms. N Engl J Med 1963;273:246

151. Ewart JM, Burke ML, Bunt TJ. Spontaneous abdominal aortic infections: essentials of diagnosis and management. Am Surg 1983;49:37-50

152. Johansen K, Devin J. Mycotic aortic aneurysms: a reappraisal. Arch Surg 1983;118:583-588

153. Cates JE, Christie RV. Subacute bacterial endocarditis. A review of 442 patients treated in 14 centres appointed by penicillin trials committee of the medical research council. Q J Med 1951;20:93-126

154. Horstkotte D. Mikrobiell verursachte Endokarditiden: Prognose und Nachsorge. Gahl K (ed) Infektiöse endokarditis. Steinkopff, Darmstadt 1994

155. Alpert JS, Krous HF, Dalen JE, O'Rourke RA, Bloor CM. Pathogenesis of Osler's nodes. Ann Intern Med 1976;85:471-473

156. Bani-Sadr F, Hamidon M, Richard P, Tiab M, Lalande S, Grollean JY. Vasculorite cutanee et insuffisance renale aigue revelant une endocardite a actinobacillus activomycetemcomitans. Presse Med 1993;22:446-448

157. Wedgewood J. Early diagnosis of subacute bacterial endocarditis. Lancet 1955;2:1058-1062

158. Weinstein L. Modern infective endocarditis. JAMA 1975;233:260-284

159. Howard EJ. Osler's nodes. Am Heart J 1960;59:633-635

160. Perronne C, Leport C, Vilde J. Complications due to septic embolism and immune-complex vasculitis. Horstkotte D, Bodnar E (eds) Infective Endocarditis. ICR, London, 1991;39-43

161. Cross PF, Ellis JG. Occurrence of the Janeway lesion in mycotic aneurysm. Arch Intern Med 1966;118:588-591

162. Kilpatrick ZM, Greenberg PA, Sanford JP. Splinter hemorrhages - their clinical significance. Arch Intern Med 1965;115:730-733

163. Platts MM, Greaves MS. Splinter hemorrhages. Br Med J 1958;2:143-144

164. Willerson JT, Moellering RC, Buckley MJ, Austen WG. Conjunctival petechiae after open-heart surgery. N Engl J Med 1971;284:539-540

165. Roth M. Über Netzhautaffektionen bei Wundfiebern. Dtsch Z Chir 1872;1:471-472

166. Litten M. Über akute maligne Endokarditis und die dabei vorkommende Retinalveränderungen. Charit Ann 1878;3:137-138

167. Doherty WB, Trubek M. Significant hemorrhagic retinal lesions in bacterial endocarditis (Roth's spots). JAMA 1931;97:308-310

168. Chulay JD, Lankerani MR. Splenic abscess. Report of 10 cases and reviews of the literature. Am J Med 1976;61:513-522

169. Chun CH, Raff MJ, Contreras L, Varghese R, Waterman N, Daffner R, Melco JC. Splenic abscess. Medicine 1980;59:50-65

170. Mammana RB, Levitsky S, Sermaque D, Beckmann CB, Silverman NA. Valve replacement for left sided endocarditis in drug addicts. Ann Thorac Surg 1983;35:436-441

171. Stinson EB, Griepp RB, Vosti K, Copeland JG, Shumway NE. Operative treatment of active endocarditis. J Thorac Cardiovasc Surg 1976;71:659-665

172. Boles JM, Michelet C, Garo B, Garre M, Cartier F. Neurologic complications of infective endocarditis. Horstkotte D, Bodnar E (eds) Infective Endocarditis. ICR, London 1991;34-38

173. Le Cam B, Guivarch G, Boles JM, Garre M, Cartier F. Neurologic complications in a group of 86 bacterial endocarditis. Eur Heart J 1984;5:97-100

174. Pruitt AM, Rubin RH, Darchmer AW, Duncan GW. Neurologic complications of bacterial endocarditis. Medicine 1978;57:329-343

175. Venezio FR, Westenfelder GO, Cook FV, Emmerman J, Phair JP. Infective endocarditis in a community hospital. Arch Intern Med 1982;789-792

176. Arendt G. Diagnostik und Therapie neurologischer Komplikationen der bakteriellen Endokarditis. Horstkotte D (ed) Bakterielle Endokarditis. SMV, Grafelfing, 1992;85-95

177. Wang K, Gobel F, Gleason DF, Edwards JE. Complete heart block complicating bacterial endocarditis. Circulation 1972;46:939-941

178. Cooke RA, Chambers JB. The role of echocardiography in the diagnosis and management of infective endocarditis. Br J Clin Pract 1992;46:111-115

179. Aguado JM, Gonzalez-Vilchez F, Martin-Duran R, Arjona R, Vazquez de Prada JA. Perivalvular abscesses

associated with endocarditis. Clinical features and diagnostic accuracy of two-dimensional echocardiography. Chest 1993;104(1):88-93

180. Ellis Sg, Goldstein J, Popp RL. Detection of endocarditis associated perivalvular abscess by two-dimensional echocardiography. J Am Coll Cardiol 1985;5:647-653

181. Neiman LF, Danchin N, Godenier JP, Villemot JP, Faivre G. Two-dimensional echocardiography recognition of aortic valve ring abscess. Eur Heart J 1984;5(Suppl C):59-65

182. Miyatake K, Yamamoto K, Park YD, Izumi S, Yamagishi M, Sakakibara H, Nimura. Diagnosis of mitral valve perforation by real time two-dimensional Doppler flow imaging techniques. J Am Coll Cardiol 1986;8:1235-1239

183. Reid CL, Chandraratna AN, Harrison E, Kawanishi DT, Chandrasoma P, Nimalasuriya A, Rahimtoola SH. Mitral valve aneurysm: clinical features, echocardiographic-pathologic correlations. J Am Coll Cardiol 1983;2:400-404

184. Ballal RS, Mahan EF, Nanda NC, Sanyal R. Aortic and mitral valve perforation: diagnosis by transesophageal echocardiography and color flow imaging. Am Heart J 1991;121:214-217

185. Bruss J, Jacobs LE, Kotler MN, Ioli AW. Utility of transesophageal echocardiography in the conservative management of prosthetic valve endocarditis. Chest 1992;102:1886-1888

186. Erbel R, Rohmann S, Drexler M, Mohr-Kahaly S, Gerharz CD, Iversen S, Oelert H. Improved diagnostic value of echocardiography in patients with infective endocarditis by transoesophageal approach. A prospective study. Eur Heart J 1988;9:43-48

187. Henderson RA, Palmer TJ. Echocardiographic diagnosis of infective endocarditis of all four cardiac valves. Int J Cardiol 1991;33:173-175

188. Karalis DG, Bansal RC, Hauck AJ, Ross JJ, Applegate PM, Jutzy DR, Mintz GS, Chandrasekaran K. Transesophageal echocardiographic recognition of subaortic complications in aortic valve endocarditis: clinical and surgical implications. Circulation 1992;86:353-362

189. Khandheria BK. Suspected bacterial endocarditis: to TEE or not to TEE. J Am Coll Cardiol 1993;21:222-224

190. Kronzon I, Tunick PA. Transesophageal echocardiography as a tool in the evaluation of patients with embolic disorders. Prog Cardiovasc Dis 1993;36:39-60

191. Murphy JG, Foster-Smith K. Management of complications of infective endocarditis with emphasis on echocardiographic findings. Infect Dis Clin North Am 1993;7:153-165

192. Rohmann S, Seifert T, Erbel R, Jakob H, Mohr-Kahaly S, Makowski T, Gorge G, Oelert H, Meyer J. Identification of abscess formation in native-valve infective endocarditis using transesophageal echocardiography - Implications for surgical treatment. Thorac Cardiovasc Surg 1991;39:273-280

193. Rohmann S, Erbel R, Gorge G, Makowski T, Mohr-Kahaly S, Nixdorff U, Drexler M, Meyer J. Clinical relevance of vegetation localization by transesophageal ecchocardiography in infective endocarditis. Eur Heart J 1992;12:446-452

194. Rohmann S, Erbel R, Darius H, Makowski T, Jensen P, Fischer T, Meyer J. Spontaneous echo contrast imaging in infective endocarditis: A predictor of complications? Int J Card Imaging 1992;8:197-208

195. Roudaut R, Barbeau P, Leherissier A, Durandet P, Gosse P, Dallocchio M. Diagnostic contribution of transesophageal echocardiography in infective endocarditis. Apropos of 101 cases. Arch Mal Coeur 1993;86:49-55

196. Sanfilippo AJ, Picard MH, Newell JB, Rosas E, Davidoff R, Thomas JD, Weyman AE. Echocardiographic assessment of patients with infective endocarditis: Prediction of risk for complications. J Am Coll Cardiol 1991;18:1191-1199

197. Shively BK, Gurule FT, Roldan CA, Legett JH, Schiller NB. Diagnostic value of transesophageal compared with transthoracic echocardiography in infective endocarditis. J Am Coll Cardiol 1991;18:391-397

198. Sochowski RA, Chan KL. Implication of negative results on a monoplane transesophageal echocardiographic study in patients with suspected infective endocarditis. J Am Coll Cardiol 1993;21:216-221

199. Taoms MA, Gussenhoven EJ, De Jaegere P, Roelandt JRTC, Sutherland GR, Bom N. Enhanced morphological diagnosis in infective endocarditis by transesophageal compared with transthoracic echocardiography in infective endocarditis. J Am Coll Cardiol 1990;18:391-397

200. Cerqueira MD. Detection of cardiovascular infections with radiolabelled leukocytes. J Nucl Med 1992;33:1493-1495

201. Melvin ET, Berger M, Lutzker LG, Goldberg E, Mildvan D. Non-invasive methods for detection of valve vegetations in infective endocarditis. Am J Cardiol 1981;47:271-272

202. Kroll J. Arterial blood culture. Danish med Bull 1965;1965:131-134

203. Washington JA. The role of the microbiological laboratory in the diagnosis and antimicrobial treatment of infective endocarditis. Mayo Clin Proc 1982;57:22-32

204. Gutuzzo E, Carillo C, Guerra J, Llosa L. An evaluation of diagnostic methods for brucellosis - the value of bone marrow culture. J Infect Dis 1986;153:122-125

205. Jones JM. Laboratory diagnosis of invasive candidiasis. Clin Microbiol Rev 1990;3:32-45

206. McKenzie R, Reimer LG. Effect of antimicrobials on blood cultures in endocarditis. Diagn Microbiol Infect Dis 1987;8:165-172
207. Washington JA. Blood cultures: An overview. Europ J Clin Microbiol Infect Dis 1989;8:803-806
208. Tarrand JJ, Guillot C, Wenglar M, Jackson J, Lajeunesse JD, Roston KV. Clinical comparison of the resin-containing BACTEC 26 Plus and the Isolator 10 blood culturing systems. J Clin Microbiol 1991;19:2245-2249
209. Barlow JF. Once is not enough. Rational use of the blood culture. S D J Med 1992;45:181
210. Pesanti E, Smith IM. Infective endocarditis with negative blood cultures. An analysis of 52 cases. Am J Med 1979;66:43-50
211. Walterspiel JN, Kaplan SL. Incidence and clinical characteristics of "culture-negative" infective endocarditis in a pediatric population. Pediatr Infect Dis 1986;5:328-332
212. Ruoff KL. Nutritionally variant streptococci. Clin Microbial Rev 1991;4:184-190
213. Gray IR. Rational approach to the treatment of culture-negative infective endocarditis. Drugs 1991;41:729-736
214. Von Graevenitz. Diagnostische und therapeutische Strategien bei kulturnegativer Endokarditis. Horstkotte D (Hrsg) Bakterielle Endokarditis. SMV, Gräfelfing 1992;35-45
215. Murray P. Determination of the optimum incubation period of blood culture broths for the detection of clinically significant septicemia. J Clin Microbiol 1985;21:481-485
216. Sapico FL, Sarma RJ. Infective endocarditis due to anaerobic and microaerophilic bacteria. West J Med 1982;137:18-23
217. Wilkins TD, West SEH. Medium-dependent inhibition of peptostreptococcus anaerobius by sodium polyanetholsufonate in blood culture media. J Clin Microbiol 1976;3:393-396
218. Jacobs F, Abramowicz D, Vereerstraeten P, Le Clerc JL, Zech F, Thys JP. Brucella endocarditis: the role of combined medical and surgical treatment. Rev Infect Dis 1990;12:740-744
219. Kolman S, Maayan MC, Gotesman G, Rozenszajn LA, Wolach B, Lang R. Comparison of the Bactec and lysis concentration methods for recovery of Brucella species from clinical specimens. Eur J Clin Microbiol Infect Dis 1991;10:647-648
220. Kasten MJ, Allerberger F, Anhalt JP. Campylobacter bacteremia: Clinical experience with three different blood culture systems at Mayo Clinic 1984-1990. Infection 1991;19:88-90
221. Wang WLL, Blaser MJ. Detection of pathogenic Campylobacter species in blood culture systems. J Clin Microbiol 1986;23:709-714
222. Jones RB, Priest JB, Kuo C. Subacute chlamydial endocarditis. JAMA 1982;247:655-658
223. Murray BE, Karchmer AW, Moellering RC. Diphtheroid prosthetic valve endocarditis. A study of clinical features and infecting organisms. Am J Med 1980;69:838-848
224. Tobin MJ, Cahill N, Gearty G, Maurer B, Blake S, Daly K, Hone R. Q fever endocarditis. Am J Med 1982;72:396-400
225. Rubinstein E, Noriega ER, Simberkoff MS, Holzman R, Rahal JJ. Fungal endocarditis. Analysis of 24 cases and review of the literature. Medicine 1975;54:331-344
226. Murray PR, Spizzo AW, Niles AC. Clinical comparison of the recoveries of bloodstream pathogens in septi-chek brain heart infusion both with saponin and the Isolator lysis-centrifugation system. J Clin Microbiol 1991;29:901-905
227. Telenti A, Roberts GD. Fungal blood cultures. Eur J Clin Microbiol Infect Dis 1989;8:825-831
228. Reimer LG, Reller LB. Gardnerella vaginalis bacteremia: a review of thirty cases. Obstet Gynecol 1984;64:170-172
229. Van Scoy RE. Culture-negative endocarditis. Mayo Clin Proc 1982;57:149-154
230. Ah Fat LNC, Patel BR, Pickens S. Actinobacillus actinomycetemcomitans endocarditis in hypertrophic obstructive cardiomyopathy. J Infect Dis 1983;6:81-88
231. Ellner JJ, Rosenthal MS, Lerner PL, McHenry MC. Infective endocarditis caused by slow-growing, fastidious, gram-negative bacteria. Medicine 1979;58:145-158
232. Tompkins LS, Roessler BJ, Redd SC, Markowitz LE, Cohen ML. Legionella prosthetic-valve endocarditis. New Engl J Med 1988;318:530-534
233. Griffith DE, Girard VM, Wallace RJ. Clinical features of pulmonary disease caused by rapidly growing mycobacteria. An analysis of 154 patients. Am Rev Respir Dis 1993;147:1271-1278
234. Kiehn TE, Cammarata R. Laboratory diagnosis of mycobacterial infections in patients with accquired immunodeficiency syndrome. J Clin Microbiol 1986;24:708-711
235. Cohen JI, Sloss SJH, Kundsin R, Golightly L. Prosthetic valve endocarditis caused by Mycoplasma hominis. Am J Med 1989;86:819-821
236. Davies S, Eggington R. Recovery of Mycoplasma hominis from blood culture media. Med Lab Sci 1991;48:110-113
237. Potts DW. Poor yield of Neisseria gonorrhoeae from blood culture. Arch Intern Med 1981;141:546-547
238. Scribner RK, Welch DF. Neutralization of the inhibitory effect of sodium polyanetholesufonate on

neisseria meningitidis in blood cultures processed with the Du Pont Isolator System. J Clin Microbiol 1984;20:40-42

239. Heiddal S, Sverrisson JT, Yngvason FE, Cariglia N, Kristinsson KG. Native-valve endocarditis due to neisseria sicca: case report and review. Clin Infect Dis 1993;16:667-670

240. Ayral X, Piette AM, Roullet-Audy JC, Gepner P, Baillet A, Baglin AC, Chapman A. Endocardite a nocardia asteroides sur bioprothese aortique compliquee d'aneurismes mycotiques hepatiques. Ann Med Interne 1989;140:652-654

241. Roberts GD, Brewer NS, Hermans PE. Diagnosis of nocardiosis by blood culture. Mayo Clin Proc 1974;49:293-296

242. Simon MW, Wilson HD. Streptobacillus moniliformis endocarditis. Clin Pediatr 1986;25:110-111

243. Stein DS, Nelson KE. Endocarditis due to nutritionally deficient streptococci: therapeutic dilemma. Rev Infect Dis 1987;9:908-916

244. Weinstein L. Infective endocarditis. Braunwald E (ed) Heart Disease. Saunders, Philadelphia 1984;1136

245. Bain RC, Edwards JE, Scheiffey CH, Geraci JE. Right-sided bacterial endocarditis and endarteritis: Clinical and pathologic study. Amer J Med 1958;24:98-104

246. King ME, Weyman AE. Echocardiographic findings in infective endocarditis. Cardiovasc Clin 1983;13:147-165

247. Pollack SJ, Felner JM. Echocardiographic identification of an aortic valve ring abscess. JACC 1986;7:1167-1168

248. Cormier B, Vitoux B, Starkman C, Enriquez-Sarano M, Kulas A, Dewilde J, Grimberg D, Acar J. Value of transesophageal echocardiography. From a preliminary experience of 532 cases. Arch Mal Coeur 1990;83:23-29

249. Hwang JJ, Shyu KG, Chen JJ, Tseng YZ, Kuan P, Lien WP. Usefulness of transesophageal echocardiography in the treatment of critically ill patients. Chest 1993;104:861-866

250. Mügge A, Daniel WG, Frank G, Lichtlen PR. Echocardiography in infective endocarditis: reassessment of prognostic implications of vegetations' size determined by the transthoracic and the transeophageal approach. JACC 1989;14:631-638

251. Gorge G, Erbel R, Heinrichs KJ, Wenchel HM, Wemer HP, Meyer J. Positive blood cultures during transesophageal echocardiography. Am J Cardiol 1990;65:1404-1406

252. Melendez LJ, Chan KL, Cheung PK, Sochowski RA, Wong S, Austin TW. Incidence of bacteriemia in transesophageal echocardiography: A prospective study of 140 consecutive patients. JACC 1991;18:1650-1654

253. Steckelberg JM, Khandheria BK, Anhalt JP, Ballard DJ, Seward JB, Click RL, Wilson WR. Prospective evaluation of the risk of bacteriemia associated with transesophageal echocardiography. Circulation 1991;84:177-180

254. Völler H, Spielberg DH, Schröder K, Gast D, Schröder R. Frequency of positive blood cultures during transesophageal echocardiography. Am J Cardiol 1991;68:1538-1540

255. Bahar RH, Mohammed MM, Dyen HA. Detection of infection of cardiac xenograft by gallium-67-scan. Int J Cardiol 1986;13:88-92

256. Cerqueira MD, Jacobson AF. Indium-111 leukocyte scintigraphic detection of myocardial abscess formation in patients with endocarditis. J Nucl Med 1989;30:703-706

257. Piper C, Horstkotte D, Arendt G, Schulte HD, Strauer BE. Akute zerebrale Embolien bei florider Endokarditis: Indikation, nicht Kontraindikation zum dringlichen klappenchrirugischen Eingriff. Intensivmed 1993;30:267

258. Lewin RF, Sidi Y, Hermoni Y, Zafir N, Dean H, Glazer Y, Pinkhas J, Agmon J. Serial two-dimensional echocardiography in infective endocarditis of the pulmonary valve. Isr J Med Sci 1983;19:53-57

259. Tak T, Rahimtoola SH, Gumage N, Kumar A, Chandraratna PAN. Streptococcus viridans endocarditis: favorable prognosis in geriatric patients. Prognosis depends on correct identification of the organism and appropriate antibiotic therapy. Geriatrics 1988;28:68-73

260. Niehues R, Piper C, Kramer H, Horstkotte D. Einflusse der Grösse von Vegetationen auf die Inzidenz konsekutiver thromboembolischer Komplikationen bei Patienten mit akuter infektiöser Endokarditis. Intensivmed 1993;30:268-269

261. Roudaut R, Barbeau P, Leherissier A, Durandet P, Gosse P, Dallocchio M. Diagnostic contribution of transesophageal echocardiography in infective endocarditis. Apropos of 101 cases. Arch Mal Coeur 1993;86:49-55

262. Horstkotte D, Schulte HD, Bircks W. Factors influencing prognosis and indication for surgical intervention in acute native valve endocarditis. Horstkotte D, Bodnar E (eds) Infective Endocarditis. ICR Publishers, London, 1991;171-197

263. Horstkotte D, Rosin H. Therapie und Prophylaxe der infektiösen Endokarditis. Schweiz Med Wschr 1984;114:1575-1581

264. Ting W, Silverman N, Levitsky S. Valve replacement in patients with endocarditis and cerebral septic

emboli. Ann Thorac Surg 1991;51:18-21

265. Daniel WG, Durst UN. Cardiological diagnosis in arterial embolism. Herz 1991;16:405-418

266. Klein RM, Horstkotte D, Niehues R, Piper C, Schulte HD, Strauer BE. Mitral kissing vegetations in acute aortic endocarditis: Frequency and therapeutic consideration. J Heart Valve Dis 1995;3:300

267. Horstkotte D, Niehues R, Klein RM, Piper C, Schultheiss HP, Schulte HD, Strauer BE. Diagnostische und therapeutische Probleme bei akuter hochgradiger Mitralinsuffizienz. Intensivmed 1992;29:288-297

268. Bone RC, Fisher CJ, Clemmer TP. A controlled clinical trial of high dose methylprednisolon in the treatment of severe sepsis and septic shock. N Engl J Med 1987;317:653-658

269. Fateh-Moghadam A, Wick M. Therapie mit polyvalenten Immunglobulinpräparaten. Auswahlkriterien und Anwendungsbereiche. Intensivmed 1989;26(Suppl II):81-89

270. Ziegler EJ, Fischer CJ, Sprung CL, Straube RC, Sadoff JC, Foulke GE, Wortel CH, Fink MP, Dellinger RP, Teng NN et al. Treatment of gram-negative bacteremia and septic shock with HA-1A human monoclonal antibody against endotoxin. A randomized, double-blind, placebo-controlled trial. The HA-1A Sepsis Study Group. N Engl J Med 1991;324:429-436

271. Hack CE, Ogilvie AC, Eisele B, Erenberg JM, Wagstoff J, Thijs LG. C1-inhibitor substitution therapy in septic shock and in the vascular leak syndrome induced by high doses of interleukin-2. Intensive Care Med 1993;19:519-528

272. Lüthy R. Principles of antimicrobial therapy in infective endocarditis. Horstkotte D, Bodnar E (eds.) Infective endocarditis. ICR Publishers, London 1991;93-96

273. Francioli P, Etienne J, Hoigne R, Thys JP, Gerber A. Treatment of streptococcal endocarditis with a single daily dose of ceftriaxone sodium for four weeks. Efficacy and outpatient treatment feasibility. JAMA 1992;267:264-267

274. Chambers HF, Mills J, Drake TA, Sande MA. Failure of a once daily regimen of cefonicid for treatment of endocarditis due to staphylococcus aureus. Rev Inf Dis 1984;6:870-874

275. Moellering RC, Krogstadt DJ, Greenblatt DJ. Vancomycin therapy in patients with impaired renal function: a nomogram for dosage. Ann Int Med 1981;94:343-346

276. Chambers HF. Antibiotic treatment of staphylococcal endocarditis. Horstkotte D, Bodnar E (eds) Infective Endocarditis. ICR Publishers, London 1991;110-117

277. Rifkin GD, Fekety FR, Silva J. Antibiotic-induced colitis: implications of a toxin neutralized by clostridium sordellii antitoxin. Lancet 1977;2:1103-1106

278. Bartlett JG. Antibiotic-associated pseudomembranous colitis. Rev Infect Dis 1979;1:530-539

279. Tedesco FJ. Clindamycin and colitis: a review. J Infect Dis 1977;135:95-98

280. George WL, Rolfe RD, Finegold SM. Treatment and prevention of antimcirobial agent-induced colitis and diarroehea. Gastroenterology 1989;79:366-372

281. Newfield P, Roizen MF. Hazards of rapid administration of vancomycin. Ann Intern Med 1979;91:581-584

282. Faber RF, Moellering RC. Retrospective study of the toxicity of preparations of vancomycin from 1974 to 1981. Antimicrob Agents Chemother 1983;23:138-141

283. Hess J, Dankert J, Durack D. Significance of penicillin tolerance in vivo: prevention of experimental streptococcus sanguis endocarditis. J Antimicrob Chemother 1983;11:555-564

284. Holloway Y, Dankert J. Penicillin tolerance in nutritionally variant streptococci. Antimicrob Agents Chemother 1982;22:1073-1075

285. Shanson DC, Tadayon M, Bakhtiar M. Bactericidal activity of netilmicin compared with gentamicin and streptomycin, alone and in combination with penicillin, against penicillin tolerant viridans streptococci and enterococci. J Antimicrob Chemother 1986;18:479-490

286. Slater GJ, Greewood D. Detection of penicillin tolerance in streptococci. J Clin Path 1983;36:1353-1356

287. Sande MA, Scheld WM. Combination antibiotic therapy of bacterial endocarditis. Ann Intern Med 1980;92:390-395

288. Report of a Working Party of the British Society for Antimicrobial Chemotherapy. Antibiotic treatment of streptococcal and staphylococcal endocarditis. Lancet 1985;2:815-817

289. Shanson BC. Antibiotic treatment of endocarditis due to penicillin-sensitive streptococci. Horstkotte D, Bodnar E (eds) Infective Endocarditis. ICR Publishers, London 1991;97-101

290. Wolfe J, Johnson WD. Penicillin-sensitive streptococcal endocarditis: in vitro and clinical observations on penicillin-streptomycin therapy. Am J Inter Med 1974;81:178-181

291. Konrad F, Wagner R, Neumeister B, Rommel H, Georgieff M. Studies on drug monitoring in thrice and once daily treatment with aminoglycosides. Intensive Care Med 1993;19:215-220

292. Schentag JJ, Plaut ME, Cerra FB. Comparative nephrotoxicity of gentamicin and tobramycin: pharmacokinetic and clinical studies in 201 patients. Antimicrob Ag Chemother 1981;19:859-866

293. Vacek V. Die hochdosierte Lincomycin-Therapie. Lincomycin-Symposium. Dustri, München-Deisenhofen 1971;71-80

294. Eliopoulos GM, Eliopoulos CT. Therapy of enterococcal infections. J Clin Microbiol Infect Dis 1990;9:118-126

295. Geraci JE, Martin WJ. Antibiotic therapy of bacterial endocarditis VI: Subacute enterococcal endocarditis, clinical, pathologic and therapeutic consideration of 33 cases. Circulation 1954;10:173-194
296. Hunter TH. Use of streptomycin in the treatment of bacterial endocarditis. Am J Med 1947;436-442
297. Moellering RC, Korzeniowski OM, Sande MA, Wennersten CB. Species-specific resistance to antimicrobial synergism in streptococcus faecium und streptococcus faecalis. J Infect Dis 1979;140:203-208
298. Wennersten CB, Moellering RC. Mechanism of resistance to penicillin-aminoglycoside synergism in streptococcus faecium. Nelson JD, Grassi C (eds): Current chemotherapy and infective disease. Am Society for Microbiol, Washington 1980;1:710-712
299. Thauvin C, Eliopoulos GM, Wennersten C, Moellering RC. Antagonstic effect of penicillin-amikacin combinations against enterococci. Antimicrob Agents Chemother 1985;28:78-83
300. Bisno AL, Dismukes DT, Durack WE, Kaplan EL, Karchmer AW, Kaye D, Rahimtoola SH, Sande MA, Sanford JP, Watanakunakorn C, Wilson WR. Antimicrobial treatment of infective endocarditis due to viridans streptococci, enterococci and staphylococci. J Am Med Ass 1989;261:1471-1477
301. Herman DJ, Gerding DN. Screening and treatment of infections caused by resistant enterococci. Antimicrob Agents Chemother 1991;35:215-219
302. Huycke MM, Spiegel CA, Gilmore MS. Bacteremia caused by hemolytic, high-level gentamicin-resistant enterococcus faecalis. Antimicrob Agents Chemother 1991;35:1626-1634
303. Wurtz R, Sahm D, Flaherty J. Gentamicin-resistant, streptomycin-susceptible enterococcus (Streptococcus) faeecalis bacteremia. J Infect Dis 1991;163:1393-1394
304. Yao JDC, Thauvin-Eliopoulos C, Eliopoulos GM, Moellering RC. Efficacy of teicoplanin in two dosage regimens of experimental endocarditis caused by a beta-lactamase-producing strain of enterococcus faecalis with high-level resistance to gentamicin. Antimicrob Agents and Chemotherapy 1990;34:827-830
305. Murray BE, Mederski-Samoraj B. Transferable beta-lactamase. A new mechanism for in vitro penicillin resistance in streptococcus faecalis. J Clin Invest 1983;72:1168-1171
306. Sabath LD, Postic B, Finland M. Methicillin treatment of severe staphylococcal disease. N Engl J Med 1962;267:1049-1052
307. Klein JO, Sabath LD, Steinhauer VW, Finland M. Oxacillin treatment of severe staphylococccal infections. N Engl J Med 1965;272:699-703
308. Egert J, Carrizosa J, Kaye D. Comparison of methicillin, nafcillin and oxacillin in therapy of staphylococcus aureus endocarditis in rabbits. J Lab Clin Med 1977;89:1262-1265
309. Turnidge J, Grayson ML. Optimum treatment of staphylococcal infections. Drugs 1993;45:353-366
310. Sande MA, Courtney KB. Nafcillin-gentamicin synergism in experimental staphylococcal endocarditis. J Lab Clin Med 1970;88:118-123
311. Watanakunakorn C, Tisons JC. Synergism between vancomycin and gentamicin or tobramycin for methicillin-susceptible and methicillin-resistant staphylococcus aureus strains. Antimicrob Agents Chemother 1982;22:903-908
312. Geraci JE, Wilson WR. Vancomycin therapy for infective endocarditis. Rev Infect Dis 1981;1981:250-255
313. Levine DP, Fromm BS, Reddy BR. Slow response to vancomycin or vancomycin plus rifampin in methicillin-resistant staphylococcus aureus endocarditis. Ann Intern Med 1991;115:674-741
314. Faville RJ, Zuske DE, Kaplan EL, Crossley K, Sabath LD, Quie PG. Staphylococcus aureus enocarditis: combined therapy with vancomycin and rifampin. J Am Med Assoc 1978;240:1963-1966
315. Zak O, Scheld WM, Sande MA. Rifampin in experimental endocarditis due to staphylococcus aureus rabbits. Rev Infect Dis 1983;5:481-485
316. Van der Auwera P, Meunier-Carpenter F, Klastersky J. Clinical study of combination therapy with oxacillin and rifampin for staphylococcal infections. Rev Infect Dis 1983;5:481
317. Bary NL, Supena RB, Fekety R. Persistent staphylococcal bacteremia in an intravenous drug abuser. Antimicrob Agents Chemother 1986;29:209-212
318. Reisberg B. Infective endocarditis in the narcotic addict. Progr Cardiovasc Dis 1979;22:193-198
319. Noriega ER, Rubinstein E, Simberkoff M. Subacute and acute endocarditis due to pseudomonas cepacia in heroin addicts. Amer J Med 1975;59:29-33
320. Pefanis A, Giamarellou H, Karayiannakos P, Donta I. Efficacy of ceftazidime and aztreonam alone or in combination with amikacin in experimental left-sided pseudomonas aeruginosa endocarditis. Antimicrob Agents Chemother 1993;37:308-313
321. Wieland M, Lederman MM, Kline-King C. Left-sided endocarditis due to pseudomonas aeruginosa. A report of 10 cases and review of literature. Medicine (Baltimore) 1986;65:180
322. Potel G, Caillon J, Fantin B, Raza J, Le Gallou F, Lepage JY, LeConte P, Bugnon D, Baron D, Drugeon H. Impact of dosage schedule on the efficacy of gentamicin, tobramycin, or amikacin in an experimental model of serratia marcescens endocarditis: in vitro-in vivo correlation. Antimicrob Agents Chemother 1991;35:111-116
323. Ena J, Amador C, Parras F, Bouza E. Ciprofloxacin as an effective antibacterial agent in serratia endocarditis. J Infect 1991;22:103-105

324. Geraci JE, Wilson WR. Endocarditis due to gram negative bacteria: Report of 56 cases. Mayo Clin Porc 1982;57:145-148
325. Da Camara CC, Weiner B, Stets JJ. Acute bacterial endocarditis due to hemophilus parainfluenzae response to ceftizoxime in an ampicillin allergic patient. Pharmacotherapy 1987;7:185-186
326. Lynn DJ, Kane JG, Parker RH. Hemophilus parainfluenzae and influenzae endocarditis: A review of forty cases. Medicine (Baltimore) 1977;56:115-120
327. Chen YC, Chang SC, Luh KT, Hsieh WC. Actinobacillus actonomycetemcomitans endocarditis: a report of four cases and review of the literature. Q J Med 1991;81:871-878
328. Deleiyhe M, Bardiau C, Huberlant P, Nelis E, Reginster M. Subacute endocarditis on a prosthetic valve due to actinobacillus actinomycetemcomitans. A new classic. Rev Med Liege 1991;46:123-130
329. Pritchard TM, Foust RT, Cantely JR, Leman RB. Prosthetic valve endocarditis due to cardiobacterium hominis occurring after upper gastrointestinal endoscopy. Am J Med 1991;90:516-518
330. Williams JD, Maskell JP, Shain H, Chrysos G, Sefton AM, Fraser HY, Hardie JM. Comparative in-vitro activity of azithromycin, macrolides (erythromycin, clarithromycin and spiramycin) and streptogramin RP 59500 against oral organisms. J Antimicrob Chemother 1992;30:27-37
331. Landis SJ, Korver J. Eikenella corrodens endocarditis: case report and review of the literature. Can Med Assoc J 1983;128:882
332. Goutzmanis JJ, Gonis G, Gilbert GL. Kingella kingae infection in children: ten cases and a review of the literature. Pediatr Infect Dis J 1991;10:677-683
333. Drouket E, DuPont B. Evolution of antifungal agents: past, present and future: Rev Infect Dis 1987;9:4-14
334. Leaf HL, Simerkoff MS. Fungal endocarditis. Horstkotte D, Bodnar E (eds) Infective Endcarditis. ICR Publishers, London 1991;118-134
335. Naidoo DP, Singh B, Haffejee A. Cardiovascular complications of parenteral nutrition. Postgrad Med J 1992;68:629-633
336. Wilson HA, Downes RT, Julian JS, White WL, Haponik EF. Candida endocarditis. A treatable form of pacemaker infection. Chest 1993;103:283-284
337. Bogers AJJC, Vanvreeswijk H, Verbaan CJ, Kappetein AP, Vanherwerden LA, Mochtar B, Bos E. Early surgery for active infective endocarditis improves early and late results. Thorac Cardiovasc Surg 1991;39:284-288
338. Dinuhile MJ. Surgery in active endocarditis. Ann Int Med 1982;96:650-655
339. Haydock D, Barratt-Boyes B, Macedo T, Kirklin JW, Blackstone E. Aortic valve replacement for active infective endocarditis in 108 patients. J Thorac Cardiovasc Surg 1992;103:130-139
340. Nakamura K, Koyanagi H, Hirosawa K. Spectrum of the infective endocarditis in the past five years. Jpn Circ J 1982;46:352-361
341. Mills J, Utlay J, Abbott J. Heart failure in infective endocarditis: predisposing factors, course and treatment. Chest 1974;66:151
342. Reitz BA, Baumgartner WA, Oyer PE, Stinson EB. Surgical treatment of infective endocarditis. Bisno AL (ed) Treatment of infective endocarditis. Grune & Stratton, New York pp. 193-207
343. Stinson EB. Surgical treatment of infective endocarditis. Prog Cardiovasc Dis 1979;22:145-152
344. Utley JR, Mills J, Roe B. The role of valve replacement in the treatment of fungal endocarditis. J Thorac Cardiovasc Surg 1975;69:255-259
345. Yoshida K, Yoshikawa J, Akasaka T, Hozumi T, Maeda K, Okumachi F, Shiratori K, Koizumi K, Kato H, Okada YY, Shomuura T. Infective endocarditis - Analysis of 116 surgically and 26 medically treated patients. Jpn Circ J 1991;55:794-798
346. Acar J, Cabrol C, Carter F, Fouchard J. Cure chirurgicale d'une endocardite bacterienne avec insuffisane aortique. Arch Mal Coeur 1966;59:757-767
347. Michel PL, Vitoux B, Hage A, Ghanem G, Dybantsa P, Acar J. Early or delayed surgery in acute native aortic valve endocarditis. Horstkotte D, Bodnar E. Infective Endocarditis. London, ICR Publishers 1991;220-228
348. Acar J, Michel PL. Chirurgie de l'endocardite bacterienne. Arch Mal Couer 1993;86:1863-1867
349. Michel PL, Iung B, Drissi F, Dadez E, Cormier B, Acar A, Deloche A, Vahanian A, Acar J. Conservative mitral valve surgery in the treatment of mitral regurgitation due to infective endocarditis. Arch Mal Coeur 1994;87:349-355
350. Arvay A, Lengyel M. Incidence and risk factors of prosthetic valve endocarditis. Eur J Cardioth Surg 1988;2:340-342
351. Turina M. Prosthetic valve endocarditis. Thorac Cardiovasc Jury 1986;30:350-353
352. Slaughter L, Morris JE, Starr A. Prosthetic valvular endocarditis: a 12-year review. Circulation 1973;47:1319
353. Karchmer AW. Prosthetic valve endocarditis; Mechanical valves. Maggilian DJ, Quinn EL (eds): Endocarditis - medical and surgical management, M Dekker New York-Basel 1986;241-252
354. Klosters FE. Infective prosthetic valve endocarditis. Rahimtoola ShH (ed): Infective Endocarditis, Grune

& Stratton, New York 1978;291-305

355. Paneth M. Native and prosthetic valve endocarditis. Thorac Cardiovasc Surg 1982;30:302-308
356. Karchmer AW, Archler GL, Dismukes WE. Staphylococcus epidermidis causing prosthetic valve endocarditis: microbiologic and clinical observations as guides to therapy. Ann Intern Med 1983;98:447-452
357. Saffle JR, Gardner P, Schoenhausen SC, Wild W. Prosthetic valve endocarditis: a case for prompt valve replacement. J Thorac Cardiovasc Surg 1977;73:416-421
358. Karchmer AW, Dismukes WE, Buckley MJ, Austen WG. Late prosthetic valve endocarditis, clinical features infuencing therapy. Am J Med 1978;64:199-204
359. Ferrans VJ, Boyce SW, Billingham M, Spray TL, Roberts WC. Infection of glutaraldehyde-preserved porcine valve heterografts. Am J Cardiol 1979;43:1123-1136
360. Zussa C, Galloni MR, Zattera GF, Pansini S, Di-Summa M, Poletti GA, Ottino G, Morea M. Endocarditis in patients with bioprostheses: pathology and clinical correlations. Int J Cardiol 1984;6:719-723
361. Barnhart GR, Jones M, Ishihara T, Chavez AM, Rose DM, Ferrans VJ. Bioprosthetic valvular failure. Clinical and pathological observations in an experimental animal model. J Thorac Cardiovasc Surg 1982;83:618-631
362. Brodie B, Grossman W, McLaurin L. Diagnosis of prosthetic valve malfunction with combined echo-phonocardiography. Circulation 1976;54:93-98
363. Cunha CLP, Guiliani ER, Callahan JA, Pluth JR. Echo-phonocardiographic findings in patients with prosthetic heart valve malfunction. Mayo Clin Proc 1980;55:231-239
364. Horstkotte D, Aul C, Seipel L, Körfer R, Budde T, Schulte HD, Bircks W, Loogen F. Einflusse von Klappentyp und Klappenfunktion auf die chronische intravasale Hämolyse nach Mitral- und Aortenklappenersatz. Z Kardiol 1983;72:119-131
365. Horstkotte D, Curtius JM, Bircks W, Loogen F. Non-invasive evaluation of prosthetic valves. Rabago G (ed) Heart valve replacement. Current status and future trends. New York, Futura Publishing 1987
366. Kotler MN, Mintz GS, Panidis J, Morganroth J, Segal BL, Ross J. Non-invasive evaluation of normal and abnormal prosthetic valve function. J Am Coll Cardiol 1983;2:151-173
367. Sands MJ, Lachman AS, O'Reilly DJ, Leach CN, Sappington JB, Katz AM. Diagnostic value of cinefluoroscopy in the evaluation of prosthetic heart valve dysfunction. Am Heart J 1982;104:622-627
368. Veyrat C, Witchiz S, Lessana A, Ameur A, Abitbol G, Kalmanson D. Valvular prosthetic dysfunction. Localisation and evaluation of the dysfunction using the Doppler technique. Br Heart J 1985;54:273-284
369. Arora R, Jolly N, Singh B, Mohan JC, Kalra GS, Sethi KK, Khalilullah M. Clinical utility of transoesophageal echocardiography - preliminary experience of 100 cases. Indian Heart J 1991;43:357-360
370. Gussenhoven EG, Taams MA, Roelandt JRT, Ligtvoet KM, McGhie J, Van-Herwerder LA, Cahalan MK. Transoesophageal two-dimensional echocardiography: ets role in solving clinical problems. JACC 1986;8:975-979
371. Khan SS, Gray RJ. Valvular emergencies. Cardiol Clin 1991;9:689-709
372. Cormier B, Vitoux B, Starkman C, Enriquez-Sarano M, Kulas A, Dewilde J, Grimberg D, Acar J. Value of transesophageal echocardiography. From a preliminary experience of 532 cases. Arch Mal Coeur 1990;83:23-28
373. Chambers J, Monaghan M, Jackson G. Colour flow Doppler mapping in the assessment of prosthetic valve regurgitation. Br Heart J 1989;62:1-9
374. Horstkotte D, Loogen F. The natural history of aortic valve stenosis. Eur Heart J 1988;9(Suppl E):57-64
375. Horstkotte D, Niehues R, Strauer BE. Pathomorphological aspects aetiology and natural history of acquired mitral valve stenosis. Eur Heart J 1991;12(Suppl B):55-60
376. Stollerman GH. Rheumatic fever and streptococcal infection. Grune & Stratton, New York 1975
377. Stollerman GH. Streptococci and rheumatic heart disease. De Vries RRP, Cohen IR, Van Rood JJ (eds) The role of micro-organisms in non-infective diseases. Springer, London 1990;9-20
378. Goldstein I, Halpert B, Robert L. Immunological relationship between streptococcus A polysaccharide and the the structural glycoproteins of the heart valves. Nature 1967;213:44-53
379. Dale JB, Beachey EH. Epitopes of streptococcal M proteins shared with cardiac myosin. J Exp Med 1985;162:583-587
380. Tomai M, Kolb M, Majundar G, Beachey EH. Superantigenicity of streptococcal M protein and their relationship to rheumatic fever. J Exp Med 1990;169:269-275
381. Rammelkamp C, Wannamoker LW, Denny FW. Studies on epidemiology of rheumatic fever in armed services. Thomas 1956;19-38
382. Burch GE, Giles TD, Colcolough HL. Pathogenesis of rheumatic heart disease: critique and theory. Am Heart J 1970;80:556-501
383. Feinstein AR, DiMassa M. Prognostic significance of valvular involvement in acute rheumatic fever. New Engl J Med 1959;260:1001-1012
384. Taranta A, Kleinberg E, Feinstein AR. Rheumatic fever in children and adolescents. A long term

epidemiologic study of subsequent prophylaxis, streptococcal infections and clinical sequelae V. Relation of the rheumatic fever recurrence rate per streptococcal infection to pre-existing clinical features of patients. Ann Intern Med 1964;60(Suppl 5):58-68

385. Jones Criteria (revised) for guidance in the diagnosis of rheumatic fever. Circulation 1965;32:664-666
386. Vaisman S, Guasch J, Vignau A. The failure of penicillin to alter acute rheumatic valvulitis. JAMA 1965;194:1284-1287
387. United Kingdom and United States Joint Report on Rheumatic Heart Disease. The natural history of rheumatic fever and rheumatic heart disease. Ten year report of cooperative clinical trial of ACTH, cortisone and aspirin. Circulation 1965;32:457-459
388. American Heart Association Committee on rheumatic fever and bacterial endocarditis. Prevention of rheumatic fever. Circulation 1988;78:1082-1084
389. Kim HS, Suzki M, Lie JT, Titus JL. Non-bacterial thrombotic endocarditis (NBTE) and disseminated intravascular coagulation (DIC) - Autopsy study of 36 patients. Arch Pathol Lab Med 1977;101:65-68
390. Oppenheimer EH, Esterley JR. Non-bacterial thrombotic vegetations. Am J Pathol 1968;53:63-81
391. Rosen P, Armstrong D. Infective endocarditis in patients treated for malignant neoplastic disease. A postmortem study. Am J Clin Pathol 1973;60:241-250
392. Hodgson S, Child A, Dyson M. Endocardial fibroelastosis possible X linked inheritance. J Med Genet 1987;24:210-214
393. Schryer MJP, Karnauchow PN. Endocardial fibroelastosis: Etiologic and pathogenic considerations in children. Am Heart J 1974;88:557-561
394. Moller JN, Sucas RV, Adams P. Endocardial fibroelastosis. A clinical and anatomic study of 47 patients with emphasis on its relationship to mitral insufficiency. Circulation 1964;30:759-765
395. Sellers FJ, Keith JD, Manning JA. The diagnosis of primary endocardial fibroelastosis. Circulation 1964;29:49-52
396. Griffin ML, Hernandez A, Martin TC, Goldring D, Bolman RM, Spray TL, Strauss AW. Dilated cardiomyopathy in infants and children. J Am Coll Cardiol 1988;11:139-144
397. Davies J, Spry CJF, Vijayaraghavan G, de Souza JA. A comparison of the clinical and cardiological features of endomyocardial disease in temperate and tropical regions. Postgrad Med J 1983;59:179-185
398. Frustaci A, Abdulla AK, Possati G, Manzoli U. Persisting hypereosinophilia and myocardial activity in the fibrotic stage of endomyocardial disease. Chest 1989;96:674-675
399. Löffler W. Endocarditis parietalis fibroplastica mit Bluteosinophilien. Ein eigenartiges Krankheitsbild. Schweiz Med Wschr 1936;66:817-821
400. Olsen EGJ, Path FRC. Pathological aspects of endomyocardial fibrosis. Postgrad Med J 1983;59:135-139
401. Spry CJF. The pathogenesis of endomyocardial fibrosis: the role of the eosinophil. Semin Immunopathol 1989;11:471-477
402. Valithan MS, Bala Krishnan KG, Kortha CC. A profile of endomyocardial fibrosis. Indian J Pediatr 1987;54:229-233
403. Child JS, Perloff JK. The restrictive cardiomyopathies. Cardiol Clin 1988;6:289-316
404. Connor DH, Somers K, Hutt MSR, Manion WC, d'Arbela PG. Endomyocardial fibrosis in Uganda (Davies' disease). Part II. Am Heart J 1968;75:107-120
405. Ive FA, Willis AJP, Ikeme AC, Brockington JF. Endomyocardial fibrosis and filiariasis. Q J Med 1967;36:495-502
406. Olsen EGJ, Spry CJF. The pathogenesis of Loeffler's endomyocardiac disease and its relationship to endomyocardial fibrosis. Yu PN, Goodwin JF (eds) Progress in Cardiology, Vol 8, Lea & Fetriger, Philadelphia 1979;281-303
407. Becker BJP, Chatgidakis CB, Von Lingen B. Cardiovascular collaganosis with parietal endocardial thrombosis. Circulation 1953;7:345-356
408. Hardy WR, Anderson RE. The hypereosinophilic syndromes. Ann Intern Med 1968;68:1220-1229
409. Cushid MJ, Dale DC, West BC, Wolff SM. The hypereosinophilic syndrome: analysis of fourteen cases with review of the literature. Medicine (Baltimore) 1975;54:1-27
410. Niehues R, Horstkotte D, Aul C, Strauer BE. 76-jähriger patient mit Herzinsuffizienz und Bluteosinophilie. Internist 1992;33:188-192
411. Rohrbach MS, Wheatley CL, Slifman NR, Gleich GJ. Activation of platelets by eosinophil granule proteins. J Exp Med 1990;172:1271-1274
412. Kroegel C, Costabel U, Barness PF, Matthys H. Die pathologische Bedeutung der eosinophilen Granulozyten. Dtsch Med Wochenschr 1988;36:1405-1411
413. Sasano H, Virmani R, Patterson RH, Rabinowitz M, Guccion JG. Eosinophilic products lead to myocardial damage. Hum Pathol 1989;20:850-857
414. Report of the WHO/ISFC Task Force on the definitions and classification of cardiomyopathies. Br Heart J 1980;44:672-673
415. Olsen EGJ. Restrictive cardiomyopathy. Postgrad Med J 1986;62:607-608

416. Fauci AS. The idiopathic hypereosinophilic syndrome: clinical, pathophysiological and therapeutic considerations. Ann Intern Med 1982;97:78-92
417. Olsen EGJ, Spry CJF. Relation between eosinophilia and endomyocardial disease. Prog Cardiovasc Dis 1985;27:241-254
418. Parrillo JE, Lawley TJ, Frank MM, Kaplan AP, Fauci AS. Immunologic reactivity in the hypereosinophilic syndrome. J Allergy Clin Immun 1979;64:113-121
419. Spry CJF, Tai PC, Davies J. The cardiotoxicity of eosinophils. Postgrad Med J 1983;59:147-151
420. Kim CH, Vliestra RE, Edwards WD, Reeder GS, Gleich GJ. Steroid-responsive eosinophilic myocarditis. Diagnosis by endomyocardial biopsie. Am J Cardiol 1984;53:1472-1473
421. Spry CJF, Davies J, Tai PC. Yoshida T, Torisu M (eds) Immunbiology of the eosinophil. Elsevier, North Holland Philadelphia 1983;229-244
422. Parrillo JE. Heart disease and the eosinophil. N Engl J Med 1990;323:1560-1561
423. Stierle U, Schwarting K, Rinast E, Spicher V, Sheikhzadeh A. Rechtsventrikuläre Endomyokardfibrose. Z Kardiol 1987;76:445-450
424. Tai PC, Ackerman SJ, Spry CJF, Dunnette S, Olsen EGJ, Gleich GJ. Deposits of eosinophil granule in cardiac tissues of patients with cosinophilic endomyocardial disease. Lancet. 1987;1:643-647
425. De Mello DE, Liapis H, Jureidini S, Nouri S, Kephart GM, Gleich GJ. Cardiac localisation of eosinophil-granule major basic protein in acute necrotizing myocarditis. N Engl J Med 1990;323:1542-1545
426. Jones EL, Hendren MD, Smith MD. Aortic and mitral replacement in IHES. Am Thorac Surg 1988;46:570-571
427. Rodger JC, Irvine DJ, Lerski RA. Echocardiography in Loffler's endocarditis. Br Heart J 1981;46:110-112
428. Acquatella H. Two-dimensional echocardiography in endomyocardial disease. Postgrad Med J 1983;59:157-158
429. Gottdiener JS, Maron BJ, Schooley RT, Harley JB, Roberts WC, Fauci AS. Two-dimensional echocardiographic assessment of the idiopathic hypereosinophilic syndrome. Circulation 1983;67:572-578
430. Chew CJ, Ziady GM, Raphael MJ, Nellen M. Primary restrictive cardiomyopathy. Non-tropical endomyocardial fibrosis and hypereosinophilic heart disease. Br Heart J 1977;39:399-413
431. Gilbert GJ. Churg-Strauss syndrome: determining adequacy of corticosteroid dosage by the eosinophil count. South Med J 1987;80:266-268
432. Cupps TR, Fauci AS. The vasculitis syndromes. Arch Intern Med 1982;27:315-319
433. Roberts WC, Liegler DC, Carbone PP. Endomyocardial disease and eosinophilia. A clinical and pathological spectrum. Am J Med 1969;46:28-42
434. Parrillo JE, Fauci AS, Wolff SM. Therapy of the hypereosinophilic syndrome. Ann Intern Med 1978;89:167-172
435. Haas R, Mundinger A, Bohn T, Schaz K, Hunstein W. Therapiemoglichkeiten beim Hypereosinophilie-syndrom mit endomyocarditis fibroplastica Löffler. Dtsch Med Wochenschr 1985;41:1573-1576
436. Eakins DL, Gill DP, Weiss GB. Response of hypereosinophilic syndrome to six-thioguanin and cytarabin. Cancer Treat Rep 1982;66:545-552
437. Murphy PT, Fennelly DF, Stuart M, O'Donnell JR. Alpha-Interferon in a case of hypereosinophilic syndrome. Br J Hemotal 1990;75:619-620
438. Prigent C, Baculard P, Carpentier A, Passelecq J, Dubost C. Endocardite fibreuse du ventricule gauche chez un filarien. Cure chirurgicale. Arch Mal Coeur Vaiss 1973;66:101-104
439. Martinez EE, Ventrui M, Buffalo E, Carvalho AC, Alexopoulos D, Bocanegra J, Andrade JL, Kambara A, Portugal OP, Ambrose JA. Operative results in endomyocardial fibrosis. Am J Cardiol 1989;63:627-629
440. Gramsch-Zabel H, Bircks W, Preusse C, Putz B. Zur Problematik der operativen Behandlung der Löffler-Endomyokardfibrose. Z Herz Thorax Gefasschir 1990;4:130-135
441. Oliveira SA, Pereira-Baretto AC, Mady C, Oliveira-Dallan LA, Da Luz PL, Jatene AD, Pileggi F. Surgical treatment of endomyocardial fibrosis. A new approach. J Am Coll Cardiol 1990;16:1246-1251
442. Liberthson RR, Homey C, Fallon JT. Systemic lupus erythematosus and heart disease. Primary Cardiol 1983;9:77-83
443. Bourel G, Gouffault J, Boudesseul B. Cardiovasular manifestations of SLE. Coeur Med Interne 1971;10:535-544
444. Gross L. Cardiac lesions in Libman-Sacks disease with consideration of its relationship to acute diffuse lupus erythematosus. Am J Pathol 1940;16:375-379
445. Leung WH, Wong KL, Lau CP, Wang CK, Cheng CH. Cardiac abnormalities in systemic lupus erythematosus: A prospective M-mode, cross-sectional and Doppler echocardiographic study. Int J Cardiol 1990;27:367-375
446. Libman E, Sacks B. A hitherto undescribed form of valvular and mitral endocarditis. Arch Intern Med 1924;33:701-703
447. Wood PHN. The incidence of RA and SLE in Great Britain. Wood PHN (ed) The challenge of arthritis and rheumatism British League against rheumatism, London 1977

448. Ebling FM, Hahn BH. Pathogenic subsets of antibodies to DNA. International Reviews in Immunology. H Kohler, C. Bonce (eds) 1989;5:7995
449. Reichlin M. Antibodies to cytoplasmic antigens in systemic lupus erythematosus. RG Lahita (ed) New York, Wiley 1987;257-269
450. Nihoyannopoulos P, Gomez PM, Joshi J, Loizou S, Walport MJ, Oakley CM. Cardiac abnormalities in systemic lupus erythematodes. Circulation 1990;81:369-375
451. Roldan CA, Shively BK, Lau CC, Gurule FT, Smith EA, Crawford MH. Systemic lupus erythematosus valve disease by transesophageal echocardiography and the role of antiphospholipid antibodies. JACC 1992;20:1127-1134
452. Rawsthorne L, Ptacin MJ, Choi H, Olinger GN, Bamrah VS. Lupus valvulitis necessitating double valve replacement. Arthritis Rheum 1981;24:561-564
453. Doherty NE, Siegel RJ. Cardiovascular manifestations of systemic lupus erythematodes. Am Heart J 1985;110:1257-1260
454. Enomoto K, Kaji Y, Mayumi T, Tsuda Y, Kanayas S, Nagasawa K, Fujino T, Niho Y. Frequency of valvular regurgitation by color Doppler echocardiography in systemic lupus erythematodes. Am J Cardiol 1991;67:209-211
455. Harris EN, Chan JK, Asherson RA, Aber VR, Gharavi AE, Hughes GR. Thrombosis, recurrent foetal loss, thrombocytopenia: Predictive value of the anticardiolipin antibody test. Arch Intern Med 1986;146:2153-2154
456. Chartash EK, Lans DM, Paget SA, Qamar T, Lockshin MD. Aortic insufficiency and mitral regurgitation in patients with systemic lupus erythematosus and the antiphospholipid syndrome. Am J Med 1989;86:407-412
457. Stollerman GH. Rheumatic fever and other rheumatic diseases of the heart. Heart Disease. E Braunwald (ed) 1992;1721-1741
458. Strickmann NE, Rossi PA, Massumkhani GA, Hall RJ. Carcinoid heart disease: a clinical pathological and therapeutic update. Curr Probl Cardiol 1982;6:1-42
459. Ross EM, Roberts WC. The carcinoid syndrome: Comparison of 21 necropsy subjects with carcinoid heart disease to 15 necropsy subjects without carcinoid heart disease. Am J Med 1985;79:339-343
460. May B. Karzinoid: Diagnostik und Therapie. Dtsch Med Wochenschr 1975;100:2163-2165
461. Lundin L, Norheim J, Landelius J, Oberg K, Theodorsson-Norheim E. Carcinoid heart disease: Relationship of circulating vasoactive substances to ultrasound-detectable cardiac abnormalities. Circulation 1988;77:264-270
462. Lundin L, Landelius J, Andren B, Oberg K. Transesophageale echocardiography improves the value of cardiac ultrasound in patients with carcinoid heart disease. Br Heart J 1990;64:190-193
463. Lundin L, Funa K, Hansson HE, Wilander E, Oberg K. Histochemical and immunohistochemical morphology of carcinoid heart disease. Pathol Res Pract 1991;187:73-78
464. Roberts WC, Sjoerdsma A. The cardiac disease associated with the carcinoid sydrome. Am J Med 1964;36:5-35
465. Tornebrandt K, Eskilsson J, Nobin H. Heart involvement in metastatic carcinoid disease. Clin Cardiol 1986;9:13-17
466. Reid CL, Chandraratna PA, Kawanishi DT, Pitha JV, Rahimtoola SH. Echocardiographic features of carcinoid heart disease. Am Heart J 1984;107:801-803
467. Hendel N, Leckie B, Richards J. Carcinoid heart disease: eight-year survival following tricuspid valve replacement and pulmonary valvotomy. Ann Thorac Surg 1980;30:391-395
468. Oberg K, Norheim I, Lind E, Alm G, Lundquist G, Wide L, Jonsdottin B, Magnusson A, Wilander E. Treatment of maligant carcinoid tumors with human leukocyte interferon: Long term results. Cancer Treatment Rep 1986;70:1297
469. Feldman JM. Carcinoid tumors and sydrome. Semin Oncol 1987;14:237-252
470. Kvols LK, Moertel CG, O'Connell MJ, Schutt AJ, Rubin J, Hahn RG. Treatment of the malignant carcinoid sydrome: Evaluation of a long-acting somatostatin analogue. N Engl J Med 1986;315:663
471. Lundin L, Hansson HE, Landelius J, Oberg K. Surgical treatment of carcinoid heart disease. J Thorac Cardiovasc Surg 1990;100:552-554
472. Kahn AH, Spodick DH. Rheumatoid heart disease. Semin Arthritis Rheum 1972;1:327-335
473. Roberts WC, Kehoe JA, Carpenter DF. Cardiac valvular lesions in rheumatoid arthritis. Arch Intern Med 1968;122:141
474. Linch DC, Gillmer DH, Whimster WF, Keates JRW. Rheumatoid aortic valve prolapse requiring emergency valve replacement. Br Heart J 1980;43:237-240
475. Gene H, Stollerman HD. Rheumatic fever and other rheumatic diseases of the heart. Heart Disease. Braunwald E (ed) 1992;1721-1741
476. Kelly CA, Bourke JP, Malcolm A, Griffiths JD. Chronic pericardial disease in patients with rheumatoid arthritis. A longitudinal study. Q J Med 1990;75:461-464

477. Morris PB, Imber MJ, Heinsimer JA, Hlatky MA, Reimer KA. Rheumatoid arthritis and coronary arthritis. Am J Cardiol 1986;57:689-671

478. Mac Donald WJ, Crawford MH, Klippel JH, Zvaifler FNJ, O'Rourke RA. Echocardiographic assessment of cardiac structure and function in patients with rheumatoid arthritis. Am J Med 1977;63:890-892

479. Gottdiener JS, Katin MJ, Borer JS, Bacharach SL, Green MV. Late cardiac effects of therapeutic mediastinal irridiation: Assessment by echocardiography and radionuclide angiography. N Engl J Med 1983;308:569-574

480. Shashaty GG. Aortic insufficiency following mediastinal radiation for Hodgkin's disease. Am J Med Sci 1984;287:46-51

481. Detrano RC, Yiannikas J, Salcedo EE. Two dimensional echocardiographic assessment of radiation-induced valvular heart disease. Am Heart J 1984;107:584-588

482. O'Donnell L, O'Neill T, Toner M, O'Brian S, Graham I. Myocardial hypertrophy fibrosis and infarction following exposure of the heart to radiation for Hodgkin's disease. Postgrad Med J 1986;62:1055-1060

483. Gomez GA, Park JJ, Panahon AM, Pathasarathy KL, Pearle J, Reese P, Bakshi S, Hendeoon ES. Heart size and function after radiation therapy to the mediastinum in patients with Hodgkins disease. Cancer Treat Rep 1983;67:1099-1103

484. Cilliers GD, Harper JS, Lochner A. Radiation-induced changes in the ultrastructure and mechanical function of the rat heart. Radiotherapy Oncol 1989;16:311-318

485. Rosenthal DS, Braunwald E. Hematological-oncological disorders and heart disease. Heart Disease. Braunwald E (ed) 1992;1742-1766

Chapter 6.4

Antibiotic Prophylaxis for Infective Endocarditis

Catherine Leport, Jean-Louis Vilde

Antibiotic prophylaxis of infective endocarditis (IE) has recently been the subject of several national (1-3) and international (4) discussions. Though its practice is not based on well established scientific grounds, the poor prognosis of the disease and data from experimental models (5-6) have led to the consideration that the prevention of IE is desirable and possible. For more than thirty years several countries have published and regularly updated recommendations for the prophylaxis of IE (2,7- 14). Thus, the national recommendations at the present time vary slightly from one country to another. They have been elaborated in most countries by panels of experts, and less frequently by a consensus conference which involves a wider population of participants.

The important issue with prophylaxis of IE is its efficacy, which has recently been questioned. In fact, from the few available data, its seems that the incidence of the disease is not decreasing, despite these world wide recommendations for prevention. Thus it was recently suggested that rather than improving the content of the recommendations, further efforts should be directed towards improving the diffusion and the applicability of these prophylactic measures (4).

Administration of antibiotics to cardiac patients at risk before they undergo a procedure that carries a risk is the basis of the recommendations. It is expected to reduce the risk of valvular seeding of bacteria circulating in the blood after a procedure which has induced a break through the mucocutaneous barrier. It is addressed to a subgroup of patients who are known to have a valvular heart disease predisposing to bacterial seeding, and is designed to cover a subgroup of procedures which are supposed to be at high risk of valvular seeding. Antibiotics are selected to be active against the most frequent bacteria causing IE. From these data, it appears that prophylactic antibiotics can be defined for certain conditions. The French committee has especially underlined that 1) prophylactic antibiotics cannot prevent every case of IE occurring in predisposed patients following risk procedures, 2) they are distinct from the antibiotic treatment of infectious episodes and foci of infection, which require rigorous treatment in cardiac patients at risk, 3) they do not apply to early postoperative IE, for which different antibiotic regimens are required and which is excluded from this review, and finally, 4) antibiotic prophylaxis is only one aspect of the general prevention of IE (2).

The aim of this report is to present the current opinion in prophylaxis of IE based on the updated recommendations from several countries (2,7- 14) and the summary of the international and European discussions which have taken place over the last two years (4), on behalf of the International Society for Chemotherapy and the Working Group on Valvular Heart Disease of the European Society of Cardiology. The first part of this report will discuss the opportunity to further recommend antibiotic prophylaxis of IE.

Table 6.4-I: Cardiac conditions at risk requiring antibiotic prophylaxis for infective endocarditis - European Consensus

---

Cardiac diseases with the highest risk
-Prosthetic valves
-Congenital heart disease causing cyanosis
-Previous infective endocarditis

Other cardiac diseases at risk
-Valvular heart disease: AR, MR, AS, including MVP with MR, and bicuspid aortic valve
-Congenital heart disease which does not cause cyanosis, except IAC
-Hypertrophic obstructive cardiomyopathy

AR: aortic regurgitation MR: mitral regurgitation,
AS: aortic stenosis, MVP: mitral valve prolapse
IAC: interatrial communication

The population and the procedures at risk will be then defined. Finally the antibiotic schedules will be presented.

RATIONALE FOR ANTIBIOTIC PROPHYLAXIS OF IE

Infective endocarditis remains a severe disease with a mortality rate of approximately 20%, requiring prolonged administration of antibiotics and hospitalization, and cardiac surgery in 30% of cases (15). The average cost was estimated at approximately 130,000 FF per case for initial hospital care alone in France (2).

Risk factors for the occurrence of IE have long been established based on experimental data and clinical experience, although rigorous assessment of these risk factors is limited. Some cardiac conditions are associated with an increased risk of IE, as are some invasive procedures. The combination of these two types of predisposing factors further increases the risk. Thus administration of antibiotics to cardiac patients undergoing invasive procedures is one measure which can prevent IE. The efficacy of this strategy has been assessed through a limited number of studies, ranging from 49% to 91% (16-19). From these estimates, it can be expected that routine use of antibiotic prophylaxis would lead to a 5% to 10% decrease in the overall incidence of IE, i.e. 60 to 130 cases would be avoided each year in France. Whether such a strategy would be cost efficient should be studied further.

However, a remaining number of cases of IE occur in patients with no previously known cardiac disease or in the absence of any invasive procedure. Clearly other preventive measures are required to prevent these cases. These measures should be addressed to the general population; the public should be aware of the importance of good oral hygiene, which might have more beneficial consequences than just prevention of IE. Clear assessment of the impact of such measures is difficult.

Thus, at the present time, recommending antibiotic prophylaxis of IE appears worthwhile, with special attention being paid to the patients at the highest risk i.e. those with prosthetic valves, and to dental procedures (3,4).

Table 6.4-II: Cardiac diseases not at risk for infective endocarditis - European Consensus

---

IAC
MVP without MR, functional MR, mitral ring calcifications,
Coronary artery bypass grafting
Cardiac pacemakers
Implantable defibrillators
Corrected left to right shunts

IAC: interatrial communication
MVP: mitral valve prolapse
MR: mitral regurgitation

CARDIAC PATIENTS AT RISK

The estimation of the relative risk of IE according to cardiac condition is based on limited scientific data. The risk of bacterial seeding on cardiac valves remains difficult to assess since rigorous epidemiologic data are limited. Only patients with a prosthetic valve constitute a well defined population at risk (20-22). In these patients, as in patients with previous endocarditis, the risk seems approximately five to 10 times higher than in those with native valve disease. According to the different countries, the cardiac conditions predisposing to endocarditis which require antibiotic prophylaxis are very similar. Some countries have distinguished the cardiac diseases at risk and those which are not at risk. Some countries have identified a subgroup of cardiac diseases which are considered at high risk among those at risk (Table 6.4-I). It is suggested that a single antibiotic regimen be scheduled for all cardiac patients at risk, with a flexible formulation allowing the optimal regimen to be strongly recommended for the patients with the highest risk. Furthermore, it appears worthwhile establishing the list of cardiac conditions which do not constitute a predisposing condition for IE and do not require specific prophylaxis (Table 6.4-II).

PROCEDURES AT RISK

The risk of IE associated with various procedures was not assessed in prospective studies until recently. Most of the recommendations rely on anecdotal clinical reports and data from experimental models (23). First, it must be recalled that regular survey and dental care is mandatory in all cardiac patients at risk. It is widely accepted that dental procedures are the main risk factors for IE (24) and should all be covered with antibiotic prophylaxis, with the only exclusions being procedures without any risk of bleeding such as cure of a superficial caries and bloodless supragingival prosthetic preparations. Application of a local antiseptic is recommended, as an adjunct to antibiotic prophylaxis. Apart from the mouth, it is difficult to identify with any accuracy the procedures which carry a risk of IE and to quantify this risk. The procedures considered at risk are those responsible for bacteremia with a consistent frequency. However, it does not necessarily predict the risk of IE (25). The micro-organism likely to appear in blood following the procedure is an important factor; the procedures causing Gram negative bacilli and anaerobe bacteremia are less likely to induce IE than those causing streptococcal or enterococcal bacteremia. The duration of the procedure is a

---

Table 6.4-III: Procedures at risk for infective endocarditis requiring antibiotic prophylaxis - European Consensus

Dental	All procedures
Upper respiratory tract	Tonsillectomy - adenoidectomy
Gastrointestinal	- Oesophageal dilatation or surgery
	- Esophageal laser procedures,
	- Sclerosing procedures of esophageal varices
	- Abdominal surgery
Urologic	- Instrumental procedures involving the ureter or the kidney
	- Biopsy or surgery of prostate or urinary tract

Procedures for which the risk of infective endocarditis is controversial

Upper respiratory tract	- Fiberoptic fibroscopy
	- Endotracheal intubation
Gastrointestinal	- Coloscopy ± biopsy
Genital	- Vaginal hysterectomy, vaginal delivery*
	- Caesarean section

*However antibiotic treatment is required in case of concomitant infection

---

possible factor which has to be considered. Some procedures are supposed to be covered in all countries (Table 6.4-III). It is especially important to underline that a negative urine culture should be obtained before urologic procedures. Gynecologic and obstetric procedures are not in general considered at risk (26). The fitting of an intra-uterine device is not encouraged in female cardiac patients at risk, except in developing countries, where the risk of pregnancy should be weighted against the risk of IE. Also, patients undergoing a transesophageal echocardiography should not be given antibiotic prophylaxis (27). For these controversial procedures, no recommendation can be made for routine use. However in particular situations, the physician may wish to give a patient some antibiotics.

ANTIBIOTIC SCHEDULES

In general, antibiotics for dental and upper respiratory tract procedures are given to prevent IE caused by viridans streptococci, which are usually highly susceptible to penicillin, while antibiotics for gastrointestinal and urologic procedures are given to prevent IE caused by enterococci, which are less susceptible to penicillin. For dental and upper respiratory tract procedures, there are different regimens for patients who can take oral medications, which is the most frequent situation, and for patients under general anesthesia, who require parenteral antibiotics. In all countries, antibiotic regimens are based on penicillin, and alternative regimens have been defined for patients who are allergic to penicillin. It is a common agreement that antibiotics should be started one hour before the procedure is performed (5,6,28). The duration has to be adapted according to the healing process after the procedure.

Table 6.4-IV - Antibiotic prophylaxis for infective endocarditis - European consensus

	1 hour before the procedure	6 hours later
Minimal Regimen		
No allergy to penicillin	Amoxicillin 3g orally	No second dose
Allergy to penicillin	Clindamycin 300-600 mg orally	No second dose
Flexible modifications from minimal to maximal regimen		
	- additional doses after the procedure - adjunction of aminoglycosides - use of parenteral route of administration	
Maximal Regimen		
No allergy to penicillin	Amoxicillin (ampicillin) 2g IV + gentamicin 1.5 mg/kg IM or IV	1-1.5 g orally
Allergy to penicillin	Vancomycin 1g ≥ 1 hour IV infusion + gentamicin 1.5 mg/kg IM or IV	1g ≥ 1 hour IV infusion[*]

[*]12 hours later instead of 6 hours later

Oral prophylaxis for dental and upper respiratory tract procedures

The regimen consists of three gram amoxicillin given orally one hour before the procedure in most countries. In some countries, oral penicillin V is an alternative. A second or several additional doses of amoxicillin are recommended in some countries, specially for high risk patients. For patients allergic to penicillin, clindamycin is the most common recommendation, the dose varying from 300 to 600 mg. Alternative antibiotics, erythromycin or pristinamycin are proposed in other countries.

Parenteral prophylaxis for dental and upper respiratory tract procedures

The common proposition is based on ampicillin or amoxicillin given by intravenous infusion one hour before the procedure, completed with a second oral dose six hours later. There are differences in the dosages of ampicillin used in the different countries. Aminoglycosides are not added in some countries, while they are recommended in

---

Table 6.4-V: Criteria to select the most appropriate antibiotic regimen for prophylaxis of infective endocarditis - European Consensus

Minimal regimen	Maximal regimen
Cardiac risk	High cardiac risk
Dental procedure	Gastrointestinal or urologic procedure
Single procedure	Multiple procedures
Out-patients	Hospitalised patients
Local anesthesia	General anesthesia

others, especially in high risk patients. For allergic patients, one gram vancomycin intravenous infusion is proposed. Teicoplanin, which can be given as a 400 mg intravenous bolus, or intravenous clindamycin, are possible alternatives to vancomycin in some countries.

Gastrointestinal and urologic procedures

In general, parenteral prophylaxis is recommended. However, in some countries, low risk patients may be given oral antibiotics. The antibiotic regimens are similar to those used for parenteral prophylaxis of dental procedures, except that adjunction of an aminoglycoside is recommended in all countries in order to have a maximal activity against enterococci, and clindamycin is not suitable because it is not sufficiently active against intestinal streptococci.

Consensus propositions

At the present time, comparison of the various national recommendations shows clearly that there are very slight differences from one country to another (4). It appears that the different regimens from the national guidelines vary within two limits. The minimal and simplest regimen consists of a single oral dose of antibiotic. The maximal regimen relies upon the synergistic and prolonged (multiple doses) effect of a cell wall acting antibiotic and an aminoglycoside, and offers the widest margin of efficacy (Table 6.4-IV). The antibiotic regimen for a given patient should be selected between these two limits. It can be proposed that criteria to select the appropriate regimen for a given patient should include the type of cardiac condition at risk, the type, number and duration of the procedure, and the conditions of anesthesia required to perform the procedure (Table 6.4-V). This presentation allows a flexible modulation of the antibiotic prophylaxis to be adapted to each individual situation, and preserves the discretionary nature of the recommendations, the physician being responsible for his own patient in a given situation.

CONCLUSIONS

Antibiotic prophylaxis is recommended for cardiac patients at risk who undergo a procedure carrying a risk. Presently, recommendations are close to the maximum that can be done and minimal additional benefits can be obtained by changing these guidelines. Attention has to concentrate on patients and procedures with the highest risk, i.e. those with prosthetic valves undergoing dental procedures. Major efforts and future research remain to be done to improve the compliance of the recommendations, which are usually made by the experts and used by physicians and dentists (29). Diffusion of the information to the appropriate users, assessment of the knowledge, and application of the guidelines by both dentists and patients is required.

References
1. Editorial. Chemoprophylaxis for infective endocarditis, faith, hope and charity challenged. Lancet 1992;339:525-526
2. Consensus conference on antibiotic prophylaxis of infective endocarditis. Summary. Med Mal Infect

1992;22:1112-1118

3. Simmons NA, Ball AP, Cawson RA, et al. Dental prophylaxis for endocarditis. Lancet 1992;340:1353

4. Leport C, Horstkotte D, Burckhardt D, and the Group of Experts of the International Society for Chemotherapy. Antibiotic prophylaxis for infective endocarditis. From an international group of experts towards a European consensus. Eur Heart J 1995;16(Suppl B):126-131

5. Glauser MP, Bernard JP, Moreillon P, Francioli P. Successful single dose amoxicillin prophylaxis against experimental endocarditis: evidence for two mechanisms of protection. J Infect Dis 1983;145:568-575

6. Francioli P, Glauser P. Comparison of single doses of amoxicillin or of amoxicillin-gentamicin for the prevention of endocarditis caused by Streptococcus faecalis and by viridans streptococci. J Infect Dis 1985;152:83-89

7. American Heart Association Committee on Prevention of Bacterial Endocarditis - Prevention of bacterial endocarditis. Circulation 1984;70:1123A-1126A

8. Empfehlungen der Schweizerishen Arbeitsgruppe fur endokarditisprophylaxe. Prophylaxe der bakteriellen endokarditis. Schweiz Med Wochenschr 1984;114:1246-1252

9. Delaye J, Etienne J, Feruglio A, et al. Prophylaxis of infective endocarditis for dental procedures. Report of a Working Party of the European Society of Cardiology. Eur Heart J 1985;6:826

10. Empfehlungen zur Prophylaxe bakterieller Endokarditiden. Herausgegeben von der Kommmission fur Klinische Kardiologie der Deutschen Gesellschaft fur Herz - und Kreislaufforschung. Z Kardiol 1987;76:451- 453

11. Working Party of the British Society for Antimicrobial Chemotherapy - The antibiotic prophylaxis of infective endocarditis. Lancet 1990;335:88-89

12. Dajani AS, Bisno AL, Chung KJ, et al. Prevention of bacterial endocarditis. Recommendations by the American Heart Association JAMA 1990;260:2919-2922

13. Endocarditis prophylaxis in the Netherlands. Hartbulletin 1992;23:249-253

14. Simmons NA. Recommendations for endocarditis prophylaxis. J Antimicrob Chemother 1993;31:437-438

15. Delahaye F, Goulet V, Lacassin F, et al. Characteristics of infective endocarditis in France in 1991: a one-year survey. Eur Heart J 1995;16:394-401

16. Horstkotte D, Fridrichs W, Pippert H, Bircks W, Loogen F. Nutzen der endokarditispropphylaxie bei patienten mit prosthetischen herklappen. Z Kardiol 1986;75:8-11

17. Imperiale TF, Horwitz RI. Does prophylaxis prevent postdental infective endocarditis? A controlled evaluation of protective efficacy. Am J Med 1990;88:131-136

18. Van der Meer J, Van Wijk W, Thompson J, Vanderbroucke J, Walkerburg H, Michel M. Efficacy of antibiotic prophylaxis for prevention of native valve endocarditis. Lancet 1992;339:135-139

19. Hoen B, Lacassin F, Briancon S, et al. Gestes a risque d'endocardite infectieuse. Une enquete cas-temoins. Med Mal Infect 1992;22:1010-1022

20. Calderwood SB, Swinski LA, Waternaux CM, Karchmer AW, Buckley MJ. Risk factors for the development of prosthetic valve endocarditis. Circulation 1985;72(1):31-37

21. Leport C, Vilde JL, Bricaire F, et al. Fifty cases of late prosthetic valve endocarditis: improvement in prognosis over a 15 year period. Br Heart J 1987;58:66-71

22. Burckhardt D, Striebel E, Vogt S, et al. Heart valve replacement with St. Jude Medical valve prothesis - Long term experience in 743 patients in Switzerland. Circulation 1988;78(Suppl.I):18-24

23. Moreillon P, Overholser CD, Malinverni R, Bille J, Glauser MP. Predictors of endocarditis in isolates from cultures of blood following dental extractions in rats with periodontal disease. J Infect Dis 1988;157:990-995

24. Bayliss R, Clarke C, Oakley C, Somerville W, Whitfield AGW. The teeth and infective endocarditis. Br Heart J 1983;50:513-519

25. Everett ED, Hirschmann JV. Transient bacteremia and endocarditis prophylaxis: a review. Medicine 1977;56:61-77

26. Sugrue D, Blake S, Troy P, Mc Donald D. Antibiotic prophylaxis against infective endocarditis after normal delivery - is it necessary? Br Heart J 1980;44:499-502

27. Steckelberg JM, Khandheria BK, Anhalt JP, et al. Prospective evaluation of the risk of bacteremia associated with transoesophageal echocardiography. Circulation 1991;84:177-180

28. Berney P, Francioli P. Successful prophylaxis of experimental streptococcal endocarditis with single-dose amoxicillin administered after bacterial challenge. J Infect Dis 1990;161:281-285

29. Gutschik E, Lippert S. Dental procedures and endocarditis prophylaxis in patients with prosthetic heart valves: results of a questionnaire to 220 patients. Scand J Infect Dis 1989;21:665-668

30. Lacossin F, Hoen B, Leport C et al. Procedures at risk for infective endocarditis in adults. A case control study. Eur heart J 1996 (in press)

Chapter 6.5

Concomitant Coronay Heart Disease

Bernard Iung and Philippe Luxereau

With the introduction of coronary surgery, and the increasing number of patients suffering concomitant valvular and coronary heart disease, the concept of simultaneous surgical repair has become apparent and generally accepted. After the first cases were reported at the beginning of the 1970's (1), the improvement in the results of this combined valvular and coronary surgery led to its widespread use (2-9).

The coexistence of valvular and coronary lesions still poses a certain number of questions though, which can be summarized as follows:

- What is the relationship between coronary damage and valvulopathy, and what is the incidence of this association?
- In the preoperative review of valvular cardiopathy, how does the coexistence of coronary stenosis manifest itself, and is it possible to predict the outcome without almost inevitably resorting to coronary arteriography?
- What are the results of combined valvular and coronary surgery and to what extent does information from the literature enable the therapeutic needs of these patients to be optimized?

THE RELATIONSHIP BETWEEN ISCHEMIC AND VALVULAR CARDIOPATHIES

The coexistence of an ischemic and a valvular cardiopathy should be viewed in two different ways; in aortic and mitral valvulopathies of non-ischemic origin two different pathologies co-exist, whilst in ischemic mitral insufficiency the valvulopathy is the direct consequence of the coronary lesions.

Co-existence of coronary artery disease and valvulopathy

The estimation of the incidence of coronary artery disease associated with valvulopathy obtained from autopsy data can be inaccurate because of a selection bias at post-mortem (10-12). Clinical studies in which indications for coronary arteriography are independent of the presence of angina usually represent 20% to 40% of associated coronary lesions (2,5,7,13-34). These differences can in part be explained by the differences between the study populations (22), medical or surgical recruitment, geographic origin of patients and vascular risk factors, especially age (35). This association therefore tends to become more frequent because patients undergoing surgery for valvular cardiopathy are increasingly elderly, in part due to the overlapping incidence of degenerative etiology (36,37).

Some autopsy studies have suggested a "protective" role for aortic stenosis in coronary atheroma from the observation of an inverse relationship between the severity of valvulopathy and that of coronary damage (38). Clinical studies do not seem to confirm this. There are no significant differences in the incidence of coronary artery disease depending upon the valve affected (15-17,19,22,24,26). It is possible that the coexistence of aortic stenosis leads to an earlier diagnosis of coronary lesions and in turn to a greater incidence of single-vessel disease, but the interpretation of this association as a protective effect of the valvulopathy is debatable. Moreover, in several recent series, a majority of patients had multiple vessel disease (9,27,32,34,39). Several authors have reported an incidence of 19% to 25% of left predominance in cases of aortic stenosis, whilst it is about 10% in the general population (17,18,40).

Non-atheromatous coronary lesions associated with valvular cardiopathies have practically disappeared. They were the syphilitic ostial stenoses and the ostial fibroses seen in the past after coronary canulation during open heart surgery (41). The possibility of coronary emboli should be remembered, especially in the case of mitral stenosis.

Ischemic mitral regurgitation

The incidence of significant ischemic mitral incompetence among ischemic cardiopathies has been estimated to be between 4% and 7% (42-46). It results in spatial changes between different parts of the mitral valve apparatus by three main mechanisms:

- Rupture of the papillary muscle most often affects the posterior muscle supplied by the right coronary or the circumflex artery. It leads to prolapse of the mitral valve into the left atrium, massive mitral incompetence and hemodynamic failure (47), whilst the extent of the adjacent necrosis is often moderate (48,49);
- Papillary dysfunction without rupture results from an ischemic necrosis of the papillary muscle, most often the posterior muscle. The function of the subvalvular apparatus is modified by necrosis and/or papillary fibrosis. The mechanism of the incompetence was initially considered to be mitral valve prolapse (47), but ultrasonic studies seem to show that the restriction in valve movement is associated with a displacement of the point of coaptation on the ventricular side of the annular plane (50).
- Ischemic mitral incompetence can be seen in the absence of a lesion of the papillary muscle. It is the result of areas of adjacent necrosis which alter the geometry of the left ventricle and therefore that of the subvalvular mitral apparatus by displacement of the papillary muscles (47,51). These cases are often associated with extensive necrosis (52) resulting in left ventricular and mitral annular dilation (44).

The differentiation between these three mechanisms is well-established and is widely used in clinical reports (8,43,53,54), even though recent experimental and clinical studies seem to indicate that the abnormalities in parietal kinetics are responsible rather than the papillary muscles themselves (55,56).

DIAGNOSIS

Angina

The positive predictive value of angina is especially poor in the case of aortic stenosis since it may be caused by both coronary lesions and left ventricular hypertrophy. Its value is estimated to be between 30% and 50% of cases (13-19,22-24,26-28,30,33). The figures are similar for aortic incompetence (2,14,20,29,31). The positive predictive value is greater in mitral valvulopathy, but usually remains below 70% (16,19,22,26,57). Analysis of the circumstances of its occurrence or its severity and the distinction between typical angina pain and atypical pain may improve its diagnostic value (19-21,23,33). The indication for coronary arteriography in the presence of angina is not disputed.

On the other hand, the indications for coronary arteriography in the absence of angina have been disputed for a long time; some authors have reported that in the absence of angina valvular cardiopathies, especially aortic stenosis, are not associated with coronary lesions (23,58-61). However, numerous studies have shown the likelihood of significant coronary stenosis in the absence of angina (2,18,19,21,22,24-33,57). In one series (62) triple vessel or left main stenosis was observed in 14% of cases in patients suffering from aortic valve disease in the absence of angina and completely asymptomatic triple vessel disease has also been reported in cases of mitral valve disease (17,19). It is therefore now established that severe coronary lesions may be overlooked if coronary arteriography is not performed in anyone of the patients without angina.

Vascular risk factors

The incidence of coronary artery stenosis associated with aortic or mitral valvulopathy increases with age (19,22,28,35) and is higher in men than in women. Other vascular risk factors, such as family history of coronary artery disease, smoking, arterial hypertension, hypercholesterolemia and diabetes, when considered in isolation, are generally more common in the case of associated coronary illness, but the trend does not always reach (statistical) significance (2,23,31,35). The relationship between the number of risk factors and the incidence of coronary lesions is clearer (63); in a prospective study, the incidence of coronary stenosis increased from 6.2% in the absence of risk factors to 34.9% when at least one risk factor was present, and there was a relationship between the extent and the severity of coronary lesions and the number of risk factors, both for aortic valvulopathy and mitral disease (22).

Electrocardiogram at rest

Repolarization analysis is of no help in the prediction of coronary lesions (16). The presence of coronary Q waves does not appear to be a specific sign of coronary stenosis. Some studies have reported the existence of Q waves in patients without significant coronary stenosis (20,35), especially in the anterior region (35).

Coronary calcification

Coronary calcification on fluoroscopy is found more often in the case of significant coronary stenosis, but it can be seen in its absence (20,24,28).

Hemodynamic data

The aortic gradient is usually lower when coronary stenosis is associated with aortic stenosis than it is when the coronary vessels are normal (20,28,35,39). In mitral stenosis, no significant relationship between hemodynamic parameters and coronary stenosis have been found (21,64).

Myocardial ischemia provocation tests

The diagnostic value in valvulopathy of ECG exercise testing is poor since the frequency of abnormalities in repolarization render the interpretation of their possible changes equivocal (65). Several studies have reported the results of myocardial exercise scintigraphy in the case of aortic stenosis, but the indications remain controversial. Due to the age of patients and their valvulopathy, the level of effort required cannot always be attained, resulting in a reduction in the sensitivity of the test (66). The major problem is the inherent risk of the effort test itself. Studies which have reported a good tolerance of effort tests in the case of aortic stenosis often included only a small number of patients (61,67-70), and rarely involved large numbers (71,72). However, the risk of a mishap occurring on effort exists (73); severe aortic stenosis remains a standard contraindication to the effort test (74) and we do not recommend the widespread use of this technique in these patients.

Moreover, the results do not appear to be completely satisfactory; the specificity is poor since reversible hypofixation frequently occurs in the absence of coronary lesions (65,75), mainly when myocardial hypertrophy is prominent (68). Furthermore, the sensitivity is insufficient, leading to a risk of false negative findings (67-69). Recourse to tomography appears to improve the diagnostic performance, but to the detriment of specificity (70). The alternative of myocardial scintigraphy using dipyridamole has been put forward with the argument that it results in better safety compared with the effort test. One case of death has however been reported in a patient suffering from aortic stenosis (76). The series published by Aubry et al. (77) suggested a specificity of 69% with strict diagnostic criteria and a sensitivity of 95%, inadequate, according to the authors themselves. Myocardial scintigraphy using dipyridamole can be associated with an isometric (hand-grip) test; it is also credited with a specificity and a sensitivity greater than 80% in the case of mitral and aortic valvulopathies (66,78,79). Sensitivity remains inadequate for a routine detection test for coronary disease, however, and can result in false negative findings, even in the case of left main stenosis (66).

Finally, isotope angiographic research on segmental left ventricular kinetic abnormalities on effort do not appear to contribute to the diagnosis of associated coronary disease (80), even though one study showed good sensitivity (81). Thus, due to uncertainty regarding their potential risk and their less than perfect diagnostic value, isotope studies alone cannot be used at the present time for the detection of coronary disease associated with valvular cardiopathy.

Multifactorial analysis

The inadequate diagnostic value of the different published data can be compensated for by taking several of them into account simultaneously; predictive scores for coronary disease have been established in this way, using discriminatory analysis taking several variables into account (28,30,31,39,82). Discriminatory thresholds are generally chosen

Table 6.5-I: Results of aortic valve replacement combined with CABG for patients with aortic valve disease associated with coronary artery disease.

Series	Years of Surgery	No. of Patients AVR+ CABG	AS+ CABG	Mean Age (yr)	Sign.Cad (% diam.)	No of Dis. Vessels*	No of Grafts	Op.death (%)	Peri-op MI (%)	Late Survival (%)
Loop (88)	67-73	80		57	70	1.8(29)	1.3	8.7	-	5 (3.5 yr)
(1977)			54	-	70	1.8(30)	1.3	9.3	-	-
Lundell (91)	73-78	82		60	70	1.9	1.6	19.5	7	-
(1978)			49	-	-	-	-	-	-	-
McManus (100)	70-77	80		63	50	-	1.5	6.3	7.5	75 (5 yr)
(1978)			44	-	-	-	-	-	-	-
Miller (2)	72-77	101		64	60	2.4	1.6	8.9	12	92 (3.5 yr)**
(1979)			87	65	60	2.5	1.6	10.3	12	-
Richardson	70-77	220		59	70	2.1(26)	1.8	5.4	11	74(4 yr)
(1979) (3)			138	-	-	-	-	6	10	-
Reed (92)	78-81	66		63	70	-	3.2	7.6	7.6	-
(1983)										
Nunley (5)	69-81	197		64(26%> 70 yr)	50	(19)	1.6	10.2	8.1	52(10 yr)
(1983)			52	-	-	-	-	-	-	-
Lytle (3,105)	67-81	500		62	70	(23)	1.7	5.8	6.5	52(10 yr)**
(1983-88)			294	-	-	-	-	-	-	-
Cohn (6)	72-83	233		-	-	-	-	9.0	-	58 (9 yr)
(1984)			178	-	-	-	-	7.8	-	-
Donzeau-Gouge	70-81		56	64	-	2(34)	1.3	16	9	68(3 yr)
(1984) (89)										
Magovern (90)	78-84	89		67(34%> 70 yr)	70	-	-	13.5	-	-
(1987)			64	-	70	-	-	14.1	-	-
Mullany (62)	67-76	112	-	-	50	2(34)	1.5	6.3	-	49(10 yr)
(1987)	82-83	99	-	-	50	2.3(48)	2.1	4	-	-
Czer (9)	69-84	233		67(15%> 70 yrs)	50	2.3(52)	2.2	8.2	-	41(10 yr)
(1988)			126	-	-	-	-	-	-	-
Jones (32)	74-82	69		58	50	1.9(39)	1.5	13	17	76(3 yr)
(1989)			18	-	-	-	-	-	-	-
Lund (39)	75-86		55	64	50	2.1(47)	-	3.6	2	62(10 yr)
(1990)										
Iung (34)	79-92		144	69(51%> 70 yrs)	60	2(31)	1.7	10.4	6.9	67(9 yr)
(1993)										

* : mean number of diseased vessels (% of left main stem or 3 vessel disease)
**: among post-operative survivors
AVR: aortic valve replacement; AS: aortic stenosis; CAD: coronary artery disease (minimum % of vessel diameter considered as significant CAD); CABG: coronary artery bypass graft; OP: operative; MI: myocardial infarction.

in order to obtain maximum sensitivity, reducing the number of coronary arteriography investigations without overlooking the coronary lesion. In aortic and mitral valvulopathy (82) and aortic incompetence (31), such scores can decrease the number of coronary arteriography by 30%. In aortic stenosis, studies have concluded that age and sex are predominant factors and that there is therefore a need for coronary arteriography in men over 40 years and in women over 50 (28,30).

Indications for coronary arteriography in the preoperative evaluation of valvular cardiopathy

It is not intended to discuss a possible tolerance threshold for overlooking coronary lesions either in general terms or from an economic point of view (30,83). If one considers that it is not acceptable to overlook coronary stenosis before intervention, an analysis of the literature shows that it is only possible to dispense with coronary arteriography in young patients without angina or any vascular risk factor. Echocardiography often enable a correct recognition of the valvular defect, especially the degree of aortic stenosis. However, the evaluation of the coronary arteries remains dependent upon coronary arteriography (84,85). Moreover, the risk of invasive exploration is very low if it is limited to coronary arteriography.

Thus, according to current American guidelines (86), coronary arteriography is indicated in the preoperative review of valvular cardiopathy; routinely in male patients over 35 years of age and in women following the menopause, irrespective of age, if thoracic pain is present or if the ECG suggests coronary artery disease, or if at least one major vascular risk factor is present. The exception to these rules is a patient with a particularly unstable hemodynamic state requiring urgent surgery (87).

THERAPY

Aortic valve disease

Combined aortic and coronary surgery

Table 6.5-I shows the principal characteristics of patients included in the combined aortic and coronary surgical series comprising more than 50 patients. The main differences between the patients studied were the following:

- most often, it was a global evaluation of aortic valvulopathies including stenosis, insufficiency and mixed disease; few studies report specifically on aortic stenosis (2,34,39,88-90);
- the severity of coronary lesions varied with respect to the degree of stenosis (50% to 70% of the diameter) and especially with regard to the number of stenosed vessels;
- the mean age of patients varied between 57 years (88) and 69 years (34);
- the calendar date of surgery was important; perioperative combined surgical mortality diminished during the 1970's (4-6,32,62,89), notably due to the widespread use of cold potassium induced cardioplegia (89,91). During the 1980's, this tendency was counterbalanced by the increased number of older patients with more severe whose coronary lesions. This explains the persistence of a surgical mortality of about 10% in some recent series (32,34,90).

Several series have compared the immediate results of combined aortic and coronary surgery with those of isolated aortic valve replacement in patients with normal coronary vessels. Operative mortality in combined surgery is often a little higher than it is when the coronary arteries are normal, both in the case of mixed aortic valve disease (9,32,62,90,92) and aortic stenosis (2,34,89,93).

In the majority of comparative series patients with aortic valvulopathy and coronary

Table 6.5-II: Results of aortic valve replacement without CABG for patients with aortic valve disease associated with coronary artery disease.

Series	Years of Surgery	No. of Patients AVR+ CABG	AS+ CABG	Mean Age (yr)	Sign.Cad (% diam.)	No of Dis Vessels	3V or LM Disease[*]	Op.Death (%)	Peri-Op MI (%)	Late Survival (%)
Miller (2) (1979)	72-77	31		63	60	1.7	-	6.5	-	82 (3.3 yr)[**]
Bonow (102) (1981)	72-78	56		59	50	-	18	4	9	74 (4 yr)
Donzeau-Gouge (1984) (89)	70-81		9	65		1.8	30	0	11	78 (2 yr)
Mullany (62) (1987)	67-76	78		-	50	1.7	14	10.3	-	36 (10 yr)
	82-83	32		1	50	1.6	25	9.4	-	-
Czer (9) (1988)	69.84	56	-	67	50	1.6	14	7.1	-	67 (5 yr)
Jones (32) (1989)	74-82	55		61	50	1.3	7.3	16	15	62 (3 yr)
Lund (39) (1990)	75-86		28	66	50	-	14	17.9	7.1	51 (5 yr)
Iung (34) (1993)	79-92		39	71	40(1)	1.4	10	7.7	2.6	91 (5 yr)
			46	67	60(2)	1.5	15	13	2.2	64 (5 yr)

[*] : % of left main stem or 3 vessel disease; [**]: among postoperative survivors. Abbreviations as in Table 6.5-I; (1) moderate coronary artery stenosis (40 to 60%); (2) severe coronary artery stenosis (>60%) non-suitable for CABG.

lesions are older than those with normal coronary vessels (2,9,32,89,90) and sometimes differ in their functional class and left ventricular ejection fraction (9), both known to be independent predictors of surgical outcome (94-97). We have compared patients who had calcified aortic stenosis with or without concomitant coronary heart disease, and who were matched for comparable age, sex, functional class, left ventricular ejection fraction and the year of surgery. Despite matching, a tendency towards greater surgical mortality persisted in the presence of bypassed coronary lesions (10.4% versus 4.9%) (34,98).

The incidence of perioperative infarction mainly depends on the diagnostic criteria used (3,99). It has diminished with cold potassium induced cardioplegia (3,6,9,100).

Long term survival has been improving and recent studies have suggested a survival rate greater than 60% at nine and 10 years (34-39) despite the worsening risk in the patient populations (Table 6.5-I). The functional results are good; more than 70% of patients are in functional class I or II of the NYHA, and the incidence of recurrent angina and coronary events remains low (2,3,32,34,90,92,100).

Published data are more at variance when the long term results of combined surgery are compared with those of isolated aortic valve replacement in the presence of normal coronary arteries. Several series report no increased late mortality after combined surgery (2,3,32) but this observation is not uniform (6,39,88). As with early results, the comparison is biased by the differences between the patient characteristics, mainly by the greater age of those with coronary lesions. In our comparison of a matched series late mortality was not increased in the group undergoing combined surgery compared with those with normal coronary vessels (34). The relationship between the late results and the complete or incomplete nature of coronary revascularization is difficult to establish;

an incomplete revascularization is often associated with less satisfactory late results than a complete revascularization, but patients in whom revascularization is incomplete generally have more severe coronary artery disease (9,34).

Aortic valve disease with non-revascularized coronary lesions

The main series are listed in Table 6.5-II. The absence of revascularization in coronary stenosis can be due to to very different reasons: moderate coronary stenosis (around 50%), tight stenosis unsuitable for bypass for technical reasons, including multiple stenoses with poor runoff, small and/or calcified arteries, and finally the deliberate refusal of revascularization. However, the majority of series do not mention the reason why coronary stenoses in certain patients were not bypassed or do not detail their outcome as a function of these different causes of non-revascularization (2,9,32,39,62,101). The absence of bypass was deliberate only in the series of Bonow (102). Results in the event of technical difficulties are rarely specified (34,89).

When surgical mortality of aortic valve replacement (AVR) without coronary bypass is compared to that of combined surgery, the trend is variable and often not significant (2,9,32,34,93); two series reported a significantly higher surgical mortality in the absence of coronary bypass (39,103). However, the numbers are often small and patients whose coronary stenoses have not been bypassed have a lower number of affected coronary branches than those who have been bypassed (2,9,34). The absence of a significant difference in favor of combined surgery should not therefore be an argument against performing coronary bypass surgery in association with aortic valve replacement, since the patients are not comparable. In the populations under study, the risk of a perioperative infarct remains moderate even in the absence of associated coronary revascularization (2,32,34).

Several authors have noted a tendency towards an increased mortality in the case of isolated AVR compared with combined surgery (2,9,32,34). The functional results are however satisfactory (2,32,34) with, in particular, a frequent disappearance of angina after isolated AVR despite the absence of coronary revascularization (34,89).

Late survival after AVR without coronary surgery in the presence of concomitant caronary heart disease has also been compared to survival after AVR in patients with normal coronary vessels. In the majority of series, survival is significantly lower in the presence of non-bypassed diseased coronary vessels (9,32,34,39,101). The only study finding an identical survival in the two groups was that of Bonow (102) in which the absence of coronary bypass was deliberate. These results must however be interpreted with care as the majority of patients had limited coronary lesions (24 patients with single vessel disease out of 55) and the survivors were only followed up for four years. These limitations of this study have been underlined by several authors (5,104,105).

Finally, the need for coronary bypass can be questioned in the case of moderate coronary stenosis. In a series of combined surgery, the degree of stenosis at which coronary lesions were bypassed varied from 50% to 70%. In our series, the absence of bypass for moderately stenosed coronary vessels (40 to 60%) did not appear to have any detrimental effect on the early and late results, which were comparable to those seen after AVR in aortic stenosis in the absence of coronary lesions (34,106).

Indications for combined aortic and coronary surgery

Only a prospective study with randomization of coronary revascularization in patients presenting with coronary stenosis associated with aortic valvulopathy can provide scientifically indisputable evidence; all published data are retrospective and their interpretation must take into account the different populations studied. However, despite these methodologic limitations, it seems that:

- the principle of the revascularization of left main stenosis is accepted even by those who dispute the benefit of coronary bypass in other settings (102);
- compared with aortic surgery in patients with normal coronary vessels, surgical mortality often tends to be a little higher, but these patients are at greater risk;
- late outcome of combined surgery, whether in terms of survival or functional result, favors bypass for tight coronary stenosis, especially when compared with non-bypassed coronary artery disease.

These observations led us to recommend revascularization for tight coronary stenoses whenever possible in the case of AVR, in keeping with the conclusions of many authors (2-5,100). When coronary lesions cannot be bypassed for technical reasons, the indications for AVR remain the same. In our experience, aortocoronary bypass is not encouraged in the case of moderate (50% or less) coronary stenoses.

Special cases of combined aortic and coronary surgery

Moderate aortic stenosis with tight coronary lesions

The problem of a possible associated AS is present when the indication for coronary bypass exists and the degree of aortic stenosis is between 0.75 cm^2 and 1.5 cm^2. One must therefore take into account the risk linked to a more complex surgical intervention and late morbidity associated with the aortic prosthesis on the one hand and, in the absence of valvular surgery, the risk of the progression of stenosis leading to reintervention in a patient already having undergone bypass surgery on the other (107).

The combination of AVR with coronary bypass seems logical when one can assume a potentially rapid progress of the aortic stenosis, such as stenosis of degenerative origin and major valve calcification (108). However, the progression of stenosis remains, in part, unpredictable, and the indications for AVR must therefore be wide, taking into account the problems posed by reoperation in patients previously bypassed.

Aortic insufficiency

The results of combined surgery in aortic insufficiency with coronary lesions have been more frequently studied, but few series have presented the results according to the type of valvulopathy (2,3,88,90) and comparison of the results with combined surgery for aortic stenosis has given variable results. In one series of 500 AVR with coronary bypasses, 89 of whom had aortic insufficiency, Lytle (4), using multivariate analysis, isolated aortic insufficiency as one of the predictors of higher operative mortality, independent of other factors.

The left ventricular ejection fraction is often a major element in the indications for surgery in the case of aortic insufficiency. When coronary lesions co-exist, the problem

Table 6.5-III: Results of mitral valve replacement associated with CABG for patients with mitral valve disease associated with coronary artery disease.

Series	Years of Surgery	No. of Patients	Etiology (%)	Mean Age (yr)	Sign.Cad (% diam.)	No of Dis Vessels[*]	No of Grafts	Op.Death (%)	Peri-Op MI (%)	Late Survival (%)
Berger (138) (1975)	70-74	16	rh. 50 isch. 50	56	70	1.8	1.5	6.2	6.2	75[**] (1.5 yr)
Rossiter (116) (1975)	71-74	22	-	-	-	-	-	4.5	5	-
Miller (57) (1978)	71-78	97	rh. 36 deg. 37 isch. 27	61 63 60	60 60 60	2.3 } 3.1 } 2.7	1.5	14 17 23	11 3 4	70 (5 yr) 50 (5 yr) 40 (4 yr)
Chaffin (115) (1979)	68-77	12	-	-	-	-		8.3		50 (9 yr)[**]
Wisoff (139) (1979)	70-78	33	-	61	-	-		3.3	-	73 (1.5 yr)
Di Sesa (111) (1982)	72-81	100	rh. 45 isch. 55	62 82	- -	- -	- -	17.8 18.2	- -	- -
Reed (92) (1983)	78-81	28[***]	-	-	70	-	2.4	3.5	25	-
Czer (7) (1984)	69-82	179	rh. 31 } isch. 54 } other 15	63	50	2.5 (71)	-	13.9	-	44 (8 yr)
Lytle (8) (1985)	70-83	300	rh. 34 } isch. 16 } other 50	(54%>60 yr)	70	1.8(25)	1.8	8.8 } 10.6 } 5.3	8.4	33 (10 yr)[**]
Magovern (112) (1985)	77-82	28	-	-	-	-	-	17.8	-	-
Arcidi (128) (1988)	77-83	20	rh. 35 } isch. 30 } other 35	61	-	-	2.3	25		31 (5 yr)
Stahle (110) (1991)	80-88	75	-	63	-	-		16	5.5	-
He (54) (1991)	79-89	135	rh. 35 } isch. 27 } other 38	61	70	2 (55)	2.3	11.8	3	50 (10 yr)[**]

[*] : mean number of diseased vessels (% of left main stem or 3 vessel disease); [**]: among post-operative survivors; [***]: 21 valve replacement + 7 valve repair; CAD: coronary artery disease (minimum % of vessel diameter considered as significant CAD); CABG: coronary artery bypass grafting; OP: operative; MI: myocardial infarction; rh: rheumatic fever; isch: ischemic mitral regurgitation; deg: degenerative mitral valve disease (other include endocarditis, congenital and mainly degenerative mitral valve disease).

may arise of the respective role of aortic incompetence and coronary pathology in the interpretation of left ventricular dysfunction.

In dystrophic aortic insufficiency with aneurysm of the ascending aorta, tissue fragility may compromise the anastomoses of the coronary grafts. Internal mammary graft is desirable in these cases.

Mitral valvulopathies

The relationship between coronary heart disease and mitral valve disease is more complex than it is in the case of aortic valve disease, because

- the coronary disease may not only be associated with mitral valve disease, but might

be the cause in the case of ischemic mitral incompetence;
- valve repair plays a dominant role within the different surgical options.

Combined surgery for mitral valvulopathy: all causes combined

The main data from published series are shown in Table 6.5-III. The data are heterogenous due to the frequent regrouping of different etiologies (109). Surgical mortality is generally higher in the case of ischemic mitral insufficiency than for mitral valvulopathy of non-ischemic origin (7,57,110), especially when the surgery is urgent (110-112).

There is little data on the results of surgery for mitral repair combined with coronary bypass surgery in non-ischemic mitral insufficiency. In a series of 39 cases of mitral surgery with associated coronary bypass (113), surgical mortality was nil in the group consisting of 27 valve repairs and 8.3% in the 12 valve replacements, even though the patients were older in the valve repair group. These observations are in keeping with results of mitral valve repair results in patients with non-ischemic mitral incompetence (114).

When the immediate results of combined mitral and coronary surgery are compared with those of isolated mitral surgery in patients with normal coronary vessels, the operative mortality is higher in the former case (7,57,110,112,115). However, as in the case of aortic valvulopathy, patients without a coronary lesion are generally younger, less symptomatic and have better left ventricular ejection fractions than those with coronary lesions (7,57,110,112), which might explain in part the difference in mortality independent of the state of the coronary vessels.

Isolated mitral valve replacement in the presence of non-bypassed coronary stenosis is accompanied in general by a higher operative mortality than in the case of combined surgery (9,57,115). The number of coronary vessels affected is generally less in non-revascularized patients (7,57).

The use of cold cardioplegia seems to be accompanied by a less clear cut improvement in surgical results in combined mitral surgery than in aortic surgery (7,111). It is possible that the myocardium might be less sensitive to ischemia in mitral than in aortic valvulopathy, where hypertrophy is more commonplace (116). However, in some series, when emergencies are excluded, cold potassium cardioplegia is associated with a significant improvement in short term results in combined mitral and coronary surgery (111).

The poor prognosis for ischemic etiology re-emerges, in general, beyond the period of hospitalization, with a less satisfactory long term survival than in rheumatic or degenerative disease (7,8,57). Functional improvement is clear cut in the majority of series whatever the cause of the valvulopathy (8,9,57,112,115). Even if the differences are not always significant, late survival after combined surgery is usually less good than that seen after isolated mitral valve replacement in patients with normal coronary vessels (9,57,115), including when matched populations are compared (9). In the case of mitral valve replacement without bypass of coronary stenosis, there is often an increased late mortality compared with patients who have undergone combined surgery (9,115).

Combined surgery in ischemic mitral insufficiency

These belong to a heterogenous group, where the different mechanisms responsible

Table 6.5-IV: Results of mitral valve surgery associated with CABG for patients with ischemic mitral regurgitation.

Series	Years of Surgery	No. of Patients	Etiology of MR (%)	Pre-op Status	Mean Age (yr)	3 V or LM Disease	Mitral Surgery	CABG (u)	Op.Death (%)	Late Survival (%)
Radford (1979) (52)	70-75	46 13 other	24 PMR 63 PMD	-	60	-	46 MVR	40	-	73EF>0.35 38 EF<0.35 (4 yrs)
Killen (1979) (49)	71-79	16	100 PMR	50% low-output other 50% CHF	64	7	16 MVR	6	19	75 (5 yr)
Pinson (1984) (117)	70-83	37	38 PMR 27 PMD 35 other	-	-	-	28 MVR 9 Repair } 37		38	44 (5 yrs)
Tepe (1985) (118)	73-83	11	45 PMR 55 PMD	100% shock	60	43	11 MVR	5	54	-
Kay (1986) (43)	70-83	141	50 PMR or PMD 50 other	48% class IV 18% MI<1 month	62	-	40 MVR 101 Repair	40 101	- -	27 (6 yr) 60 (6 yr)
Connolly (1986) (44)	80-84	16	56 PMR 31 PMD 13 other	88% CHF 38% recent MI	64	-	16 MVR	16	19	100% (5 yr)**
Carpentier (1987) (125)	76-86	44	-	25% acute MR 75% chronic MR	-	-	26 MVR 18 Repair } 22		19 11	death:5.1pt/yr death:2.7pt/yr
Hickey (1988) (45)	81-87	59	-	64% class IV	63	61	59 MVR	59	41	55 (5 yrs)
Rankin (1988) (52)	81-87	55	16 PMR 57 PMD 27 other	emergency 67%	63 62	53 83	32 MVR 23 Repair	32 23	53 26	- -

* : % of left main stem or 3 vessel disease; **: among postoperative survivors; MR: mitral regurgitation; OP: operative; MI: myocardial infarction; PMR: papillary muscle rupture; PMD: papillary muscle dysfunction (necrosis, fibrosis excluding rupture); CHF: congestive heart failure; MVR: mitral valve replacement.

for ischemic mitral insufficiency (see above) and the proportion of emergency procedures are taken into account. Results of some important series are shown in Table 6.5-IV. Emergency surgery carries a bad prognosis, whether due to acute mitral insufficiency (45,53), recent infarction (43,44), or more significantly cardiogenic shock (117). The poor hemodynamic tolerance in acute post-infarction mitral insufficiency can, on its own, be related to the volume of regurgitation only, without extensive necrosis (48,52). The prognosis is particularly poor in acute mitral insufficiency in cardiogenic shock, where operative mortality can exceed 50% (117,118). Surgery is justified, however, because of the very poor spontaneous prognosis in these patients, but it must be performed at the earliest possible moment when the hemodynamics become unstable (118).

The other main prognostic factors are left ventricular ejection fraction (52,53,119) and regurgitant volume (44,117). Estimation of the left ventricular ejection fraction is often difficult and tends to be overestimated in cases of severe mitral regurgitation (52,118).

Series which have compared the immediate results of reconstructive surgery and mitral valve replacement in ischemic mitral incompetence show a lower operative mortality with surgical repair (43,45,53), especially when the left ventricular ejection fraction is impaired (43) or when the proportion of emergency cases is high (53). Different annuloplasty techniques are used in reparative surgery for ischemic mitral insufficiency (53,119,120). The use of the semi-rigid Carpentier ring appears to give better short term results in terms of residual mitral incompetence than suture annuloplasty techniques (121). The use of intraoperative transesophageal echocardiography can be of great help (122). Surgical repair can include reimplantation of the papillary muscles (53), but few cases have been reported and the inherent problems of such repair of infarcted tissue and the possible outcome should lead to caution in this specific case.

Pre- and postoperative medical treatment can affect the immediate outcome of surgery for ischemic mitral valve insufficiency. In the acute forms with unstable hemodynamics, intra-aortic balloon counterpulsation or circulatory assistance may be necessary (112). Reperfusion of the artery responsible for the infarct by thrombolysis or angioplasty can lead to a reduction in the degree of mitral incompetence (45) and a dramatic improvement in the hemodynamic state, including patients in cardiogenic shock (123). Early coronary reperfusion could obviate in certain cases mitral valve surgery (53,123), but this remains necessary after a brief delay in the absence of a rapid improvement in the hemodynamics (46,124). A fall in the extent of mitral insufficiency has sometimes been observed in the event of late reperfusion.

One of the determinant factors of late survival in patients undergoing surgery for mitral insufficiency is left ventricular ejection fraction (43,52,53,117). Therefore, patients with mitral insufficiency due to infarction or chordal/papillary rupture have a better prognosis than those with mitral insufficiency related to extensive abnormalities of segmental kinetics of the left ventricle (46,49,52).

Late survival is better after surgical repair than after mitral valve replacement in comparative studies (43,45,53,125), especially when the preoperative left ventricular ejection fraction is altered (43), which can be related to the better preservation of left ventricular function due to the preservation of the entire valvular and sub-valvular apparatus after mitral valve repair (126).

Long term post-surgical functional improvement is often clear cut, even in the case of an initial deterioration of the left ventricular ejection fraction (43,52). When resection of a left ventricular aneurysm is associated, the results vary according to the published series, but good functional results are possible (52,127).

Indications for combined mitral valve and coronary surgery in the case of moderate mitral insufficiency

When the indication for coronary revascularization is present and mitral incompetence is moderate, the opportunity to operate on the mitral valve should be considered. Some authors have recommended avoiding mitral valve replacement due to the better long term results obtained after coronary bypass alone (128). The regurgitant volume of an ischemic mitral valve can diminish following isolated bypass (42), and late survival can therefore be good when mitral insufficiency is moderate (85% at five years) (117). Other studies have however reported an increased late mortality in the absence of the correction of mitral incompetence (44).

When the mitral insufficiency is moderate, the combination of valve replacement and coronary bypass does not therefore seem to be necessarily routine. On the other hand, the good results of surgical repair in ischemic mitral insufficiency must lead to a widening of these indications for the correction of moderate mitral incompetence (45).

Special aspects of the combined treatment of valvular and coronary lesions

Repeat cardiac surgery

Combined surgical intervention may be necessary at reoperation, following prior isolated valve surgery. The presence of associated coronary artery disease increases the risk of further surgery; Lytle found an operative mortality of 17% in 41 patients undergoing redo aortic valve replacement associated with coronary bypass prior to 1984 (129) (compared with 11% during repeated surgery in the absence of bypass) and 7.2% of 69 patients undergoing repeat surgery between 1985 and 1989 (130).

Reoperation in patients who have already undergone combined valvular and coronary surgery leads to technical difficulties related to pericardial adhesions and the risk of trauma or atheromatous emboli linked to pre-existing coronary bypass grafts (131). Coronary grafts can hamper the exposure of the aortic prosthesis. Moreover, it is necessary to ensure myocardial perfusion via the original coronaries but also from the grafts; retrograde cardioplegia is particularly beneficial in these cases (130).

Prosthesis selection

Some series of combined valvular and coronary surgery have demonstrated better survival with bioprostheses than with mechanical valves, whether in the aortic (6,105) or in the mitral (8) position, but their conclusions were not unanimous (9,90). Above all, these series consisted of a small number of patients whose follow up exceeded seven to 10 years, by which time primary degeneration of the bioprostheses occurs. There appear to be a downwards slope in overall survival (9) and/or survival without complications from the sixth year (105,132).

Taking into account the potential risk of reintervention, it seems preferable to use mechanical prostheses in the case of combined valvular and coronary surgery. The choice of a bioprosthesis on the other hand, seems to be acceptable in elderly patients aged over 75 years, taking into account their life expectancy, the iatrogenic potential of anticoagulant therapy and the lower level of primary bioprosthetic degeneration in this age group (132,133).

Selection of coronary bypass graft type

Certain series have reported the use of mammary grafts for coronary revascularization associated with valve surgery (34,44,53,54,91,110), but, the cases are not very numerous. Even if the long term advantages of internal mammary grafts are no longer disputed, their use in combined surgery is still controversial due to the length of surgery and the possible inadequate blood flow from a mammary graft to a hypertrophied myocardium in the case of an aortic stenosis (130). In a series of 102 patients who underwent combined surgery with at least one mammary graft, Lytle did not observe any change in mortality or in perioperative morbidity as compared to a matching group with saphenous grafts only (130). Long follow up information is necessary in order to evaluate the long term benefit of the use of internal mammary grafts in combined surgery, but their longevity is particularly interesting for those patients in whom reoperation would be complex.

Multiple valve replacement associated with coronary artery surgery

The results of multiple valve replacement with coronary bypass are rarely described in isolation, and the numbers are limited (134-136). Operative mortality is 12.1% in the largest series of 33 patients (136) and survival at six years is 61%. Myocardial protection is especially important in these lengthy operations (134,136).

The place of coronary angioplasty in the treatment of lesions associated with valvular cardiopathy

Coronary angioplasty can be of interest in certain aortic valvulopathies, including:

- moderate aortic stenosis associated with significant and symptomatic coronary stenosis, where coronary angioplasty, if technically feasible, has the advantage over surgery in not posing the problem of possible aortic valve replacement when the valvulopathy is of minor importance (see above);
- as a complement to surgery in certain distal non-bypassable stenoses;
- in the event of new stenoses in the native coronary arteries or within the bypass grafts in patients who have already undergone a combined procedure and in whom further surgery would be difficult.

Cases of combined dilation of the aortic valve and coronary angioplasty of single-vessel disease have been reported (137), but they should be considered only as palliative procedures.

The benefit of coronary angioplasty in mitral insufficiency of ischaemic origin has been emphasized (see above). Emergency coronary reperfusion can result in a reduction in the volume of mitral regurgitation and a dramatic and long lasting improvement in the hemodynamic state (45,123).

References

1. Flemma RJ, Johnson WD, Lepley D, Auer JE, Tector AJ, Blitz J. Simultaneous valve replacement and aorta-to-coronary saphenous vein bypass. Ann Thorac Surg 1971;12:163-170
2. Miller DC, Stinson EB, Oyer PE, Rossiter SJ, Reitz BA, Shumway NE. Surgical implications and results of combined aortic valve replacement and myocardial revascularization. Am J Cardiol 1979;43:494-501
3. Richardson JV, Kouchoukos NT, Wright JO, Karp RB. Combined aortic valve replacement and myocardial revascularization: Results in 220 patients. Circulation 1979;59:75-81
4. Lytle BW, Cosgrove DM, Loop FD et al. Replacement of aortic valve combined with myocardial revascularization: determinants of early and late risk for 500 patients, 1967-1981. Circulation 1983;68:1149-1162
5. Nunley DL, Grunkemeier GL, Starr A. Aortic valve replacement with coronary bypass grafting. J Thorac Cardiovasc Surg 1983;85:705-711
6. Cohn LH, Allred EN, DiSesa VJ, Sawtelle K, Shemin RJ, Collins JJ. Early and late risk of aortic valve replacement. A 12 year concomitant comparison of the porcine bioprosthetic and tilting disc prosthetic aortic valves. J Thorac Cardiovasc Surg 1984;88:695-705

7. Czer LSC, Gray RJ, DeRobertis MA et al. Mitral valve replacement: impact of coronary artery disease and determinants of prognosis after revascularization. Circulation 1984;70(Suppl I):198-207

8. Lytle BW, Cosgrove DM, Gill CC et al. Mitral valve replacement combined with myocardial revascularization: early and late results for 300 patients, 1970 to 1983. Circulation 1985;71:1179-1190

9. Czer LS, Gray RJ, Stewart ME, De Robertis M, Chaux A, Matloff JM. Reduction in sudden late death by concomitant revascularization with aortic valve replacement J Thorac Cardiovasc Surg 1988;95:390-401

10. Coleman EH, Soloff LA. Incidence of significant coronary artery disease in rheumatic valvular heart disease. Am J Cardiol 1970;25:401-404

11. Tadavarthy SM, Vlodaver Z, Edwards JE. Coronary atherosclerosis in subjects with mitral stenosis. Circulation 1976;54:519-521

12. Reis RN, Roberts WC. Amounts of coronary arterial narrowing by atherosclerotic plaques in clinically isolated mitral valve stenosis: analysis of 76 necropsy patients older than 30 years. Am J Cardiol 1986;57:1117-1123

13. Harris CN, Kaplan MA, Parker DP, Dunne EF, Cowell HS, Ellestad MH. Aortic stenosis, angina, and coronary artery disease interrelations. Br Heart J 1975;37:656-661

14. Graboys TB, Cohn PF. The prevalence of angina pectoris and abnormal coronary arteriograms in severe aortic valvular disease. Am Heart J 1977;93:683-686

15. Lacy J, Goodin R, McMartin D, Masden R, Flowers N. Coronary atherosclerosis in valvular heart disease. Ann Thorac Surg 1977;23;429-435

16. Baxter RH, Reid JM, McGuiness JB, Stevenson JG. Relation of angina to coronary artery disease in mitral and in aortic valve disease. Br Heart J 1978;40:918-922

17. Vacheron A Metzger JPh, Heulin A, Lafont H, Georges Ch, Di Matteo J. La coronarographie dans l'exploration pre-operatoire des valvulopathies acquises non ischemiques. Arch Mal Coeur 1978;11:1233-1238

18. Storstein O, Enge I. Angina pectoris in aortic valvular disease and its relation to coronary pathology. Acta Med Scand 1979;205:275-278

19. Morrisson GW, Thomas RD, Grimmer SFM, Silverton PN, Smith DR. Incidence of coronary artery disease in patients with valvular heart disease. Br Heart J 1980;44:630-637

20. Hakki AH, Kimbiris D, Iskandrian AS, Segal BL, Mintz GS, Bemis CE. Angina pectoris and coronary artery disease in patients with severe aortic valve disease. Am Heart J 1980;100:441-449

21. Chun PKC, Gertz E, Davia JE, Cheitlin MD. Coronary atherosclerosis in mitral stenosis. Chest 1982;81:36-41

22. Ramsdale DR, Bennett DH, Bray CL, Ward C, Beton DC, Faragher EB. Angina, coronary risk factors and coronary artery disease in patients with valvular disease. A prospective study. Eur Heart J 1984;5:716-726

23. Exadactylos N, Sugrue DD, Oakley CA. Prevalence of coronary artery disease in patients with isolated aortic valve stenosis. Br Heart J 1984;51:121-124

24. Danchin N, Khalife K, Neimann JL et al. Etude retrospective du role de la coronarographie systematique chez les patients valvulaires. Arch Mal Coeur 1984;9:1026-1032

25. Enriquez-Sarano M, Houllegatte JP, Luxereau Ph, Vahanian A, Acar J. Resultats et indications de la coronarographie dans les valvulopathies mitrales. Arch Mal Coeur 1985;78:65-71

26. Olofsson BO, Bjerle P, Aberg T, Osterman G, Jacobsson KA. Prevalence of coronary artery disease in patients with valvular heart disease. Acta Med Scand 1985;218:365-371

27. Monsuez JJ, Drobinski G, Verdiere C, Chollet D, Grosgogeat Y. Etude prospective de la frequence de l'atteinte coronarienne en cas de retrecissement aortique pur. Ann Cardiol Angeiol 1985;34:65-69

28. Acar J, Luxereau Ph, Vahanian A et al. Should coronary angiography be performed in all patients who undergo catheterization for valvular heart disease? Z Kardiol 1986;75(Suppl II):53-60

29. Pathak R, Padmanabhan VT, Tortolani AJ, Ong LY, Hall MH, Pizzarello RA. Angina pectoris and coronary artery disease in isolated, severe aortic regurgitation. Am J Cardiol 1986;57:649-651

30. Vandeplas A, Willems JL, Piessens J, De Geest H. Frequency of angina pectoris and coronary artery disease in severe isolated valvular aortic stenosis. Am J Cardiol 1988;62:117-120

31. Timmermans Ph, Willems JL, Piessens J, De Geest H. Angina pectoris and coronary artery disease in severe aortic regurgitation. Am J Cardiol 1988;61:826-829

32. Jones M, Schofield PM, Brooks NH et al. Aortic valve replacement with combined myocardial revascularisation. Br Heart J 1989;62:9-15

33. Chobadi R, Wurzel M, Teplitsky I, Menkes H, Tamari I. Coronary artery disease in patients 35 years of age or older with valvular aortic stenosis. Am J Cardiol 1989;64:811-812

34. Iung B, Drissi MF, Michel PL et al. Prognosis of valve replacement for aortic stenosis with or without coexisting coronary heart disease: a comparative study. J Heart Valve Dis 1993;2:430-439

35. Hancock EW. Aortic stenosis, angina pectoris, and coronary artery disease. Am Heart 1977;93:382-393

36. Selzer A. Changing aspect of the natural history of valvular aortic stenosis. N Engl J Med 1987;317:91-98

37. Acar J, Michel PL, Dorent R et al. Evolution des etiologies des valvulopathies operees en France sur une

periode de 20 ans. Arch Mal Coeur 1992;85:411-415

38. Nakib A, Lillehei CW, Edwards JE. The degree of coronary atherosclerosis in aortic valvular disease. Arch Pathol 1965;80:517-520

39. Lund O, Nielsen TT, Pilegaard HK, Magnussen K, Knudsen MA. The influence of coronary artery disease and bypass grafting on early and late survival after valve replacement for aortic stenosis. J Thorac Cardiovasc Surg 1990;100:327-337

40. Murphy ES, Rosch J, Rahimtoola SH. Frequency and significance of coronary arterial dominance in isolated aortic stenosis. Am J Cardiol 1977;39:505-509

41. Luxereau Ph, Vasile N, Pouget P, Duron F, Grimberg D, Acar J. Pathologie coronarienne et valvulopathies. Depistage et incidences therapeutiques. Coeur 1975;(N.special):801-809

42. Balu V, Hershowitz S, Zaki Masud AR, Bhayana JN, Dean DC. Mitral regurgitation in coronary artery disease. Chest 1982;81;550-555

43. Kay GL, Kay JH, Zubiate P, Yokoyama T, Mendez M. Mitral valve repair for mitral regurgitation secondary to coronary artery disease. Circulation 1986;74(Suppl II):88-98

44. Connolly MW, Gelbfish JS, Jacobowitz IJ et al. Surgical results for mitral regurgitation from coronary artery disease. J Thorac Cardiovasc Surg 1986;91:379-388

45. Hickey MStJ, Smith LR, Muhlbaier LH et al. Current prognosis of ischemic mitral regurgitation implications for future management. Circulation 1988(Suppl I):51-59

46. Rankin JS, Hickey MStJ, Smith LR et al. Ischemic mitral regurgitation. Circulation 1989;79(Suppl I):116-121

47. Burch GE, DePasquale NP, Phillips JH . The syndrome of papillary muscle dysfunction. Am Heart J 1968;75:399-414

48. Wei JY, Hutchins GM, Bulkley BH. Papillary muscle rupture in fatal acute myocardial infarction. Ann Intern Med 1979;90:149-153

49. Killen DA, Reed WA, Wathanacharoen S, Beauchamp G, Rutherford B. Surgical treatment of papillary muscle rupture. Ann Thorac Surg 1983;35:243-248

50. Godley RW, Wann LS, Rogers EW, Feigenbaum H, Weyman AE. Incomplete mitral leaflet closure in patients with papillary muscle dysfunction. Circulation 1981;63:565-571

51. Kono T, Sabbah HN, Stein PD, Brymer JF, Khaja F. Left ventricular shape as a determinant of functional mitral regurgitation in patients with severe heart failure secondary to either coronary artery disease or idiopathic dilated cardiomyopathy. Am J Cardiol 1991;68:355-359

52. Radford MJ, Johnson RA, Buckley MJ, Daggett WM, Leinbach RC, Gold HK. Survival following mitral valve replacement for mitral regurgitation due to coronary artery disease. Circulation 1979;60(Suppl I):39-47

53. Rankin JS, Feneley MP, Hickey MStJ et al. A clinical comparison of mitral valve repair versus valve replacement in ischemic mitral regurgitation. J Thorac Cardiovasc Surg 1988;95:165-177

54. He GW, Hughes CF, McCaughan B et al. Mitral valve replacement combined with coronary artery operation: determinants of early and late results. Ann Thorac Surg 1991;51:916-923

55. Fehrenbacher G, Schmidt DH, Bommer WJ. Evaluation of transient mitral regurgitation in coronary artery disease. Am J Cardiol 1991;68:868-873

56. Kaul S, Spotnitz WD, Glasheen WP, Touchstone DA. Mechanism of ischemic mitral regurgitation. An experimental evaluation. Circulation 1991;84:2167-2180

57. Miller DC, Stinson EB, Rossiter SJ, Oyer PE, Reitz BA, Shumway NE. Impact of simultaneous myocardial revascularization on operative risk, functional result, and survival following mitral valve replacement. Surgery 1978;84:848-857

58. Bonchek LI, Anderson RP, Rosch J. Should coronary arteriography be performed routinely before valve replacement? Am J Cardiol 1973;31:462-466

59. Berndt TB, Hancock EW, Shumway NE, Harrison DC. Aortic valve replacement with and without coronary artery bypass surgery. Circulation 1974;50:967-971

60. Basta LL, Raines D, Najjar S, Kioschos JM. Clinical, haemodynamic and coronary angiographic correlates of angina pectoris in patients with severe aortic valve disease. Br Heart J 1975;37:150-157

61. Nylander E, Ekman I, Marklund T, Sinnerstad B, Karlsson E, Wranne B. Severe aortic stenosis in elderly patients. Br Heart J 1986;55:480-487

62. Mullany CJ, Elveback LR, Frye RL et al. Coronary artery disease and its management: influence on survival in patients undergoing aortic valve replacement. J Am Coll Cardiol 1987;10:66-72

63. Ramsdale DR, Bennett DH, Bray CL, Ward C, Beton DC, Faragher EB. Coronary arteriography prior to valve replacement. Eur Heart J 1981;2:83-86

64. Mattina CJ, Green SJ, Tortolani AJ et al. Frequency of angiographically significant coronary arterial narrowing in mitral stenosis. Am J Cardiol 1986;57:802-805

65. Aronow WS, Harris CN. Treadmill exercise test in aortic stenosis and mitral stenosis. Chest 1975;68:507-509

66. Huikuri HV, Korhonen UR, Ikaheimo MJ, Heikkila J, Takkunen JT. Detection of coronary artery disease by thallium imaging using a combined intravenous dipyridamole and isometric handgrip test in patients with aortic valve stenosis. Am J Cardiol 1987;59:336-340

67. Bailey IK, Come PC, Kelly DT at al. Thallium 201 myocardial perfusion imaging in aortic valve stenosis. Am J Cardiol 1977;40:889-899

68. Pfisterer M, Muller-Brand J, Brundler H, Cueni T. Prevalence and significance of reversible radionuclide ischemic perfusion defects in symptomatic aortic valve disease patients with or without concomitant coronary disease. Am Heart J 1982;103:92-96

69. Huikuri HV, Korhonen UR, Heikkila J, Takkunen JT. Detection of coronary artery disease by thallium scintigraphy in patients with valvar heart disease. Br Heart J 1986;56:146-151

70. Kupari M, Virtanen KS, Turto H et al. Exclusion of coronary artery disease by exercise thallium 201 tomography in patients with aortic valve stenosis. Am J Cardiol 1992;70:635-640

71. Areskog NH. Exercise testing in the evaluation of patients with valvular aortic stenosis. Clin Physiol 1984;4:201-208

72. Linderholm H, Osterman G, Teien D. Detection of coronary artery disease by means of exercise ECG in patients with aortic stenosis. Acta Med Scand 1985;218:181-188

73. Atwood JE, Kawanishi S, Myers J, Froelicher VF. Exercise testing in patients with aortic stenosis. Chest 1988;93:1083-1087

74. Schlant RC, Friesinger GC, Leonard JL et al. ACP/ACC/AHA Task Force Statement. Clinical competence in exercise testing. J Am Coll Cardiol 1990;16:1061-1065

75. Candell-Riera J, Castell-Conesa J, Ortega-Alcade D. Detection of coronary artery disease by thallium scintigraphy in patients with valvar heart disease (letter). Br Heart J 1987;57:393-394

76. Friedman HZ, Goldberg SF, Hauser AM, O'Neill. Death with dipyridamole thallium imaging. Ann Intern Med 1988;109:990-991

77. Aubry P, Assayag P, Faraggi M et al. Detection d'une maladie coronarienne avant chirurgie valvulaire. Apport de la scintigraphie myocardique sous dipyridamole. Ann Cardiol Angeiol 1991;40:9-13

78. Huikuri HV, Airaksinen KEJ, Ikaheimo MJ, Korhonen UR, Heikkila J, Takkunen JT. Detection of coronary artery disease by dipyridamole thallium tomography in mitral valve stenosis. Am J Cardiol 1989;63:124-126

79. Kettunen R, Huikuri HV, Heikkila J, Takkunen JT. Preoperative diagnosis of coronary artery disease in patients with valvular heart disease using technetium-99m isonitrile tomographic imaging together with high-dose dipyridamole and handgrip exercise. Am J Cardiol 1992;69:1442-1445

80. Hecht HS, Hopkins JM. Exercise-induced regional wall motion abnormalities on radionuclide angiography: lack of reliability for detection of coronary artery disease in the presence of valvular heart disease. Am J Cardiol 1981;47:861-865

81. Milanes JC, Paldi J, Romero M, Goodwin D, Hultgren HN. Detection of coronary artery disease in aortic stenosis by exercise gated nuclear angiography. Am J Cardiol 1984;54:787-791

82. Ramsdale DR, Faragher EB, Bennett DH, Bray CL, Ward C, Beton DC. Preoperative prediction of significant coronary artery disease in patients with valvular heart disease. Br Med J 1982;284:223-226

83. Georgeson S, Meyer KB, Pauker SG. Decision analysis in clinical cardiology: when is coronary angiography required in aortic stenosis? J Am Coll Cardiol 1990;155:751-762

84. Nitter-Hauge S, Ihlen H. May non-invasive methods replace catheterization in quantification of aortic stenosis? Eur Heart J 1988(Suppl E):101-104

85. Miller FA. Aortic stenosis: most cases no longer require invasive hemodynamic study. J Am Coll Cardiol 1989;13:551-553

86. Ross J, Brandenburg RO, Dinsmore RE et al. Guidelines for coronary angiography: a report of the American College of Cardiology/American Heart Association task force on assessment of diagnostic and therapeutic cardiovascular procedures (subcommittee on coronary angiography). J Am Coll Cardiol 1987;10:935-950

87. Roberts WC. Reasons for cardiac catheterization before cardiac-valve replacement. N Engl J Med 1982;306:1291-1293

88. Loop FD, Phillips DF, Roy M, Taylor PC, Groves LK, Effler DB. Aortic valve replacement combined with myocardial revascularization. Circulation 1977;55:169-173

89. Donzeau-Gouge P, Blondeau Ph, Enriquez O et al. Retrecissement aortique calcifie et coronarographie. A propos de 115 operes. Arch Mal Coeur 1984;77:856-864

90. Magovern JA, Pennock JL, Campbell DB et al. Aortic valve replacement and combined aortic valve replacement and coronary artery bypass grafting: Predicting high risk groups. J Am Coll Cardiol 1987;9:38-43

91. Lundell DC, Laks H, Geha AS, Khachane VB, Hammond GL. The importance of myocardial protection in combined aortic valve replacement and myocardial revascularization. Ann Thor Surg 1978;28:501-506

92. Reed GE, Sanoudos GM, Pooley RW et al. Results of combined valvular and myocardial revascularization

operations. J Thorac Cardiovasc Surg 1983;85:422-426
93. Sethi GK, Miller DC, Souchek J et al. Clinical, hemodynamic and angiographic predictors of operative mortality in patients undergoing single valve replacement. J Thorac Cardiovasc Surg 1987;93:884-897
94. Scott WC, Miller DC, Haverich A et al. Determinants of operative mortality for patients undergoing aortic valve replacement. Discriminant analysis of 1479 operations. J Thorac Cardiovasc Surg 1985;89:400-413
95. Cormier B, Luxereau P, Bloch C et al. Prognosis and long term results of surgically treated aortic stenosis. Eur Heart J 1988;9(Suppl E):113-120
96. Craver JM, Weintraub WS, Jones EL, Guyton RA, Hatcher CR. Predictors of mortality, complications, and length of stay in aortic valve replacement for aortic stenosis. Circulation 1988;78(Suppl I):85-90
97. Lund O, Pilegaard H, Nielsen TT, Knudsen MA, Magnussen K. Thirty-day mortality after valve replacement for aortic stenosis over the last 22 years. A multivariate risk stratification. Eur Heart J 1991;12:322-331
98. Iung B, Michel PL, De Pamphilis O et al. Pronostic apres remplacement valvulaire aortique pour retrecissement aortique avec ou sans lesions coronaires associees. Arch Mal Coeur 1993;86:231-236
99. McGregor CGA, MacLeod MD, Muir AL, Smith AF, Hannan WJ, Miller HC. Myocardial infarction related to valve replacement surgery. Br Heart J 1984;51:612-617
100. Macmanus Q, Grunkemeier G, Lambert L, Dietl C, Starr A. Aortic valve replacement and aorta-coronary bypass surgery. J Thorac Cardiovasc Surg 1978;75:865-869
101. Copeland JG, Griepp RB, Stinson EB, Shumway NE. Long term follow up after isolated aortic valve replacement. J Thorac Cardiovasc Surg 1977;74:875-889
102. Bonow RO, Kent KM, Rosing D et al. Aortic valve replacement without myocardial revascularization in patients with combined aortic valvular and coronary artery disease. Circulation 1981;63:243-251
103. Christakis GT, Weisel RD, David TE, Salerno TA, Ivanov J and the cardiovascular surgeons at the University of Toronto. Predictors of operative survival after valve replacement. Circulation 1988;78(Suppl I):25-34
104. Kirklin JW, Kouchoukos NT. Aortic valve replacement without myocardial revascularization. Circulation 1981;61:252-253
105. Lytle BW, Cosgrove DM, Gill CC. Aortic valve replacement combined with myocardial revascularization. J Thorac Cardiovasc Surg 1988;95:402-414
106. Iung B, De Pamphilis O, Michel PL et al. Influence of moderate coronary artery disease on the prognosis of isolated aortic valve replacement for aortic stenosis (abstract). Eur Heart J 1992;13(Suppl):141
107. Sindhi R, Belisle J, Cleveland R, Diehl JT. Patch aortotomy for aortic valve replacement after previous coronary artery bypass surgery. Ann Thorac Surg 1991;51:676-677
108. Wagner S, Selzer A. Patterns of progression of aortic stenosis: a longitudinal hemodynamic study. Circulation 1981;65:709-712
109. Karp RB. Mitral valve replacement and coronary artery bypass grafting. Ann Thorac Surg 1982;34:480-481
110. Stahle E, Bergstrom R, Malm T, Nystrom SO, Hansson HE. Early results of mitral valve replacement. Scand J Thor Cardiovasc Surg 1991;25:179-184
111. DiSesa VJ, Cohn LH, Collins JJ, Koster JK, Van Devanter S. Determinants of operative survival following combined mitral valve replacement and coronary revascularization. Ann Thorac Surg 1982;34:482-489
112. Magovern JA, Pennock JL, Campbell DB, Pierce WS, Waldhausen JA. Risks of mitral valve replacement and mitral valve replacement with coronary artery bypass. Ann Thorac Surg 1985;39:346-352
113. Cohn LH, Couper GS, Kinchla NM, Collins JJ. Decreased operative risk of surgical treatment of mitral regurgitation with or without coronary artery disease. J Am Coll Cardiol 1990;16:1575-1578
114. Michel PL, Iung B, Blanchard B, Luxereau P, Dorent R, Acar J. Long term results of mitral valve repair for non-ischemic mitral regurgitation. Eur Heart J 1991;12(Suppl B):39-43
115. Chaffin JS, Daggett WM. Mitral valve replacement: a nine-year follow up of risks and survivals. Ann Thorac Surg 1979;27:312-319
116. Rossiter SJ, Hultgren HN, Kosek JC, Wuerflein RD, Angell WW. Myocardial damage in combined valvular and coronary bypass surgery. Circulation 1975;51(Suppl I):119-125
117. Pinson CW, Cobanoglu A, Metzdorff MT, Grunkemeier GL, Kay PH, Starr A. Late surgical results for ischemic mitral regurgitation. Role of wall motion score and severity of regurgitation. J Thorac Cardiovasc Surg 1984;88:663-670
118. Tepe NA, Edmunds LH Jr. Operation for acute postinfarction mitral insufficiency and cardiogenic shock. J Thorac Cardiovasc Surg 1985;89:525-530
119. Kay JH, Zubiate P, Mendez MA, Vanstrom N, Yokoyama T, Gharavi MA. Surgical treatment of mitral insufficiency secondary to coronary artery disease. J Thorac Cardiovasc Surg 1980;79:12-18
120. Carpentier A, Chauvaud S, Fabiani JN et al. Reconstructive surgery of mitral valve incompetence. J Thorac Cardiovasc Surg 1980;79:338-348
121. Czer LSC, Maurer G, Trento A et al. Comparative efficacy of ring and suture annuloplasty for ischemic mitral regurgitation. Circulation 1992;86(Suppl II):46-52

122. Sheikh KH, Bengston JR, Rankin JS, De Bruijn NP, Kisslo J. Intraoperative transoesophageal doppler color flow imaging used to guide patient selection and operative treatment of ischemic mitral regurgitation. Circulation 1991;84:594-604
123. Shawl FA, Forman MB, Punja S, Goldbaum TS. Emergent coronary angioplasty in the treatment of acute ischemic mitral regurgitation: long term results in five cases. J Am Coll Cardiol 1989;14:986-991
124. Le Feuvre C, Metzger JP, Lachurie ML, Georges JL, Baubion N, Vacheron A. Treatment of severe mitral regurgitation caused by ischemic papillary muscle dysfunction: indications for coronary angioplasty. Am Heart J 1992;123:860-865
125. Carpentier A, Loulmet D, Deloche A, Perier P. Surgical anatomy and management of ischemic mitral valve incompetence. Circulation 1987;76(Suppl IV):446
126. Bonchek LI, Olinger GN, Siegel R, Tresch DD, Keelan MH. Left ventricular performance after mitral reconstruction for mitral regurgitation. J Thorac Cardiovasc Surg 1984;88:122-127
127. Gold FL, Sharma B, Hodges M, Helseth HK. Combined left ventricular aneurysmectomy, mitral valve replacement and aortocoronary bypass grafting: results of surgery. Circulation 1980;62(Suppl I):147-152
128. Arcidi JM, Hebeler RF, Craver JM, Jones EL, Hatcher CRJr, Guyton RA. Treatment of moderate mitral regurgitation and coronary disease by coronary bypass alone. J Thorac Cardiovasc Surg 1988;95:951-959
129. Lytle BW, Cosgrove DM, Taylor PC et al. Reoperations for valve surgery: perioperative mortality and determinants of risk for 1000 patients, 1958-1984. Ann Thorac Surg 1986;42:632-643
130. Lytle BW. Impact of coronary artery disease on valvular heart surgery. Cardiol Clin 1991;9:301-314
131. Dor V, Mermet B, Kreitmann P at al. Chirurgie valvulaire et coronaire associee. Problemes tactiques, techniques et resultats. Arch Mal Coeur 1981;74:1045-1052
132. Lytle BW, Cosgrove DM, Taylor PC et al. Primary isolated aortic valve replacement. Early and late results. J Thorac Cardiovasc Surg 1989;97:675-694
133. Jamieson WRE, Rosado LJ, Munro AI et al. Carpentier-Edwards standard porcine bioprosthesis: primary tissue failure (structural valve deterioration) by age groups. Ann Thorac Surg 1988;46:155-162
134. Okies JE, Phillips SJ, Chaitman BR, Starr A. Technical consideration in multiple valve and coronary artery surgery. J Thorac Cardiovasc Surg 1974;67:762-769
135. Stephenson LW, Edie RN, Harken AH, Edmunds LH. Combined aortic and mitral valve replacement. Changes in practice and prognosis. Circulation 1984;69:640-644
136. Akins CW, Buckley MJ, Daggett WM, Hilgenberg AD, Austen G. Myocardial revascularization with combined aortic and mitral valve replacements. J Thorac Cardiovasc Surg 1985;90:272-277
137. Hamad N, Pichard A, Lindsay J. Combined coronary angioplasty and aortic valvuloplasty. Am J Cardiol 1988;60:1184-1185
138. Berger TJ, Karp RB, Kouchoukos NT. Valve replacement and myocardial revascularization. Results of combined operation in 59 patients. Circulation 1975;51(Suppl I):126-131
139. Wisoff BG, Fogel R, Weisz D, Garvey J, Hamby R. Combined valve and coronary artery surgery. Ann Thorac Surgery 1980;29:440-443

Chapter 6.6

Asymptomatic Heart Valve Disease

Jean Acar, Jean-Pierre Laborde, Jean-Pierre Delahaye, Guy De Givegney

The advances in cardiac surgery in terms of myocardial protection, conservative surgical techniques, and replacement devices lead one to envisage early surgery for certain patients while valvular dysfunction is severe but remains asymptomatic.

It is important, however, clearly to state what is defined under the terms asymptomatic or minimally symptomatic patients. This group should include patients without any functional disorder and those who only have a slight limitation in their physical activity (NYHA classes I and II). This selection, based on questioning the patient, is subject to certain errors due to the cardiologist (questioning which is too fast, not objective, or badly orientated) or to the patient (memory gaps, or difficulty of expression for various reasons). Therefore, specific information from the patient and family, and sometimes near relations, on the patient's professional activities and daily life is indispensable before any functional classification is made.

Another cause of error is to be avoided; certain patients considering themselves to be without symptoms are, in fact, falsely asymptomatic and should be excluded from this group. The physician must take into account not only the current period but the clinical history. The patient may have had a transient pulmonary oedema but has been able to resume his activity as previously without symptoms. In our opinion he should not be included in NYHA functional class I or II because a pulmonary oedema attack, even if it is transient, has, with certain valvular lesions, a well-defined prognostic value.

Other patients do not complain because they have reduced their activity as the disease advanced and adapted it to their capacity. This is often the case among the elderly with valvular lesions. In these difficult cases, an exercise test may be useful (treadmill and bicycle ergometry or more practically simple stair climbing) but valvular lesions must be taken into account; severe aortic stenosis is for most authors a contraindication to these tests.

SURGERY IN ASYMPTOMATIC PATIENTS WITH MITRAL VALVE DISEASE

Jean Acar, Jean-Pierre Laborde

Different problems present themselves according to the type of cardiopathy and the therapy proposed, whether it is percutaneous valvulotomy, conservative surgery or valve replacement. We will discuss, successively, the therapeutic possibilities that one might consider for isolated mitral incompetence, tight mitral stenosis requiring a commissurotomy, and severe valvular pathology which necessitates valve replacement (1).

Pure and isolated mitral incompetence

In the absence in the literature of comparable randomized series of surgically or medically treated patients with asymptomatic mitral incompetence, the indications for surgery must rest upon indirect arguments. A certain number of considerations lead one to consider that conservative surgery, undertaken at an early stage, is desirable in isolated and severe mitral incompetence.

The results of surgery in mitral incompetence depend to a great degree on the stage to which it has progressed at the time of surgery. In our group, 342 patients had valve repair replacement for pure mitral incompetence between 1970 and 1992. Operative mortality for the entire series was 3.8%. It did not vary significantly according to NYHA functional class; 1.9% for classes I and II and 4.6% for classes III and IV (p=NS). However, the actuarial survival was very different at 15 years; 75% for classes I and II and 49% for classes III and IV.

If the preoperative predictive parameters for long term surgical outcome are analyzed not only in terms of late death but also left ventricular dysfunction, they can be classified into two types (1-3). One is related to the stage of cardiopathy, rhythm, cardiothoracic ratio, the degree of dilatation and systolic function of the left ventricle; the other depends upon the type of surgery (replacement or repair), with a clear advantage in favour of conservative surgery. Some authors (4) also underline the prognostic value of the size of the left atrium in five-year postoperative survival.

Other left ventricular functional indices have been proposed, such as endsystolic volume or the endsystolic stress/volume index of the left ventricle, but their prognostic value has been contested (5,6).

It has now been proven that *repair procedures* produce better results in terms of operative mortality and long term outcome than prosthetic replacement (1,2,7-11). This finding arises out of multivariate studies already cited which analyze the predictive preoperative factors for surgical outcome and compare repair series with prosthetic replacement. Undertaken by a team with wide experience of this method, repair represents only a slight operative risk (less than 2%) and gives good long term results. In more than 80% of cases in our series, the valve was competent or presented a discrete regurgitation at the time of the last echo Doppler examination (1,2).

Three factors determine the outcome (1-3,9,11):

- etiology; the best results are obtained in non-rheumatic regurgitation;
- type of surgery; surgery on the anterior leaflet leads to the highest number of residual leakages;
- experience of the surgical team; in the hands of certain surgical teams the results of repair improved and technical advances now enable the cure of complex lesions.

If the *outcome of surgery* in asymptomatic or minimally symptomatic patients with mitral regurgitation is analyzed, it should be borne in mind that this patient group is not homogenous regarding etiology or morphology of the lesions; degenerative causes, irrespective of the functional class, remain the most frequent (58% in our series) (1).

The comparison, in relation to the functional class, for preoperative parameters (1) shows that the surgical patients in functional class I or II have the least advanced cardiopathies; they are younger, have smaller cardiothoracic ratio, less dilated left atrium and fewer atrial fibrillation than the other categories. Likewise, pulmonary pressures are lower and cardiac index and left ventricular ejection fraction are higher. Also note that in the absence of significant functional disability, few patients (10% approximately) have ejection fractions lower than 50%, a very pathologic figure, nevertheless, for this type of valvular lesion (1).

Finally, *conservative surgery* seems appropriate if two conditions are met: the presence of severe mitral incompetence assessed by echo, sometimes by angiography, and the potential for a low-risk repair procedure with good short term and long term results. Several factors must be taken into consideration, including:

- experience of the surgical team;
- etiology; it is clear that certain types of mitral incompetence (chordae tendineae rupture through degenerative disease or bacterial endocarditis) have a more serious spontaneous outcome than chronic mitral incompetence of rheumatic origin, and justify, therefore, more rapid intervention (12);
- type of anatomical lesions assessed by transthoracic and transoesophageal echo Doppler; surgery will be earlier considered if the regurgitation can be treated by a repair procedure, like in the case of rupture or elongation of the chordae tendineae of the posterior mitral leaflert. If these lesions affect the anterior leaflet or both leaflets, surgical repair is still feasible and results will depend on the experience of the surgical team;
- degree of cardiopathy; it is desirable to operate before the appearance of a complete arrhythmia, pronounced cardiomegaly (cardiothoracic ratio > 0.60), major left ventricular dilatation (VTDI > 200 ml/m^2), change in systolic function (ejection fraction < 0.55), or the development of major left atrial dilatation, although in the latter case the exact values which should not be exceeded are still to be determined;
- age; advanced age increases the surgical risk, therefore, the older the patient the less likely that early surgery is to be envisaged, and if so, only reluctantly with the expectation of complications. Beyond 75 years, a chronic asymptomatic or minimally symptomatic mitral incompetence should not be operated except in special circumstances.

Mitral stenosis

If the mitral stenosis (MS) is tight, asymptomatic or with few symptoms, should it undergo commissurotomy? The problem was resolved by the introduction in 1984 of percutaneous valvulotomy (PV).

Do the risks and benefits that one can expect from the technique compared to the spontaneous progression of the illness justify its use and for which types of mitral stenosis? In the experience of our group (1,14-16), 22% of the first 810 patients were in functional classes I or II and 78% in class III or IV. These 810 cases can be subdivided into three groups by echo Doppler and fluoroscopy; Group 1: 192 patients (24%) with flexible, non-calcified valves and a barely altered subvalvular apparatus; Group 2: 417 patients (51%) with no calcification but with major changes to the subvalvular apparatus; and Group 3: 201 patients (25%) with calcification.

The results of PV in terms of mortality during or after procedure, severe mitral

Table 6.6-I: Risk of percutaneous mitral valvulotomy (810 cases).

	Grade I %	Grade II %	Grade III %
Mortality	0	0.2	1.5
Severe MI	0	4	6
Poor immediate results	3	9	30

MI: mitral insufficiency.

incompetence and poor immediate outcome (mitral surface < 1.5 cm^2 and/or regurgitation ≥ 3/4) are given in Table 6.6-I. The risk of poor outcome is very slight in Group 1 with good immediate results, noticeably greater in Group 3 and intermediate in Group 2. The mortality, however, remains low. The medium term results are a function of the anatomical lesions and the immediate outcome (15,16).

On the other hand, should we not be satisfied with a simple *periodic surveillance of a tight mitral stenosis* in patients in class I or II? The risk of delay is embolism; that was the initial event in 21% of 105 patients with mitral stenosis, asymptomatic or slightly symptomatic, followed up for a mean of four to five years by Bannister et al. (17). These emboli in mitral stenosis are serious due to their frequency (1.5% to 4% per patient-year), the second most frequent cause of death in mitral stenosis (20%) after cardiac failure (1,18).

Can one predict the embolic risk in a patient suffering from mitral stenosis? Atrial fibrillation is the principal clinical sign to fear and all the more so with advancing age.

Spontaneous echo contrast in the left atrium, common in arrhythmia but not so in mitral stenosis with sinus rhythm, is considered to be a thromboembolic risk factor (19). However, only its negative predictive value is high, its positive predictive value is slight. Recently, laboratory signs of increased fibrinolytic activity following hypercoagulability in a cardiac cavity have been described (14), such as plasma levels of fibrinopeptide A, fibrinopeptide B, β 15-42, thrombin-antithrombin III complex and D-dimer, but this laboratory contribution still requires confirmation.

Does mitral valvulotomy prevent embolism? It can be presumed from several facts that

- The embolic risk is slight during the two years following a PV; in our series it was 1.1% per patient-year against 2.7% for the two years preceding valvulotomy (1). In our experience, the risk of embolism is 3.7% during PV, but the majority of these emboli are gaseous in origin, transient and without sequelae. Of 810 cases, only three patients had emboli with sequelae;
- Spontaneous contrast in sinus rhythm very often disappears after effective PV (20). Experience in surgical commissurotomy (14) demonstrates a reduction in the frequency of emboli in the majority of reported series (0.3/1.8 per patient-year).

Our suggestions are as follows; in Group 1, for optimal valvular lesions, PV will be the best treatment. In Group 2, non-calcified mitral stenosis with subvalvular lesions, PV can be undertaken in patients at risk of either hemodynamic or thromboembolic (atrial fibrillation, spontaneous contrast on TEE) complications, and open commissurotomy

Table 6.6-II: Long term results of mitral valve replacement.

	Prosthesis	Survival 8 - 10 yrs %	Survival > 10 yrs %
1st generation prosthesis			
MILLER 1983	SE 6120	47 (10 yrs)	37 (14yrs)
SCHOEVAERDTS 1987	SE 6120	65 (10 yrs)	54 (19yrs)
GRUNKEMEIER	SE 6120	54 (10yrs)	26 (20 yrs)
LINDBLOM 1988	BS	58 (10 yrs)	
COHN 1989	Hancock	61 (10 yrs)	43 (15 yrs)
JAMIESON 1990	CE	55 (10 yrs)	
2nd generation prosthesis			
NITTER-HAUGE 1989	MH	56 (10 yrs)	
ROQUES 1988	St. J	79 (8.5 yrs)	
CZER 1990	St. J	41 (9 yrs)	
NAIR 1990	St. J	57 (8 yrs)	
AROM 1989	St. J	58 (10 yrs)	

SE: Starr Edwards; BS: Björk-Shiley; CE: Carpentier-Edwards Standard; St. J: St. Jude; MH: Medtronic Hall.

proposed in the event of left auricular thrombosis detected by TEE. In Group III, with calcified mitral valves, the approach will differ according to the patient, medical surveillance or prosthesis. Percutaneous valvulotomy can only be justified in very special cases due to a definite risk, such as valves with discrete calcification and hemodynamic or thromboembolic risk factors (complete arrhythmia, spontaneous contrast).

Valve disorders not suitable for conservative treatment

Some lesions cannot be corrected by PV or conservative surgery, only mitral valve replacement (MVR). This is often the case in mitral disease with severe valvular pathology, in highly calcified mitral stenosis and some cases of mitral incompetence.

Valve replacement is more hazardous than valve repair. Table 6.6-II shows the long term results that one can hope to achieve after MVR (21-31) with first and second generation prostheses. The 8-10 year survival rates vary from 41% to 79%. Generally, they lie between 50% and 65%. Late mortality related to the valve is lower with second generation prostheses. It accounts for less than 20% of late deaths with Saint Jude and Medtronic Hall valves, versus 25% to 40% with Starr-Edwards 6120 and Björk-Shiley Standard valves.

The long term prognosis depends more on the stage of cardiopathy than on the type of prosthesis. This fact is clearly shown in the series undertaken by the Logeais team and recently published by Vidal et al. Out of 790 MVR cases using a variety of prostheses, the 15 year survival for patients preoperatively in functional class III or IV was less than

40%, whereas it was 71% for class I and II patients (32). Independent preoperative predictors of late outcome after MVR were found to be functional class (NYHA), concomitant coronary heart disease, age, type of valvulopathy (isolated mitral incompetence or mixed lesion), left ventricular function, tricuspid incompetence and right ventricular failure, left atrial size in mitral incompetence and cardiomegaly (29,32-35).

Valve replacement may be considered for certain patients in functional class II if (a) the hemodynamic consequences of the valve lesion are serious, (b) the mitral valve is not suitable for repair, (c) the patient cannot adapt to the functional limitation and (d) the age is less than 75 years.

Surgical intervention must be planned before the appearance of left ventricular dysfunction (EF < 50%), major left atrial dilatation, right ventricular failure and/or tricuspid incompetence. The indication is always individual.

References

1. Acar J, Vahanian A, Michel PL, Luxereau P, Cormier B, Iung B. Faut-il opérer les valvulopathies mitrales a - ou paucisymptomatiques? Arch Mal Coeur 1992;85:1837-1843
2. Michel PL, Enriquez Sarano M, Cazaux P, et al. Facteurs influencant la survie aprés chirurgie de l'insuffisance mitrale pure non ischémique. Arch Mal Coeur 1990;83:45-51
3. De Gevigney G, Volpelliere N, Grare JP, Masin J, Milon H, Delahaye JP. Postoperative prognosis of mitral regurgitation (Abstract). Eur Heart J 1989;10(Suppl):375
4. Reed D, Abbott RD, Smucker ML, Kaul S. Prediction of outcome after mitral valve replacement in patients with symptomatic chronic mitral regurgitation. Circulation 1991;84:23-34
5. Carabello BA, Nolan SP, McGuire LB. Assessment of preoperative left ventricular function in patients with mitral regurgitation: value of the end-systolic volume ratio. Circulation 1981;64:1212-1217
6. Corin WJ, Murakami T, Monrad ES, Hess OM, Krayen- buehl HP. Inability of the end-systolic stress/end systolic volume index ratio to predict post-operative outcome in chronic mitral regurgitation (Abstract). J Am Coll Cardiol 1987;9:85A
7. Galloway AC, Colvin SB, Baumann FG, et al. A comparison of mitral valve reconstruction with mitral valve replacement: intermediate-terms results. Ann Thorac Surg 1989;47:655- 662
8. Deloche A, Jebara VA, Relland JY, et al. Valve repair with Carpentier techniques. The second decade. J Thorac Cardiovasc Surg 1990;99:990-1002
9. Michel PL, Iung B, Blanchard B, Luxereau P, Dorent R, Acar J. Long term results of mitral valve repair for non ischaemic mitral regurgitation. Eur Heart J 1991;12(Suppl. B):39- 43
10. Lessana A, Carbone C, Romano M, et al. Mitral valve repair: results and the decision-making process in reconstruction. J Thorac Cardiovasc Surg 1990;99:622-630
11. Duran CMG, Gmetza B, Balasundaram S, Al Halees Z. A feasibility study of valve repair in rheumatic mitral regurgita- tion. Eur Heart J 1991;12(Suppl. B):34-38
12. Delahaye JP, Gare JP, Viguier E, Delahaye F, De Gevigney G, Milon H. Natural history of severe mitral regurgitation. Eur Heart J 1991;12(Suppl. B):5-9
13. Vahanian A, Slama M, Cormier M, Michel PL, Savier CH. Valvuloplastie mitrale percutanée chez l'adulte. Arch Mal Coeur 1986;79:1896-1902
14. Acar J, Vahanian A, Michel PL, et al. Percutaneous aortic and mitral valvuloplasty. Cardiologia 1989;(Suppl. I):289-297
15. Vahanian A, Michel PL, Cormier B, et al. Results of percutaneous mitral commissurotomy in 200 patients. Am J Cardiol 1989;63:847-852
16. Vahanian A, Michel PL, Cormier B, et al. Immediate and mid-term results of percutaneous mitral commissurotomy. Eur Heart J 1991;12(Suppl. B):84-89
17. Bannister R. The risks of differring valvotomy in patients with moderate mitral stenosis. Lancet 1960;2:329-333
18. Acar J, Cormier B, Laborde JP. Rétrécissement mitral. In: Cardiopathies valvulaires acquises. Flammarion Médecine Sciences, 1986
19. Daniel WG, Nellessen O, Schroder E, et al. Left atrial spontaneous echo contrast in mitral valve disease. An indication for an increased thromboembolic risk. J Am Coll Cardiol 1988;11:204-211
20. Cormier B, Vahanian A, Iung B, et al. Influence of percutaneous mitral commissurotomy on left atrial

spontaneous contrast of mitral stenosis. J Am Coll Cardiol 1993;71:842-847

21. Miller DC, Oyer PE, Stinson EB, et al. Ten to fifteen year reassessment of the performance characteristics of the Starr-Edwards Model 6120 mitral valve prosthesis. J Thorac Cardiovasc Surg 1983;85:1-20

22. Schoevaerdts JC, Buche M, El Gariani A, et al. Twenty years' experience with the model 6120 Starr-Edwards valve in the mitral position. J Thorac Cardiovasc Surg 1987;94:375-382

23. Grunkemeier LG, Starr A. Twenty-five year experience with Starr-Edwards heart valves: follow-up methods and results. Can J Cardiol 1988;4:381-385

24. Lindblom D, Lindblom U, Qvist J, Lundstrom H. Long term relative survival rates after heart valve replacement. JACC 1990;15:566-573

25. Cohn LJ, Collins JJ, Disesa ST, et al. Fifteen year experience with 1678 Hancock porcine bioprosthetic heart valve replacements. Ann Surg 1989;210:435-443

26. Jamieson WRE, Allen P, Miyagishima RT, et al. The Carpentier Edwards standard porcine bioprosthesis. A first generation tissue valve with excellent long term clinical performance. J Thorac Cardiovasc Surg 1990;99:543-561

27. Nitter-Hauge S, Abdelnoor M. Ten year experience with the Medtronic Hall valvular prosthesis. A study of 1104 patients. Circulation 1989;80(Suppl. I):43-48

28. Roques X, Oca C, Daviaud M, Collot M, Laborde N, Baudet N. Complications thromboemboliques aprés remplacement valvulaire par la prothése de Saint Jude Médical. Résultats á long terme (9 ans) chez 1072 malades opérés de 1200 remplacements valvulaires. Coeur 1987;18:443-450

29. Czer LSC, Chaux A, Matloff JM, et al. Ten-year experience with the St. Jude Medical valve for primary valve replacement. J Thorac Cardiovasc Surg 1990;100:44-55

30. Nair CK, Mohiuddin SM, Hilleman DE, et al. Ten-year results with the St. Jude Medical prosthesis Am J Cardiol 1990;65:217-225

31. Arom KM, Nicoloff DM, Kersten TE, Worthrup WF, Lindsay WG, Emery RW. Ten years' experience with the St. Jude Medical valve prosthesis. Ann Thorac Surg 1989;47:831-837

32. Vidal V, Langanay T, Lelong B, et al. Résultats immédiats et éloignés de 790 remplacements valvulaires mitraux. Arch Mal Coeur 1992;85:169-174

33. Burckhardt D, Striebel D, Vogt S, et al. Heart valve replacement with St Jude mechanical valve prosthesis: long term experience in 743 patients in Switzerland. Circulation 1988;(Suppl. I):118-124

34. Abdelnoor M, Fjeld BB, Svennevig JL, Klingen G, Wickstrom E. Risk factors for morbidity and mortality in mitral valve replacement. Eur J Thorac Surg 1990;4:425-430

35. Ben Ismail M, Abid F, M'Zah N, Derbel F, Binon JP. Devenir des valvulopathies mitrales évoluées et opérées par prothäses mécaniques. Coeur 1988;19:141-147

ASYMPTOMATIC AND MINIMALLY SYMPTOMATIC AORTIC VALVE DISEASE

Jean-Pierre Delahaye, Guy De Gevigney

Asymptomatic or minimally symptomatic aortic stenosis and regurgitation present different problems.

Aortic regurgitation

Natural history

Excellent functional tolerance of important asymptomatic aortic regurgitation (AR) has been reported in many studies. For rheumatic AR, Segal et al. (1) reported that the mean delay between the diagnosis of hemodynamically important AR and the appearance of the first symptoms was 10.3 years. Bland and Wheeler (2) in their study on severe rheumatic AR in children and adolescents reported that 10 years after diagnosis, 35% of the patients had remained asymptomatic. Degeorges and Delzant (3) in a retrospective study of 105 patients with important chronic AR with a diastolic blood pressure of ≤ 50 mmHg found that 54 of them were asymptomatic. Goldschlager et al. (4) following 126 patients with chronic AR, noted that the percentage of subjects with asymptomatic or minimally symptomatic AR decreased from 100% below 30 years of age to 44% in those over 60 years old.

The early studies concerned mainly rheumatic AR, and their conclusions cannot be extrapolated to dystrophic AR, which is more widely found today in developed countries. However, these studies specified the predictive value of some simple variables. Massell et al. (5), in a long term prospective study in 323 patients with AR, reported no deaths among those with no or moderate cardiomegaly, a diastolic blood pressure greater than 40 mmHg and positive T-waves in D2 and V4 to V6. Spagnuolo et al. (6), in a study involving 174 young patients followed up for a mean of 10 years, identified three factors with a poor prognosis: cardiomegaly, hypertrophy (systolic strain of the left ventricle on electrocardiogram), systolic hypertension and/or diastolic hypotension. Froment et al. (7) and Smith et al. (8), added arrhythmias and conduction disorders to these classical poor prognostic factors.

Recent large prospective studies confirm the good prognosis of asymptomatic AR when the left ventricular function remains normal or only slightly impaired. Bonow et al. (9) followed 104 patients with important asymptomatic or minimally symptomatic AR (scored 3 or 4 on angiography), and normal or almost normal left ventricular systolic function (ejection fraction ≥ 45%, and echocardiographic shortening fraction ≥ 29%) from 1973 to 1988, and they observed that after 11 years of follow up, 79 patients had remained asymptomatic or minimally symptomatic and had good left ventricular function.

The percentage of patients who have to undergo surgery due to the appearance of symptoms and/or a silent left ventricular dysfunction is about 5% per year; Bonow et al. (9,10) and Siemienczuk et al. (11) report a slightly lower, and Turina et al. (12) a slightly higher percentage. Yousof et al. (13) reported a markedly higher percentage, 9% per year, in patients with mainly rheumatic AR (39/60).

A patient with AR presenting no symptoms or only very discrete symptoms is not free from risk. Studies performed over the last 15 years have attempted to identify the best way to evaluate this risk, which is mainly hemodynamic, but can also involve aortic wall and rhythm risks. We will not discuss infectious risk here since this is the same for both asymptomatic and symptomatic AR.

Evaluation of the hemodynamic risk

The appearance of left ventricular dysfunction following the volume overload due to AR can be free from any functional disorder, and there is no correlation between the hemodynamic severity of the AR and the degree of functional disability (14). Recent surgical statistics show that a non-negligible percentage of asymptomatic or minimally symptomatic patients have undergone surgery for left ventricular dysfunction, which is severe in some cases. Clark et al. (15) observed that nine out of 17 patients who underwent surgery with an ejection fraction of <0.50 were in NYHA functional class I or II. In the study by Luxereau et al. (16) 15 of the 73 patients in NYHA I or II had an ejection fraction lower than 0.40.

However, the fact that left ventricular dysfunction is a poor postoperative prognostic factor in patients with AR has been well demonstrated in the studies by the groups of Acar (17) and Bonow (18-21). Therefore, it is very important to evaluate the left ventricular function in patients with important AR while they are still asymptomatic or minimally symptomatic.

Which are the most reliable indicators of left ventricular dysfunction in AR, and can we distinguish between reversible and irreversible dysfunction? There is no consensus for the answer to the first question. Evaluation of exercise capacity (14,18,22) and maximal oxygen uptake (23) are a first approach in this assessment. The echocardiographic determination of left ventricular diameters and shortening fractions (18,19,24-28), the estimation of left ventricular ejection fraction at rest and during exercise using isotope ventriculography (9,19,29-32), and the volumetric and functional indicators from invasive examinations (11,17,33,34) have all been widely used in the screening and monitoring of left ventricular dysfunction in patients with AR. From these studies it can be concluded that

- no single isolated anomaly can be considered to be a sufficiently reliable indicator of left ventricular dysfunction and its potential progress. Echocardiographic measurements, in addition to the unavoidable inter- and intra-observer differences (35), do not provide categorical criteria for use in the decision whether to operate or not (24-26);
- the variations in the isotopic ejection fraction during exercise do not provide additional useful information (for the prognosis of left ventricular dysfunction) to that obtained at rest (9,36);
- it is essential to combine information obtained during successive evaluation of left ventricular function using several tests, such as echocardiographically and radiologically determined cardiac diameters, and echocardiographic and isotope indicators of left ventricular systolic function (21,37).

It is not possible to predict the reversibility of myocardial dysfunction for a given patient. Bonow et al. (18) observed that the risk of irreversibility of the dysfunction increases with the length of time of its evolution before surgery. Patients with a very dilated left ventricle (endsystolic diameter ≥55 mm) have a persistently dilated left ventricle after surgery (15,25,26). This persistent dilatation carries a higher risk of cardiac failure and subsequent mortality (22,27).

Evaluation of the aortic wall risk

The aortic wall risk arises from dystrophic disorders. Several possibilities exist.

Annulo-aortic ectasia: the risk of aortic dissection is very high in patients with annulo-aortic ectasia (38,39), and it is, without doubt, higher in those with Marfan's syndrome than in its "formes frustes" (40), although the risk is not predictable for a given patient. Thus in asymptomatic patients where an annulo-aortic ectasia is diagnosed, it is necessary to propose aortic valve and root replacement. This is true also for patients in whom surgery would not be otherwise justified, i.e. on the basis of the current aortic regurgitation and its effects on the left ventricle.

Surgery cannot be deferred in the event of aortic parietal risk if echocardiographic and nuclear magnetic resonance results show a progressive increase in the volume of the aneurysm (41) and/or when the diameter of the proximal aorta is at least twice the size of the distal aorta (42). Treasure (43) recommends that surgery be undertaken in all patients with Marfan's syndrome when the diameter of the ascending aorta reaches 55 mm, and perhaps even earlier.

Cylindrical dilatation of the aortic root: the aortic parietal risk is less well known for the cylindrical dilatation of the aortic root than for the annulo-aortic ectasia. A recent French co-operative study (44) compared two groups of patients who had undergone aortic valve replacement without aortic root replacement. One group had cylindrical dilatation of the aortic root (41 to 55 mm: n=49), and the other did not (n=40). This study showed that

- clear signs of aortic media necrosis are more often shown by histology of a sample of aortic wall taken during the operation from patients with a dilated aorta;
- the actuarial survival rate of patients after isolated aortic valve replacement (at seven years) is lower in those with a dilated aorta (54% vs. 74%), but this difference is not statistically significant (p=0.08);
- complications related to the aortic root (aneurysm and/or dissection) are significantly more frequent in patients with a dilated aorta (at seven years; 44% in those with a dilated aorta vs. 5% in those without; p<0.01).

It is more difficult to define the therapeutic attitude in this case than in the case of annulo-aortic ectasia. The difficulty of coronary reimplantation when a true aneurysm of the aorta does not exist leads to the recommendation of regular surveillance of the patient with transthoracic and transoesophageal echography, and/or by nuclear magnetic resonance.

Surgery is also indicated in the case of progressive dilatation of the diameter of the aorta. Replacement of the aortic root with coronary reimplantation is performed only if there is evidence of dystrophy in the aortic root (thin walls, and/or intimal tears observed during intervention, and/or histological evidence of lesions in biopsy material taken during surgery). Current trends in using a homograft or a pulmonary autograft for aortic root replacement may change this surgical attitude (see Chapters 9.2 and 9.3).

Isolated valve dysplasia: the co-operative study by Michel et al. (44) confirmed the low aortic parietal risk of valve dysplasia in the absence of aortic root dilatation. In this case the therapeutic indications are the same as those related to the myocardial risk.

Risk of sudden death

As early as 1956, Segal et al. (1) brought to attention the risk of sudden death in patients with severe AR; 5% of their patients with non-decompensated AR died suddenly, and many of these patients had ventricular premature beats. Spagnuolo et al. (6), in a study on 31 high-risk patients (see above), reported seven deaths, four of which were sudden. Smith et al. (8) reported that sudden death was exceptional in patients with a cardiothoracic ratio lower than 0.60. This was confirmed by Turina et al. (45,46), who observed that sudden death can occur in asymptomatic patients with a dilated left ventricle. Bonow et al. (9) observed only two cases of sudden death in a study on 104 asymptomatic patients with intact left ventricular function during a mean follow up of eight years (i.e. a risk of 0.4%/pty). The two patients who died had a highly dilated left ventricle (enddiastolic diameter ≥ 80 mm; endsystolic diameter ≥ 55mm).

Several recent studies (47-50) have concentrated on ventricular arrhythmias in AR detected by Holter monitoring. Complex ventricular arrhythmias (Lown class 3 or 4) were observed in five out of 21 asymptomatic or minimally symptomatic patients in a study by Hochreiter et al. (47). Von Olshausen et al. (48) reported a fairly close correlation (r=-0.78) between the degree of severity of the premature beats (expressed as Lown class) and the left ventricular ejection fraction. This correlation was not observed in the study by Hochreiter et al. (47), but was observed in the study by Michel et al. (50), where the mean value of the ejection fraction was 41% in patients with Lown class 3 or 4 arrhythmias and 51% in those with Lown class 0 to 2 arrhythmias. Severe arrhythmias were less frequent as the postoperative interval increased (50). Periodic Holter monitoring of patients with AR and left ventricular dysfunction or dilatation may help to determine the best time to operate.

Monitoring and treatment of asymptomatic AR patients and timing of surgery

The aortic wall risk and the rhythm risk should be considered when deciding when to operate. We presented above the surgical indications linked to the risk in aortic root dystrophies. The rhythmic risk is not independent of the hemodynamic risk, and requires additional monitoring, using Holter monitoring and high- amplification ECG in patients with asymptomatic AR and complex ventricular arrhythmias (Lown class ≥ 3).

Monitoring of patients with asymptomatic AR is focused on left ventricular systolic function. Can treatment with vasodilators delay the occurrence of ventricular dysfunction? It has been shown that nifedipine (51-53) and hydralazine (54,55) can decrease left ventricular dilatation and increase the ejection fraction (54,55). It is perhaps too early to decide, as Scognamiglio et al. (53) have said, if "such therapy has the potential to delay the need for valve replacement in asymptomatic patients", but ACE-inhibitors may open new possibilities in this respect.

We have pointed out that asymptomatic patients with intact left ventricular function (ejection fraction ≥0.50) have an excellent spontaneous prognosis (9,10). These patients, while they remain asymptomatic, and/or their left ventricular function is intact, and/or their left ventricular dilatation is stable should not undergo surgery (56). They should be regularly seen for clinical, echocardiographic and isotope examinations. This is necessary because the left ventricular function may alter without any apparent major functional disability. To allow the left ventricular dysfunction to progress without taking action, under the pretext that the patient is not experiencing any discomfort, results in a risk of persistence or worsening of the dysfunction after surgery is performed too late.

The data to be taken into consideration in during the medical follow up are the following:

- Functional disability, which is rarely seen without altered left ventricular function, and therefore the first signs of this should lead to close monitoring of the left ventricular functional and dimensional indicators, and to action being taken when the limits defined above are reached. It should be pointed out that functional disorders are initially not very disabling, and that the patients are not always worried by their appearance, which is why regular monitoring (yearly or, even better, every six months) of the variables studied above is necessary;

- Left ventricle echocardiographic data and their evolution. In the study by Bonow et al. (9,10), significant left ventricular dilatation (with endsystolic diameter greater than 55mm and enddiastolic diameter greater than 80mm) carried a risk (in particular of sudden death) even before a decrease in the left ventricular systolic function. The progressive increase of the ventricular diameters is to be taken into account, as shown by the following limits (10); when the initial endsystolic diameter is less than 50mm, and this increases by at least 1 mm per year, the annual risk of the occurrence of any event (appearance of symptoms and/or left ventricular dysfunction, surgery, death) is less than 1%. This risk reaches 27% when the initial endsystolic diameter is ≥50 mm and it increases by more than 1 mm a year;
- Left ventricular ejection fraction estimated by isotope examination. The spontaneous risk of evolution is higher in asymptomatic patients with an initial ejection fraction lower than 0.45 (9), and there is good reason not to defer surgery for such patients. A progressive decrease in the ejection fraction at rest also gives rise to an indication for surgery. The study of changes in the ejection fraction during exercise does not add anything to the predictive value of the parameters obtained at rest. Finally, in a multivariate analysis of the prognostic factors for asymptomatic AR, Bonow et al. (9) identified only four independent prognostic factors; age, initial left ventricular endsystolic diameter, its progressive increase, and the progressive decrease of left ventricular ejection fraction determined at rest.

In summary, there are three indications for aortic valve replacement in patients with initially asymptomatic AR (9,57): appearance of symptoms, appearance and progression of echocardiographic and/or isotopic signs of left ventricular dysfunction at rest, and significant dilatation of the left ventricle (enddiastolic diameter >70mm, enddiastolic volume >200 ml/m^2).

Results of surgery in asymptomatic AR patients

The results of aortic valve replacement, when performed for the indications defined above, are excellent. There are no perioperative deaths for these patients (9,58,59). Long term results are good; at five years, 88.4% (58), and at eight years 87% (59) of the patients are alive. In the long term, 82% of the patients are either asymptomatic or minimally symptomatic after surgery (59). Failure due to myocardial dysfunction is rare and difficult to predict before surgery. The poor prognostic factors for symptomatic patients do not have the same predictive value in asymptomatic patients (57,58), and this may be because only a few patients progressing to left ventricular dysfunction undergo surgery before any symptoms are seen (57).

Aortic stenosis

In the last 25 years, numerous studies have shown that the risk of progress was very low in patients with asymptomatic aortic stenosis (AS). Ross and Braunwald (60) reported this in 1968, when they noted that no more than 5% of deaths due to AS were in asymptomatic patients. Chizner et al. (61) confirmed the excellent prognosis of asymptomatic AS in patients under 30 years old. Horstkotte and Loogen (62) corroborated the low risk for asymptomatic patients, but noted that the risk depends on the first symptom to appear. Thus, the risk is low when angina pectoris is the first symptom, higher when the first symptom is syncope, and even higher when it is congestive heart failure.

Kelly et al. (63) followed up 51 asymptomatic patients with AS, with a maximum transvalvular Doppler gradient of ≥ 50 mmHg, for a mean of 17 months; two cardiac deaths, one of which was sudden, were reported. In both patients symptoms appeared before death occurred, heart failure in one, and angina pectoris in the other. Turina et al. (46), in a study on 73 patients with AS who had not undergone surgery, reported that 90.2% of the asymptomatic or minimally symptomatic patients were still alive after five years.

In the recent study by Pellikka et al. (64) 143 asymptomatic patients with AS, (including 113 patients who had not undergone surgery) were followed up for a mean of 20 months. A total of 14 deaths were reported, six of which were attributed to cardiovascular causes. In all patients, including the two who died suddenly, symptoms appeared several months before death.

Although the low risk for asymptomatic patients should lead to deferring surgery until the first symptom occurs, in several recent surgical studies on large numbers of patients, about 30% of the patients were asymptomatic or minimally symptomatic.

In the Mayo Clinic study (64), 30 of the 143 asymptomatic patients underwent surgery. This attitude can be defended if the data concerning the history of patients with AS after surgery are considered in the light of the pre-operative degree of functional discomfort. Cormier et al. (65) reported that 59% of operated patients in NYHA class III, and 39% of those in NYHA IV were alive ten years after surgery, compared with 78% of those classed as NYHA I or II.

The attitude to recommend surgery for asymptomatic patients with AS is primarily based on the degree of stenosis; if the AS is not very tight (aortic surface > 0.75 cm^2 measured with Doppler echocardiography), surgery is not recommended. Is the same attitude to be recommended for tight AS, which is silent in a third of patients (46)? Here we should consider some factors which can help to determine the optimum time for surgery.

The rate of progression of the stenosis: There is initially no way of separating "fast progressors", with a mean aortic surface decrease of 0.15 cm^2 per year, from the "slow progressors" with a mean aortic surface decrease of 0.02 cm^2 per year (66). It is, therefore, advisable that patients with AS should be regularly examined by Doppler echocardiography when their aortic surface area approaches the critical limit (63).

The patient's age and level of physical activity: It is justified not to delay surgery in patients who are exposed to a high level of physical activity, and in elderly patients. For these latter patients perioperative morbidity-mortality increases with age.

Objective evaluation of functional disability: Many elderly patients with AS are only false asymptomatic patients, who avoid effort and lead a slow life. The evaluation of functional disability with an exercise test, under controlled conditions, may be useful for these patients.

The quality of left ventricular systolic function assessed using echocardiography and/or isotopic ventriculography: Pellikka et al. (64) reported that the risk of progress is higher in patients with a left ventricular ejection fraction lower than 0.50 and in those with a peak of maximum aortic flow velocity higher than 4.5 m/sec (measured using Doppler echocardiography).

The rhythm risk: Ventricular arrhythmias are frequent in patients with AS (48-50). One-third of the patients in the study by Michel et al. (50) presenting with ventricular arrhythmias scored ≥ 3 on the Lown scale. There is a relation between the severity of the arrhythmia recorded and the risk of sudden death (48,67), but this is not seen in asymptomatic patients. In one study on preoperative mortality (unpublished data), we observed six deaths in 150 patients, three of which were sudden (five of these patients were in functional class III and the other was in class IV).

Specific problems

Mixed aortic regurgitation and stenosis

It is not necessary to single out the subgroup of patients presenting with both a significant aortic stenosis and an important regurgitation. In these patients it is still possible to evaluate the aortic surface with Doppler echocardiography, and also to quantify a regurgitation associated with a significant stenosis. The indication to operate is not based on the relative importance of the stenosis and the regurgitation, but on their effects on the left ventricular function, which is evaluated using the same methods and parameters and leads to the same indication irrespective of the predominant dysfunction.

Associated pathologies

Associated pathologies are frequently observed, and these are sometimes as silent as the valve disease itself. Significant coronary lesions have been observed in 20% to 30% of patients in Europe and in 30% to 40% in the United States. Coronary artery disease probably increases the risk of progression (68), so it is important during an invasive examination of the aorta, even in asymptomatic patients, to perform coronarography in order to identify silent coronary disorders.

Visceral deficiencies, in particular respiratory or renal failure, are, like atherosclerotic coronary, aortic or carotid disorders, to be taken into consideration in asymptomatic patients. If their condition allows it, aortic valve surgery should be performed (69).

Multiple-orifice involvement

Cardiologists are often faced with the problem of multiple-orifice involvement with both rheumatic and dystrophic etiologies. Surgery may be justified for one orifice but not for the other. The fear of seeing the latter orifice evolve, and imposing a second operation sooner or later, should not lead to correction of a valve dysfunction which itself does not yet justify surgery. The attitude of delaying surgery for the principal orifice affected so as to allow the other lesion to develop is also irrational and carries the risk of poor results due to surgery being performed too late (see also Chapter 6.2).

Finally in patients with valve disease, as in those with coronary disease, we should no longer wait for symptoms to appear before performing examinations and considering surgery. Regular examinations should be performed during the pre-symptomatic period to determine when surgery should be considered. This monitoring should not become troublesome for patients without symptoms, and it should be kept in mind that surgical indications are rare in patients with strictly asymptomatic aortic stenosis and are not to be considered as often as for patients with asymptomatic aortic regurgitation.

References

1. Segal J, Harvey WP, Hufnagel C. A clinical study of one hundred cases of severe aortic insufficiency. Am J Med 1956;21:200-210
2. Bland EF, Wheeler EO. Severe aortic regurgitation in young people. A long-term perspective with reference to prognosis and prosthesis. N Engl J Med 1957;256:667-672
3. Degeorges M, Delzant JF. Eléments de pronostic de l'insuffisance aortique isolée recueillis chez 206 malades agés de moins de 50 ans. Sem Hop Paris 1966;42:1171-1182
4. Goldschlager N, Pfeifer J, Cohn K, Popper R, Selzer A. The natural history of aortic regurgitation. A clinical and hemodynamic study. Am J Med 1973;54:577-588
5. Massell BF, Amezcua FJ, Czonieczer G. Prognosis of patients with pure or predominant aortic regurgitation in the absence of surgery. Circulation 1966;164(Suppl. III):33-34
6. Spagnuolo M, Kloth H, Taranta A, Doyle E, Pasternack B. Natural History of rheumatic aortic regurgitation. Criteria predictive of death, congestive heart failure, and angina in young patients. Circulation 1971;44:368-380
7. Froment R, Perrin A, Normand J, Saint-Pierre A, Besset C. Bases anatomo-cliniques des indications opératoires pour insuffisance aortique pure ou prédominante (d'après 201 observations personnelles). Actualités Cardio Vasc Med Chir 1964;1:120-170
8. Smith HJ, Neutze JM, Roche AHG, Agnew TM, Barratt-Boyes BG. The natural history of rheumatic aortic regurgitation and the indications for surgery. Br Heart J 1976;38:147-154
9. Bonow RO, Lakatos E, Maron BJ, Epstein SE. Serial long-term assessment of the natural history of asymptomatic patients with chronic aortic regurgitation and normal left ventricular systolic function. Circulation 1991;84:1625-1635
10. Bonow RO, Rosing DR, McIntosh CL, et al. The natural history of asymptomatic patients with aortic regurgitation and normal left ventricular function. Circulation 1983;68:509-517
11. Siemienczuk D, Greenberg B, Morris C, et al. Chronic aortic insufficiency: factors associated with progression to aortic valve replacement. Ann Int Med 1989;110:587-592
12. Turina J, Hess OM, Krayenbühl HP. Spontanverlauf der Aortenvitien und Indikationen für den Aortenklappenersatz. Schweiz med Wschr 1988;118:508-516
13. Yousof AM, Mohammed MMJ, Khan N, Shuhaiber H, Cherian G. Chronic severe aortic regurgitation: a prospective follow-up of 60 asymptomatic patients. Am Heart J 1988;116:1262-1267
14. Kraus F, Dacian S, Hall D, Klein U, Rudolph W. Relationship between symptoms and hemodynamics associated with regurgitant lesions of the aortic or mitral valve. Z Kardiol 1986;75(Suppl 2):137-140
15. Clark DG, McAnulty JM, Rahimtoola SH. Valve replacement in aortic insufficiency with left ventricular dysfunction. Circulation 1980;61:411-421
16. Luxereau P, Vahanian A, Ducimetiere P, Bottineau G, Kassab R, Acar J. L'heure de la chirurgie dans le traitement de l'insuffisance aortique chronique. Ann Cardiol Angeiol 1983;32:473-478
17. Luxereau P, Vahanian A, Ducimetiere P, et al. Mortalité opératoire et évolution à distance des remplacements valvulaires aortiques. Incidence de la dysfonction myocardique. Arch Mal Coeur 1982;75:1137-1147
18. Bonow RO, Rosing DR, Maron BJ, et al. Reversal of left ventricular dysfunction after aortic valve replacement for chronic aortic regurgitation: influence of duration of preoperative left ventricular dysfunction. Circulation 1984;70:570-579
19. Bonow RO, Picone AL, McIntosh CL, et al. Survival and functional results after valve replacement for aortic regurgitation from 1976 to 1983: impact of preoperative left ventricular function. Circulation 1985;72:1244-1256
20. Bonow RO. Asymptomatic patients with significant aortic or mitral incompetence and left ventricular dysfunction should undergo operation. Z Kardiol 1986;75(Suppl 2):124-132
21. Bonow RO, Epstein SE. Is preoperative left ventricular function predictive of survival and functional results after aortic valve replacement for chronic aortic regurgitation? J Am Coll Cardiol 1987;10:713-716

22. Bonow RO, Borer JS, Rosing DR, et al. Preoperative exercise capacity in symptomatic patients with aortic regurgitation as a predictor of post operative left ventricular function and long-term prognosis. Circulation 1980;62:1280-1290

23. Scriven AJI, Lipkin DP, Fox KM, Poole-Wilson PA. Maximal oxygen uptake in severe aortic regurgitation: a different view of left ventricular function. Am Heart J 1990;120:902-909

24. Henry WL, Bonow RO, Rosing DR, Epstein SE. Observations on the optimum time for operative intervention for aortic regurgitation. II. Serial echocardiographic evaluation of asymptomatic patients. Circulation 1980;61:484-492

25. Daniel WG, Hood WP, Siart A, et al. Chronic aortic regurgitation: reassessment of the prognostic value of preoperative left ventricular end-systolic dimension and fractional shortening. Circulation 1985;71:669-680

26. Fioretti P, Roelandt J, Sclavo M, et al. Postoperative regression of left ventricular dimensions in aortic insufficiency: a long-term echocardiographic study. J Am Coll Cardiol 1985;5:856-861

27. Gaasch WH, Andrias CW, Levine HJ. Chronic aortic regurgitation: the effect of aortic valve replacement on left ventricular volume, mass and function. Circulation 1978;58:825-836

28. Gaasch WH, Carroll JD, Levine HJ, Criscitiello MG. Chronic aortic regurgitation: prognostic value of left ventricular end-systolic dimension and end-diastolic radius/thickness ratio. J Am Coll Cardiol 1983;1:775-782

29. Bassand JP, Faivre R, Becque O, et al. Les anomalies de fonction systolique ventriculaire gauche dévoilées par l'effort dans l'insuffisance aortique chronique. Arch Mal Coeur 1986;79:1555-1561

30. Tissot A, Veillas G, Lasne Y, Besson JE. Fonction ventriculaire gauche dans l'insuffisance aortique chronique asymptomatique. Etude par angioscintigraphie. Arch Mal Coeur 1989;82:223-230

31. Bonow RO, Dodd JT, Maron BJ, et al. Long-term serial changes in left ventricular function and reversal of ventricular dilatation after valve replacement for chronic aortic regurgitation. Circulation 1988;78:1108-1120

32. Bonow RO. Radionuclide angiography in the management of asymptomatic aortic regurgitation. Circulation 1991;84(Suppl I):296-302

33. Borow KM, Green LH, Mann T, et al. End-systolic volume as a predictor of postoperative left ventricular performance in volume overload from valvular regurgitation. Am J Med 1980;68:655-663

34. Delaye J, Durand JP, Convert G, et al. Pronostic des insuffisances aortiques chroniques asymtomatiques ou paucisymptomatiques. Arch Mal Coeur 1982;75:439-448

35. Szlachcic J, Massie BM, Greenberg B, et al. Intertest variability of echocardiographic and chest X-ray measurements: implications for decision making in patients with aortic regurgitation. J Am Coll Cardiol 1986;7:1310-1317

36. Nishimura RA, McGoon, Schaff HV, Giuliani ER. Chronic aortic regurgitation: indications for operation 1988. Mayo Clin Proc 1988;63:270-280

37. Borow KM. Surgical outcome in chronic aortic regurgitation: a physiologic framework for assessing preoperative predictors. J Am Coll Cardiol 1987;10:1165-1170

38. Michel PL, Chapelon C, Vahanian A, Chomette G, Boustani F, Acar J. Potentiel évolutif des lésions de l'aorte ascendante dans les insuffisances aortiques dystrophiques. Arch Mal Coeur 1986;79:1460-1465

39. Beaune J, Nony P, Chassignolle J, Loire R, Gros P, Delaye J. Les insuffisances aortiques par anévrysme dystrophique de l'aorte ascendante: étude évolutive de 95 observations. Intéret de la biopsie cutanée dans le diagnostic étiologique. Arch Mal Coeur 1989;82:1389-1396

40. Acar J, Michel PL, Chomette G, Iung B, Starkman C. Les insuffisances aortiques dystrophiques. Arch Mal Coeur 1991;84:105-111

41. De Belder MA, Child AH, Pumphrey W. The timing of aortic root replacement in Marfan's syndrome. Cardiovasc Med 1989;8:57-70

42. Svensson LG, Crawford E, Coselli JS, Safi HJ, Hess KR. Impact of cardiovascular operation on survival in the Marfan patient. Circulation 1989;80(Suppl I):233-242

43. Treasure T. Elective replacement of the aortic root in Marfan's syndrome. Br Heart J 1993;69:101-103

44. Michel PL, Hanania G, Chomette G, et al. Insuffisance aortique dystrophique: influence de la dilatation de l'aorte ascendante sur l'évolution secondaire. Arch Mal Coeur 1991;84:477- 482

45. Turina J, Turina M, Rothlin M, Krayenbuehl HP. Improved late survival patients with chronic aortic regurgitation by earlier operation. Circulation 1984;70(Suppl I):147-152

46. Turina J, Hess O, Sepulcri F, Krayenbuehl HP. Spontaneous course of aortic valve disease. Eur Heart J 1987;8:471- 483

47. Hochreiter C, Jeffrey S, Borer M, Kligfield P. Complex ventricular arrhythmias in patients with valvular regurgitation: a potentially important, clinically overlooked phenomenon? (Abstract). Am J Cardiol 1982;49:910

48. Von Olshausen K, Schwarz F, Apfelbach J, Röhrig N, Krämer B, Kübler W. Determinants of the incidence and severity of ventricular arrhythmias in aortic valve disease. Am J Cardiol 1983;51:1103-1109

49. Klein RC. Ventricular arrhythmias in aortic valve disease: analysis of 102 patients. Am J Cardiol 1984;53:1079- 1083
50. Michel PL, Mandagout O, Vahanian A, et al. Ventricular arrhythmias in aortic valve disease before and after aortic valve replacement. Acta Cardiologica 1992;47:145-156
51. Fioretti P, Benussi B, Scardi S, Klugmann S, Brower RW, Camerini F. Afterload reduction with nifedipine in aortic insufficiency. Am J Cardiol 1982;49:1728-1732
52. Montemurro D, Ronzani G, Gozzelino G, Spadaccini, Panataro C, Brusca A. Studio doppler ad analisi spettrale e a codice di colori delle modificazioni del rigurgito aortico indotte da vasodilatatori in pazienti asintomatici affetti da insufficienza aortica grave. G Ital Cardiol 1990;20:842-849
53. Scogamiglio R, Rahimtoola SH, Fasoli G, Nistri S, Dalla Volta S. Nifedipin in asymptomatic patients with severe aortic regurgitation and normal left ventricular function. N Engl J Med 1994; 331:689-692
54. Greenberg B, Massie B, Bristow JD, et al. Long-term vasodilator therapy of chronic aortic insufficiency. A randomized double-blinded, placebo-controlled clinical trial. Circulation 1988;78:92-103
55. Dumesnil JG, Tran K, Dagenais GR. Beneficial long-term effects of hydralazine in aortic regurgitation. Arch Intern Med 1990;150:757-760
56. Schwarz F, Ehrmann J, Olschewski P, Scheurlen H, Saggau W, Kübler W. Patients with significant aortic incompetence should not be operated on until they are symptomatic. Z Kardiol 1986;75(Suppl 2):133-136
57. Acar J. Quel traitement pour l'insuffisance aortique chronique? Arch Mal Coeur 1987;80:1297-1303
58. Tissot A, Delahaye JP, Milon H, Normand J, Age C. Pronostic des insuffisances aortiques chroniques opérées. Arch Mal Coeur 1986;79:1168-1175
59. Cormier B, Vahanian A, Luxereau P, Acar J. Résultats du replacement valvulaire dans l'insuffisance aortique chronique a ou paucisymptomatique. Arch Mal Coeur 1987;80:66-73
60. Ros J, Braunwald E. Aortic stenosis. Circulation 1968;37-8(Suppl V):61-67
61. Chizner MA, Pearle DL, Deleon AC. The natural history of aortic stenosis in adults. Am Heart J 1980;99:419-424
62. Horstkotte D, Loogen F. The natural history of acquired aortic stenosis. Eur Heart J 1988;9(Suppl E):57-64
63. Kelly TA, Rothbart RM, Morgan Cooper C, Kaiser DL, Smucker ML, Gibson RS. Comparison of outcome of asymptomatic to symptomatic patients older than 20 years of age with valvular aortic stenosis. Am J Cardiol 1988;61:123-130
64. Pellikka PA, Nishimura RA, Bailey KR, et al. The natural history of adults with asymptomatic, hemodynamically significant aortic stenosis. J Am Coll Cardiol 1990;15:1012-1017
65. Cormier B, Luxereau P, Bloch C, et al. Progression and long-term results of surgically treated aortic stenosis. Eur Heart J 1988;9(Suppl E):113-120
66. Davies SW, Gershlick AH, Balcon R. Progression of valvar aortic stenosis: a long-term retrospective study. Eur Heart J 1991;12:10-14
67. Von Olshausen K, Witt T, Schmidt G, Meyer J. Ventricular tachycardia as a cause of sudden death in patients with aortic valve disease. Am J Cardiol 1987;59:1214-1215
68. Erichetti A, Greenberg JM, Gaasch WM. Is valve replacement indicated in asymptomatic patients with aortic stenosis or aortic regurgitation? Cardiovasc Clin 1990;21:199-210
69. Gare JP, Kosmider A, Delahaye F, De Gevigney G, Michaud C, Delahaye JP. Chirurgie valvulaire et pathologies associées chez les sujets agés. Arch Mal Coeur 1992;85:973-979

Chapter 7.1

Non-Invasive Medical Treatment

Luc A. Pierard, Henri E. Kulbertus

Properly timed correction of valvular dysfunction by surgery or interventional catheterization is the corner-stone of the treatment of valvular heart disease. The role of medical therapy is therefore limited in this field. Nonetheless, whatever the nature and severity of the lesion, patients with heart valve disease need careful medical attention. In this chapter we shall first discuss two problems which apply to most cases with valvular heart disease, such as prevention of recurrences of rheumatic fever when the valvular lesion is of rheumatic origin, and treatment of the early stages of heart failure.

We shall then envisage the problems of cardiac and non-cardiac surgery and of pregnancy in patients with valvular heart disease, and finally consider each form of valvular heart disease separately and discuss their hemodynamic consequences and treatment in greater details. Two important aspects of non-invasive medical treatment are anticoagulation and prevention of infective endocarditis, both having an entire chapter devoted to the respective subject. The reader is therefore referred to Chapter 6.4 and 10.3 regarding these issues.

PREVENTION OF RECURRENCES OF RHEUMATIC FEVER

Rheumatic fever is now extremely rare in industrialized countries. It still remains a major problem in the developing world and, to some extent, in the lower socio-economic classes all over the world. Prevention of recurrences of rheumatic fever in a patient presenting with rheumatic valvular disease thus remains necessary (1).

The most widely recommended technique consists of monthly intramuscular injection of 1,200,000 Units of benzathine-penicillin G. Alternatives have been proposed such as 1.0 g of sulfadiazine once daily (500 mg for patients with a body weight lower than 30 kg) or 200,000 Units of oral penicillin twice daily.

In cases of intolerance or allergy, erythromycin 250 mg twice daily may be used. The optimal duration of this prophylactic therapy is as yet subject of debate. The risk of recurrence decreases with age and with the length of time elapsed since the last attack. The risk remains significant during the first 5-10 years following the acute episode. In general, the preventive treatment is maintained for a minimum of five years and, at least, until the age of twenty. Adult patients at high risk of infection by streptococci may benefit from prolonged prophylaxis (poor socio-economic conditions, personnel of nursery schools, military personnel, paramedical staff, etc.). Special attention must be paid to all sporadic streptococcal infections for example of the ear, throat or nose, which must prompt appropriate antibiotic therapy for at least one week. Enlarged and cryptic amygdaline should preferably be removed.

PREVENTION OF BACTERIAL ENDOCARDITIS

The risk of bacterial endocarditis is different depending on the nature of the valvular lesions. It is highest in aortic valve disease and in mitral incompetence. To the contrary, it is low in pure mitral stenosis. A significant effort is made world wide in an attempt to prevent infective endocarditis (2-8) (see Chapter 6.4).

TREATMENT OF THE EARLY STAGES OF HEART FAILURE

Currently, an intervention is performed in most cases before the patient experiences significant symptoms of overt heart failure. Sometimes, however, the patient is already decompensated when first referred to the cardiologist; medical therapy of heart failure may also become necessary when surgery must be delayed or is refused.

Well compensated and NYHA class I patients

As a rule, patients with valvular heart disease will be advised to refrain from exhausting exercise and physically demanding competitive sport activities.

NYHA class II patients

Medical treatment as such is generally instituted when symptoms of NYHA class II develop, i.e. when the patient complains of fatigue, dyspnea and palpitations during common life activities such as rapid climbing of stairs, rapid walk, intensive gardening, etc. The patient will then be advised to maintain a regular moderate level of exercise but to avoid heavy activities. These patients will be encouraged to lose weight, and salt intake will be restricted to no more than 4.0 g of NaCl per day. Concomitant hypertension will be carefully treated.

Administration of digitalis should then be considered. Digitalis is primarily indicated to control the ventricular rate in atrial fibrillation. Its value in the presence of sinus rhythm is controversial but its use is recommended by some in the presence of echocardiographic evidence of left atrial enlargement. Digoxin may be prescribed without loading dose at a maintenance daily dose of 0.25 mg (0.125-0.5 mg) and digitoxin at the dose of 0.1 mg/day. Digoxin is generally preferred if renal function is normal and, even more, in the presence of hepatic disorders. In case of renal insufficiency, digitoxin which is metabolized in the liver is the drug of choice. Before starting digitalis and as along as it is administered, the level of serum potassium should be carefully checked and corrected if needed. Particular care is needed in elderly patients who are sometimes extremely sensitive to digitalis glycosides. Determination of serum levels of digoxin or digitoxin may be helpful to check the patient's compliance and good absorption of the drug. If despite this symptoms persist or worsen, greater attention will be paid to salt intake and a thiazide will be added.

NYHA classes III and IV patients

The treatment of patients in advanced stage of heart failure depends on the nature of the valvular lesions and will be discussed separately (vide infra).

SURVEILLANCE OF ANTICOAGULANT THERAPY

Patients in atrial fibrillation or in overt heart failure with enlarged heart or dilated left atrium, especially if spontaneous echo contrast is present ,or if antecedents of stroke are noted should be anticoagulated (9,10). Although the efficacy of anticoagulants in valvular heart disease has not been proven by randomized clinical trials, it is suggested by several reports (9). The optimal target INR (International Normalized Ratio) range has not been evaluated but it is generally considered that a moderate anticoagulant effect i.e. an INR of 2.0 - 3.0 is appropriate (10). However, a higher level of anticoagulation (INR 3.0 - 4.5) should be advised in patients with high thromboembolic risks (mitral stenosis with atrial fibrillation or previous systemic embolism even with sinus rhythm).

Warfarin or acenocoumarol may be started at a daily dose of 4.0 mg with the INR measured weekly. The dose may be adjusted by increments of 1.0 mg so as to maintain the patient in the desired therapeutic range. Phenprocoumone may also be used, its action lasts longer and is considered to be more stable. For details of risk factors, management and complications see Chapter 10.3

VALVULAR HEART DISEASE AND SURGERY

Preparation of the patient for valvular surgery

Prior to valvular surgery, all patients should be submitted to a careful dental examination and receive appropriate therapy. Digitalis should be stopped because of the risk of digitalis intoxication which is frequent postoperatively. All electrolyte disturbances should be carefully corrected. Diuretics may also be interrupted a few days before surgery because the blood volume can easily be controlled during anesthesia. Oral anticoagulants should also be interrupted three or four days before the operation and replaced by intravenous heparin.

Valvular heart disease and non-cardiac surgery

The operative risk associated with non-cardiac surgery in a patient with valvular heart disease depends on the nature of the surgical operation and on the functional status of the myocardium. For example, surgical correction of a hernia or transuretral prostate resection are generally well tolerated and may be performed provided antibiotic prophylaxis of bacterial endocarditis is applied. In contrast, major abdominal intervention (cholecystectomy, gastrectomy, intestinal resection) or thoracic surgery (pneumectomy) carry a higher risk, especially in patients in NYHA classes III or IV. The risk is highest in patients with severe aortic stenosis or mitral stenosis. In such cases, the risk of sudden death or of acute pulmonary edema during the perioperative period is so serious that it seems preferable to correct the valvular problem before undertaking such severe surgical procedure. Despite the fact that the risk is lower in the case of valvular insufficiency, it may also be preferable to correct the valvular dysfunction before any serious surgical undertaking. The presence of heart failure significantly aggravates the risk of non-cardiac surgery. Heart failure must be carefully treated and hypovolemia or hypokalemia must by all means be avoided.

The surgical intervention may precipitate atrial fibrillation related to heart failure, mitral valve disease, hypovolemia or a pulmonary disorder (emboli, infection, atelectasis). The atrial fibrillation should be treated with digitalis possibly in combination with verapamil or a beta-blocking agent. If the arrhythmia persists after the triggering factor has been cured, DC-shock will be considered. Atrial flutter may also develop during or after major surgery. It generally induces a rapid ventricular response which is badly tolerated. This rhythm disorder may be treated by DC-shock or by atrial overdrive pacing. The latter technique may be repeated without discomfort to the patient. It generally transforms atrial flutter to fibrillation which allows an easier pharmacologic control of the heart rate. In any case, the anesthetist must be well aware of the underlying cardiac problem to choose the parameters to be monitored during the operation and the optimal techniques of anesthesia.

Decision regarding continuation or interruption of long term anticoagulation may be difficult. The reader is referred to Chapter 10.3 for details of this issue.

PREGNANCY AND VALVULAR HEART DISEASE (11,12)

Hemodynamic consequences of pregnancy and delivery

Pregnancy induces significant hemodynamic consequences. The cardiac output increases; this increase, already present during the first trimester, reaches its peak (30 to 50%) between weeks 20-24. Until the 20th week the increase in cardiac output is due only to an increase in the heart rate (+10 beats/minute). Later the stroke volume also increases.

Blood volume starts to increase after six weeks. Initially rapid, this increase continues more slowly after the 14th week. The maximal difference reaches 50% on average. Exchangeable sodium increases on average by 500 to 600 mmoles and total water by about eight liters.

Uterine contractions induce an elevation of systemic blood pressure (+10%), the injection of 300-500 ml blood into the maternal circulation and a 15 to 20% increase in cardiac output. Immediate blood losses vary from 500 ml after a normal delivery to 1,000 ml after a Caesarean operation. During the days following delivery, a relative bradycardia accompanied by a further increase in cardiac output is often observed. It is attributed to the autotransfusion related to uterine contractions and to re-absorption of some of the liquid which has accumulated in the extracellular spaces during pregnancy.

The risk of pregnancy in valvular heart disease

Pregnancy carries a particularly high risk in patients with mitral stenosis. The increase in cardiac output, the rapid heart rate and the retention of water and salt are all deleterious in this condition: they cause left atrial pressure elevation and pulmonary congestion. These consequences may, in turn, provoke hemoptysis or pulmonary edema.

The elevated left atrial pressure can induce atrial fibrillation which aggravates the risk of heart failure, the development of atrial thrombi and systemic emboli. This may partly account for the increased fetal and maternal mortality which has been reported in the presence of mitral stenosis. In addition, the patient with mitral stenosis needs a high left atrial pressure to ensure a proper ventricular filling. Both pregnancy and delivery may induce abrupt variations in the distribution of blood volume. These manifest themselves by sudden lowering of atrial pressure and rapid fall of cardiac output. These considerations imply that a significant mitral stenosis in a young woman should better be relieved by surgery or percutaneous mitral valvuloplasty before she becomes pregnant.

No treatment is needed when symptoms are absent. A limitation in physical activities and salt intake will however, be recommended. If arrhythmia or pulmonary congestion develop, the classical therapy will be undertaken. If necessary a balloon valvulotomy may be performed with a low risk (13). If this is not possible, surgical valvulotomy should be completed. Surgery is possible during pregnancy, preferably during the first four months but it is possible until the seventh.

The risks of a close commissurotomy are low for the mother (less than 1%) and acceptable for the fetus (less than 10%). An open heart procedure can also be envisaged but it carries a higher fetal risk (25 to 33%). A normal vaginal delivery under the joint surveillance of an obstetrician, an anesthetist and a cardiologist appears to be the best possible mode of delivery.

Pregnancy is generally well tolerated in mitral insufficiency. Aortic stenosis is more frequent in man than in woman. It is therefore infrequent for a cardiologist to be confronted with the problem of a pregnancy in that disorder. If this happens, the risk is high if the stenosis is severe. In such cases the heart may be unable to provide a sufficient cardiac output because of the obstruction to left ventricular ejection. Any decrease of venous return can provoke a severe fall in cardiac output with cerebral or cardiac ischemia leading to dyspnea, angina or syncope. In these conditions it seems preferable to perform a valvotomy or implant a bioprosthesis prior to pregnancy. If a pregnancy develops in a patient with a severe aortic stenosis, the classical measures of prophylaxis against bacterial endocarditis will be applied. Hypovolemia will be avoided and physical activities limited. If symptoms develop and are difficult to control, the pregnancy should be interrupted or in exceptional conditions aortic surgery undertaken.

Aortic insufficiency is also infrequent in young women. Like mitral insufficiency, it is generally well tolerated in the presence of pregnancy. Preventive measures against bacterial endocarditis are indispensable. Should endocarditis develop and induce a severe heart failure, surgery should be promptly indicated.

Tricuspid and pulmonary valvular diseases are generally well tolerated during pregnancy and only require antibiotic prophylaxis against bacterial endocarditis.

Whatever the valvular lesion, the presence of pulmonary hypertension is extremely dangerous during pregnancy. Compression of the inferior vena cava by the enlarged uterus and blood losses during delivery may lead to the death of the mother. In such circumstances therefore pregnancy should be avoided or interrupted.

Contraception and voluntary interruption of pregnancy

In some cases contraception may have to be advised after one or several pregnancies. In patients without high thromboembolic risk (aortic insufficiency with sinus rhythm) and absence of arterial risk factors, hormonal contraception is advised. However, estrogens may induce water retention and hypercoagulability, and should be used in low doses, in association with progestatives. In patients with high thromboembolic risk due to the valvular disease (mechanical prosthesis, mitral stenosis, atrial fibrillation) or arterial risk factors, mechanical contraception should be preferred. Condom is used most frequently. Vaginal diaphragm combined with a spermicide is a less reliable method. Sterilet should be excluded because of the risk of infection (endocarditis) and of bleeding (anticoagulant). For permanent sterilization the Fallopian tubes should be ligated.

Cardiovascular drugs and pregnancy

Diuretics may be used during pregnancy in the case of heart failure. Hypovolemia and hypokalemia should be carefully avoided. Both digoxin and digitoxin cross the placenta and the plasma levels in the fetus are comparable to those observed in the mother. In general, a given dose of digoxin will lead to lower serum levels during pregnancy. Digoxin serum levels must therefore be carefully checked. It is interesting to note that digitalis reduces the duration of delivery probably because it has on the uterine muscle an effect similar to that it has on the myocardium.

Beta-blockers have been administered without difficulty to a large number of pregnant women. They decrease the umbilical blood flow and may result in a lower fetal weight. When they are administered just before delivery, a careful control of the newborn's heart rate and respiratory rate is mandatory. Quinidine has often been used without problem during pregnancy. It seems however preferable to avoid the administration of anti-arrhythmic agents at least during the first four months: some accidents have been noted with procainamide and disopyramide.

Oral anticoagulant drugs cross the placenta and can produce characteristic embryopathy, central nervous system abnormalities or fetal bleeding. The embryopathy consists of nasal hypoplasia, stippled epiphysis or both and seems to occur only after exposure during the first trimester. The central nervous system abnormalities (agenesis of the corpus callosum, Dandy-Walker malformations and ventral midline dysplasia with characteristic optic atrophy) have been reported with exposure to coumarin during the first trimester. Fetal bleeding appears primarily after the third month. The alternative consists of the administration of subcutaneous heparin which does not cross the placenta. Despite this feature, it appears that heparin treatment increases both maternal and fetal mortality.

Reports linking captopril to possible craniofacial defects and oligohydramiose and the results of toxicity studies in animals have convinced physicians that captopril should be avoided or used with caution in pregnancy. The use of other ACE-inhibitors have the same restriction although documentation of this danger is incomplete. It has to be underlined that the original captopril reports were at the time of high captopril doses and that it is not certain that with current lower doses the same danger would apply.

Obstetric medications and valvular heart disease

Low doses of prostaglandin E2 and F2 generally have no hemodynamic effects. Betamimetic drugs which are given to stop premature work all induce sinus tachycardia and an increase in ventricular work. They are contra-indicated in the case of compromised cardiac function. Finally, synthetic oxytocin is preferred for bleeding control, because it has no vasopressor effect.

SPECIFIC HEART VALVE DISORDERS

Whatever the valvular heart disease, bacterial endocarditis and (potentially) recurrent rheumatic fever should be meticulously prevented.

Aortic regurgitation

Acute aortic regurgitation

Acute severe aortic insufficiency carries a high risk of death from fulminant pulmonary edema and/or myocardial ischemia. It is always a medical emergency and aortic valve replacement should be indicated rapidly. The etiology influences the timing of surgery. Immediate intervention is warranted in aortic dissection. Aortic infective endocarditis raises difficult medical decisions during the first few days or weeks, because of a dilemma between a tendency to postpone surgery 10 to 15 days in the hope of controlling infection by intense antibiotic therapy on the one hand, and a continuous risk of sudden hemodynamic deterioration from perforation or rupture of valve cusps on the other. Awaiting microbiology results frequently causes an inappropriate delay that may result in irreversible myocardial damage. Early surgery is indicated in the presence of congestive heart failure and is not associated with high surgical risk (14-17). Early valve replacement is also needed when the valve is infected with organisms like serratia or candida, because sterilization is rarely accomplished medically (18,19).

Medical therapy may help to stabilize patients before operation. Vasodilators are the most useful drugs in acute aortic insufficiency because they can acutely decrease the amount of regurgitation and increase stroke volume. In such an unstable clinical situation, the vasodilator of choice must have a rapid but especially short action and should be given intravenously. The ideal agent in this setting is nitroprusside, which dilates both arteriolar and venous vessels and has a short half-life (20). It should be given in the intensive care unit with continuous monitoring of systemic arterial pressure and preferably pulmonary artery and wedge pressures. The initial dose is 0.5 Mg/kg/min and it can be increased stepwise (0.5 Mg/kg/min to 2.0 Mg/kg/min). The optimal individual perfusion rate is adjusted to normalize pulmonary artery wedge pressure without significant reduction of systolic and importantly diastolic arterial pressure.

Nitroprusside should not be discontinued abruptly to avoid rebound vasoconstriction (21). Its main side effects are methemoglobinemia and thiocyanate toxicity with an increased incidence when renal function is impaired or when high doses of the drug are given for a long period.

In addition to vasodilator drugs, a loop diuretic such as furosemide will be given if pulmonary congestion is present. Inotropic agents are not useful, because systolic function is usually normal until myocardial ischemia appears with its extremely bad prognosis. Any agent that increases systemic vascular resistance is of course contra-indicated because it would increase regurgitant fraction.

Chronic aortic regurgitation

The most difficult problem in the management of chronic aortic regurgitation is the optimal timing of valve replacement when symptoms are mild (NYHA functional classes I and II).

Asymptomatic patients with mild aortic regurgitation do not require any medication. In the rare setting of syphilitic aortic regurgitation, complete anti-syphilitic therapy is warranted.

Patients with systemic arterial hypertension should be treated if the diastolic blood pressure is increased, indicating high systemic vascular resistance that can worsen the severity of regurgitation. Vasodilators combined if necessary with a diuretic are the agents of choice. Beta-blockers must be avoided because they prolong diastolic time and may induce heart failure. Beta-blockade is also inappropriate in angina pectoris which is better treated by nitrates and/or calcium channel blockers. Asymptomatic patients with aortic regurgitation should be followed annually.

Many asymptomatic patients with chronic aortic regurgitation and normal left ventricular systolic function remain clinically stable for many years, others develop left ventricular dysfunction or symptoms and require operation. Surgery should be performed before the occurrence of irreversible myocardial damage (22,23). Symptoms usually appear before, or coincide with the onset of impaired left ventricular function (24). Echocardiographic and radionuclide angiographic studies, both initially and serially, are useful methods to identify patients at risk of complications or sudden death. Quantitative Doppler echocardiography allows accurate measurement not only of regurgitant fraction but more importantly of regurgitant volume (25). Radionuclide angiography aims to assess left ventricular volumes and ejection fraction both at rest and during exercise. Patients at risk of developing symptoms and requiring operation may be identified by initial end-systolic dimension, and rate of change in end-systolic dimension and rest ejection fraction during serial studies (24). Asymptomatic patients should undergo valve replacement if left ventricular systolic dysfunction is observed or if marked left ventricular dilatation develops (end-systolic dimension ≥80 mm or end-systolic dimension ≥55 mm on echocardiography).

In degenerative aortic regurgitation, surgery should not be postponed if the valvular lesion is associated with an ascending aortic aneurysm. Surgical indications should also be extended in cases of enlarged aorta particularly in patients with Marfan's syndrome (26).

Vasodilators are useful in chronic severe aortic regurgitation. Their unloading action reduces regurgitant fraction and increases forward stroke volume. Long term vasodilator therapy with hydralazine (27) or nifedipine (28) reduces left ventricular end-diastolic volume and improves cardiac performance. Such therapy could have a beneficial effect on the natural history of the disease and possibly delay the need for operation (28). The ideal vasodilator is unknown. Hydralazine has many side effects. Nifedipine causes neurohormonal activation. Other calcium antagonists could be more indicated. Angiotensin-converting enzyme inhibitors could have a better efficacy vs. side effect profile, but results only on the short time effect of captopril are at present available (29).

Once patients become symptomatic, surgery should be considered without delay. Temporary medical treatment before operation includes digoxin or digitoxin, diuretics and a vasodilator. In patients who are considered to be inoperable because of advanced ventricular dysfunction, similar treatment should be given and surgical intervention should again be discussed a few months later. Careful hemodynamic evaluation is then required with preferably a combined analysis of left ventricular performance using the time varying elastance concept and myocardial performance using circumferential stress-shortening relations (30).

Aortic stenosis

Medical treatment is of limited value because, when the patient with aortic stenosis becomes symptomatic, surgery is clearly indicated.

If the aortic stenosis is significant, the asymptomatic patient should avoid strenuous exercise, although sudden death during heavy exercise has been rarely reported in aortic stenosis. Doppler echocardiography allows assessment of physiologic changes with exercise (31) and could become a valuable approach for estimating the extent of possible sporting activities. Patients with moderate aortic stenosis are at significant risk for the development of complications (32). Therefore, optimal management is a regular annual follow up, with a careful history taking, an electrocardiogram and a Doppler echocardiogram. Before the onset of symptoms, survivorship is nearly normal (33). In contrast, after the onset of symptoms there is a rapid decline in survival. If surgery is not performed, half of the patients are dead within five years after the onset of angina, within three years after onset of syncope and in two years if heart failure is present. The patient should know that these three symptoms are prognostically important and must be rapidly reported to the physician as soon as they develop.

Surgery should not be recommended in the absence of symptoms only on the basis of a high transvalvular gradient because, in this situation, death occurring before the onset of symptoms is extremely uncommon (34). However, any postponement of operation once symptoms occur is associated with an increased risk of mortality (35). Surgery should therefore be performed in the early symptomatic stage, before the advent of cardiac enlargement and pulmonary vascular congestion (36). In infancy, balloon valvuloplasty has proved to be helpful in congenital severe aortic stenosis, as a substitute of surgical valvotomy. It provides safe and effective intermediate term gradient relief aiming to postpone valve replacement until adult life (37). This contrasts with the moderate and temporary results of balloon aortic valvulotomy in elderly patients, which is only a palliative treatment that should be reserved for poor candidates for valve replacement because of the high incidence of restenosis (80%) (38) and a significant, although infrequent (6%) incidence of life-threatening complications (39).

Aortic stenosis in the elderly is frequent and deserves some comments. The most common cause of aortic stenosis has become degenerative calcification of aortic valve. Moderate aortic stenosis may remain well tolerated until the patient remain in sinus rhythm but may cause rapid heart failure in the occurrence of atrial fibrillation or atrioventricular block. Therefore, frequent atrial ectopic beats recorded in the elderly patient with aortic stenosis should be treated preferably first with digitalis glycosides with the addition, if necessary, of an anti-arrhythmic drug (a class I agent, such as quinidine or flecainide, or even amiodarone). If atrial fibrillation develops, digitalis glycosides will be given to control ventricular rate, and cardioversion will be considered followed, if successful, by long term anti-arrhythmic therapy to avoid recurrence. The preservation of properly timed atrial contribution to left ventricular filling and cardiac output is indeed important in these patients. Therefore, when cardiac pacing is required, dual-chamber pacing providing atrioventricular synchrony is appropriate.

In the old patient, carotid stenosis may be difficult to detect from auscultatory findings, because of radiation of the cardiac murmur to the neck. Non-invasive evaluation of carotid arteries with duplex scanning (Doppler and echo) should be systematically performed, particularly before valve operation.

Most medications - nitrates, vasodilators and even diuretics - are potentially harmful in patients with severe aortic stenosis who may require high filling pressure to keep adequate cardiac output. In the presence of angina, nitrates should be used with great caution, because of the risk of hypotension or syncope. Heart failure complicating critical aortic stenosis is a dramatic, often unstable clinical situation which can be reversed by emergent valve replacement (40) after aggressive medical treatment under careful hemodynamic monitoring. Because of the fixed afterload, many drugs are however of limited value.

Diagnosis of heart failure secondary to critical aortic stenosis may be difficult, because cardiac murmur may be weak or absent. Doppler echocardiography is helpful in this setting to demonstrate thickened, calcified aortic valves and to measure aortic valve gradient and aortic valve area. When left ventricular performance is severely reduced, transvalvular gradients may be low, and in this situation it is not easy to distinguish between severe aortic stenosis and a coincident cardiomyopathy with a mild aortic stenosis. This distinction is however crucial because the latter situation is best treated by vasodilators and the former by early surgery. Calculation of transaortic gradient and valve area should be performed in this clinical setting under conditions that may increase cardiac output, such as a low dose catecholamine infusion.

Mitral stenosis

When mitral stenosis is severe, the only solution is to increase valve area by surgical intervention - valve replacement or valvotomy - or by balloon dilatation. Percutaneous mitral valvulotomy is currently an excellent alternative to surgical commissurotomy, with equally good results (41,42). Not every mitral stenosis is severe enough to require an intervention. Medical management has an important role to improve symptoms, and to prevent and/or correct atrial fibrillation and systemic embolism.

Control of symptoms

Dyspnea results from the effects of increased left atrial pressure on the lungs. Patients with pulmonary congestion or edema may considerably benefit from diuretic therapy. The effectiveness of currently used diuretics has made severe salt restriction unnecessary, but a no-added-salt diet is still required. Digitalis is of limited value if sinus rhythm is still present. It does not improve heart failure and does not prevent exercise-induced tachycardia. Digitalis could however be considered in the presence of right ventricular dysfunction or of enlarged left atrium which may foreshadow atrial fibrillation.

Chest pain suggesting angina pectoris should be properly investigated: it can be related to coronary atherosclerosis, coronary embolism or right ventricular dysfunction. Nitrates should be used with caution, as all vasodilators.

Management of atrial fibrillation (43)

Atrial fibrillation is a frequent complication of mitral stenosis and may precipitate acute pulmonary edema or increase the risk of systemic embolism. The onset of atrial fibrillation is often preceded by the occurrence of atrial premature complexes. Such an observation requires preventive therapy by digitalis alone or in conjunction with quinidine or disopyramide which should not be given alone because of the risk of increased ventricular response if atrial fibrillation develops.

The high pulse rate of new onset atrial fibrillation requires rapid control of the ventricular rate with intravenous digitalis followed by oral digitalization. Anticoagulation should begin immediately. Electric cardioversion should be considered at the initial presentation only in the presence of serious hemodynamic deterioration because of the risk of embolization. Preliminary data suggest that early cardioversion can be performed safely if transesophageal echocardiography excludes the presence of atrial thrombi (44). It is however premature to recommend this approach in all patients (45). The classic management requires administration of anticoagulants for two to four weeks prior to cardioversion in order to allow time for friable thrombi to be organized. Anticoagulation should also be continued after cardioversion because the restoration of atrial function may detach a clot and also because recovery of atrial function is usually progressive, allowing the development of new thrombi. For many physicians, the onset of atrial fibrillation in the course of mitral stenosis represents an indication for long term anticoagulation. Because of the risk of serious ventricular arrhythmias induced by cardioversion if there is digitalis toxicity, digoxin is usually discontinued two days and digitoxin one week before the procedure. This remains however controversial.

Following its restoration, long term therapy is needed to maintain sinus rhythm. The combination of digitalis-quinidine or digitalis-disopyramide is frequently used. Other anti-arrhythmic agents may be considered in this situation: class Ic agents - flecainide, propafenone -, beta-blockers - preferably sotalol, verapamil or amiodarone.

Cardioversion is usually unsuccessful if the left atrium is very large (>50 mm on echocardiography) or if atrial fibrillation has been present for more than six months. Conversion of atrial fibrillation to sinus rhythm can be usually considered again after correction of the mitral stenosis by surgery or balloon valvulotomy. If permanent atrial fibrillation cannot be avoided, ventricular rate must be controlled not only at rest - this is obtainable using digitalis-, but also during physical activities. This frequently requires the addition of another drug. In mitral stenosis, the benefit of prolonging diastole and increasing left ventricular filling time overcomes the negative inotropic effect of beta-blockers or verapamil. Small doses, such as 10 to 20 mg propranolol two to four times a day or 80 mg verapamil three times a day may suffice. Adequate control of heart rate can be assessed by 24 hour Holter monitoring and/or an exercise test. If the heart rate remains high, hyperthyroidism is to be excluded.

Anticoagulation

Systemic embolism, in two-third of cases stroke, is sometimes the first clinical manifestation of mitral stenosis (46,47). It may occur in the presence of sinus rhythm, although paroxysmal or chronic atrial fibrillation increases the risk (48) which is highest soon after the onset of atrial fibrillation. This explains why some centers suggest the systematic use of warfarin in every patient with significant mitral stenosis. The benefit must be weighed against the risk of bleeding in patients with advanced age, impaired liver function or known sources of serious bleeding. Risk factors of systemic emboli to be considered are history of previous embolism, enlarged left atrium (>45 mm on echocardiography), atrial fibrillation, congestive heart failure or reduced cardiac output and spontaneous echo contrast within the left atrium indicating stasis (49). The degree of mitral stenosis is also a promoting factor. Spontaneous echo contrast disappears after percutaneous balloon valvulotomy (50).

Antiplatelet agents, such as aspirin, dipyridamole or ticlopidine have not been shown to be possible substitutes for warfarin. Their addition to warfarin could reduce the incidence of emboli, but proper indications are not well defined.

Mitral regurgitation

Management of atrial fibrillation follows the same guidelines as for mitral stenosis. In the presence of dyspnea, orthopnea and fatigue, medical treatment is necessary and should include a diuretic and a vasodilator. The value of digitalis is more limited. Vasodilator therapy has an important role in patients with mitral regurgitation and leads to a considerable improvement, even if left ventricular function is still normal. The reduction of peripheral vascular resistance reduces regurgitant fraction and reduces left ventricular volume, thus the size of the regurgitant orifice (51). A number of vasodilators have been used: nitrates, arterial vasodilators, such as hydralazine, or angiotensin-converting enzyme inhibitors - captopril, enalapril, lisinopril and so on (52,53). The vasodilator effect of captopril is parasympathetically meditated (54). ACE-inhibitors must be used initially in small doses because of their hypotensive effects. The starting dose of 6.25 or 12.5 mg for captopril - or 2.5 or 5 mg for enalapril or lisinopril - should be progressively increased. Right heart catheterization is not warranted to monitor early response to the drug. Renal function and serum potassium must be monitored. In some patients, the dose of diuretic must be increased because of fluid retention, but this increase in diuretic requirement is often temporary.

The most difficult problem is the optimal time for surgical correction (55), and this issue is discussed in detail in Chapter 4.2. In brief, patients with NYHA class III or IV should be operated without delay. The presence of preoperative markers of suboptimal response to corrective surgery (LV endsystolic dimension >50 mm, ejection fraction <50%) should prompt to perform mitral valve repair or mitral valve replacement with preservation of the chordae tendinae if possible. This technique reduces the risk for the development of LV dysfunction which is concealed preoperatively by the particular loading conditions - reduced afterload, increased preload - associated with chronic mitral regurgitation.

Patients with no or minimal symptoms should be followed regularly and undergo exercise testing and Doppler echocardiography. Radionuclide angiography at rest and during exercise has been shown to be useful in this condition (56). The onset of atrial fibrillation warrants surgery. It is essential to perform surgery before the development of irreversible LV dysfunction. The good late results of mitral valve repair (57) and the recent advances in this type of surgery (58) have changed our timing of surgical correction in asymptomatic patients. An early surgery is advisable in cases of severe valve regurgitation whenever a valve repair is possible (59).

Calcification of the mitral annulus

Mitral regurgitation due to mitral annular calcification is frequent in the elderly. Heart failure is rare if mitral annular calcification is the only cardiac abnormality (60) and is managed as presented earlier. Attention should be paid to the development of conduction abnormalities: bundle branch block or atrioventricular block (61). Rarely, massive mitral annular calcification can produce functional mitral stenosis (62).

Antibiotic prophylaxis should be considered for dental or surgical procedures in patients with mitral annular calcification, as infective endocarditis may occur and is frequently fatal because of the development of abscesses in the annular ring (63). Systemic embolism has also been reported in this condition.

Mitral valve prolapse

Most patients with asymptomatic and mild mitral valve prolapse have a long term uncomplicated clinical course and should be reassured. If the electrocardiogram is normal, the murmur short and the valve leaflets not redundant, a follow up examination every three years is sufficient. In other cases, an annual follow up is required. Holter ECG monitoring and exercise testing are indicated in patients who have palpitations or dizziness (64). Long Q-T interval may be present (65). Arrhythmias are usually well controlled with propranolol or another beta-blocker. Second-time agents are sotalol, disopyramide or amiodarone. Interesting results have been obtained on arrhythmias with the use of barbiturates. Sudden death is rare (66): the mechanism is ventricular tachycardia or fibrillation in most cases. Persons with isolated mitral valve prolapse dying suddenly tend to be relatively young women without mitral regurgitation (67).

Chest pain is best treated with a beta-blocking drug and less frequently relieved by nitrates which can increase the valvular prolapse by reducing left ventricular volume. Embolic events have been reported, but the incidence is very low and aspirin should be considered only in patients who have experienced suggestive symptoms. Infective endocarditis is not uncommon and antibiotic prophylaxis should be performed at least in patients with mitral regurgitation determined by clinical examination or echocardiography. Some authors also recommend prophylaxis even for an isolated click, especially if the leaflets are redundant (see also Chapter 4.3).

Rupture of the chordae tendinae

Spontaneous rupture of chordae tendinae may be observed in mitral valve prolapse syndrome, Marfan's syndrome, fibroelastic degeneration, infective endocarditis or secondary to trauma. Mitral regurgitation may be acute and severe, depending on the number of ruptured chordae.

The unprepared left atrium transmits systolic pressure to the pulmonary veins resulting in the sudden onset of dyspnea or pulmonary edema. The lesions are very well defined by echocardiography, particularly from the transesophageal window. Intensive care may be warranted and drugs may be administered intravenously, similarly as for acute aortic regurgitation. In such a severe situation emergency surgery is frequently necessary: repair is usually possible and successful, but mitral valve replacement may be necessary.

In other patients, acute mitral regurgitation is easily treated with vasodilators, diuretics and digitalis, and valve repair is not required if the left ventricle is not significantly enlarged (see also Chapter 4.2).

Mitral regurgitation and coronary artery disease

Mitral regurgitation is common in patients with coronary artery disease. It can be related to dyskinesia of the inferior wall, postinfarction fibrosis of a papillary muscle, left ventricular aneurysm or congestive cardiomyopathy. It may be episodic, caused by reversible ischemia, or dramatic in the setting of papillary muscle rupture complicating acute myocardial infarction, especially in inferior infarction. This latter situation usually leads to acute pulmonary edema, hypotension and cardiogenic shock. Immediate surgery should be undertaken as more than 50% of patients die within 24 hours (68). Transient hemodynamic improvement may be obtained by intra-aortic balloon pumping, intravenous sodium nitroprusside and/or dobutamine allowing coronary arteriography and transesophageal echocardiography to be performed before operation.

Acute severe mitral regurgitation secondary to ischemic posterior papillary dysfunction without rupture can be treated by emergency coronary angioplasty with favorable long term outcome in selected cases (69). Reversible ischemia may sometimes induce papillary muscle dysfunction and acute reversible mitral regurgitation, causing rarely pulmonary edema (70). In cases of severe chronic mitral regurgitation caused by papillary dysfunction, valve surgery (repair or valve replacement) should be envisaged with coronary artery bypass grafting, when possible.

In other patients with coronary artery disease, mitral regurgitation may be only moderate. Treatment of atrial fibrillation or heart failure is as earlier described (see also Chapter 6.5).

Tricuspid and pulmonary lesions

Rheumatic tricuspid valve disease is not rare. Prevention of endocarditis is necessary. Salt restriction, digitalis, diuretics - loop diuretic and spironolactone - are useful. If significant, tricuspid stenosis is generally an indication for valve repair and, occasionally, balloon valvulotomy or valve replacement. Management of tricuspid regurgitation depends on organic or functional origin of the regurgitation. Severe organic tricuspid regurgitation usually requires surgery. If tricuspid regurgitation is related to pulmonary hypertension, the relief of pulmonary hypertension by mitral valve replacement, repair or reconstruction may correct the functional incompetence. In the presence of dilated but normal tricuspid valve annuloplasty may be indicated.

In the absence of pulmonary hypertension, tricuspid regurgitation is often well tolerated and easily controlled by diuretics and digitalis. In the case of tricuspid endocarditis in drug abusers, total excision of the valve without replacement may well be tolerated for a long period of time (71), but valve repair seems to be the best treatment.

Traumatic severe tricuspid regurgitation secondary to flail leaflet is best treated by tricuspid valve repair. Isolated right valvular lesions (tricuspid regurgitation, pulmonary stenosis and regurgitation) may be related to carcinoid syndrome; this diagnosis should be confirmed by the presence of vasoactive amines and their metabolites.

References:
1. American Heart Association. Committee on rheumatic fever and bacterial endocarditis: prevention of rheumatic fever. Circulation 1977;55:1
2. Canson RA. Infective endocarditis as a complication of dental treatment. Br Dent J 1981;151-409

3. Endocarditis Working Party of the British Society for Antimicrobial Chemotherapy. Antibiotic prophylaxis of infective endocarditis. Lancet 1990;335:88-89
4. Working Party of the European Society of Cardiology. Prophylaxis of infective endocarditis for dental procedures. Eur Heart J 1985;6:826-828
5. Dajani AS, Bisno AL, Chung KJ, et al. Prevention of bacterial endocarditis. Recommendation by the American Heart Association. JAMA 1990;264:2919-2922
6. Phrophylaxie de l'Endocardite Infectieuse. Recommendations Jury de la Conference de Consensus du 27 mars 1992. Arch Mal Coeur 1993;86 (Suppl.12):1897-1902
7. Sadosky D, Kunzel C. Recommendations for prevention of bacterial endocarditis: compliance by dental general practitioners. Circulation 1988;77:1316-1318
8. Vuille C, Bloch A. Les dentistes appliquent-ils correctement les recommendations pour la prophylaxie des endocardites bacteriennes? Arch Mal Coeur 1992;85:227-232
9. Dadez E. Fibrillation auriculaire et traitments antithrombotiques. in: Samama M, Acar J. Traitements antithrombotiques. Masson, Paris 1993 p 153
10. Hirsch J. Oral anticoagulant drugs. N Engl J Med 1991;324:1865-1875
11. Perloff JK. Pregnancy and cardiovascular disease. In E Braunwald: Heart disease. A textbook of cardiovascular medicine. WB Saunders, Philadelphia, 2nd Edition 1984:1763
12. McAnulty SH, Metcalfe J, Ueland K. Heart disease and pregnancy. In: J Willis Hurst: The Heart. McGraw-Hill, New York, 5th Edition, 1982:1521
13. Iung B. Cormier B, Elias J, et al. Les commissurotomie mitrale percutanee durant la grossesse. Arch Mal Coeur 1993;86:995-999
14. Middlemost S, Wisenbaugh T, Meyerowitz C, et al. A case for early surgery in native left-sided endocarditis complicated by heart failure: results in 203 patients. J Am Coll Cardiol 1991;18:663-667
15. Aufiero TX, Waldenhausen JA. Editorial comment: early surgery for native left-sided endocarditis. J Am Coll Cardiol 1991;18:668
16. Michel PL, Vitoux B, Hage A, Ghanem G, Dybantsa P, Acar J. Early or delayed surgery in acute native aortic valve endocarditis. in: "Current Issues in Heart Valve Disease" Infective Endocarditis. Horstkotte D, Bodnar E (eds). London, ICR Publishers 1991;220-228
17. Acar J, Michel PL. Chirurgie de l'endocardite bacterienne. Quand? Arch Mal Coeur 1993;86(Suppl. 12):1863-1867
18. Richardson JV, Karp RB, Kirklin JW, Dismukes WE. Treatment of infective endocarditis: a 10 year comparative analysis. Circulation 1978;58:589-597
19. Rapaport E. Editorial: the changing role of surgery in the management of infective endocarditis. Circulation 1978;58:598-599
20. Miller R, Vismara LA, De Maria AN, Salel AF, Mason DT. Afterload reduction therapy with nitroprusside in severe aortic regurgitation: improved cardiac performance and reduced regurgitant volume. Am J Cardiol 1876;38:564-567
21. Packer M, Meller J, Medina N, Gorlin R, Herman MV. Rebound hemodynamic events after the abrupt withdrawal of nitroprusside in patients with severe chronic heart failure. N Engl J Med 1979;301:1193-1197
22. Bonow RO, Picone AL, McIntosh CL, et al. Survival and functional results after valve replacement for aortic regurgitation from 1976 to 1983: Impact of preoperative left ventricular function. Circulation 1985;72:1244-1256
23. Acar J, Luxereau P, Vahanian A, et al. L'insuffisance aortique chronique operee. Arch Mal Coeur 1978;71:1387-1396
24. Bonow RO, Lakatos R, Maron BJ, Epstein SE. Serial long-term assessment of the natural history of asymptomatic patients with chronic aortic regurgitation and normal left ventricular systolic function. Circulation 1991; 84:1625-1635
25. Enriquez-Sarano M, Bailey KR, Seward JB, Tajik AJ, Krohn MJ, Mays JM. Quantitative Doppler assessment of valvular regurgitation. Circulation 1993;87:841-848
26. Michel PL, Acar J, Chomette G, Iung B. Degenerative aortic regurgitation. Eur Heart J 1991;12:875-882
27. Greenberg B, Massie B, Bristow JD, Cheitlin M, Siemienczuk D, Topic N, Wilson RA, Szlachcic J, Thomas D. Long-term vasodilator therapy of chronic aortic insufficiency: a randomized double-blinded, placebo-controlled clinical trial. Circulation 1988;78:92-103
28. Scognamiglio R, Rahimtoola SH, Fasoli G, Nistri S, Dalla Volta S. Nifedipine in asymptomatic patients with severe aortic regurgitation and normal left ventricular function. N Engl J Med 1994;331:689-694
29. Reske SN, Heck I, Kropp J, et al. Captopril mediated decrease of aortic regurgitation. Br Heart J 1985;54:415-419
30. Starling MR, Kirsch MM, Montgomery DG, Gross MD. Mechanisms for left ventricular systolic dysfunction in aortic regurgitation: importance for predicting the functional response to aortic valve replacement. J Am Coll Cardiol 1991;17:887-897

31. Otto CM, Pearlman AS, Kraft CD, Miyake-Hull CY, Burwash IG, Gardner CJ. Physiologic changes with maximal exercise in asymptomatic valvular aortic stenosis assessed by Doppler echocardiography. J Am Coll Cardiol 1992;20:1160-1167

32. Kennedy KD, Nishimura RA, Holmes Dr Jr, Bailey KR. Natural History of moderate aortic stenosis. J Am Coll Cardiol 1991;17:313-319

33. Ross J Jr, Braunwald E. Aortic stenosis. Circulation 1968;38(Suppl V):V61-V67

34. Kelly TA, Rothbart RM, Cooper CM, Kaiser DL, Smucker ML, Gibson RS. Comparison of outcome of asymptomatic to symptomatic patients older than 20 years of age with valvular aortic stenosis. Am J Cardiol 1988;61:123-130

35. Lund O. Preoperative risk evaluation and stratification of long-term survival after valve replacement for aortic stenosis. Reasons for earlier operative intervention. Circulation 1990;82:124-139

36. Hancock EW. Timing of valve replacement for aortic stenosis. Circulation 1990;82:310-312

37. O'Connor BK, Beekman RH, Rocchini AP, Rosenthal A. Intermediate-term effectiveness of balloon valvuloplasty for congenital aortic stenosis. A prospective follow-up study. Circulation 1991;84:732-738

38. Block PC, Palacios IF. Clinical and hemodynamic follow-up after percutaneous aortic valvuloplasty in the elderly. Am J Cardiol 1988;62:760-763

39. Isner JM and the Mansfield Scientific aortic valvuloplasty registry investigators. Acute catastrophic complications of balloon aortic valvuloplasty. J Am Coll Cardiol 1991;17:1436-1444

40. Smith N, McAnulty JH, Rahimtoola SH. Severe aortic stenosis with impaired left ventricular function and clinical heart failure. Results of valve replacement. Circulation 1878;58:255-264

41. Vahanian A, Michel PL, Cormier B, et al. Results of percutaneous mitral commissurotomy in 200 patients. Am J Cardiol 1989;63:847-852

42. Turi ZG, Reyes VP, Raju BS, et al. Percutaneous balloon versus surgical closed commissurotomy for mitral stenosis: a prospective, randomized trial. Circulation 1991;83:1179-1185

43. Mancini GBJ, Goldberger AL. Cardioversion of atrial fibrillation: consideration of embolization, anticoagulation, prophylactic pacemaker and long-term success. An Heart J 1982;104:617-621

44. Manning WJ, Silverman DI, Gordon PF, Krumholz HM, Douglas PS. Cardioversion from atrial fibrillation without prolonged anticoagulation with use of transesophageal echocardiography to exclude the presence of atrial thrombi. N Engl J Med 1993;328:750-755

45. Daniel WG. Should transesophageal echocardiography be used to guide cardioversion? N Engl J Med 1993;328:803-804

46. Dally R, Mattingly TW, Holt CL, Bland FF, White PD. Systemic arterial embolism in rheumatic heart disease. Am Heart J 1951;42:566

47. Bannister R. The risk of differing valvotomy in patients with moderate mitral stenosis. Lancet 1960;2:329-333

48. Szekely P. Systemic embolism and anticoagulant prophylaxis in rheumatic heart disease. Br Med J 1964;1:209-212

49. Daniel WG, Nellessen U, Schroder E, et al. Left atrial spontaneous echo contrast in mitral valve disease: an indicator for an increased thromboembolic risk. J Am Coll Cardiol 1988;11:1204-1211

50. Cormier B, Vahanian A, Iung B, et al. Influence of percutaneous mitral commissurotomy on left atrial spontaneous contrast of mitral stenosis. Am J Card 1993;71:842-847

51. Yoran C, Yellin EL, Becker RM, Gabbay S, Frater RWM, Sonnenblick EH. Mechanism of reduction of mitral regurgitation with vasodilator therapy. Am J Cardiol 1979;43:773-777

52. Greenberg BH, De Mots H, Murphy E, Rahimtoola SH. Arterial dilators in mitral regurgitation: effects on rest and exercise hemodynamics and long-term clinical follow-up. Circulation 1982;65:181-187

53. Greenberg BH, Massie BM, Brundage BH, Botvinick EH, Parmley WW, Chatterjee K. Beneficial effects of hydralazine in severe mitral regurgitation. Circulation 1878;58:273-279

54. Wisenbaugh T, Essop R, Sareli P. Short-term vasodilator effect of captopril in patients with severe mitral regurgitation is parasympathetically mediated. Circulation 1991;84:2049-2053

55. Zile MR. Chronic aortic and mitral regurgitation. Choosing the optimal time for surgical correction. Cardiology Clinics. Valvular heart disease 1991;239-253

56. Boucher CA, Okadu RD, Pohost GM. Current status of radionuclide imaging in valvular heart disease. Am J Cardiol 1980;46:1153-1163

57. Michel PL, Iung B, Blanchard B, Luxereau P, Dorent R, Acar J. Long-term results of mitral valve repair for non-ischaemic mitral regurgitation. Eur Heart J 1991;12(Suppl B):39-43

58. Deloche A, Jebara VA, Relland JY, et al. Valve repair with Carpentier's techniques. The second decade. J Thorac Cardiovasc Surg 1991;89:990-1102

59. Acar J, Michel PL, Luxereau P, Vahanian A, Cormier B. Indications for surgery in mitral regurgitation. Eur Heart J 1991;12(Suppl B):52-54

60. Gabor GE, Mohr BD, Goel PC, Cohen B. Echocardiographic and clinical spectrum of mitral annular calcification. Am J Cardiol 1876;38:836-842

61. Nair CK, Aronow WS, Sketch MH, et al. Clinical and echocardiographic characteristics of patients with mitral annular calcification: comparison with age- and sex- matched control subjects. Am J Cardiol 1983; 51:992-995
62. Osterberger LE, Goldstein S, Khaja F, Lakier JB. Functional mitral stenosis in patients with massive mitral calcification. Circulation 1981;64:472-476
63. Burnside JW, De Sanctis RW. Bacterial endocarditis on calcification of the mitral annulus fibrosus. Am J Med 1972;76:615-619
64. Winkle RA, Copes MG, Popp RL, Hancock EW. Life-threatening arrhythmias with mitral valve prolapse syndrome. Am J Med 1976;60:961-967
65. Puddu PE, Pasternac A, Tubau JF, Krol R, Farly L, Champlain J. QT interval prolongation and increased catecholamine levels in patients with mitral valve prolapse. Am Heart J 1983;105:422-428
66. Chesler E, King RA, Edwards JE. The myxomatous mitral valve and sudden death. Circulation 1983;67:632-639
67. Dollar AL, Roberts WC. Morphologic comparison of patients with mitral valve prolapse who died suddenly with patients who died from severe valvular dysfunction or other conditions. J Am Coll Cardiol 1991;17:921-931
68. Wei JT, Hutchins GM, Bulkley BH. Papillary muscle rupture in fatal acute myocardial infarction: a potentially treatable cause of cardiogenic shock. Ann Intern Med 1979;90:149-153
69. Shawl FA, Forman MB, Punja S, Goldbaum TS. Emergent coronary angioplasty in the treatment of acute ischemic mitral regurgitation: long-term results in five cases. J Am Coll Cardiol 1989;14:986-991
70. Brody W, Criley JM. Intermittent severe mitral regurgitation. Hemodynamic studies in a patient with recurrent acute left-sided heart failure. N Engl J Med 1970;283:673-676
71. Arbulu A, Holmes RJ, Asfaw I. Surgical treatment of intractable right sided infective endocarditis in drug addicts: 25 years experience. J Heart Valve Dis 1993;2:129-137

Chapter 7.2

Percutaneous balloon valvulotomy

Alec Vahanian, Olivier Nallet and Joseph Elias

Percutaneous dilation techniques have been in use for more than 15 years for the treatment of peripheral and coronary ar terial stenosis, with subsequent application in congenital and, since 1984, acquired valvular stenosis.

The percutaneous dilation of acquired valvular stenosis is therefore a relatively "young" technique in comparison with surgical procedures which date back several decades. The advantage of this recent evolution of the method is that it benefits from the rapidly advancing technology, particularly as regards dilation equipment and echocardiography. The disadvantage is that the clinical experience is limited and long term outcome is yet to be established. We shall examine in succession in this section mitral, aortic and tricuspid dilation procedures, and finally the dilation of bioprostheses.

PERCUTANEOUS MITRAL COMMISSUROTOMY

Up to the time of the first publication by Inoue on "Percutaneous Mitral Commissurotomy" (PMC) in 1984 (1), surgery was the only treatment available for patients suffering from mitral stenosis.

The majority of articles reporting experiences and results with PMC have been published from 1986 onwards. During the same period considerable technical changes have taken place and large patient cohorts have undergone treatment. Therefore, the efficacy of the treatment, its risks and the results obtained in the medium term can be reasonably well assessed.

Potentials and limitations

The original publication by Inoue (1), based on findings during and immediately after intervention, and supported later by anatomic, radiologic and echocardiographic observations (2- 8), was able to show that PMC achieved an effect equivalent to surgical commissurotomy in obtaining the release of commissural fusions.

PMC, like closed surgical commissurotomy, has only a limited effect in the case of gross fibrosis, calcification or advanced, extensive changes in the subvalvular apparatus. Particularly in this latter situation, PMC is less effective than open heart commissurotomy, which permits a complete repair at the valvular and subvalvular levels under visual control. The considerable similarity between the mechanisms of action of PMC and closed commissurotomy suggests that these two techniques would yield comparable results, both immediately and probably in the long term.

Technique

There are two main routes of access: the transarterial and the transvenous routes.

The transarterial or retrograde approach

Two different transarterial procedures are available depending on whether or not a transseptal catheterization technique is used.

The transarterial retrograde technique described by Babic (9,10) requires the insertion of a guide in the left ventricle via the transseptal route, subsequently passing through the aortic valve down to the descending aorta. The guide is then caught by a catheter introduced through the femoral artery. The balloon or balloons are then moved along the transarterial, retrograde route through the mitral valve. The advantage of this technique is that it reduces the risk of lesion to the interatrial septum. Its drawback is the risk of traumatic injury to the femoral artery, especially when using the double balloon technique. This procedure, however, is difficult to perform, requires several trained operators and is seldom used at present.

With the retrograde technique without transseptal catheterization (11-14), the balloon or balloons are introduced through the femoral or, less frequently, the brachial artery (13). Catheters and steerable guides are used for passing the balloons from the left ventricle to the left atrium. The specific advantage of this approach is that it obviates the need for transseptal catheterization. Nevertheless, retrograde catheterization of the left atrium is not always easy and involves a certain risk in the positioning of the guides through the subvalvular apparatus and a further risk of causing severe mitral insufficiency during inflation of the balloon. It has been used with good results and with a complication rate comparable to that of other techniques (14), but only in a limited number of cases, and further studies will be necessary to evaluate its true value in clinical practice.

The transvenous or anterograde approach

This approach is the most widely used currently. Transseptal catheterization is the first and undoubtedly one of the most important steps in the procedure and the development of PMC has rekindled interest in this technique. Holmes (15) recently described the conditions required for the successful performance of transseptal catheterization: (1) good knowledge of the cardiac anatomy, (2) compliance with the contraindications, and (3) adequate operator experience, which is without doubt the essential factor. A floating catheter is used (16) to facilitate passage through the mitral valve. It should reduce the number and extent of manipulations within the left atrium and provide help in avoiding iatrogenic, catheter induced lesions to the subvalvular apparatus.

Heparin is usually given after the transseptal catheterization.

Balloons

Two main techniques are used; the double balloon technique and the Inoue technique.

The double balloon technique

Many publications report experiences with this technique (17-20). Where the left ventricle has been catheterized with a floating balloon, two long change-over guides are positioned in the left ventricular apex or, less frequently, in the ascending aorta. The interatrial septum is dilated using a 5-8 mm peripheral angioplasty balloon (21). The final stage is the positioning of the balloons across the mitral valve. Two round balloons of conventional design are used, or a combination of one trifoil balloon and a conventional balloon in our case. The lengths of the balloons vary between 3 cm and 5.5 cm.

The Inoue technique

This technique was the first to be introduced, but for a long time its use was limited to Japan and the Far East (22). More widespread experience has been gained since the commercial marketing of the balloon. The Inoue balloon is made of nylon and rubber micro-mesh. It is self-positioned and its extensibility depends on the inflating pressure. Its inflated diameter varies between 24 mm and 30 mm, although it has a low profile (4.5 mm). The balloon comprises three main elements, each having its own individual elasticity, thus enabling them to be inflated in sequence. The characteristics of this balloon permit a rapid positioning and stable orientation across the mitral valve. Inoue (23) has recommended the use of a progressive dilation technique under echocardiographic control to monitor valve orifice area and changes in the degree of mitral insufficiency.

It is still difficult to compare the efficacy of the double balloon and Inoue techniques. Results of a number of retrospective studies have been published (24-30), but experience drawn from prospective randomized trials is scant, not more than two publications involving only small numbers (31-32). The following comparisons may however be made:

1. The Inoue technique is easier to use since it involves fewer manipulations. This in turn results in shorter procedure and fluoroscopy times, a factor of considerable importance for the cardiologist and also for the patient in the case of a pregnant woman.
2. The data available to us do not reveal any significant difference in terms of efficacy, although there is a tendency for slightly greater valve orifice areas to be obtained (30) and a greater frequency of bi-commissural opening with the double balloon technique (29).
3. In terms of the risks involved, the incidence of ventricular perforation is less with the Inoue balloon, since no guide is inserted in the left ventricle due to the geometry of the balloon (24-27). The incidence of severe mitral insufficiency with the Inoue technique varies according to whether or not progressive dilation is used; this procedure appears to reduce the risk of severe mitral insufficiency (33,34). Where a maximum inflation is used with the Inoue balloon straight away (22), the risk is equivalent to or even greater than that incurred with the double balloon technique. The low profile of the Inoue balloon during its insertion and withdrawal via the interatrial septum should, in theory, reduce the magnitude of interatrial shunts, but this has not yet been confirmed in the literature. The risk of balloon rupture and its associated

complications, for example embolism, appears to be less with the Inoue technique (24,27,35).
4. The main disadvantage of the Inoue technique is its price, plus the need for echocardiographic control during dilation. A final factor is the structural complexity of the materials with the consequent possibility of technical failure; the failure rate appears to be very low (36) but has yet to be definitively established.

The available data therefore suggest that the Inoue technique, as compared to the double balloon technique, makes the procedure easier, is equally effective or only slightly less so and reduces the risk of complications. Any definitive conclusion on the relative merits of these two techniques will have to be based on the outcome of controlled randomized studies involving large numbers with a long enough follow up. Nonetheless, the Inoue technique is the most widely used world-wide today.

In addition to these two techniques, there is a third technique which makes use of a balloon of large diameter.

Large diameter balloon technique

The single balloon technique was used in initial experimental series, with balloon diameters between 20 and 25 mm; this did not however permit adequate dilation since the excessive profile of these balloons caused difficulties in positioning and imposed an increased risk of damage to the interatrial septum. More recently, several preliminary series of experiments have been carried out with good results and with a low complication rate using low-profile single balloons of up to 30 mm in diameter (37,38). This technique is attractive in that it is relatively easy to carry out, but it necessitates the use of rigid guides with a consequent potential risk of left ventricular perforation.

In parallel with this, a number of authors have used a variation of the double balloon technique in the form of the bifoil balloon, which consists of two balloons with a common shaft. This approach has the same advantages as a single balloon of large diameter. In preliminary series these bifoil balloons were found to have an excessive profile (39-40), but recent developments have enabled low-profile balloons to be designed which are capable of passing through the interatrial septum without causing damage (41). The addition of a "pigtail" termination may further reduce the incidence of ventricular perforations. However, the data available on these recent models are scant and will have to be confirmed in larger series.

Choice of balloon dimension

Irrespective of the model used, the choice of balloon dimension is still a matter of argument. The desire to obtain the greatest possible increase in valve orifice area has to be set against the risk of causing a severe mitral insufficiency. The dimensions of the balloon are normally selected as a function of patient characteristics; stature (23), body surface area (a ratio between the effective dilation surface of the balloon and body surface area larger than 3.9 is predictor of a possible increase in mitral insufficiency (42)), or the mitral ring diameter (an increase in mitral insufficiency may occur if the ratio between the sum of the balloon diameters and those of the mitral ring is greater than 1.1 (43)).

Evaluation of the immediate results

There are two main techniques for evaluation of the immediate results in the hemodynamic laboratory; hemodynamic analysis and echocardiography.

Immediate hemodynamic analysis may be subject to error as a result of hemodynamic instability, for example due to hypovolemia or a vago-vagal reaction. Furthermore, the Gorlin formula may provide erroneous results because of the incorrect determination of the cardiac output in the presence of an interatrial shunt or as the result of overestimation of the valve orifice area in the event of an associated mitral insufficiency. Occlusion of the septal defect with a floating balloon (44), or with the Inoue balloon itself, enables a more exact calculation of the orifice area on conclusion of the procedure.

Echocardiographic evaluation

Echocardiography may be useful occasionally in determining the site of the transseptal puncture. This can be done by TTE and more recently by TEE, which permits a better visualization of the interatrial septum (45,46). Transesophageal echocardiography is, however, not always easy to perform in the hemodynamic laboratory, and should be restricted to cases in which significant technical difficulties arise with other techniques. A recent trial (47), carried out on a small number of patients, suggested the possibility of performing a PMC monitored only by transesophageal echocardiography, but the large number of hemopericardial accidents that occurred in this series precludes any general recommendation of the method in its present state.

Echocardiographic monitoring is of critical importance when using the Inoue technique with progressive dilation. The criteria we apply for ending balloon dilation are the obtaining of a satisfactory orifice area (> 1 cm^2/m^2) in conjunction with a commissural opening and/or the appearance or increase of more than 1/4 of a mitral insufficiency, in particular at the site of the commissure. The correlation between Doppler measurements, two- dimensional echo and hemodynamic analysis is much less satisfactory after a PMC than before. Thomas (48) has suggested that the drastic changes in atrial and left ventricular compliance accompanying PMC may prejudice the validity of the Doppler measurement using the pressure half- time after the dilation. Wisenbaugh (49) recently showed that the validity of the pressure half-time may be improved by an acute volume load.

The two-dimensional echo permits a qualitative evaluation of the results by visualizing the commissural opening, accompanied by a quantitative evaluation by planimetric methods wherever possible. The use of intracardiac echocardiography may in the future assist in the monitoring and implementation of PMC (50).

Failures

The failure rate varies from 1% to 20% (20-22,27,51,54). Failures are most often due to an inability to obtain a successful transseptal puncture or to position the balloon

Table 7.2-I: Immediate hemodynamic results: Tenon Hospital experience.
n = 810

	Before PMC	After PMC	P
Mean left atrial pressure (mmHg)	22 ± 7	13 ± 5	0.0001
Mean pulmonary artery pressure (mmHg)	33 ± 11	23 ± 9	0.0001
Cardiac index (1/mn/m^2	3 ± 0.7	3.1 ± 0.7	0.01
Mean gradient (mmHg)	15 ± 6	6 ± 3	0.0001
Valve area (cm^2)	1.1 ± 0.3	2.1 ± 0.5	0.0001

correctly across the mitral valve. The majority of technical failures occur during the early part of the experience, but they are also possible at any time under particularly unfavorable anatomic conditions such as extreme dilation of the left atrium, which complicates the transseptal puncture and intra-atrial manipulations, or a predominantly subvalvular stenosis, which prevents correct positioning of the balloon. The use of an Inoue balloon is worth considering in the latter case because of its geometry (55).

Immediate results

Several thousand patients have already undergone percutaneous mitral commissurotomy. Preliminary series had already demonstrated the efficacy of the technique, especially in young adults or children (56), and subsequently in older patients (57-59). Multicenter trials (51,54) or reports from centers which specialize in the technique (20,22,27,52,53) are now available and provide information on widely varying groups of patients, ranging from young adults with flexible mitral valves, who are excellent candidates for surgical commissurotomy, to very much older patients with more severe anatomical lesions, for whom the only surgical alternative is valve replacement, if indeed surgery is not contraindicated on other than cardiac grounds (60).

Hemodynamic results

The PMC procedure, if it is successful, achieves an ap proximate 100% increase in valve area (Table 7.2-I). This improvement in valve function causes an immediate fall in

Table 7.2-II: Valve area before and after PMC.
(Hemodynamics (cm^2))

	Number of patients	Valve Area	
		Before PMC	After PMC
Babic (10)	72	1.2 ± 0.2	2.3 ± 0.6
Hung (53)	216	1 ± 0.3	2 ± 0.7
Noboyushi (22)	106	1.4 ± 0.4	2 ± 0.5
Ruiz (52)	281	0.9 ± 0.2	2.4 ± 0.5
Tuczu (21)	311	0.9 ± 0.03	2 ± 0.1

Table 7.2-III: Major complications of PMC (%).

	Number of patients	Mortality	Hemo-pericardium	Embolism	Severe MR
Noboyushi (22)	106	0	2	0	5
Ruiz (52)	285	1	2	1.4	7
Tuczu (21)	311	1.7	-	-	8.7 (> 2 + increase)
NHLBI (54) (M)	738	3	4	3	3
French Coop Study (51) (M)	114	0	5.3	1.8	2.6
M'Heart (79)(M)	75	2.7	6.7	2.7	13 (> 2 + increase)
Herrmann (M)	200	0.5	1	1.5	2.4
Personal series	810	0.5	0.9	3.6	2.4

(M) = Multicenter study MR = Mitral Regurgitation

the left atrial and pulmonary arterial pressures (Table 7.2-II). The fall in pulmonary resistance is observed immediately and continues during the days immediate after intervention (61).

Dilation also improves the exercise hemodynamics (62-63). The results regarding the recovery of left ventricular function after dilation have been the subject of argument. Mehta and Goto (64-65) were able to show that the left ventricular ejection fraction was improved, whereas Wisenbaugh (66) concluded that elimination of the mitral obstruction did not produce an immediate improvement in this respect. Liu (67) found that PMC restored ventricular compliance almost completely, whereas Harrison (68) was unable to detect any marked changes in left ventricular relaxation or compliance after PMC.

Several recent series (69-73) have compared the results of PMC with those of surgical commissurotomy (open heart commissurotomy in two and closed heart commissurotomy in five series) in patient groups with unfavorable anatomic conditions. The conclusions were that PMC and surgical commissurotomy were comparable in terms of safety and efficacy as assessed one week after the operation and in the medium term. One non-randomized trial compared the results of closed commissurotomy and PMC in patients with less favorable anatomic conditions and arrived at the same conclusion (73). These results will have to be confirmed by larger series and longer follow up information. It would also be of interest to have information on comparative series of PMC and open commissurotomies in patients with more severe anatomic lesions, and in particular with major changes in the subvalvular apparatus.

Echocardiographic results

Echocardiographic measurements have in general confirmed the good results demonstrated by hemodynamic analysis, although after dilation the valve orifice area calculated by planimetry or determined by Doppler measurements is normally smaller than that revealed by hemodynamic measurements. At the present time, it would appear that echocardiographic evaluation, in particular by planimetric techniques, represents the most reliable method of evaluating the immediate results. Ideally, echocardiographic measurements should be carried out between 24 and 48 hours after dilation in order to eliminate the effects of elastic "recoil" (76) and to improve the accuracy of pressure half-time measurements (77). Preliminary results have emphasized the value of exercise Doppler measurements in the evaluation of the immediate results and the follow up of patients after PMC (78).

Complications

Data from large clinical series permit a sound assessment of the risks involved in the PMC technique (Table 7.2-III). The mortality rate varies between 0% and 3% in the majority of series (20,22,27,51,54,79). The main causes of death are ventricular perforations or the poor clinical state of the patients. The mortality rates are higher in multicenter trials than in those emanating from centers specializing in the treatment of large numbers of PMC patients, thus reflecting the importance of experience in the technique.

The incidence of hemopericardial accidents varies between 0.5% and 7%. Intrapericardial hemorrhages may occur in connection with transseptal catheterization or as a result of perforation of the apex by the guides or by the balloon itself (80). Here again a lower incidence of hemopericardial accidents has been reported in single-center than in multicenter trials.

Various modifications to the technique have been proposed in order to reduce the risk of perforation of the apex and its dramatic consequences, for example the use of previously shaped guides or their positioning in the aorta (18), the adoption of a "pigtail" catheter and the use of the Inoue balloon.

These hemopericardial effusions are on occasion well tolerated, but they often cause cardiac tamponade, requiring rapid drainage by pericardial puncture or surgical drainage and repair of the ventricular perforation. Puncture of the ventricle by the tip of the balloon is more serious.

Embolisms have been observed in 0.5% to 5% of cases (2,19,21,22,27,52,54,81,82), although they seldom cause a permanent deficit or have a fatal outcome. They may be either cerebral or coronary embolisms, located in particular in the right coronary artery. They may also consist of gas emboli (27,82), which occur in the case of a balloon rupture and have in general moderate and transient clinical consequences, or they may be due to the presence of intracardiac thrombi, or occasionally to calcium (81). Although the incidence of embolism is not very great, their potential consequences are serious. Therefore, all possible precautions have to be taken for their prevention before and during PMC, since recent observations made by transesophageal echocardiography have revealed the occurrence of thrombosis at the site of catheterization during the procedure (83).

In the majority of cases the degree of mitral insufficiency remains stable or increases slightly after dilation. Minor cases of mitral insufficiency have been satisfactorily detected by transesophageal and color Doppler echocardiography (84). Regurgitant jets are normally localized in the commissural opening zone. They may be due to small lacerations of the valves, localized ruptures of the chordae tendineae responsible for minor valvular prolapse (85), or an incomplete closure of rigid valves. It has been suggested, but not proved, that traumatic or ischemic malfunction of the papillary muscles may also play a role. On the other hand, mitral insufficiency may in some cases decrease or even disappear after the PMC procedure as a result of increased valve mobility.

Cases of severe traumatic mitral insufficiency are rare, with an estimated frequency between 2% and 19%, around 5% in most series (10,20-22,27,42,51-54). Surgical evidence (86,89) has shown such cases to be linked with extracommissural lacerations of the valves. In these cases the commissures are usually not opened. Very rarely, mitral insufficiency may be due to an excessive commissural opening, exceptionally to papillary muscle rupture (86,90). In our experience with serious mitral insufficiency, unfavorable anatomic conditions accompanied by severe calcifications in half of the cases and major changes in the subvalvular apparatus in all cases were found at surgery (86,89). However, severe mitral insufficiency has also been found to occur in patients with a priori favorable anatomic conditions (85), or where excess mixoid tissue is present at the site of rupture (88).

Severe mitral valve insufficiency may be well tolerated in some cases but in our experience not in the long term. Therefore, a necessary surgical intervention must be properly timed (86). This is in agreement with the results of surgical series, which have indicated an unfavorable outcome in cases of severe traumatic mitral insufficiency occurring after commissurotomy (91,92). In the majority of cases, valve replacement is necessary due to the severity and extent of the valvular lesions. A recent publication (89) has reported cases of successful repair after severe traumatic mitral insufficiency following PMC. It appears that the need for valve replacement in experienced hands is more likely to be due to underlying valvular lesions than to the actual laceration of the valve.

The incidence of interatrial shunts varies between 10% and 90% (20,22,27,84,93,96) depending on the technique used for their detection. Oximetric measurements have recorded interatrial shunts in 10%-30% of cases, but this technique is known to be less sensitive than the dye-dilution method (95). Transthoracic or transesophageal color flow echo-Doppler can detect shunts in 38%-90% of cases (36,84,94), but these are mainly minor, localized and high velocity shunts (93). Oximetry confirmed that these are separate and moderate shunts; in our experience, the left-to-right shunt is over 1.5 in only 5%, and over 2 in only 0.2% of cases. Right/left shunts have been observed in patients suffering from an independent pulmonary condition which is partly responsible for the pulmonary arterial hypertension (97).

The occurrence of a post-dilation shunt is related to clinical variables such as age, cardiac output, valvular calcifications, a high echo score, a prior history of surgical commissurotomy, to the surface area of the valve after dilation, and lastly to a number of technical factors such as the site of the transseptal puncture, the duration of the procedure and the type and dimensions of the balloons used (95,96). Surgical findings (89) have revealed vertical tears a few millimeters in height and 1-2 mm in width.

Conduction disorders, in particular complete atrioventricular block, are infrequent (< 1%), necessitating a final recourse to electric stimulation on very rare occasions (98). Vascular complications are exceptional where the transvenous approach is used.

Emergency surgical intervention (within 24 hours following PMC) is seldom necessary (20,51,54,79,89). It may, however, be indicated in the case of a massive hemopericardium due to left ventricular perforation, or less frequently for the treatment of a severe mitral insufficiency which does not respond to adequate medical therapy.

One may conclude that where percutaneous mitral commissurotomy is carried out by trained teams on carefully selected patients, the risks are relatively small.

Prediction of the immediate results

Considerable difficulty has long been experienced in selecting factors which are of use in predicting mortality attributable to the procedure in view of the relatively low mortality risk. The most recent NHLBI report (99), covering the experience of 24 centers and including 738 patients, indicated a 3% mortality immediately following the procedure; multivariate analysis has shown that experience (< 25 cases), the initial area of the valve ($\leq$ 0.5 cm^2) and the patient's age (> 70 years) are independent predictive factors of immediate mortality and of a 30 day functional improvement.

The definition of good immediate results, based on hemodynamic or echocardiographic criteria, varies from one series to another. The most widely used definitions are: a final surface area of the valve > 1.5 cm^2 and an increase in valve area of at least 25%, or a final surface area of the valve > 1.5 cm^2 without mitral insufficiency in excess of 2/4. The valvular and subvalvular anatomy, evaluated by the calculation of an echocardiographic score (100) or a classification into anatomic groups of increasing severity (20,22), are useful factors in predicting the immediate results. The rigidity and mobility of the valve appear to be the most important predictive factors among the various echocardiographic variables available (6,101).

The predictive value of echocardiographic scores has recently been disputed in a number of trials which found only a low correlation between the echocardiographic parameters and the quality of the immediate result (99,102,103). These findings suggest that the anatomy of the valve is only a relative predictive factor and that individual results may vary considerably (104); the PMC procedure normally yields good results in patients with a good valvular anatomy, but an unfavorable anatomy does not exclude the possibility of a satisfactory result. This latter point has been demonstrated by in vitro and in vivo studies in which a good immediate result was reported both in patients with an echocardiographic score in excess of 8; and in patients with valvular calcification (105-106).

The factors predicting the occurrence of a severe mitral insufficiency after PMC are even more controversial. Abascal (107) found no factors capable of predicting the occurrence of a severe mitral insufficiency on the basis of purely morphologic criteria. More recently, Essop (85) and Nair (108) arrived at the same conclusion after examining a group of patients with a favorable valvular anatomy in most cases. On the other hand, other authors (109,111) have emphasized that an unfavorable prognosis due to the extent of valvular and subvalvular lesions can be derived from anatomic or angiographic findings. It must be emphasized that in patients with calcified valves the location of the calcifications, in particular commissural calcifications, may be a more unfavorable factor than the extent of the calcifications in predicting the occurrence of a severe mitral insufficiency (7).

The influence of balloon dimensions on the occurrence of severe mitral insufficiency has also been the subject of argument (18,42,43,107). Feldman (112), for example, maintains that there is no correlation between the extent of the valvular lesions and the immediate result of dilation when using the Inoue technique. This finding may perhaps be explained by the geometry of the Inoue balloon and the use of progressive dilation. This lack of agreement on the prognostic value of echocardiographic parameters may be due to problems of reproducibility, the fact that these are only semi- quantitative measurements, that echocardiography may underestimate the dimensions of the lesions, in particular in the subvalvular apparatus, or that the most widely used classification systems disregard focal and in particular commissural changes, the prognostic value of which was stressed recently (112).

Therefore, it appears that, although valvular anatomy determined by echocardiography exerts a significant influence on the immediate results, other factors must also be taken into account. A number of studies (20,101,102,103) have demonstrated that, apart from morphologic factors, preoperative variables (age, prior surgical commissurotomy, reduced valve surface area, left atrial dimensions (113), the presence or absence of sinus rhythm and pulmonary hypertension) and the dimensions of the balloon are also useful independent factors in the prediction of the immediate result.

Medium term results

The first PMC series now have several years of follow up, permitting a medium term assessment of the results (114-131). However, a number of provisos must be made before attempting to compare these results with those of surgical commissurotomy series:

- The available follow up period after PMC is very much shorter than it is after surgical commissurotomy (132).
- The PMC series include older patients.
- The results of surgical commissurotomy have been assessed mainly, though not entirely, on the basis of clinical variables, whereas the PMC results also take into account an evaluation of valve function on the basis of hemodynamic or echocardiographic criteria.

Taken overall, the dilation procedure has achieved good results in the medium term - up to about five years. In our own experience, the actuarial results after 42 months were as follows: 87% ± 6% of the patients survived, 81% ± 3% had not required surgery and 72% ± 6% were in a good functional state (NYHA class I or II) (116). The medium term results depend on the population examined. For example, the five year results are less satisfactory in the Cohen series (122) than in the Pan series (123), in which the patients were younger; survival after five years: 76% ± 5% vs. 94% ± 1%; survival without cardiac episodes or surgery: 51% ± 6% vs. 85% ± 2%.

These results are closely related to the immediate results and to the valvular anatomy. If the dilation procedure was initially successful, the survival rates were excellent, the need for secondary surgery was rare and a functional improvement was observed in 75%-90% of cases three years after dilation (116). These favorable results were associated with a continuing improvement in valve function in the majority of cases. Echocardiographic techniques are ideally suited to a sequential evaluation of the dilation results, whereas repeated hemodynamic analyses are difficult to perform and

Table 7.2-IV: Mid-term results/anatomy in the Tenon Hospital ex perience: Actuarial results after 36 months
(n = 431)

	Survivors (%)	Not operated on (%)	NYHA class I-III (%)
Gr I	100	98 ± 2	97 ± 1
Gr 2	100	86 ± 4	86 ± 4
Gr 3	80 ± 6	68 ± 6	58 ± 6

Gr 1: Patients with pliable valves and mild subvalvular disease
Gr 2: Patients with pliable valves but extensive subvalvular disease
Gr 3: Patients with calcified valves

undoubtedly less valuable because of the overestimated valve area immediately after dilation. Determination of the incidence of a recurrent stenosis is complicated by the absence of any clear definition of this condition. The definition most frequently adopted is a > 50% loss of the initial gain after the restoration of a valve area to > 1.5 cm². The incidence of restenosis after a successful dilation is normally low at the four year point, between 10% and 20% (115,116,118,119,122,124) as assessed by echocardiography.

Age, the surface area of the valve after dilation and the anatomy of the valve are regarded as the main factors responsible for recurrence of the stenosis, but it must be pointed out that the relatively small number of patients in whom the stenosis recurs and the limited follow up period available do not permit any final conclusion to be drawn on this question.

Where the valve anatomy is unfavorable, the only form of treatment for a recurrent stenosis is valve replacement. Where the valve anatomy is still satisfactory, repeat dilations have been carried out in a number of patients with good results (124). This form of treatment is tempting where a recurrence of symptoms occurs after several years, especially in young patients. The true value of this approach remains to be determined, but the satisfactory results obtained by dilation procedures after surgical commissurotomy suggest that it might constitute a major field of application.

Where the immediate results have not been good, the medium term functional results are likely to be poor. In the case of severe mitral insufficiency, surgery is often necessary during the months following PMC. Also, if the initial opening was insufficient, subsequent surgery is often necessary. In such cases, valve replacement is the only alternative in almost all patients as a result of the unfavorable valve anatomy which was responsible for the poor initial result. In some patients, however, the moderate improvement in valve function leads to a general functional improvement which persists for several years.

The anatomy of the valve is another independent predictor of the medium term results (116,125). The results obtained in patients with a favorable or intermediate valve anatomy are good, comparable in all respects with those obtained in surgical commissurotomy series (Table 7.2-IV). In the case of valvular calcifications, on the other hand, a functional deterioration is often observed, calling for surgical intervention (106). Despite numerous individual variations, the degree of mitral insufficiency remains stable overall or falls slightly during the follow up period (118,119,122,123,125). Septal dehiscences close in the majority of cases as the interatrial pressure gradient decreases. Sequential hemodynamic analyses, and/or more frequently, echocardiographic measurements have demonstrated that 45%-80% of the shunts disappear after follow up periods varying from three months to three years (128-130). The persistence of shunts is linked with the scale on which they initially occur (QP/QS > 1.5), the defect diameter (> 0.5 cm) or a recurrence of the mitral valve obstruction, giving rise to a variant of the Lutembacher syndrome (131).

Finally, the very low incidence of embolism during the follow up period (we observed only one embolism in a series of more than 400 patients over a maximum follow up period of six years) and the progressive decrease in the intensity, or the complete disappearance of the spontaneous left atrial echo contrast, suggests that the PMC procedure reduces the risk of embolism.

In summary, the experiences gained up to now suggest that the medium term results obtained with PMC are comparable to those of closed heart surgical commissurotomy. It is however too early to assess the long term results of this technique, since it is generally known that a deteriorating valve function after surgical commissurotomy is usually observed only after a period of 8-10 years (132).

Special applications of PMC

PMC after surgical commissurotomy

Several series of observations have reported the results of PMC after surgical commissurotomy (133-138). This patient category is of particular interest for several reasons:

- in Western countries, the prevalence of mitral restenosis after surgical intervention is increasing as compared to that of primary mitral stenosis;
- the risk of a hemopericardial accident associated with PMC appears to be lower in these patients as a result of dense postoperative pericardial adhesions;
- repeated surgical intervention is associated with increased mortality, morbidity and the need for valve replacement in the majority of cases (139).

PMC has been most frequently carried out 10-15 years after the initial surgical intervention, which was a closed rather than open mitral commissurotomy in most cases.

PMC can be complicated occasionally if the interatrial septum is thickened, in particular where the transseptal approach was used for the prior surgical intervention. Another source of complication is presented by "tunnel" restenosis with a significant subvalvular involvement. Usually, the immediate improvement is satisfactory in terms of valve function, although slightly less than that obtained in the case of a primary mitral stenosis. The medium term results are good, since further surgery can be delayed for at least two years in 70%-80% of cases. These encouraging results therefore suggest that PMC can delay the need for further surgical intervention in a considerable number of patients who have suffered a recurrence of stenosis after commissurotomy. Echocardiographic assessment should be carried out with particular care prior to PMC to identify those patients in whom the recurrence of the stenosis is essentially due to a rigid valve without any significant commissural refusion.

One isolated case of a successful PMC has been reported in a patient who had mitral valve repair with ring annuloplasty for mitral insufficiency and had subsequently developed a clinically significant mitral stenosis (140).

PMC in high risk surgery patients

In Western countries a large number of patients suffering from mitral stenosis are believed to represent a high surgical risk or are even contraindicated for surgery. There are various reasons for this, including age over 75 years, respiratory insufficiency, multi-organ failure, psychiatric disorders, cancer, a very low ejection fraction, diffuse coronary disease or severe pulmonary hypertension; these aggravating factors may be present alone or in combination. In addition to the poor clinical condition, these patients often have an unfavorable valvular pathology, including rapidly calcifying valves and very narrow stenosis.

Preliminary series (60,141-145) have demonstrated that dilation can be performed under these circumstances, producing a significant although moderate improvement in valve function and imposing only an acceptable risk. These results are nevertheless clearly less satisfactory than those obtained in other patients, a deterioration usually occurs during the follow up and the medium term benefit may be limited by the associated conditions (141,144).

Wisenbaugh (146) recently reported some encouraging preliminary results in 24 percutaneous mitral commissurotomies in patients with severe pulmonary arterial hypertension. He noted, however, a high incidence of marked mitral insufficiency after dilation, which may have been due to the severity of the valvular stenosis resulting in a severe reduction of orifice area, and/or to the extent of further anatomical lesions.

PMC during pregnancy

Pregnancy may bring on serious complications in mitral stenosis. Surgery involves the risk of a fatal outcome and of high fetal morbidity, especially where extracorporeal circulation is used. Although only limited experience is currently available on PMC during pregnancy (147-154), the following comments may nevertheless be made.

For technical reasons PMC may present problems during the last weeks of pregnancy because of the size of the uterus. The Inoue technique appears to have many advantages, since it can reduce to a minimum the time spent on fluoroscopy, while at the same time the shortness of the balloon inflation/ deflation cycle limits the hemodynamic consequences of the inflation process. The procedure is effective and permits a normal term of pregnancy and date of delivery in the majority of cases; only one neonatal death out of 30 cases of administration during pregnancy has been reported in the literature.

The risk of irradiation is low if the abdomen is protected with a lead screen and if the duration of the examination is reduced to a minimum. This risk is less than with the radiation dose authorized for pregnant women exposed to ionizing radiations for occupational reasons. A number of case reports in which the fetal heart rhythm was monitored during the dilation process revealed no evidence of significant harm to the fetus during the procedure.

These good results, in particular the good tolerance, should not diminish the awareness of the potential risk of complications, which always exists during dilation and may necessitate emergency surgery.

PMC and left atrial thrombosis

Left atrial thrombosis is generally regarded as a contraindication to PMC. Two small series (155,156) have demonstrated that PMC with the Inoue balloon is feasible under such circumstances without causing systemic embolism. Similarly, we have carried out dilation procedures in 86 patients who had suffered an embolic accident more than two months previously and in whom no thrombosis had been detected by transesophageal echo before dilation. One of the 86 patients suffered an embolic accident during dilation, but no other events occurred during the follow up period (157).

Patient selection

Four factors have to be taken into account when selecting candidates for PMC: clinical condition, valvular anatomy, the level of experience of the medical and surgical teams in the institution in question - and the cost.

Evaluation of the clinical condition

Evaluation of the patient's clinical condition should take into account the degree of functional disability, the surgical risk in terms of cardiac reserve and the function of other major organs, and the presence of any contraindications to transseptal catheterization.

The indication for PMC is easy in patients with typical symptoms. The decision becomes more difficult in symptomless patients or where only a few symptoms are present. The primary difficulty in this group is to make an objective assessment of the functional disability caused by the mitral valve disease, and an exercise test is of great value before deciding whether a patient is genuinely asymptomatic. Because of the low but indisputable risk inherent in PMC, asymptomatic patients, even with a tight mitral stenosis, are regarded as candidates for balloon dilation only in the following situations: the need for emergency and/or major extracardiac surgery, the desire for, or presence of pregnancy, the presence of a significant spontaneous left atrial contrast on transesophageal echocardiography, or arrhythmia with paroxysmal atrial fibrillation. Apart from a "salvage" indication when faced with a major extracardiac emergency, the PMC procedure should only be envisaged if it is to be carried out by an experienced team on a low risk basis and in cases where the valvular anatomy is favorable.

The presence of an absolute contraindication to surgery is an obvious indication for PMC. In such cases, however, the patient's life expectancy and general condition should be considered before the intervention is indicated or refused. Where the high surgical risk is the consequence of a cardiac factor, PMC appears to be preferable to surgery, at least initially. PMC may delay the need for further surgical intervention in some patients who have already undergone surgical commissurotomies or had an aortic valve replacement (158).

The surgical risk may also be increased by an extracardiac disease. A large proportion of patients suffering from mitral stenosis in Western countries are elderly or have an associated extracardiac condition. In such patients, and in particular in the elderly, the decision must be made on an individual basis. In clinical practice PMC may be proposed, as a palliative procedure, if the surgical risk is very high.

Major cardiothoracic deformations constitute a classical contraindication to transseptal catheterization and PMC. In the case of a moderate deformation dilation may be carried out in a highly symptomatic patient where surgery is contraindicated, provided the PMC is performed by an experienced team, using transesophageal echocardiography where necessary to facilitate the transseptal puncture.

Valve anatomy

Evaluation of the valvular anatomy is necessary (a) to determine the degree of valvular pathology, (b) to exclude any contraindications to PMC, and (c) to detect any associated pathologic condition of the valve.

It is difficult - and no doubt arbitrary - to determine the maximum orifice area above which PMC is not indicated, and exercise testing is necessary in contested cases. In one series (159), PMC was successfully performed in patients suffering from moderate mitral stenosis with the aim of slowing down the natural course of the disease. We do not undertake dilation if the mitral orifice area is larger than 1.5 cm2, except in special cases with large body surface area. Beyond this threshold value, the potential risk is certainly greater than the benefit and these patients can normally be treated successfully by medical means.

A left atrial thrombus is generally regarded as a contraindication to PMC. Recently, however, two small series (13,14) demonstrated that successful dilation can be achieved without systemic embolism using the Inoue balloon. The following policy might reasonably be followed:

If the clinical condition calls for emergency treatment, surgery is to be preferred. This recommendation is obvious in the event of a floating thrombus located in the left atrial cavity at the level of the interatrial septum. Where the thrombus is located in the left atrial appendage, the danger of embolism is undoubtedly less marked but still present even with the Inoue technique, and we believe that surgery is the intervention of choice in these cases. If the patient is in a stable clinical condition without significant pulmonary hypertension, as is the case with the majority of our patients with mitral stenosis, oral anticoagulation may be instituted for a period of two months. Subsequently PMC may be carried out if control transesophageal echo indicates that the thrombus is no longer present.

Percutaneous mitral commissurotomy can be carried out on patients with a history of prior systemic embolism if at least two months oral anticoagulation has followed the last embolic episode and left atrial thrombus cannot be detected by TEE.

The majority of authors agree that a mitral valve insufficiency of 2/4 or more is a contraindication to balloon dilation. However, it is not always easy to determine the degree of mitral regurgitation even using TEE. In borderline cases the patient's general condition and the potential for a successful surgical repair should influence the decision.

Several attempts have been made to classify mitral stenosis according to the valvular/subvalvular pathology, which is con sidered to be a significant predictor of the outcome of PMC. According to Cormier (2) the following criteria should be observed.

When the valve is pliant and there is no major subvalvular pathology (equivalent of an echo score of 8 or less), PMC appears to be the method of choice; good results can be expected and the risk is low. In comparison with surgery, PMC is also more comfortable, less painful, leaves no scar and requires a shorter hospital stay. Furthermore, should the stenosis recur, patients treated by PMC may undergo a second PMC or have surgery without the difficulties resulting from pericardial adhesions.

Where the valves are highly calcified (or with an echo score between 12 and 16), the results of the dilation are doubtful and not durable. Surgery is the better solution in the absence of a contraindication of extracardiac origin.

In the intermediate groups (or with an echo score between 9 and 12) there are several choices. If major subvalvular changes have taken place, open commissurotomy affords the advantage of a complete anatomic repair at the valvular and subvalvular levels, but the results of conservative surgery depend very much on the surgeon and cannot always be foreseen during the preoperative phase. On the other hand, surgery carries higher mortality and morbidity rates. We have been able to obtain good immediate results with PMC in this group, which have been maintained into the medium term. It appears to us reasonable to advise percutaneous dilation as a first approach, reserving surgery for cases of failure due to insufficient opening of the valve or in the event of a traumatic mitral insufficiency. Where the valves are only moderately calcified or where the calcifications are localized in a commissural zone, dilation may also be proposed, with the aim of delaying valve replacement, provided that a very progressive dilation technique is used.

A tight mitral stenosis is very frequently accompanied by a minor aortic insufficiency; this is not a contraindication to PMC. Several cases of successful double aortic and mitral dilation have been reported in conjunction with a critical aortic stenosis (160-161), but this procedure should, in our view, be regarded as an exceptional indication reserved for absolute contraindications to surgery, because of the unsatisfactory results of aortic dilation. The similarly rare finding of a substantial aortic insufficiency tips the balance in favor of surgery.

Several cases of simultaneous dilation with initial success for mitral and tricuspid stenosis have been reported (162), but this situation is exceptional in Europe. The combination with tricuspid insufficiency, on the other hand, is a very commonplace finding and does not constitute a contraindication to PMC. In the case of an organic combined tricuspid disease the decision may not be easy, and it may be reasonable to recommend surgery if the clinical symptoms persist despite adequate medical treatment. Finally, two cases of triple valvular dilation have been reported by Savas and Konugres (163-164), but this must be considered an exceptional situation.

Experience of the medical and surgical teams

The importance of experience in PMC and/or surgical repair procedures can be demonstrated by comparing the initial and subsequent results obtained by the same group (learning curve), or by comparing the results of large series by a single, experienced team with those based on multicenter trials. The incidence of technical failures and complications, in particular those associated with transseptal catheterization, is clearly linked with the experience of the operators. In addition to improving skills, patient selection also improves with experience. The excellent results obtained by surgical commissurotomy make it clear that the "standard" for PMC must be high in terms of the results which must be achieved with a low complication rate. It follows that PMC should be confined to teams who have a wide experience in transseptal catheterization and are able to undertake this procedure on a regular basis and on a sufficient number of patients.

The choice will also depend on the "preference" and experience of surgical teams in the successful performance of conservative surgery in cases of mitral stenosis. In centers where conservative surgery is not generally practiced, the indications for PMC may well be broadened.

Cost

The economic aspect must also be taken into account, a problem which varies from country to country. In India, for example, the cost of dilation is six times greater than that of a closed commissurotomy, mainly because of the price of the balloons. In Western countries, on the other hand, open heart surgery and - even more so - valve replacement are very much more expensive than dilation in view of the high costs of hospitalization.

In conclusion, the good results obtained with PMC suggest that this technique is here to stay in the treatment of mitral stenosis. A significant number of indications have already been established, others are yet to be confirmed, particularly in the Western countries, where the majority of candidates are elderly and have an unclearly defined or unfavorable valvular anatomy. It is expected that the critical evaluation of mid- and long term results will provide help in clarifying the respective indications for PMC and surgery. It must be stressed, however, that PMC and surgery should not be regarded as rival methods for the treatment of mitral stenosis, but rather as complementary procedures which, in many cases, may be carried out in succession.

PERCUTANEOUS AORTIC VALVULOTOMY

The first surgical valvulotomies in the treatment of adult aortic stenosis were reported between 1950 and 1960 (165,166). Percutaneous aortic valvulotomy (PAV) was successfully performed for the first time in 1986 by Alain Cribier and coworkers on patients with absolute contraindications to surgery (167). The first results were encouraging and aroused enthusiasm, but the follow up revealed a high recurrence rate of the stenosis, resulting in a less clearly marked benefit in the medium term. PAV is currently not regarded as an alternative to valve replacement, but rather as a palliative treatment, the indications for which are limited to a few particular cases (168,169).

Mechanism of action

In Western countries, degenerative calcified aortic stenosis is the primary cause of aortic stenosis in the adult. Calcific accumulations interfere with the excursion of the aortic leaflets and create a left ventricular outflow tract obstruction. Clinically manifest aortic stenosis may develop on congenitally bicuspid valves as a result of fibrosis and progressive calcification. Less frequently the lesions are of rheumatic origin, with commissural fusion and fairly extensive calcification of the valves. The usually advanced stage of valvular pathology casts doubt on the claim that inflation of the balloon can have any beneficial effect at all (169). The absence of efficacy has also been observed by Robicsek with balloon inflations during open heart surgery (170).

Further anatomic, microscopic and on occasion radiologic studies have revealed two different mechanisms of action of the dilation, depending on the etiology of the disease (171- 178).

PAV has a very limited effect in the case of degenerative stenoses where the only consequence of balloon inflation is a series of microcracks in the calcified stroma of the aortic valve. In the case of rheumatic stenoses, on the other hand, the morphologic result is more satisfactory since the balloon performs a commissurotomy function (176,177).

Little is known of the pathology of re-stenosis. There appear to be two different mechanisms, one relating to early and the other to a late recurrence. Early recurrence can be observed within hours or days following the procedure, and it is secondary to an elastic recovery in the valve and/or aortic structures which have been stretched during inflation of the balloon (173,178). Late recurrence occurs months or years after PAV, and it is a true restenosis with the characteristic pathologic features as part of the progression of the disease reducing the orifice area by 0.03-0.15 cm^2 per annum (179).

Technique

Routes of access

Percutaneous aortic valvulotomy may be carried out both retrograde or anterograde.

The retrograde route, as described by A. Cribier is used most frequently (167), mainly via the femoral artery (167,180). Brachial access (181) is used only if ileofemoral or aortic sclerotic lesions prevent the retrograde advancement of the catheter, or in the case of double balloon intervention, which combines a femoral and a brachial approach. The latter necessitates the exposure of the brachial artery through which passage of the aortic valve is often easier than through the femoral approach, but the dimensions of the brachial artery may prevent the use of large balloons. Vascular damage may also be caused during withdrawal of partially deflated balloons. Irrespective of which artery is used, the most difficult part of the procedure is passing the balloon through the aortic valve. Once this is completed, a long change-over guide with a preshaped distal end is posi tioned in the left ventricular apex.

The anterograde route (182) requires transseptal catheterization, followed by anterograde passage of the aortic valve using a floating catheter. A long change-over guide is then positioned in the descending aorta. The interatrial septum is dilated with a 6-8 mm peripheral angioplasty balloon and finally the aortic dilation balloon is introduced via the femoral vein. The anterograde approach is more difficult than the retrograde because of the need for transseptal catheterization. It is nevertheless an attractive alternative to the brachial route in the event of an obliterating arterial disease of the lower limbs or of the abdominal aorta.

	NHLBI (189)	Mansfield Registry (190)	Safian (184)
Table 7.2-V: Aortic valvulotomy: Clinical characteristics.			
Mean age (years)	78 ± 9	79 ± 8.4	77 ± 5
Age range (years)	NA	22-95	35-94
NYHA III,IV class (%)	76	81.5	78
Angina (%)	58	54	42
Syncopes (%)	34	22.4	36
Prior infarction (%)	22	10.4	13
Ejection fraction (%)	48 ± 19	47.9 ± 19.2	> 55% in 41% of cases
Severe coronary artery disease (%)	7	18.7	11
Associated illness (%)	45	69.1	20
Cancer (%)	17	14.8	2
Renal insufficiency (%)	14	8.7	NA
Respiratory insufficiency (%)	23	14.8	4
Stroke (%)	9	0	0

Balloons

Aortic dilation is most frequently performed with a balloon of 15-25 mm diameter and 3-5 cm length with a round, bifoil or trifoil shape. More recently, A. Cribier introduced a low profile balloon (9F) which can be inserted into a 14F arterial introducer. The dimensions of the proximal section of this balloon are 20-23 mm and the distal section 15-18 mm, thus permitting progressive dilation (180). The double balloon technique (183) is used, but less frequently, to increase the effective dilation dimensions and to improve tolerance. This technique is more complex, increases the risk of vascular lesions and exposes the patient to the danger of aortic insufficiency or rupture of the aortic ring.

The choice of balloon dimensions is still a subject of argument. It would appear that the dimensions of the balloon or balloons should not exceed 1.2-1.3 times the diameter of the aortic ring in order to avoid rupture of the ring and/or aortic insufficiency (183).

Methods of evaluating the immediate results

The immediate result of the procedure is evaluated by calculating the hemodynamic area of the aortic valve. However, this evaluation during the procedure is subject to errors due to the unstable circulation and the presence of vagal or hypervolemic symptoms. The "elastic recoil" occurring hours after the procedure is responsible for the apparent differences between immediate hemodynamic results and echo- Doppler data recorded days later (178).

Results

Percutaneous aortic valvulotomy has now been carried out on several hundred

Table 7.2-VI: Aortic valvulotomy - immediate hemodynamic results.

	n patients	VA before	VA after	MG before	MG after	CO before	CO after
Mansfield	492	0.5 ± 0.18	0.82 ± 0.30	60 ± 23	30 ± 13	3.86 ± 1.26	4.05 ± 1.31
Safian	170	0.6 ± 0.2	0.9 ± 0.3	56 ± 19	31 ± 12	4.6 ± 3.4	4.8 ± 1.4
NHLBI	674	0.5 ± 0.2	0.8 ± 0.3	55 ± 21	29 ± 13	4.0 ± 1.2	4.1 ± 1.3
LETAC	506	0.55 ± 0.20	0.96 ± 0.32	$71 \pm 25^*$	$29 \pm 14^*$	NA	NA
Nishimura **	55	$0.54 + 0.15$	$0.85 + 0.23$	$48 + 18$	$33 + 12$	NA	NA

VA: valve area (cm^2; MG: mean gradient (mm Hg); CO: cardiac output (l/mm)
before: before valvulotomy; after: after valvulotomy;
*: peak to peak aortic gradient; **; Doppler study

patients and it is possible to evaluate the results on the basis of large single-center series and multi center records (180-192). The experience relates essentially to aortic stenosis in the elderly, and any analysis of the results must take into account the serious cardiac and extracardiac condition of this population (Table 7.2-V).

Immediate results

Hemodynamic results (Table 7.2-VI)

The aortic transvalvular gradient falls by 50% immediately after a successful procedure, although the cardiac output remains unchanged or increases slightly. There are considerable individual variations in the final valve area, but it is fair to say that the PAV procedure transforms a tight stenosis into a moderate stenosis with final surface areas ranging from 0.7 to 1.1 cm^2. These values are lower than those provided by mechanical or bioprosthetic valves currently in clinical use. The percentage of patients in whom the final surface area exceeds 1.0 cm^2 is variable; 25% according to Block (182) and 47% for Cribier (180), and the proportion with an orifice area of less than 0.7 cm^2 was found to be 39% and 22% by these authors, respectively. The predictors gained from the immediate hemodynamic results are the initial valve orifice area, age, sex and the degree of calcification. In addition to these clinical variables, balloon inflation times of more than 30 sec, the use of the double balloon technique and the number of inflations have been found to have a predictive value in the Mansfield register (186). Doppler measurements recorded hours or days following the procedure have revealed considerably lower values (Table 7.2-VII).

Table 7.2-VII: Aortic valvulotomy - echocardiographic results.

	No patients	Follow up (months)	Valve area before (cm^2)	Valve area after (cm^2)	Valve area follow up (cm^2)
Bernard (188)	45	2	0.53 ± 0.8	0.74 ± 0.23	0.69 ± 0.27
Nishimura (187)	31	2	0.54 ± 0.1	0.85 ± 0.2	0.67 ± 0.19
Slama (181	10	6	0.5 ± 0.1	0.7 ± 0.2	0.64 ± 0.09

(*) Valve area is derived from a combined Doppler echocardiographic (measurement of gradient) and hemodynamic method (measurement of cardiac output)

Table 7.2-VIII: Immediate complications of aortic valvulotomy.				
	NHLBI n = 674	Mansfield n = 492	Cribier n = 363	Safian n = 170
Hospital mortality %	10	7.5	4	3.5
Tamponade %	1.5	1.8	1	1.8
Acute aortic regurgitation %	1	1	0	1.2
Stroke %	3	2.2	1.4	0
Arrhythmias %	7	0.6	1	1
Myocardial infarction %	2	0.2	0.3	0.6
Vascular events * %	7	5.5	5	10

(*: Vascular events requiring surgical treatment)

Clinical results

Despite the relatively modest increase in valve area, an immediate improvement in valve function has been frequently reported (167,180,181,184,189,190). According to the NHLBI register (189), the condition of 86% of the surviving patients had improved after 30 days and 75% had moved up at least one NYHA class.

Nonetheless, the mortality and morbidity of the procedure still remain considerable (Table 7.2- VIII). In major series, the hospital mortality varied between 3.5% and 13.5% (180-182,184- 186,189,190), and 20%-25% of the patients suffered serious complications during the first 24 hours (180,182 184,186,189,191).

The main factors responsible for the mortality are poor left ventricular function, low systolic left ventricular pressure, low cardiac output and the presence of diffuse coronary lesions (189,191). A valve orifice area of less than 0.7 cm^2 on conclusion of the procedure is a further unfavorable factor (186,189).

The most frequent complication is vascular injury at the site of entry (17%-15%), which may cause major bleeding or necessitate surgical intervention in half of the complicated cases. The risk is increased with the double balloon technique, whereas the use of an arterial introducer appears to reduce the incidence of this complication (180,182-184,191). Ventricular perforation (1-2%) may cause massive pericardial tamponade (191). Acute aortic insufficiency is an infrequent complication (1-2%), but one which may necessitate an emergency valve replacement (180,185,191). Embolic complications are relatively rare (2%)(172,180,189,191). They are seldom due to the migration of calcific material since such deposits are covered with endothelium, preventing the migration of small particles into the systemic circulation (172).

There are two complications which are exceptional but extremely serious; mitral valve insufficiency (193) and pericardial tamponade as a result of rupture of the aortic ring (194), which may be the result of using excessively large balloons, especially in patients of small stature.

Medium term results

As in the case of the PMC procedure, only medium term results are available.

	No Patients	Age (years)	Follow up (months)	Restenosis (%)	1-year Survival	2-year Survival
Mansfield (197)	492	79 ± 8.4	6.2 ± 3.3	72	64	NA
Safian (184)	170	77 ± 5	6.4 ± 3.1	44	74	NA
Harrison (224)	112	75.9 ± 7.7	6	76	NA	NA
Block (195)	90	79 ± 1	5.5 ± 0.3	56	NA	NA
Bernard (216)	46	79.7 ± 3.6	21.5	NA	75	47
Chevalier (199)	48	78 ± 6.9	17 ± 12	NA	70	55

Table 7.2-IX: Long term results of aortic valvulotomy.

Clinical results

The overall survival after 12 months varies between 64% and 75% (195,197,199,216) and survival without cardiac episodes between 43% (197) and 50% (184). After two years, the survival rate is close to 50% (Table IX)(199,200).

Although PAV does not extend life expectancy, it improves the quality of life for a few months (184,185,197). The predictive factors of the medium term results are patient related and influenced by the immediate results. The following variables predict a poor prognosis.

The clinical variables include age, NYHA class III and IV, left ventricular failure, and coronary heart disease with or without previous history of myocardial infarction (189,197).

This was illustrated in a series reported by Cribier (180), who reported a two year mortality of 13% in patients who were considered to be suitable for surgery, 33% in high risk surgical patients and 63% in patients with an absolute contraindication to surgery.

The hemodynamic variables include increased left ventricular diastolic pressure, decreased cardiac output, and decreased left ventricular systolic pressure (184, 197).

The sole morphologic variable is extensive calcification. The presence of major calcification predicts a poor prognosis (180). The etiology of the condition is also a prognostic factor (171), with less satisfactory results in bicuspid valve cases, although predictions based on etiology are regarded as rather unreliable in the case of highly calcified aortic stenosis in the elderly.

The initial result of the PAV plays an important part in the prognosis. Block (195) found a six month mortality rate of 45% or 23%, depending on whether the patients had a valve surface area smaller or greater than 0.7 cm^2 on conclusion of the procedure.

The reason for the poor medium term results are the generally poor clinical condition, the limited improvement in valve function and the frequent recurrence of the stenosis.

Recurrence of the stenosis

It must be emphasized that it is very difficult to determine the true frequency of this complication. The definition is somewhat ambiguous. Systematic re- catheterization is very difficult and in these elderly patients the reported incidence of recurrent stenosis varies considerably according to whether catheterization has been carried out in all patients (the incidence of a recurring stenosis was 62% in the Mansfield register) or only in those with symptoms (with an incidence varying between 80% and 100% in the

Mansfield register (201) or as reported by Block (195) and Safian (184)). The frequency of recurrent stenosis increases with time.

Due to these uncertainties, the frequency of restenosis has been estimated to be between 50% and 100% after 12 months, thus clearly indicating the scale of the problem (182,184,195,201,224). The prognostic factors appear to be mainly patient related (age and sex) whereas the parameters linked with the procedure do not appear to have any predictive value (201).

A new intervention may be necessary in the case of a symptomatic restenosis; where the patient's condition permits, a valve replacement should be undertaken. Most frequently a single but in exceptional cases multiple dilations have also been reported in cases of repeated dilation. In the Mansfield register (202), 45 patients underwent a second and four patients a third dilation. In Block's series of 90 patients who were kept under close observation for six months, 15 had one and three had two repeat dilations. The risks and the immediate results of the repeated dilation are comparable, although very slightly inferior to those obtained at the time of the initial procedure, and the risk of a subsequent recurrence of the stenosis remains the same (180,195,202,203). Re-dilation may be recommended as an exceptional measure in the special case of the inoperable patient, even though it represents a not very satisfactory therapeutic solution.

Patient selection

In the selection of possible candidates for percutaneous balloon aortic valvulotomy three alternatives must be considered; medical treatment, surgical intervention and percutaneous valvulotomy.

Series in which the natural course of aortic stenosis has been evaluated often date back a long way (204), but two studies have been published more recently on populations similar to those used in the aortic dilation series. The Mayo Clinic series (205), which included 50 patients (mean age 77 years) who were potential candidates for aortic valvulotomy, reported a poor spontaneous prognosis, that is actuarial survival rates of 57% after 12 months and 37% after two years. Working with younger patients (mean age 43 years), Turina (206) found an actuarial survival rate of 27% after two years in the case of narrow aortic stenosis with severe symptoms where surgery was not carried out. Comparison of the data available on the dilation process suggest that this procedure improves the prospects of survival up to 12 months, but from then on the benefit becomes progressively reduced. On the other hand, dilation improves the quality of life during the survival period (180,184,189,197).

Long term experience with aortic valve replacement for aortic stenosis is good, maybe the best in the whole field of valve replacement (207). Recent improvements in surgical procedures provide for improvement in the results of surgery in the elderly (208-214). The mortality rate for elderly subjects in the most recent series varies from 3% to 28% (210,211). When the high risk operative period has been passed, the surgical results are good, with a mortality of 38% after two years for Edmunds (210) and 35% after five years for Levinson, the majority of the survivors being in a good functional state (213). Furthermore, surgery provides for the treatment of associated coronary lesions, which are frequently present in this age group (207,210).

Any comparison of the results of surgery and dilation, based on published series, are without doubt subject to bias since the patients included in the dilation series will have been in a more serious clinical condition (215). Comparative results from randomized prospective trials are not available, but the retrospective series recently published by Bernard (216) summarizes the situation very clearly. This author gave 69 patients aged over 75 years the choice between surgery and PAV; 46 patients opted for dilation while 23 patients received a bioprosthetic valve replacement. The two groups were comparable in terms of age, functional state and hemodynamic indices. The mortality figures during hospitalization were 6.5% for the dilation group and 8.7% for surgery. The actuarial survival rates at 12 months, two years and five years were 75%, 47% and 33% respectively after PAV, while the actuarial survival rates after valve replacement were 83% after 12 months and two years and 75% after three and four years.

These results, like those of our own personal series, make it clear that, although surgery involves a greater immediate risk, the subsequent results are definitely superior in terms of life expectancy and quality of life, approximating to those of normal populations of the same age and sex.

The indication must be decided on an individual basis jointly by the cardiologist and surgical teams, taking into account age, general condition, cardiac status and extracardiac concomitant degenerative diseases, and it should be discussed with the patient and his/her family. Aortic valve replacement is the treatment of choice for symptomatic, narrowed aortic stenoses (217). Age is not a contraindication to surgery, apart from extreme cases. On the other hand, if the patient is suffering from a concomitant disease and has a poor short term prognosis, or in the case of serious intellectual deterioration, the most reasonable attitude appears to be to refrain from either form of treatment.

Percutaneous aortic valvulotomy (PAV) may be envisaged under the following circumstances:

1. In the event of refusal of surgery; the number of occasions on which surgery is refused will of course vary according to the way in which the case is presented and may amount to 10% in this elderly population.
2. Where there is a major functional defect and an absolute contraindication to surgery, even if the condition is not life-threatening in the short term. A functional improvement can be expected in this case as a result of PAV without any real improvement in life expectancy.
3. The need for major non-cardiac emergency surgery in a patient with a tight aortic stenosis may justify PAV as a means of reducing the the operative risk. Aortic valve surgery may be considered as a secondary procedure.
4. PAV may be considered for patients in a critical condition, i.e. in functional stage IV or in cardiogenic shock. Signs of overall cardiac insufficiency, and a fortiori, cardiogenic shock are immediate risk factors which argue in favor of aortic valve replacement (207). In a number of short series PAV has been completed in patients in terminal cardiac insufficiency or cardiogenic shock (218, 219), with a hospital mortality varying between 6% and 49%. The place of PAV in this patient group has not been clearly established, but it can be envisaged as a bridging intervention to reduce the risk of subsequent surgery. The therapeutic value of this approach, however, will have to be confirmed by a prospective randomized comparison of surgery alone with

a two-stage approach combining dilation with surgery.
5. Dilation has also been proposed in patients with poor left ventricular function, low transvalvular gradient and a sig nificantly reduced valve orifice area calculated by the Gorlin formula (which is known to lack precision in this situation) (220).

Several series have demonstrated (221-224), even though this view is not unanimous (225,226), that PAV can improve left ventricular function, particularly when it is very depressed. In such cases, the dilation could facilitate the differential diagnosis between a tight aortic stenosis with secondary left ventricular dysfunction and cardiomyopathy with a moderate aortic stenosis; in the former case the ventricular function should improve, enabling surgery to be performed, in the latter the absence of any improvement would signify that either the PAV had failed or an underlying cardiomyopathy was present. Confirmation of this argument should come from large series with good follow up information.

Conclusion

Seven years after its introduction, it would appear that PAV is a palliative therapeutic intervention in the case of calcified aortic stenosis, with a limited number of indications.

PERCUTANEOUS TRICUSPID VALVULOTOMY

Isolated tricuspid stenosis is a rare disease, presenting mainly as part of a multiple valvular disease of rheumatic origin (227-228). So far the only treatment was surgery, consisting essentially of commissurotomy or, less frequently, valve replacement. Currently, only a few publications have reported on balloon tricuspid valvulotomy.

Anatomy and mechanism of action

Unlike mitral stenosis, tricuspid stenosis seldom occurs on its own, but is generally associated with moderate or major valvular insufficiency, because the tricuspid ring is larger and the valve leaflets are more fragile than their mitral counterparts. The expected effect of percutaneous tricuspid valvulotomy is the splitting of the commissures.

Technique

Dilation of the tricuspid valve is technically easier than that of the aortic or mitral valve. A percutaneous femoral approach is used in all cases. Where the conventional single balloon or double balloon technique is used, one or more long change-over guides with preshaped ends are introduced into the apex of the right ventricle - more frequently than into the right ventricular outflow tract. One or more often two balloons - because of the large dimensions of the tricuspid ring - are then placed across the tricuspid valve (the techniques used are summarized in Table 7.2-X). In most cases conventional balloons with a diameter within the 15-25 mm range are used. Shaw is the only author who reported a case of dilation using a 30 mm Inoue balloon (237).

Tricuspid dilation has been carried out alone in nine cases (229,231,233-237) and in

	Valve area (cm^2)		Balloon size	
	Before	After	(mm)	Follow up
Khalilullah (1 case) (229)	1.2	2.6	20	Good clinical results (8 weeks)
Ribeira (4 cases) (231)	1 ± 0.2	2.2 ± 0.2	15 + 20 18 + 20 18 + 20 20 + 20	Good clinical results + hemodynamics (3 years) VA: 2.2 ± 0.1 cm ^{2}
Bourdillon (1 case) (233)	0.78	0.95	20 + 20	Double valve replacement mitral + tricuspid (6 months)
Berland (3 cases) (162)	1.1	2.2	20 "Trefoil" 18 + (3 x 10) 19	Good clinical results + hemodynamics (6 months) VA: 2 cm^2
Goldenberg (1 case) (234)	0.82	1.64	20	Good clinical results (3 months)
Mullins (1 case) (235)	0.9	1.4	18 + 15	No follow up
Konugres (1 case) (164)	1	4	23	No follow up
Robalino (1 case) (236)	0.97	2.08	20	No follow up
Shaw (1 case) (237)	0.7	1.56	Inoue 30	Death (13 months) congestive heart failure
Savas (1 case) (164)	0.9	1	18 + 18	Good clinical results (6 months)

Table 7.2-X: Valvuloplasty of tricuspid stenosis

conjunction with mitral dilation in four cases (162,231), while Savas and Konugres (163-164) reported two cases of triple dilation (aortic, mitral and tricuspid), one of which was performed during pregnancy (164).

Where a mitral and tricuspid dilation is envisaged, it appears logical to start with the mitral stenosis, since this is technically more difficult, and to reduce the pulmonary hypertension in the case of significant tricuspid insufficiency complicating the dilation of that valve (162).

Results

To our knowledge, only 15 cases of tricuspid dilation have been published (229-237). The results are summarized in Table 7.2-X. The percutaneous dilation generally causes a significant increase in the orifice area of the valve and a significant reduction in the tricuspid gradient. The main risk is the occurrence of a tricuspid insufficiency, two cases of which have been reported (233,237). No cases of hemopericardium have been reported so far.

The information on long term results is limited. The good initial results reported by Goldenberg (234) persisted for three months, in the three observations by Berland (162) for six months and in the four cases described by Ribiero (232) for three years. The hemodynamic follow up in the short series of Ribiero and Berland showed that the good initial results had remained stable. Of the two cases of major tricuspid insufficiency (233,237), one necessitated valve replacement six months later, while the other patient died one year after the intervention due to gross cardiac insufficiency.

In addition to dilations for the treatment of tricuspid stenoses of rheumatic origin, which are the most frequent, we may note one case of dilation for congenital tricuspid stenosis in a 46 year old woman (235) and one dilation for tricuspid stenosis of carcinogenic origin (234). Both procedures were successful.

Indications

The very small number of published cases does not permit any satisfactory analysis of the immediate and medium term results of percutaneous tricuspid dilation. The indications for this method will undoubtedly be infrequent, reserved for patients suffering from poorly tolerated tight tricuspid stenosis (< 2 cm^2), either alone or in conjunction with a minor regurgitation. In all other cases, where the tricuspid stenosis is accompanied by moderate or considerable regurgitation, or is combined with another valve lesion necessitating surgical treatment, the treatment of choice will remain surgery.

PERCUTANEOUS DILATION OF BIOPROSTHESES

Percutaneous dilations have been successfully performed since 1982 on all natural valves. This technique has recently been extended to failed bioprostheses since primary tissue failure with calcification and consecutive stenosis is a frequent mode of structural failure (238-240).

Procedure

Experimental balloon valvulotomies (239-240) on removed porcine bioprostheses demonstrated that the balloons are capable of splitting the commissures in the same way as the native valves. However, the dilation may be accompanied in this case by a series of undesirable consequences, including the mobilization of friable calcific fragments or blood clots at the time of insertion, during inflation or on withdrawal of the deflated balloon, and fracturing and tearing of portions of the rigid leaflets.

These anatomic findings explain the very limited part which this procedure is liable to play in the treatment of the stenosing degeneration of bioprostheses.

Technique

The technique used for the dilation of bioprostheses is identical to that used for the dilation of native valves.

Table 7.2-XI: Valvuloplasty of bioprostheses in the mitral position.

	Valve area (cm^2) Before	After	Type and size of the bioprosthesis	Follow up
Calvo (243)	1.1	1.3	Hancock (No. 31)	N.A
	1.3	2.5	Carpentier Edwards (No. 29)	N.A
Cox (244)	1.1	1.7	Hancock (No. 33)	Good clinical results (12 months)
Arie (245)	1.0	2.6	Dura mater bioprosthesis	Good clinical results (2 months)
Orbe (246)	1.1	1.4	Hancock (No. 31)	Death (12 months)
	1.3	2.5	Carpentier (No. 29)	Operation for restenosis (12 months)
	0.9	1.7	Carpentier (No. 29)	Operation for restenosis (7 months)
Pellberg (247)	0.36	1.1	Ionescu Shiley (No. 29)	Death (8 months)
Babic (248)	0.7	1.7	Ionescu Shiley	Good clinical results + hemodynamics (10 months)

Results

Experience with dilation of stenosing bioprostheses reported in the literature is limited to 17 cases. MacKay (241) reported the first two cases of a dilation of a bioprosthesis in the aortic position. Both these cases resulted in failure, one due to massive aortic insufficiency which proved fatal, while in the second case the hemodynamic improvement was only limited (an increase of 0.7-0.8 cm^2 in the surface area of the valve), necessitating a further surgical intervention at a subsequent stage.

Ramondo (242) published a further paper on the dilation of a Hancock bioprosthesis in the aortic position, resulting in an increase in the orifice area from 0.59 to 1.07 cm^2 without the occurrence of aortic insufficiency; no follow up information was given.

Nine examples of the dilation of mitral valve bioprostheses have been published (243-248) (Table 7.2-XI). In six of these cases there was a significant increase in the surface area of the valve in excess of 1.5 cm^2. No complications occurred during the procedure, but the subsequent course was unfavorable in four patients; two died due to cardiac insufficiency (246-247) and two required surgical intervention (246). The remaining patients were in a good functional state two to 12 months after the dilation (244,245,248). Eight examples of the dilation of a tricuspid bioprosthesis have been reported. These were essentially young patients undergoing surgery for tricuspid endocarditis (250-253) (Table 7.2-XII). The immediate hemodynamic improvement was in most cases moderate; the orifice area became larger than 1.5 cm^2 in only three cases. Nevertheless, an immediate, in some cases spectacular clinical improvement was observed. There were no immediate complications.

Table 7.2-XII: Valvuloplasty of bioprostheses in the tricuspid position.

	Valve area (cm^2)		Type and size of balloon	Follow up
	Before	After		
Feit (249)	0.69	1.22	Hancock (No. 31)	Good clinical results (1 month)
Wren (250)	0.52	0.65	Ionescu Shiley (No. 29)	Restenonis (4 months) ≥ revalvulotomy
(2 procedures in a single patient)	0.43	0.58	Ionescu Shiley	Restenosis (9 months) ≥ operation
Chow (251) (6 months)	0.93	4.42	Carpentier Edwards (No. 29)	Good clinical results
Attubato (252)	0.6	1.5	Carpentier Edwards	N.A.
	1.0	1.6	(No. non precise)	N.A.
Slama (253)	0.65	1.15	Carpentier Edwards (No. 31)	Right atrial thrombosis (14 months) → operation
	0.9	1.65	Hancock (No. 33)	Restenosis (21 months) → operation

Medium term results are known in five cases. Feit and Chow (249,251) reported continuing functional improvement after one and six months, respectively. In the other cases the outcome was unfavorable. Wren (250) reported a repeat dilation of an Ionescu-Shiley bioprosthesis in the tricuspid position with a moderate increase in the surface area of the valve, which re quired repeat surgery nine months after the redilation. Two cases reported by M. Slama (253) had to undergo further surgery 14 and 21 months after the dilation as a result of right atrial thrombosis or progressive recurrence of the stenosis, respectively.

Indications

It is concluded from the anatomic findings and/or the results of dilation experiments that bioprosthesis dilations do not yield good results. They may give rise to serious immediate complications in the left heart and unsatisfactory medium term results in the tricuspid position. It may however be possible to consider this procedure for palliative purposes in the case of a stenosing degeneration of a bioprosthesis in the tricuspid position.

CONCLUSION

Our overall conclusion is, more than 10 years after the performance of the first percutaneous dilations for acquired valvular stenoses, that the general balance is positive. The first reason for this is that percutaneous mitral valvular dilation is effective and undoubtedly has an important part to play in the treatment of mitral stenosis of rheumatic origin. On the other hand, despite the very considerable initial enthusiasm, aortic dilation will certainly occupy only a limited place. This applies to tricuspid and bioprosthesis dilations also.

A number of questions remain to be answered, one of the most important being the financial aspects: will it ever be possible for the developing countries, where mitral stenoses of rheumatic origin are very frequent but where financial and technical resources are limited, to obtain widespread access to this technique?

Percutaneous mitral dilation won a place, side by side with surgery, in the treatment of mitral stenosis of rheumatic origin, where it provides a useful complement to surgery.

References

1. Inoue K, Owaki T, Nakamura T, et al. Clinical application of transvenous mitral commissurotomy by a new balloon catheter. J Thorac Cardiovasc Surg 1984,87:394- 402
2. McKay RG, Lock JE, Safian RD, et al. Balloon dilatation of mitral stenosis in adults patients: postmortem and percutaneous mitral valvulotomy studies. J Am Coll Cardiol 1987;9:723-731
3. Kaplan JD, Isner JM, Karas RH, et al. In vitro analysis of mechanisms of balloon valvulotomy of stenotic mitral valves. Am J Cardiol 1987;59:318-323
4. Block PC, Palacios IF, Jacobs ML, et al. Mechanism of percutaneous mitral valvotomy. Am J Cardiol 1987;59:178-179
5. Ribeiro PA, Zaibag M, Rajendran V, et al. The manner of achieving mitral valve area increase by in-vitro single and double balloon mitral valvotomy. Am J Cardiol 1988;62:264-270
6. Reid CL, McKay CR, Chandranata P, et al. Mechanisms of increase in mitral valve area and influence of anatomic features in double balloon catheter balloon valvulotomy in adults with rheumatic mitral stenosis: a Doppler and two-dimensional echocardiographic study. Circulation 1987;76:628- 636
7. Reifart N, Nowak B, Baykut D, et al. Experimental balloon valvulotomy of fibrotic and calcific mitral valves. Circulation 1990;81:1105- 1111
8. Martucelli E, Romeo F, Rosano G, et al. Intra-operative percutaneous double-balloon valvulotomy versus surgical commissurotomy for mitral stenosis. Am J Cardiol 1992;70:553-554
9. Babic UU, Pejcic P, Djurisic Z, et al. Percutaneous transarterial balloon valvulotomy for mitral valve stenosis. Am J Cardiol 1986;57:1101-1104
10. Babic UU, Dorros G, Pejcic P, et al. Percutaneous mitral valvulotomy: retrograde, transarterial double-balloon technique utilizing the transseptal approach. Cathet Cardiovasc Diagn 1988;14:229-237
11. Buchler JR, Assis SF, Braga SLN, et al. Percutaneous mitral valvulotomy in rheumatic mitral stenosis by isolated transarterial approach. A new and feasible technique. Am Heart J 1987;28:791-798
12. Orme EC, Wray RB, Mason JW. Balloon mitral val vulotomy via retrograde left atrial catheterization. Am Heart J 1989;117;680-683
13. Zureikat HY, Karsheh IE, Naber NM, et al. Mitral balloon valvulotomy using a retrograde transventricular approach via the brachial artery. Cathet Cardiovasc Diagn 1989;17:183-185
14. Stefanidis C, Stratos C, Pitsavos C, et al. Retrograde non-transseptal balloon mitral valvulotomy: immediate and long-term follow-up. Circulation 1992;85:1760- 1767
15. Holmes D. Transseptal catheterization 1992 - It is here to stay. Cathet Cardiovasc Diagn 1992;26:264-265
16. Bagger JP, Sennels F, Vejby-Christensen H, et al. Transseptal left heart catheterization with a Swan-Ganz flow- directed catheter: review of 173 studies. Am Heart J 1985;109:332-337
17. Zaibag M, Al Kasab S, Ribeiro PA, et al. Percutaneous double balloon mitral valvotomy for rheumatic mitral valve stenosis. Lancet 1986;1:757-761
18. Palacios IF, Block PC, Brandi S, et al. Percutaneous balloon valvotomy for patients with severe mitral stenosis. Circulation 1987;75:778- 784
19. McKay CR, Kawanishi DT, Rahimtoola SH. Catheter balloon valvulotomy of the mitral valve in adults using a double-balloon technique: early hemodynamic results. JAMA 1987;257:1753-1761
20. Vahanian A, Michel PL, Cormier B, et al. Results of percutaneous mitral commissurotomy in 200 patients. Am J Cardiol 1989;63:847-852
21. Tuzcu EM, Block PC, Palacios IF, et al. Comparison of early versus late experience with percutaneous mitral balloon valvulotomy. J Am Coll Cardiol 1991;17:1121-1124
22. Nobuyoshi M, Hamasaki N, Kimura T, et al. Indications, complications, and short-term clinical outcome

of percutaneous transvenous mitral commissurotomy. Circulation 1989;80:782-792

23. Inoue K. Percutaneous transvenous mitral commis surotomy using the Inoue balloon. Eur Heart J 1991;12(Suppl D):1-9

24. Chen CR, Huang ZD, Lo ZX, et al. Comparison of single rubber-nylon balloon and double polyethylene balloon valvulotomy in 94 patients with rheumatic mitral stenosis. Am Heart J 1990;119:102-111

25. Shim WH, Jang YS, Cho SY, et al. Comparison of outcome among double, bi-foil and Inoue balloon techniques for percutaneous mitral valvulotomy in severe mitral stenosis (Abstract). Circulation 1990;82(Suppl III):498

26. Ramaswamy K, Losordo DW, Rosenfield K, et al. Inoue balloon mitral valvulotomy vs. double balloon technique: procedure duration and radiation exposure (Abstract). J Am Coll Cardiol 1991;17:253A

27. Bassand JP, Schiele F, Bernard Y, et al. The double-balloon and Inoue techniques in percutaneous mitral valvulotomy: comparative results in a series of 232 cases. J Am Coll Cardiol 1991;18:982-989

28. Ribeiro PA, Fawzy ME, Arafat MA, et al. Comparison of mitral valve area results of balloon mitral valvotomy using the Inoue and double-balloon techniques. Am J Cardiol 1991;68:687-688

29. Fernandez Ortiz A, Macaya C, Alfonso F, et al. Mono versus double- balloon technique for commissural splitting after percutaneous mitral valvotomy. Am J Cardiol 1992;69:1100-1101

30. Ruiz CE, Zhang HP, Macaya C, et al. Comparison of Inoue single-balloon versus double-balloon technique for per cutaneous mitral valvotomy. Am Heart J 1992;123:942-947

31. Shim WH, Jang YS, Cho SY, et al. Comparison of outcome between double and Inoue balloon techniques for percutaneous mitral valvulotomy (Abstract). J Am Coll Cardiol 1991:17:83A

32. Park SS, Kim JJ, Park SM, et al. Immediate and one year results of percutaneous mitral balloon valvulotomy using Inoue and double balloon techniques. Am J Cardiol 1993;71:938- 943

33. Dietz WA, Waters JB, Ramaswamy K, et al. Use of Inoue balloon catheter to perform staged balloon inflations in combination with serial evaluation by color-flow doppler minimizes mitral regurgitation as a complication of percutaneous mitral valvulotomy (Abstract). J Am Coll Cardiol 1991;17:83A

34. Vahanian A, Michel PL, Cormier B, et al. A prospective evaluation of stepwise mitral balloon dilatation using the Inoue technique (Abstract). Circulation 1991;84(Suppl II):27

35. Weinhaus L, Labadidi Z, et al. Catheter rupture during balloon valvulotomy. Am Heart J 1987;113:1035-1036

36. Ishikura F, Nagata S, Yasuda S, et al. Residual atrial septal perforation after percutaneous transvenous mitral commissurotomy with Inoue balloon catheter. Am Heart J 1990;120:873-878

37. Hermann HC, Kussmaul WG, Hirshfeld JW, et al. Single large-balloon percutaneous mitral valvulotomy. Cathet Cardiovasc Diagn 1989;17:59-61

38. Angel J, Anivarro I, Evangelista A, et al. Percutaneous mitral valvulotomy with low profile balloon inserted through a transseptal sheath (Abstract). Circulation 1990;82(Suppl III):498

39. Patel J, Vythilingum S, Mitha AS, et al. Balloon dilatation of the mitral valve by a single bi-foil (2 x 19 mm) or trefoil (3 x 15 mm) catheter. Br Heart J 1990;64:342-346

40. Meier B, Friedli B, Von Segesser L, et al. Valvuloplasty: technical aspects, congenital heart disease. Herz 1988;13:1-13

41. Berland J, Choussat A, Fernandez F, et al. Percutaneous mitral valvotomy using a new bi-foil balloon (Abstract) Circulation 1989;80(Suppl II):358

42. Roth BR, Block PC, Palacios IF. Predictors of in creased mitral regurgitation after percutaneous mitral balloon valvulotomy. Cathet Cardiovasc Diagn 1990;20:17-21

43. Chen C, Wang X, Wang Y, et al. Value of two-dimensional echocardiography in selecting patients and balloon sizes for percutaneous balloon mitral valvulotomy. J Am Coll Cardiol 1989;14:1651-1658

44. Petrossian GA, Tuzcu EM, Ziskind AA, et al. Atrial septal occlusion improves the accuracy of mitral valve area determination following percutaneous mitral balloon valvotomy. Cathet Cardiovasc Diagn 1991;22:21- 24

45. Pandian NG, Isner JM, Hougen TJ, et al. Percutaneous balloon valvulotomy of mitral stenosis aided by cardiac ultrasound. Am J Cardiol 1987;59:380-381

46. Vilacosta I, Iturralde E, San Roman IA, et al. Transesophageal echocardiography monitoring of percutaneous mitral balloon valvulotomy. Am J Cardiol 1992;70:1040-1044

47. Kultursay H, Turkoglu C, Payzin S, et al. Mitral balloon valvulotomy with transesophageal echocardiography without using fluoroscopy (Abstract). Eur Heart J 1992;13:227

48. Thomas JD, Weyman AE. Doppler mitral half-time: a clinical tool in search of theoretical justification. J Am Coll Cardiol 1987;10:923-929

49. Wisenbaugh T, Berk M, Essop R, et al. Effect of mitral regurgitation and volume loading on pressure half-time before and after balloon valvotomy in patients with mitral stenosis. Am J Cardiol 1991;67:162- 168

50. Schwartz S, Pandian N, Kumar R, et al. Intracardiac echocardiography during simulated aortic and mitral balloon valvulotomy: in vivo experimental studies. Am Heart J 1992;123:665-674

51. Petit J, Vahanian A, Michel PL, et al. Percutaneous mitral valvotomy: French Co-operative Study: 114

patients (Abstract). Circulation 1987;76(Suppl IV):496

52. Ruiz CE, Allen JW, Lau FYK. Percutaneous double balloon valvotomy for severe rheumatic mitral stenosis. Am J Cardiol 1990;65:473-477

53. Hung JS, Chen MS, Wu JJ, et al. Short and long- term results of catheter balloon percutaneous transvenous mitral commissurotomy. Am J Cardiol 1991;67:854-862

54. The National Heart, Lung, and Blood Institute Balloon Valvuloplasty Registry. Complications and mortality of percutaneous balloon mitral commissurotomy. Circulation 1992;85:2014-2024

55. Rocha P, Berland J, Lefebvre JM, et al. Inoue balloon usefulness in case of failure to stabilize bi-foil catheter balloons during percutaneous mitral valvotomy: preliminary report. Cathet Cardiovasc Diagn 1992;26:323- 326

56. Lock JE, Khalilullah M, Shrivastava S, et al. Per cutaneous catheter commissurotomy in rheumatic mitral stenosis. N Engl J Med 1958;313:1515-1518

57. Palacios IF, Lock JE, Keane JF, et al. Percutaneous transvenous balloon valvotomy in a patient with severe calcific mitral stenosis. J Am Coll Cardiol 1986;7:1416-1419

58. Vahanian A, Slama M, Cormier B, et al. Valvuloplastie mitrale percutanée chez l'adulte. Arch Mal Coeur 1986;79:1896-1902

59. Ubago JLM, Coleman T, Figueroa A, et al. Percutaneous mitral valvulotomy in calcific and fibrotic rheumatic mitral stenosis. Am J Cardiol 1987;59:1007-1008

60. Lefevre T, Bonan R, Serra A, et al. Percutaneous mitral valvulotomy in surgical high risk patient. J Am Coll Cardiol 1991;17:348- 354

61. Levine MJ, Weinstein JS, Diver DJ, et al. Progressive improvement in pulmonary vascular resistance after percutaneous mitral valvulotomy. Circulation 1989;79:1061- 1067

62. McKay CR, Kawanishi DT, Kotlewski A, et al. Improvement in exercise capacity and exercise hemodynamics 3 months after double balloon, catheter balloon valvulotomy treatment of patients with symptomatic mitral stenosis. Circulation 1988;77:1013-1021

63. Ohshima M, Yamazoe M, Tamura Y, et al. Immediate effects of percutaneous transvenous mitral commissurotomy on pulmonary hemodynamics at rest and during exercise in mitral stenosis. Am J Cardiol 1992;70:641-644

64. Mehta PM, Wynne J, Reyes VP, et al. Abnormal left ventricular function in patients with mitral stenosis improves following valvulotomy (Abstract). J Am Coll Cardiol 1991;17:161A

65. Goto S, Handa S, Akaishi M, et al. Left ventricular ejection performance in mitral stenosis, and effects of successful percutaneous mitral commissurotomy. Am J Cardiol 1992;69:233-237

66. Wisenbaugh T, Berk M, Middlemost S, et al. Immediate effects of balloon valvotomy on depressed LV performance in mitral stenosis: is it abnormal loading or a myocardial factor? (Abstract) J Am Coll Cardiol 1991;17:162A

67. Liu CP, Ting CT, Yang TM, et al. Reduced left ventricular compliance in human mitral stenosis: role of reversible internal constraint. Circulation 1992;85:1447- 1456

68. Harrisson JK, Davidson CJ, Hermiller JB. Left ventricular filling and ventricular diastolic performance after percutaneous balloon mitral valvotomy. Am J Cardiol 1992;63:108-112

69. Turi ZG, Reyes VP, Soma Raju B, et al. Percutaneous balloon versus surgical closed commissurotomy for mitral stenosis. Circulation 1991;83:1179- 1185

70. Patel JJ, Shama D, Mitha AS, et al. Balloon valvulotomy versus closed commissurotomy for pliable mitral stenosis: a prospective hemodynamic study. J Am Coll Cardiol 1991;18:1318-1322

71. Reyes VP, Soma Raju B, Turi ZG, et al. Percutaneous balloon vs. open surgical commissurotomy for mitral stenosis: a randomized trial (Abstract). Circulation 1990;82(Suppl III):545

72. Reddy PS, Ziady G, Dayem K, et al. Balloon dilatation vs. closed commissurotomy in mitral stenosis (Abstract). Circulation 1989;80(Suppl II):358

73. Ben-Fahrat M, Ayari M, Betbout F, et al. Percutaneous balloon versus surgical closed and open mitral commissurotomy (Abstract). J Am Coll Cardiol 1993;21:488A

74. Raju BS, Turi Z, Raju R, et al. Three and one-half year follow-up of a randomized trial comparing percutaneous balloon and surgical closed mitral commissurotomy. J Am Coll Cardiol 1993;21:429A

75. Ziady G, Sudhakar Reddi P, Sayed H, et al. Comparison of early results of balloon mitral valvotomy to closed mitral commissurotomy in complex mitral stenosis (Abstract). J Am Coll Cardiol 1990;15:247A

76. Nakatani S, Nagata S, Beppu S, et al. Acute reduction of mitral valve area after percutaneous balloon mitral valvulotomy: assessment with doppler continuity equation method. Am Heart J 1991;121:770-775

77. Chen C, Wang Y, Guo B, et al. Reliability of the doppler pressure half-time method for assessing effects of percutaneous mitral balloon valvulotomy. J Am Coll Cardiol 1989;13:1309-1313

78. Tamai J, Negata S, Akaike M, et al. Improvement in mitral flow dynamics during exercise after percutaneous trans venous mitral commissurotomy: non-invasive evaluation using continuous wave doppler technique. Circulation 1990;81:46- 51

79. Herrmann HC, Kleaveland P, Hill JA, et al. The M-Heart percutaneous balloon mitral valvulotomy

registry: initial results and early follow-up. J Am Coll Cardiol 1990;15:1221-1226

80. Berland J, Gerber L, Gamra H, et al. Percutaneous balloon valvulotomy for mitral stenosis complicated by fatal pericardial tamponade in a patient with extreme pulmonary hypertension. Cathet Cardiovasc Diagn 1989;17:109-111

81. Drobinski G, Montalescot G, Evans J, et al. Systemic embolism as a complication of percutaneous mitral valvulotomy. Cathet Cardiovasc Diagn 1992;25:327-330

82. Vahanian A, Ghanem G, Michel PL. The risks of embolism during percutaneous mitral commissurotomy (Abstract) J Am Coll Cardiol 1993;21:350A

83. Milner MR, Goldtein SA, Lindsay J, et al. Transesophageal echocardiographic guidance for percutaneous balloon mitral valvulotomy (Abstract). Circulation 1990;82(Suppl III):81

84. Cormier B, Vahanian A, Michel PL, et al. Transesophageal echocardiography in the assessment of percutaneous mitral commissurotomy. Eur Heart J 1991;12(Suppl B):61-65

85. Essop MR, Wisenbaugh T, Skoularigis J, et al. Mitral regurgitation following mitral balloon valvotomy: differing mechanisms for severe versus mild-to-moderate lesions. Circulation 1991;84:1669-1679

86. Vahanian A, Cormier B, Chanem G. Anatomic features and surgical treatment of severe mitral regurgitation after percutaneous balloon valvotomy (Abstract). Circulation 1992;86(Suppl I):1-594

87. Black MD, Campagna M, Bedard P, et al. Severe mitral insufficiency post-balloon valvotomy: the late changes found in a disrupted mitral valve. Cathet Cardiovasc Diagn 1990;21:99-102

88. Serra A, Bonan R, Vanderperren O, et al. Anatomical and pathological study of mitral valve rupture following balloon valvulotomy (Abstract). Circulation 1990;82(Suppl III):449

89. Acar C, Deloche A, Tibi PR, et al. Operative findings after percutaneous mitral dilation. Ann Thorac Surg 1990;49:959-963

90. O'Shea JP, Abascal VM, Wilkins GT, et al. Unusual sequelae after percutaneous mitral valvulotomy: a Doppler- Echocardiographic study. J Am Coll Cardiol 1992;19:186-191

91. Smith WM, Neutze JM, Baratt-Boyes BG, et al. Open mitral valvotomy: effect of preoperative factors on result. J Thorac Cardiovasc Surg 1981;82:738-751

92. John S, Bashi VV, Jairap PS, et al. Closed mitral valvotomy: early results and long-term follow-up of 3274 consecutive patients. Circulation 1983;68:891-896

93. Bernard Y, Schiele F, Bassand JP, et al. Characteristics of flow though the atrial septal defect following percutaneous mitral valvulotomy (Abstract). Circulation 1989;80(Suppl II):569

94. Yoshida K, Yoshikawa J, Akasaka T, et al. Assessment of left-to-right atrial shunting after percutaneous mitral valvulotomy by transesophageal color doppler flow-mapping. Circulation 1989;80:1521-1526

95. Cequier A, Bonan R, Dyrda I, et al. Atrial shunting after percutaneous mitral valvulotomy. Circulation 1990;81:1190-1197

96. Casale P, Block PC, O'Shea JP, et al. Atrial septal defect after percutaneous mitral balloon valvulotomy: immediate results and follow-up. J Am Coll Cardiol 1990;15:1300-1304

97. Goldberg N, Roman CF, Do Cha S, et al. Right to left interatrial shunting following balloon mitral valvulotomy. Cathet Cardiovasc Diagn 1989;16:133-135

98. Carlson MD, Palacios I, Thomas JD, et al. Cardiac conduction abnormalities during percutaneous balloon mitral or aortic valvotomy. Circulation 1989;79:1197-1203

99. The National Heart, Lung and Blood Institute Balloon Valvuloplasty Registry Participants. Multicenter experience with balloon mitral commissurotomy: NHLBI balloon valvulotomy registry report on immediate and 30- day follow-up results. Circulation 1992;85:448-461

100. Wilkins GT, Gillam LD, Weyman AE, et al. Percutaneous balloon dilatation of the mitral valve: an analysis of echocardiographic variables related to outcome and the mechanism of dilatation. Br Heart J 1988;60:299- 308

101. Abascal V, Wilkins GT, O'Shea JP, et al. Prediction of successful outcome in 130 patients undergoing percutaneous balloon mitral valvotomy. Circulation 1990;82:448-456

102. Herrmann HC, Ramaswamy K, Isner JM, et al. Factors influencing immediate results, complications, and short-term follow-up status after Inoue balloon mitral valvotomy: a North-American multicenter study. Am Heart J 1992;124:160-166

103. Feldman T, Carroll JD, Isner JM, et al. Effect of valve deformity on results and mitral regurgitation after Inoue balloon commissurotomy. Circulation 1992;85:180-187

104. Reid CL, Rahimtoola SH. The role of echocardiography/Doppler in catheter balloon treatment of adults with aortic and mitral stenosis. Circulation 1991;84(Suppl I):240-249

105. Palacios IF, Block PC. Percutaneous mitral balloon valvotomy (PMV) in patients with calcific mitral stenosis (Abstract). Circulation 1989;80(Suppl II):359

106. Vahanian A, Michel PL, Iung B, et al. Should balloon valvotomy be performed for severely calcified mitral stenosis? (Abstract). Circulation 1990;82(Suppl III):79

107. Abascal VM, Wilkins GT, Choong CY, et al. Mitral regurgitation after percutaneous balloon mitral valvulotomy in adults: evaluation by pulsed doppler echocardiography. J Am Coll Cardiol 1988;11:257-263

108. Nair M, Agarwala R, Kalra GS, et al. Can mitral regurgitation after balloon dilatation of the mitral valve be predicted? Br Heart J 1992;67:442-444

109. Barraud P, Serra A, Bonan R, et al. Effect of subvalvular disease on mitral regurgitation after balloon valvulotomy (Abstract). Circulation 1990;82(Suppl III):499

110. Sadee AS, Becker AE. The significance of subvalvular involvement as a cause for mitral valve insufficiency, as assessed during in vitro balloon valvulotomy of rheumatic mitral valve stenosis (Abstract). J Am Coll Cardiol 1990;15:97A

111. Nabel EG, Bergin PJ, Kirsh MM, et al. Morphological analysis of balloon mitral valvulotomy: intra-operative results (Abstract). J Am Coll Cardiol 1990;15:97A

112. Fatkin D, Roy P, Morgan JJ, et al. Percutaneous balloon mitral valvotomy with the Inoue single balloon catheter: commissural morphology as a determination of outcome. J Am Coll Cardiol 1993;21:390-397

113. Alfonso F, Macaya C, Iniguez A, et al. Comparison of results of percutaneous mitral valvulotomy in patients with large ((gt)6 cm) versus those with smaller left atria. Am J Cardiol 1992;69:355-360

114. Palacios IF, Block PC, Wilkins GT, et al. Follow-up of patients undergoing percutaneous mitral balloon valvotomy. Circulation 1989;79:573- 579

115. Zaibag M, Ribeiro PA, Al Kasab S, et al. One year follow-up after percutaneous double balloon mitral valvotomy. Am J Cardiol 1989;63:126-127

116. Vahanian A, Michel PL, Cormier B, et al. Immediate and mid-term results of percutaneous mitral commissurotomy. Eur Heart J 1991;12(Suppl B):84-89

117. Kawanishi DT, Reid CL, Stellar WA, et al. Serial long-term follow-up of patients undergoing double-balloon catheter balloon commissurotomy for mitral stenosis (Abstract). J Am Coll Cardiol 1991;17:253A

118. Block PC, Palacios IF, Block EH, et al. Late (two-year) follow-up after percutaneous balloon mitral valvotomy. Am J Cardiol 1992;69:537-541

119. Desideri A, Vanderperren O, Serra A, et al. Long-term (9 to 33 months) echocardiographic follow-up after successful percutaneous mitral commissurotomy. Am J Cardiol 1992;69:1602-1606

120. Babic UU, Grujicic S, Popovic Z, et al. Percutaneous transarterial balloon dilatation of the mitral valve: five year experience. Br Heart J 1992;67:185-189

121. Abascal VM, Wilkins GT, Choong CY, et al. Echocardiographic evaluation of mitral valve structure and function in patients followed for at least 6 months after percutaneous balloon mitral valvulotomy. J Am Coll Cardiol 1988;12:606-615

122. Cohen DJ, Kuntz RE, Gordon SPF, et al. Predictors of long-term outcome after percutaneous balloon mitral valvulotomy. N Engl J Med 1992;327:1329-1335

123. Pan M, Medina A, Lezo JJ, et al. Factors determining late success after mitral balloon valvulotomy. Am J Cardiol 1993;71:1181-1186

124. Vahanian A, Iung B, Elias J, et al. Restenosis after successful percutaneous mitral commissurotomy (Abstract). J Am Coll Cardiol 1993;21:350A

125. Palacios IF, Tuzcu EM, Newell JB, et al. Four-year clinical follow-up of patients undergoing percutaneous mitral balloon valvotomy (Abstract). Circulation 1990;(Suppl III):545

126. Pan JP, Lin SL, Go JU, et al. Frequency and severity of mitral regurgitation one year after balloon mitral valvulotomy. Am J Cardiol 1991;67:264-268

127. Hernandez R, Macaya C, Benuelos C, et al. Predictors, mechanisms and outcome of severe mitral regurgitation complicating percutaneous mitral valvotomy with the Inoue balloon. Am J Cardiol 1993;70:1169-1174

128. Vanderperren O, Bonan R, Desideri A, et al. Atrial shunting after successful percutaneous mitral valvulotomy: long term follow-up (Abstract). Circulation 1990;82(Suppl III):46

129. Mahan III EF, Helmcke F, Parro A, et al. Atrial septal defect after percutaneous mitral balloon valvulotomy: estimation of shunt volume and predictors of persistence by color doppler echocardiography (Abstract). J Am Coll Cardiol 1991;17:70A

130. Reid CL, Kawanishi DT, Stellar W, et al. Long- term incidence of atrial septal defects after catheter balloon commissurotomy for mitral stenosis (Abstract). J Am Coll Cardiol 1991;17:339A

131. Sadaniantz A, Luttmann C, Shulman RS, et al. Acquired Lutembacher syndrome or mitral stenosis and acquired atrial septal defect after transseptal mitral valvulotomy. Cathet Cardiovasc Diagn 1990;21:7-9

132. Hickley MS, Blackstone EH, Kirklin JW, et al. Outcome probabilities and life history after surgical mitral commissurotomy: implications for balloon commissurotomy. J Am Coll Cardiol 1991;117:29-42

133. Rediker DE, Block PC, Abascal VM, et al. Mitral balloon valvulotomy for mitral restenosis after surgical commissurotomy. J Am Coll Cardiol 1988;11:252-256

134. Serra A, Bonan R, Cequier A, et al. Mitral restenosis after surgical commissurotomy. Is percutaneous mitral valvulotomy an alternative to reoperation? (Abstract). Circulation 1989;80(Suppl II):72

135. Medina A, Delezo JS, Hernandez E, et al. Balloon valvulotomy for mitral restenosis after previous surgery: a comparative study. Am Heart J 1990;120:568-571

136. Vahanian A, Michel PL, Cormier B, et al. Mid-term results of mitral balloon valvotomy for re-stenosis after

surgical commissurotomy (Abstract). Circulation 1990;82(Suppl III):80

137. Rath PC, Berland J, Gamra H, et al. Balloon mitral valvotomy for mitral restenosis after surgical commissurotomy: immediate result and follow- up (Abstract). J Am Coll Cardiol 1991;17:253A

138. Davidson CJ, Bashore TM, Mickel M, et al. Balloon mitral commissurotomy after previous surgical commissurotomy. Circulation 1992;86:91- 99

139. Rutledge R, McIntosh CL, Morrow AG, et al. Mitral valve replacement after closed mitral commissurotomy. Circulation 1982;66(Suppl I):162-166

140. Saenz CB, Nocero M, Weauer CJ. Percutaneous valvulotomy in a patient with mitral stenosis following surgical annuloplasty. Cathet Cardiovasc Diagn 1990;21:18-22

141. Michel PL, Vahanian A, Maroni JP, et al. Percutaneous mitral commissurotomy in patients over 70 years of age (Abstract). Eur Heart J 1990;11:223

142. Scortichini D, Bonan R, Mickel M, et al. Balloon mitral commissurotomy in surgical high risk patients: results from the NHLBI balloon valvulotomy registry (Abstract). Circulation 1991;84(Suppl II):203

143. Shaw TRD, McAreavey D, Essop AR, et al. Percutaneous balloon dilatation of the mitral valve in patients who were unsuitable for surgical treatment. Br Heart J 1992;67:454-459

144. Tuzcu EM, Block PC, Griffin BP, et al. Immediate and long-term outcome of percutaneous mitral valvotomy in patients 65 years and older. Circulation 1992;85:963-971

145. Le Feuvrec C, Bonan R, Lachurie ML, et al. Balloon mitral commissurotomy in patients aged >70 years. Am J Cardiol 1993;71:233-236

146. Wisenbaugh T, Essop R, Middlemost S, et al. Is severe pulmonary hypertension a risk factor for poor outcome with balloon mitral valvotomy? (Abstract). J Am Coll Cardiol 1992;19:363A

147. Safian R, Berman A, Sachs B, et al. Percutaneous balloon mitral valvulotomy in a pregnant women with mitral stenosis. Cathet Cardiovasc Diagn 1988;15:103-108

148. Palacios IF, Block PC, Wilkins G, et al. Percutaneous mitral balloon valvotomy during pregnancy in a patient with severe mitral stenosis. Cathet Cardiovasc Diagn 1988;15:109-111

149. Smith R, Brender D, McCredie M. Percutaneous transluminal balloon dilatation of the mitral valve in pregnancy. Br Heart J 1989;61:551-553

150. Mangione JA, De Mzuliani MF, Delcastillo JM, et al. Percutaneous double balloon mitral valvulotomy in pregnant women. Am J Cardiol 1989;64:99- 102

151. Esteves CA, Ramos AI, Braga SN, et al. Effectiveness of percutaneous balloon mitral valvotomy during pregnancy. Am J Cardiol 1991;68:930-934

152. Drobinski G, Fraboulet P, Montalescot G, et al. Valvuloplastie mitrale au quatrieme mois de grossesse: protection foetale par un manteau de plomb. Arch Mal Coeur 1991;84:249-251

153. Ribeiro P, Fawzy M, Awad M, et al. Balloon valvotomy for pregnant patients with severe pliable mitral stenosis using the Inoue technique with total abdominal and pelvic shielding (Abstract). J Am Coll Cardiol 1992;19(Suppl A):143A

154. Gangbar EW, Watson KR, Howard RS, et al. Mitral balloon valvulotomy in pregnancy: advantages of a unique balloon. Cathet Cardiovasc Diagn 1992;25:313-316

155. Hung JS, Lin FC, Chiang CW. Successful percutaneous transvenous catheter balloon mitral commissurotomy after warfarin therapy and resolution of left atrial thrombus. Am J Cardiol 1989;64:126-128

156. Chen WJ, Chen MF, Liau CS, et al. Safety of percutaneous transvenous balloon mitral commissurotomy in patients with mitral stenosis and thrombus in the left atrial appendage. Am J Cardiol 1992;70:117-119

157. Vahanian A, Michel PL, Ghanem G, et al. Percutaneous mitral balloon valvotomy in patients with a history of embolism (Abstract). Circulation 1991;84(Suppl II):205

158. Bernard Y, Bassand JP, Schible F. Percutaneous mitral valvulotomy in non-optimal candidates. Eur Heart J 1991;12(Suppl B):90-94

159. Pan M, Medina A, Suarez De Lezo J, et al. Balloon valvulotomy for mild mitral stenosis. Cathet Cardiovasc Diagn 1991;24:1-5

160. Berman AD, Weinstein JS, Safian RD, et al. Combined aortic and mitral balloon valvulotomy in patients with mitral aortic and mitral valve stenosis: results in six cases. J Am Coll Cardiol 1988;1213-1218

161. Kritzer GL, Block PC, Palacios I. Simultaneous percutaneous mitral and aortic balloon valvotomies in an elderly patient. Am Heart J 1987;114:420-423

162. Berland J, Rocha P, Melhemelhe R. Percutaneous valvulotomy for combined mitral and tricuspid stenosis: results in 3 cases. Arch Mal Coeur 1990;83:1585-1589

163. Savas V, Grines CL, O'Neill W. Percutaneous triple-valve balloon valvulotomy in a pregnant woman. Cathet Cardiovasc Diagn 1991;24:288-294

164. Konugres G, Lau F, Ruiz L. Successive percutaneous double-balloon mitral, aortic and tricuspid valvotomy in rheumatic trivalvular stenoses. Am Heart J 1990;119:663-666

165. Bailey CP, Glover RP, O'Neill TJE, et al. Experiences with the experimental surgical relief of aortic stenosis. J Thorac Surg 1950;20:516

166. Bailey CP, Bolton HE, Jamison WL, et al. Commissurotomy for rheumatic aortic stenosis. Surgery.

Circulation 1954;9:23
167. Cribier A, Savin T, Saoudi N, et al. Percutaneous transluminal valvulotomy of acquired aortic stenosis in elderly patients: an alternative to valve replacement? Lancet 1986;11:63-67
168. Wayne Isom O, Rosengart TK. Editorial comment. Percutaneous aortic valvulotomy: off the bandwagon, again. J Am Coll Cardiol 1992;20:804- 805
169. Hostetler MD, Dunn MI. Editorial comment. Percutaneous aortic valvulotomy: Dr. Bailey revisited. J Am Coll Cardiol 1992;20:802-803
170. Robicsek F, Harbold NB. Limited value of balloon dilatation in calcified aortic stenosis in adults: direct observations during open heart surgery. Am J Cardiol 1987;60:857-864
171. McKay RG, Safian RD, Lock JE et al. Balloon dilatation of calcific aortic stenosis in elderly patients: post-mortem, intra-operative, and percutaneous valvulotomy studies. Circulation 1986;74:119-125
172. Safian RD, Mandell VS., Thurer RE, et al. Post- mortem and intra- operative balloon valvulotomy of calcific aortic stenosis in elderly patients: mechanisms of successful dilatation. J Am Coll Cardiol 1987;9:665-660
173. Kennedy KD, Hauck AJ, Edwards WD, et al. Mechanism of reduction of aortic valvular stenosis by percutaneous transluminal balloon valvulotomy: report of five cases and review of literature. Mayo Clin Proc 1988;63:769- 776
174. Letac B, Gerder LI, Konig R. Insights on the mechanism of balloon valvulotomy in aortic stenosis. Am J Cardiol 1988;62:1241-1247
175. Vahanian A, Guerinon J, Michel PL, et al. Experimental balloon valvulotomy of calcified aortic stenosis in the elderly (Abstract). Circulation 1986;74(Suppl II):365
176. Ribeiro PA, Al Zaibag M, Halim M, et al. Percutaneous single and double balloon aortic valvotomy in adolescents and young adults with congenital aortic stenosis. Eur Heart J 1988;9:866-874
177. Ribeiro PA, Al Zaibag M, Rajendran V. Double balloon aortic valvotomy for rheumatic aortic stenosis: in vitro studies. Eur Heart J 1989;10:417-423
178. Desnoyers MR, Isner JM, Pandian NG, et al. Clinical and non-invasive hemodynamic results after aortic balloon valvulotomy for aortic stenosis. Am J Cardiol 1988;62:1078-1084
179. Wagner S, Selzer A. Patterns of progression of aortic stenosis: A longitudinal hemodynamic study. Circulation 1982;65:709-712
180. Cribier A, Gerber L I, Letac B. Aortic valvulotomy. In: Topol EJ (ed). Update 3. Textbook of interventinal cardiology. WB Saunders Co. 1992:43- 58
181. Slama M, Vahanian A, Michel PL et al. Valvuloplasties percutanees des stenoses aortiques de l'adulte. Resultats immediats et a moyen terme: a propos de 78 tentatives. Arch Mal Coeur 1989;82:307-312
182. Block PC, Palacios IF. Comparison of hemodynamic results of anterograde versus retrograde percutaneous balloon aortic valvulotomy. Am J Cardiol 1987;60:659-662
183. Mullins CE, Nihill MR, Vick GW, et al. Double balloon technique for dilatation of valvular or vessel stenosis in congenital and acquired heart disease. J Am Coll Cardiol 1987;10:107-110
184. Safian RD, Berman AD, Diver DJ, et al. Balloon aortic valvulotomy in 170 consecutive patients. N Engl J Med 1988;319:125-130
185. Letac B, Cribier A, Koning R. Le traitement du rétrécissement aortique acquis de l'adulte par valvuloplastie percutanée par cathéter à ballonnet. Expérience de 245 cas. Arch Mal Coeur 1989;82:17-25
186. McKay and the Mansfield Scientific Registry Experience. Overview of acute hemodynamic results and procedural complications. J Am Coll Cardiol 1991;17:485-491
187. Nishimura RA, Holmes DR Jr, Reeder GS, et al. Doppler evaluation of results of percutaneous aortic balloon valvulotomy in calcific aortic stenosis. Circulation 1988;78:791-799
188. Bernard Y, Bassand JP, Anguenot T, et al. Aortic valve area evolution after percutaneous aortic valvulotomy. Eur Heart J 1990;11:98-107
189. NHLBI Balloon Registry Participants. Percutaneous balloon aortic valvulotomy. Acute and 30-day follow-up results in 674 patients from the NHLBI balloon valvulotomy registry. Circulation 1991;84:2383-2387
190. Holmes DR Jr, Nishimura RA, Reeder GS and the Mansfield Scientific Registry Experience. In hospital mortality after balloon aortic valvulotomy: frequency and associated factors. J Am Coll Cardiol 1991;17:189- 192
191. Isner JM and the Mansifeld Scientific Registry Experience. Acute catastrophic complications of balloon aortic valvuloplsty. J Am Coll Cardiol 1991;17:1436-1444
192. Reeder GS, Nishimura RA, Holmes DR and the Mansfield Scientific Registry Experience. Patient age and results of balloon valvulotomy. J Am Coll Cardiol 1991:17:909-913
193. De Ubago JLM, Vasquez de Prada JA, Moujir F, et al. Mitral valve rupture during percutaneous dilatation of aortic valve stenosis. Cathet Cardiovasc Diagn 1989;16:115- 118
194. Lembo NJ, King SB, Roubin GS, et al. Fatal aortic rupture during percutaneous balloon valvulotomy for valvular aortic stenosis. Am J Cardiol 1987;60:733-737
195. Block PC, Palacios IF. Clinical and hemodynamic follow-up after percutaneous aortic valvulotomy in the elderly. Am J Cardiol 1988;62:760- 763

196. Lancelin B, Chevalier B, Bourdin T, et al. Suivi à moyen terme après valvulotomy aortic per-cutanée du sujet âgé. Etude clinique à propos de 102 procéduces. Arch Mal Coeur 1989;82:1397-1404
197. O'Neill WW and the Mansfield Scientific Registry Experience. Predictors of long term survival after percutaneous aortic valvulotomy. Report of the Mansfield valvulotomy registry. J Am Coll Cardiol 1991;17:193-198
198. Serruys PW, Luitjen HE, Beatt KJ, et al. Percutaneous valvulotomy for calcific aortic stenosis. A treatment "sine cure"? Eur Heart J 1988;9:782-794
199. Chevalier B, Lancelin B, Dapelo A, et al. Long term survival rate after percutaneous aortic valvulotomy in the elderly (Abstract). Eur Heart J 1990;11(Suppl):74
200. Legrand V, Beckers J, Fastrez M, et al. Long term follow-up of elderly patients with severe aortic stenosis treated by balloon aortic valvulotomy. Importance of hemodynamic parameters before and after dilatation. Eur Heart J 1991;12:451-457
201. Bashore TM, Davidson CJ and the Mansfield Scientific Registry Experience. Follow-up recatheterization after balloon aortic valvulotomy. J Am Coll Cardiol 1991;17:1188-1195
202. Ferguson JJ, Garza RA and the Mansfield Scientific Registry Experience. Efficacy of multiple balloon aortic valvulotomy procedures. J Am Coll Cardiol 1991;17:1430-1435
203. Ross TC, Banks AK, Collins TJ, et al. Repeat balloon aortic valvulotomy for aortic restenosis. Cathet Cardiovasc Diagn 1989;18:96-98
204. Acar J, Hodara M, Maurat JP, et al. Elements de pronostic due retrecissement aortique calcifiè et indications opèratoires. Coeur et Mèdecine interne 1966;5:295-301
205. O'Keefe JH, Vlietstra RE, Bailey KR, et al. Natural history of candidates for balloon aortic valvulotomy. Mayo Clin Proc 1987;62:986-991
206. Turina J, Hess O, Sepulcri F, et al. Spontaneous course of aortic valve disease. Eur Heart J 1987;8:471-483
207. Cormier B, Luxereau P, Bloch C, et al. Prognosis and long term results of surgically treated aortic stenosis with or without insufficiency. Eur Heart J 1988;9(Suppl E):113-120
208. Rich MW, Sandza JG, Kleiger RE, et al. Cardiac operations in patients over 80 years of age. J Thorac Cardiovasc Surg 1985;90:56-60
209. Tsai TP, Matloff JM, Gray RJ, et al. Cardiac surgery in the octogenarian. J Thorac Cardiovasc Surg 1986;91:924-928
210. Edmunds LH, Stephenson LW, Edie RN, et al. Open heart surgery in octogenarians. N Engl J Med 1988;319:131-136
211. Blakeman BM, Pifarre R, Sullivan HJ, et al. Aortic valve replacement on patients 75 years old and older. Ann Thorac Surg 1987;44:637-639
212. Culliford AT, Galloway AC, Colvin SB, et al. Aortic valve replacement for aortic stenosis in persons aged 80 years and over. Am J Cardiol 1991;67:1256-1260
213. Levinson JR, Akins CW, Buckley MJ, et al. Octogenarians with aortic stenosis: outcome after valve replacement. Circulation 1989;80(Suppl I):49-56
214. Freeman WK, Schaff HV, O'Brien PC, et al. Cardiac surgery in octogenarians: perioperative outcome and clinical follow-up. J Am Coll Cardiol 1991;18:29-35
215. Letac B, Cribier A, Koning R, et al. Aortic stenosis in elderly patients aged 80 and older. Treatment by percutaneous balloon valvulotomy in a series of 92 cases. Circulation 1989;80:1514-1520
216. Bernard Y, Etievent J, Mourand JL, et al. Long term results of percutaneous aortic valvulotomy compared with aortic valve replacement in patients more than 75 years old. J Am Coll Cardiol 1992;20:796-801
217. Acar J, Vahanian A, Slama M, et al. Treatment of calcified aortic stenosis: surgery or percutaneous transluminal aortic valvulotomy. Eur Heart J 1988;9(Suppl):163-168
218. Desnoyers MR, Salem D, Rosenfield K, et al. Treatment of cardiogenic shock by emergency aortic balloon valvulotomy. Ann of Intern Med 1988;108:833-835
219. Cribier A, Lafont A, Eltchanioff, et al. La valvuloplastie aortique percutanèe en dernier recours chez les patients atteints de rètrècissement aortique en ètat critique. Arch Mal Coeur 1990;88:1783-1790
220. Gorlin R, Gorlin G. Hydraulic formula for calculation of area of stenotic mitral valve, other valves and central circulatory shunts. Am Heart J 1951;41:1-10
221. Berland J, Cribier A, Savin T, et al. Percutaneous balloon valvulotomy in patients with severe aortic stenosis and low ejection fraction. Immediate results and 1-year follow-up. Circulation 1989;79:1189-1196
222. McKay RG, Safian RD, Lock JE, et al. Assessment of left ventricular and aortic valve function after balloon valvulotomy in adult patients with aortic stenosis. Circulation 1987;75:192-203
223. Safian RD, Warren SE, Berman AD, et al. Improvement in symptoms and left ventricular performance after balloon aortic valvulotomy in patients with aortic stenosis and depressed left ventricular ejection fraction. Circulation 1988;78:1181-1191
224. Harrison JK, Davidson CJ, Leithe ME, et al. Serial left ventricular performance evaluated by cardiac catheterization before, immediately after and at 6 months after balloon aortic valvulotomy. J Am Coll Cardiol 1990;16:1351-1358

225. Davidson CJ, Harrison JK, Leithe ME, et al. Failure if aortic balloon valvulotomy to result in sustained clinical improvement in patients with depressed left ventricular function. Am J Cardiol 1990;65:72-77
226. Rodriguez AR, Minor ST, West MS, et al. Balloon aortic valvulotomy is not an effective long term therapy for calcific aortic stenosis with left ventricular dysfunction (Abstract). Eur Heart J 1990;11(Suppl):74
227. Roberts WC, Sullivan MF. Combined mitral valve stenosis and tricuspid valve stenosis. Morphologic observations after mitral and tricuspid valve, replacements or mitral replacement and tricuspid valve commissurotomy. Am J Cardiol 1986;58:850-852
228. Yousuf AM, Shafei MZ, Endrys G, et al. Tricuspid stenosis and regurgitation in rheumatic heart disease. A prospective cardiac catheterization study in 525 patients. Am Heart J 1985;110:60-64
229. Khalilullah M, Tyagi S, Yadav BS, et al. Double-balloon valvulotomy of tricuspid stenosis. Am Heart J 1987;11:1232-1235
230. Al Zaibag M, Ribeiro P, Al Kasab S. Percutaneous balloon valvotomy in tricuspid stenosis. Br Heart J 1987:57:51-53
231. Ribeiro PA, Al Zaibag M, Al Kasab S, et al. Percutaneous double-balloon valvotomy for rheumatic tricuspid stenosis. Am J Cardiol 1988;61:660- 662
232. Ribeiro PA, Al Zaibag M, Idris MT. Percutaneous double-balloon tricuspid valvotomy for severe tricuspid stenosis: 3 year follow-up study. Eur Heart J 1990;11:1109-1112
233. Bourdillon PDV, Hookman LD, Morris SN, et al. Percutaneous balloon valvulotomy for tricuspid stenosis: hemodynamic and pathological findings. Am Heart J 1989;117:492-495
234. Goldenberg I, Pedersen W, Olson J, et al. Percutaneous double balloon valvulotomy for severe tricuspid stenosis. Am Heart J 1989;118:417- 419
235. Mullins PA, Hall JA, Shapiro LM. Balloon dilatation of tricuspid stenosis caused by carcinoid heart disease. Br Heart J 1990;63:249-250
236. Robalino B, Whitlow P, Marwick T, et al. Percutaneous balloon valvotomy for the treatment of isolated tricuspid stenosis. Chest 1991;100:867-869
237. Shaw TRD. The Inoue balloon for dilatation of the tricuspid valve: a modified over-the-wire approach. Br Heart J 1992;67:263-265
238. Schoen FJ, Levy R. Bioprosthetic heart valve failure: pathology and pathogenesis. Cardiol Clin 1984;2(4):717
239. Waller BF, McKay C, Vantassel J, et al. Catheter balloon valvulotomy of stenotic porcine bioprosthetic valves: part I: anatomic considerations. Clin Cardiol 1991;14:686- 691
240. Waller BF, McKay C, Vantassel J, et al. Catheter balloon valvulotomy of stenotic porcine bioprosthetic valves: part II: mechanisms, complications and recommendations for clinical use. Clin Cardiol 1991;14:764- 772
241. McKay CR, Waller BF, Hong R, et al. Problems encountered with catheter balloon valvulotomy of bioprosthetic aortic valves. Am Heart J 1988;115:463-465
242. Ramondo A, Gamalli M, Chioin R. Balloon dilatation of a porcine bioprosthetic valve in aortic position. Int J Cardiol 1989;24:105-107
243. Calvo OL, Sobrino N, Gamallo C, et al. Balloon percutaneous valvulotomy for stenotic bioprosthetic valves in the mitral position. Am J Cardiol 1987;60:746-747
244. Cox DA, Friedman PL, Selwyn AP, et al. Improved quality of life after successful balloon valvulotomy of a stenosed mitral bioprosthesis. Am Heart J 1989;118:839-841
245. Arie S, Arato Goncalves MT, et al. Balloon dilatation of a stenotic dura mater mitral bioprosthesis. Am Heart J 1989;117:201-202
246. Orbe LC, Sobrino N, Mate I, et al. Effectiveness of balloon percutaneous valvulotomy for stenotic bioprosthetic valves in different position. Am J Cardiol 1991;68:1719- 1721
247. Spellberg RD, Mayeda GS, Flores JH, et al. Balloon valvulotomy of a stenosed mitral bioprosthesis. Am Heart J 1991;122:1785-1787
248. Babic U, Grujicic S, Vucinic M, et al. Balloon valvulotomy of mitral bioprosthesis. Int J Cardiol 1991;30:230-232
249. Feit F, Stecy PJ, Nachamie M, et al. Percutaneous balloon valvulotomy for stenosis of a porcine bioprosthesis in the tricuspid valve position. Am J Cardiol 1986;58:363-364
250. Wren C, Hunter S. Balloon dilatation of stenosed bioprosthesis in the tricuspid valve position. Br Heart J 1989;61:65-67
251. Chow WH, Cheung KL, Tai YT, et al. Successful percutaneous balloon valvulotomy of a stenotic tricuspid bioprosthesis. Am Heart J 1990;119:666-668
252. Attubato MI, Stroh JA, Bock RG, et al. Percutaneous double balloon valvulotomy of porcine bioprosthetic valves in the tricuspid position. Cathet Cardiovasc Diagn 1990;20:202-204
253. Slama MS, Drieu LH, Malergue MC, et al. Percutaneous double balloon valvulotomy for stenosis of porcine bioprosthetic in the tricuspid valve position: a report of 2 cases. Cathet Cardiovasc Diagn 1993;28:142- 148

Chapter 8.1

Special Aspects of Surgical Management of Valvular Heart Disease

P.H. Deleuze and J.P. Cachera

Surgical replacement of cardiac valves may involve many different technical and strategic procedures when concomitant pathologic conditions are present. These concomitant diseases can concern the coronary arteries, the left ventricle or atrium, the ascending aorta, the perivalvular annulus and adjacent structures; reconstructive surgery may involve combination procedures of varying complexity.

This chapter examines combined valvular replacement and coronary artery bypass grafting, combined valvular replacement and surgery of the ascending aorta, and lastly surgical management of the small aortic annulus.

COMBINED VALVULAR REPLACEMENT AND CORONARY ARTERY BYPASS GRAFTING

Mitral or aortic valve disease in association with coronary atherosclerosis has been described in Chapter 6.5 regarding etiology, pathogenesis and diagnosis. We therefore limit our remarks in this chapter to strictly surgical aspects.

Combined valvular replacement and coronary bypass grafting was first performed in France in 1971 (1) and then in the USA (2). The most important technical advance that enabled its development was deep myocardial hypothermia (3,4). Indeed, only modern techniques of myocardial protection enabling intramyocardial temperatures to be lowered to around 15° C (topical cooling, cardioplegic solutions) afford sufficient durations of ischemia required in combination procedures.

Aortic valve replacement and aortocoronary bypass grafting

The valvular lesion most commonly encountered is calcific aortic stenosis (79%); aortic regurgitation is more rarely involved (21%) (5).

The surgical techniques of valve replacement and coronary artery bypass grafting are basically the same as in the case of isolated aortic valve or coronary surgery. Of particular interest are two issues: the order in which aortic valve replacement and coronary bypass grafting are completed and the type of replacement valve to be used.

Selection of the operating sequence has been the subject of differing opinions, some of which (6-8) adhere to the valvular surgery - distal coronary anastomosis - proximal anastomosis sequence, while others investigators (2,9,10,11) advocate the completion of bypass grafting prior to valve replacement.

We recommend that the distal coronary artery anastomoses be done first, followed by valvular replacement, performed with continuous clamping of the aorta and proximal anastomoses (in case of saphenous vein grafts) performed after de-airing with the crossclamp removed (12).

Selection of the prosthetic valve depends on personal preferences of the cardiologist and cardiac surgeon: technically there is no difference between the insertion of a mechanical valve or a bioprosthesis (13). However, in this context three factors should be considered: the mean age of these patients which is about 50-60 years, the requirement of anticoagulant treatment as a result of bypass grafting and the disadvantage of repeat surgery on an ascending aorta access to which might be blocked by saphenous vein grafts. These three elements lead us to recommend mechanical prostheses in 83% of our patients in combination procedures, and use bioprostheses only when special indication(s) exist.

Mitral valve replacement and aortocoronary bypass grafting

Coexisting coronary atherosclerosis with rheumatic mitral valve disease is less frequently encountered than with an aortic valvular lesion, about 15% of operated cases. A more common condition is mitral regurgitation of ischemic origin, which can account for up to 30% of patients with mitral valve disease in some centers. We shall examine these two very different types of mitral valve disease (14).

Combined valve replacement for rheumatic mitral valve disease and aortocoronary bypass grafting do not pose very different strategic and technical problems from those discussed above in the management of aortic valvular disease. The sequence of distal coronary artery anastomosis - mitral valve replacement - proximal anastomosis also appears to be the most appropriate and reliable method. Selection of the type of prosthesis also depends on the cardiologist's or cardiac surgeon's personal preferences; the patient's age of about 60 years, the need for anticoagulant treatment required because of coronary artery lesions, and the potential risks of repeat surgery are arguments in favor of a mechanical prosthesis. In some selected cases, mitral valve repair can be proposed (15,16).

Surgery of post-ischemic mitral regurgitation poses very different problems. The pathology is much more severe, associating three types of lesions:

- severe, generally three-vessel, coronary artery disease;
- one or more recent or previous myocardial infarcts, with impaired left ventricular function,
- mitral regurgitation that is often severe due to chordal or papillary rupture, or to fibrous elongation of the papillary muscle (Fig. 8.1-1).

Mitral valve replacement can then be combined either with myocardial revascularization or with a more or less extensive resection of the left ventricle to remove a dyskinetic area or aneurysm; in some cases, a triple procedure can be performed, combining mitral valve replacement, resection of the left ventricle and revascularization of the coronaries (17) (Fig. 8.1-2).

Mitral valve replacement for treatment of post ischemic mitral regurgitation can be performed under very different clinical conditions: outside of the acute phase, that is several months after an infarction , or as a major emergency in cardiogenic shock following complete

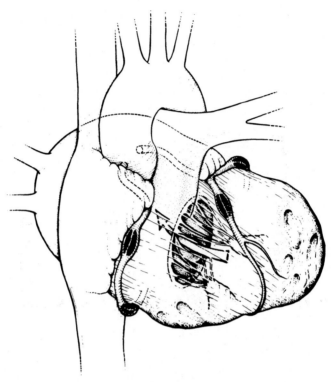

Figure 8.1-1: Ischemic mitral regurgitation; posterior papillary muscle elongation, left ventricular dilatation with 3-vessel coronary artery disease. (Reproduced with the permission of Flammarion Medicine-Sciences, Paris.)

rupture of a papillary muscle. The technical conditions for mitral valve replacement are influenced by the degenerative nature of the lesions involved (16): thin, flaccid chordae tendinae and valve cusps, and an often friable mitral annulus. These conditions favor the use of a low profile prosthesis, like the St. Jude Medical valve. Special sutures are necessary to secure the prosthesis firmly in place: mattress-sutures supported by velour pledgets in most cases, and reinforcement of the mitral annulus with velour strips.

Left ventricular resection combined with mitral valve replacement may be planned in two different ways. When a postero-basal aneurysm is involved - a possible situation commonly associated with lesions of the posterior papillary muscle - the mitral valve must be approached as usual through the left atrium, and the mitral valve is resected: then with the heart tilted, the aneurysm is resected. Surgical repair then consists successively of reconstruction of the left ventricular wall by everting sutures, followed by repair of the mitral annulus and insertion of the prosthetic valve. When an antero-apical aneurysm is involved, the first phase of the operation consists of resection of the ventricle, then, there are two possible approaches for mitral valve replacement: either by using the classical left posterior transatrial route, or through the ventricle if the resection is wide enough to enable resection of the mitral valve under good conditions, and insertion of the prosthesis from bottom to top (Fig. 8.1-3). In these two possible cases, selection of a prosthesis currently also tends to favor a low profile valve.

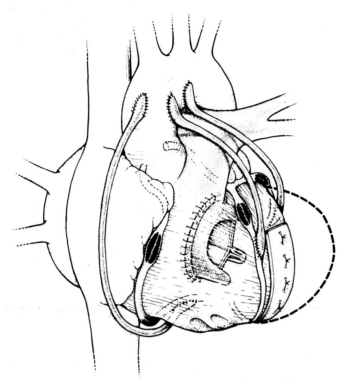

Figure 8.1-2: Triple procedure combining mitral valve replacement, left ventricular wall resection and multiple-vessel aortocoronary bypass grafting. (Reproduced with the permission of Flammarion Medicine-Sciences, Paris.)

Finally, myocardial resection as complete as possible should always be associated with this procedure; bypass grafting does not involve any particular technical aspects. When the combined triple procedure is used, the sequence of distal coronary anastomoses - ventricular resection - mitral valve replacement - proximal anastomoses, appears to be the most reliable method.

Overall results of combined surgical procedures

Operative mortality of combined valvular replacement and coronary bypass grafting, apart from ischemic mitral regurgitation, is about 4%. Operative mortality for mitral valve replacement is slightly higher (5%) than for aortic valve replacement (3%). These results are found in almost all series (18-22) even though a higher mortality rate was reported in earlier cases (23-27). Thus concomitant myocardial revascularization does not increase the risk of valve replacement (15,20,21,28,29) while valvular surgery alone with coexisting coronary artery lesions which are ignored involves a higher mortality rate (5,20,30-33). Intermediate and long term prognosis of patients undergoing surgery is also favorable: survival by life-table analysis is 91% at one year and 80% at five years (13,18,34).

Functional improvement is very good: 94% of patients are in class I or II, with a mean of 1.4 (13-15,34,35). In summary, the overall surgical prognosis of patients in this

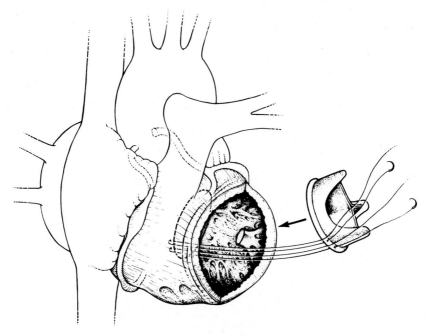

Figure 8.1-3: Insertion of a prosthetic mitral valve by left ventricular approach following resection of a left ventricular aneurysm. (Reproduced with the permission of Flammarion Medicine-Sciences, Paris.)

category does not differ from that of valvular replacement surgery alone, and should lead the surgeon to always perform a combined surgical procedure whenever a patient has concomitant valvular and coronary heart disease (1 5,20,36). More recently, combined procedures have been proposed to septuagenarians and octogenarians with an overall mortality of around 20% (37).

In the treatment of post-ischemic mitral regurgitation, the surgical risk varies considerably with the clinical presentation: in patients operated outside of the acute phase for chordal rupture or elongation of a papillary muscle, the operative risk is about 8 to 10%; in patients undergoing emergency surgery for pulmonary edema and cardiogenic shock due to the rupture of a papillary muscle, the operative mortality rises to 20 or 30%. Lastly, in patients with congestive heart failure, the combined triple procedure has an overall mortality of 40 to 50% (17,18).

These results should not appear discouraging because of the catastrophic spontaneous course of mitral regurgitation following a myocardial infarct. All in all, some risk factors have been shown to carry a bad prognosis: advanced age, low ejection fraction, pre-operative NYHA IV, severe mitral regurgitation (13-15,18,29).

AORTIC VALVE SURGERY COMBINED WITH SURGERY OF THE ASCENDING AORTA

In 1961, DeBakey and Cooley reported the first attempts at surgical correction of aortic root lesions together with aortic valve disease. Much progress has been reported since, but it should be stressed that this type of surgery remains relatively rare and its indications are debated. Although morbidity and mortality are much lower after surgery as compared to the natural course of the disease (38), they are far from negligible. The considerable number of surgical techniques proposed so far shows the difficulties in selecting the appropriate type of management.

In practice, possible repair of the ascending aorta and of the aortic valve is encountered either in the case of aneurysm of the ascending aorta or in the case of dissecting aortic aneurysm involving the first aortic segment. Both lesions may be present in Marfan's syndrome.

Surgery of the aortic valve and aneurysms of the ascending aorta

Aneurysms of the ascending aorta, outside of rare cases caused by syphilis, are caused by alterations in the media. They gradually extend to the aortic annulus, and in typical cases result in annulo-aortic ectasia, as observed in Marfan's syndrome. Annular dilation creates valvular dysfunction with development of aortic regurgitation. The latter, much more so than the risk of aneurysmal rupture, requires surgery because of the rapid impact on the left ventricle (39,40). Grossly, the root of the aorta is dilated, sometimes monstrously so in the shape of an onion bulb, with all of the arterial tissue being particularly thin and friable. Extension of the aneurysm to the aortic sinus is of capital importance, because it causes ascension of the coronary ostia separating them from the annulus. The entire valve is altered and cannot be saved, in particular in patients with Marfan's syndrome where valvular tissue is also affected.

Surgical techniques

The procedure is performed with cardiopulmonary bypass. Arterial cannulation is most commonly done via the femoral artery, as well as venous cannulation through the femoral vein in the event of a massive aneurysm blocking access to the right atrium. It is almost always possible to clamp the aorta just above the innominate artery. Myocardial protection is achieved by cardioplegia and topical cooling. Some aneurysms involving the aortic arch require elective clamping of the supra-aortic trunks with total circulatory arrest under deep hypothermia (41-45).

Correction of aortic regurgitation due to annular dilatation with or without valvular lesions leads inevitably to replacement of the aortic valve. The type of valve used is little debated because complications caused by dysfunction or thrombosis are rare and equally distributed (46-48). There is a unanimous agreement on the risk of detachment of the prosthesis and the need to secure it very firmly to the annulus, if necessary by sutures transfixing the aorta supported on Teflon velour.

There are two types of complications that are specific for this type of surgery. During surgery, the difficulty in achieving satisfactory hemostasis is the cause of immediate or early failure because a vicious circle of events rapidly develops, i.e. hemorrhage, prolonged bypass time and disturbances of hemostasis. The surgeon thus must make an air-tight repair on an aortic tissue which is in poor condition. Subsequently, recurrence of aneurysm from portions of the aorta left in place is a possible troublesome complication. This unfavorable course was demonstrated by Blondeau in 1970 (49) and

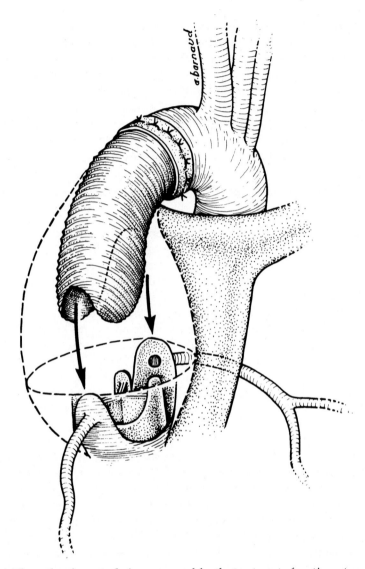

Figure 8.1-4: The authors' own technique proposed for the treatment of aortic root aneurysm. The coronary orifices are preserved and the Dacron vesculer graft tailored accordingly. (Reproduced with the permission of Flammarion Medicine-Sciences, Paris.)

led to the abandonment of simple "aortoplasties" (50). Currently, only two types of repair are carried out, but there are many technical variations.

The conventional repair consists of replacing the aortic valve and the ascending aorta above the coronary ostia. DeBakey and Cooley were the first to use this procedure. Shortly thereafter, Wheat (51) improved on it by excising all the aortic tissue except for two flaps involving the coronary ostia in order to minimize the risk of recurrence. However, suture of Dacron tubing then becomes difficult. To improve secure fixation of the proximal suture, it appears preferable to suture the Dacron tube directly into the depth of the aneurysm in the aortic sinus, circumventing the coronary ostia (Fig. 8.1-4), according to a technique which we have described. This technique, combined with preclotting by heating the Dacron tube in heparinized serum enables rapid and reliable hemostasis. Collagen-coated Dacron prosthesis which are now available gives more comfort as far as hemostasis is concerned. When the coronary orifices, in particular the right one, are displaced, Miller proposed dissection with a small aortic collar and reimplantation in the Dacron (52,53). Lastly, external wrapping of the ascending aorta after valvular replacement with or without aortoplasty described by Egloff and Robicsek (54,55) may regain its popularity with some surgeons (56).

Composite graft insertion described by Bentall in 1968 (57-59) consists of prior suturing of a valve into a Dacron tube. This composite graft is then inserted inside the aneurysm, suturing the valve to the aortic annulus and re-inserting the coronary ostia into the Dacron prosthesis (Fig. 8.1-5). The advantages of this are obvious: by closing the aneurysmal shell on the prosthesis the risk of per and post operative bleeding is minimized. In addition, all diseased aortic tissue is excluded from the circulation. However, the need to reimplant the coronary arteries is not without disadvantages and several cases where sutures have loosened or false aneurysm have formed at this level have been described (60,61). Various procedures have been used to eliminate this disadvantage, either by mounting the coronary suture on Teflon (62,63), by inserting saphenous vein bypasses (64-66), or by reimplanting the coronary arteries with an aortic collar (67). In 1978, Cabrol (68) described the use of several special techniques to prevent the above complications (Fig. 8.1-6).

Indications

They depend above all on personal preferences and experience. The published series are small and from different time frames, thus difficult to compare. Apart from the systematic approaches adopted by some investigators (69), primarily the arrangement of the lesions and their etiology are to be taken into consideration. If the *coronary ostia* have ascended considerably, it appears logical to perform a Bentall operation. In this instance, Cabrol's technique produces anastomoses which are not under tension and have little risk of being compressed under the wall of the aneurysm once it is closed (67,69). In contrast, when the coronary ostia are in place or little deviated, the technique we use is recommended.

Patients presenting with *Marfan's syndrome* are at very high risk for progression of the aneurysm. Therefore, it appears to be attractive to propose a composite graft to these patients to prevent a recurrence. However, the age of these patients, sometimes quite young, must be taken into account as it makes a late re-replacement of the inserted valve highly probable. Such a reoperation on a composite graft may pose enormous technical difficulties (70).

Anticoagulant treatment

The frequency of postoperative neurological complications resulting from cerebral embolism makes this treatment mandatory, installation of a bioprosthesis is apparently not an exception to this rule (46).

Particular cases

Crawford reported a series on the repair of aneurysms of the ascending aorta

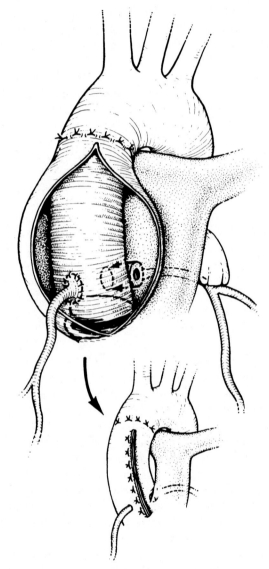

Figure 8.1-5: Bentall's technique proposed for aortic root aneurysm. The composite graft is placed inside the aneurysm; the coronary orifices are reimplanted in the Dacron tube. (Reproduced with the permission of Flammarion Medicine-Sciences, Paris.)

extending to the aortic arch with a remarkably low, 4% hospital mortality. He used cardiopulmonary bypass with deep hypothermia (71). Reported mortality figures of about 20% are much less favorable regarding reoperations for recurrent aneurysm (42).

Results

Hospital mortality rates have improved considerably, from 8 - 66% between 1965 and 1975

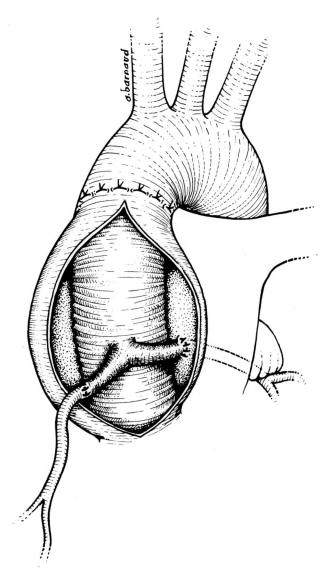

Figure 8.1-6: Bentall's technique modified by Cabrol: reimplantation of the coronary orifices is obtained through a small Dacron tube. (Reproduced with the permission of Flammarion Medicine-Sciences, Paris.)

to 3 - 15% between 1985 and 1993. The best results in large series show that the surgeon's experience is not a negligible factor: 13% of hospital mortality in 90 cases of Miller (52), 15.5% in 65 cases of MacCready (72), 11.1% in 63 cases of Liddi Coat (73), 5% in 68 patients of Cabrol (69), 9% in 717 patients of Crawford (43), 6 to 10% in 127 patients with conventional surgery versus 1.8% in 164 patients with the wrapping technique in Carrel's series (56). With regard to early complications, bleeding and low cardiac output are observed in the same proportions, i.e. 10 to 13% regardless of technique used. During long term follow up (40 months on average) there was an 8.8% rate of aneurysmal recurrence, although Miller in 90 cases, where the prosthesis was sutured at a very low level, did not observe any such complications.

MacCready reported a series of seven patients presenting with recurrent aneurysm 6.5 years on average after the first operation. Repeat surgery carried a high mortality (57%). One repeat procedure also performed for aneurysm followed by immediate post-operative death has been described by Berckman (74). For composite grafts, a large series demonstrated an occurrence of 6.4% aneurysms in coronary anastomoses, 6.1% aneurysms in the distal aorta and 2.2% compression with a mean follow up of 36 months.

Aortic valve surgery and aortic dissection

Aortic dissection results from a break or tear in the inner layer of the aortic wall which can develop in different parts of the aorta. Blood infiltrates into this tear and initiates a cleavage which extends upwards and downwards. When this cleavage reaches the branches of the aorta, these exert a certain amount of resistance to further extension of this process. Shumway classified as type A dissections any dissection which involves the ascending aorta (52). Type A dissection is the aggregate of type II (ascending aorta only) and type I (total aorta) dissections, according to DeBakey's classical terminology (47).

Several features are common in all forms of type A dissections. One is the high risk of aortic rupture into the pericardium which in any event justifies surgery. Another common factor is the frequent involvement (about 80%) of the aortic valve in these dissections. In most cases, valvular injury is caused by the dissection itself. The plane of cleavage extends upward into the aortic sinus and disinserts the valvular cusps which tilt towards the left ventricle. In 20% of cases the cusps themselves are diseased, especially in patients with Marfan's syndrome.

Surgical techniques

The procedure is performed with cardiopulmonary bypass. When the dissection involves the entire aorta, arterial cannulation may be difficult with partial perfusion of a false lumen, hindering hypothermia and increasing the risk of neurological accidents. It thus is prudent to plan multiple cannulation via the femoral and/or axillary approach (75,76).

The objective of the procedure is eliminating aortic regurgitation and excluding the ascending aorta from the circulation because in nine out of ten cases the false lumen originates from there.

Valvular repair can be achieved by conservative surgery when the cusps are normal. This can be performed by simply suspending the valvular commissures, but it appears preferable to support the sutures by Teflon pledgets both inside and outside of the aortic wall (77) Fig. 8.1-7. Some investigators prefer to use GRF glue to fasten the two layers rather than Teflon (78).

In contrast, when the valvular cusps themselves are diseased, valvular replacement is required, posing the same problems as in the case of aneurysm of the ascending aorta. *Aortic repair* is performed using a preclotted Dacron tube. There are many methods of repair, depending on the site and technique used for anastomosis. The procedure we recommend is replacement of the ascending aorta up to the origin of the innominate

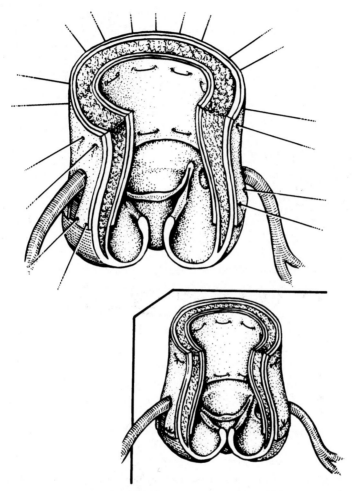

Figure 8.1-7: The authors own technique proposed for treatment of acute dissection of the ascending aorta. Reconstructive modelling of the aorta by a double velour sleeve achieves both the elimination of the plane of cleavage and conservative treatment of aortic regurgitation. (Reproduced with the permission of Flammarion Medicine-Sciences, Paris.)

artery with sutures supported by a double sleeve of velour (Fig. 8.1-8). Intraluminal prostheses may also be used with each end reinforced by a rigid cylinder; after insertion of the prosthesis into the aorta, purse strings are tied around the aorta, compressing it against the cylinders, hemostasis is thus achieved (79-81). In cases of aortic valve replacement, some investigators prefer Bentall's procedure or one of its variations.

Replacements of the aortic arch have been performed frequently but with variable results; Crawford published the first series of total replacement of the aorta, without acceptable results (71); but a more recent paper shows a dramatic improvement in survival (43). Carpentier has proposed replacing the diseased part of the aorta, cut off by an indwelling clamp, via an extra-anatomical bypass implanted into the abdominal aorta (82).

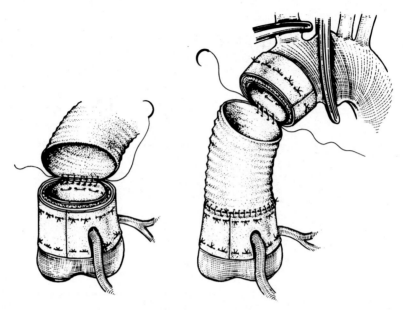

Figure 8.1-8: The area of entry of the aortic dissection is resected; aortic continuity is re-established by suturing a Dacron tube below and above to a double velour cylinder. (Reproduced with the permission of Flammarion Medicine-Sciences, Paris.)

Indications

All investigators with large series appear to agree in several points:

- Repair of the ascending aorta alone, regardless of the anatomic type of dissection, is justifiable because excision of the level of dissection no longer is an absolute dogma (multiple dissections, frequently also long term patency of the false lumen). Indications for surgery of the aortic arch must be restrained (52).
- Conservative treatment of the aortic valve is desirable whenever possible, considering that minimal aortic regurgitation is preferable to valvular replacement with a prosthetic valve.
- If valvular replacement is required, there is an ongoing debate regarding combined procedures involving the aorta and the aortic valve and/or composite grafts. However, reimplantation of the coronary orifices may be difficult because intramural dissection is frequently present in the first few millimeters of the wall of the coronary arteries. It should also be stressed that this very delicate surgery, which includes clamping the aorta and often long extracorporeal circulation, should be reserved for patients with no major neurological complications and under 70 years of age.

Results

The prognosis of spontaneous outcome in dissecting aortic aneurysm based on a study at the Mayo Clinic demonstrates a 95% rate of rupture with 7% survival at five years. These figures justified the initial attempts to correct this condition.

The largest series show in average a 25% rate of operative mortality for type I aortic dissection and 8% for type II (43,52,56,69,83). Long term follow up demonstrates good results obtained with conservative procedures for valvular disease, regardless of the surgical technique (73,83,84). In contrast, a CT scan study of outcome of the false lumen shows that it remains patent in over half of the cases accompanied by dilation of the aorta in 20%. These anatomically imperfect results, together with a few reported cases of death due to long term rupture of an aneurysm (47,77,85) show that progress remains to be made in the surgical management of dissecting aortic aneurysm or, better, in its prevention.

VALVULAR SURGERY AND ENLARGEMENT OF THE AORTIC ANNULUS

Aortic valve disease commonly coexists with a smaller than normal aortic annulus; this situation is encountered notably when calcific aortic valvular disease develops secondary to a pre-existing congenital aortic stenosis. Regardless of the type of prosthesis used, i.e. mechanical or bioprosthesis, a narrow aortic annulus forms a persistent impediment to left ventricular ejection (86). To prevent this situation, techniques for enlarging the aortic annulus have been developed. These technical solutions can be divided into two types of procedures: procedures for posterior enlargement and procedures for anterior enlargement.

Procedures for posterior enlargement

These techniques, initiated by Nicks in 1970 (87), are characterized by a common vertical incision in the posterior wall of the aorta, descending either through the posterior aortic sinus (87-91) or through the posterior commissure separating the left coronary cusp from the non-coronary cusp (92-94). This incision is then continued downwards to open the roof of the left atrium and the aortic annulus; the incision is then extended (Fig. 8.1-9) through the anterior leaflet of the mitral valve towards its geometric center.

Surgical repair consists of using a diamond-shaped Dacron or pericardial patch, sutured to the two edges of the mitral valve incision, and then to the two edges of the aortic valve incision,. The left atrial incision generally can be closed directly without a patch.

Some surgeons (92,93,95) prefer to end the incision at the root of the mitral valve, and not open the left atrium, the wall of which is only detached from the aortic annulus; the latter is enlarged using a triangular patch, the enlargement thus obtained is clearly smaller.

Procedures for anterior enlargement

These procedures were described at almost exactly the same time by Konno (96) and Rastan (97).

A vertical incision is made on the left anterolateral wall of the aorta, the aortic annulus is then opened by making an incision extending either in the anterior aortic sinus between the right coronary ostium and the left commissure, or through the left commissure between the right and left coronary valves. Then the incision is continued

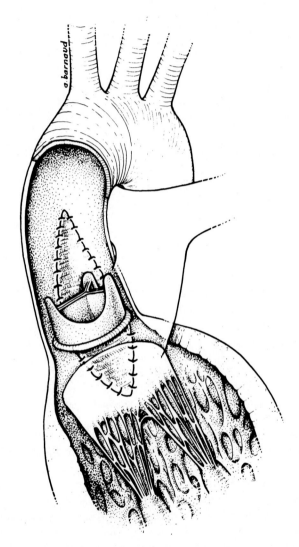

Figure 8.1-9: Technique for posterior enlargement of the aortic annulus; an incision can be made in the posterior sinus Valsalva or in the adjacent commissure; the enlargement patch can be extended into the anterior leaflet of the mitral valve. (Reproduced with the permission of Flammarion Medicine-Sciences, Paris.)

through the anterior muscle structures, simultaneously opening the anterior wall of the conus arteriosus of the right ventricle and the interventricular septum (Fig. 8.1-10). The more the incision is extended downwards the greater the enlargement, involving not only the aortic annulus and the aorta, but also the area below the aorta.

Repair is made using a diamond-shaped Dacron or pericardial patch. The patch is sutured successively to the edges of the incision of the muscular septum, and then to the edges of the aortotomy. The prosthetic valve is thus sutured to the aortic annulus in its posterior 2/3 and to the enlargement patch in its anterior 1/3. The conus arteriosus of

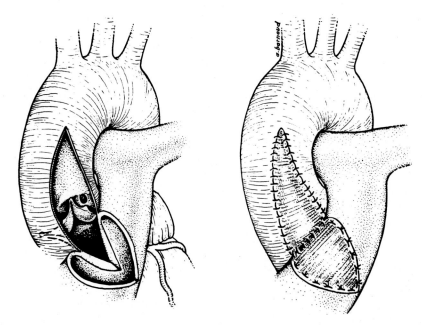

Figure 8.1-10: Technique for anterior enlargement described by Konno and Rastan. Two superimposed patches are required: the first enlarges the aortic annulus and the left ventricular outflow tract, the second enlarges the conus arteriosus of the right ventricle. (Reproduced with the permission of Flammarion Medicine-Sciences, Paris.)

the right ventricle is reconstructed using a second triangular patch secured at its base to preceding one (Fig. 8.1-10).

Simple in principle, this technique is not easy to perform; the lateral point of union where the two patches are sutured together to the aortic wall at the annular level must be put together perfectly, otherwise there will be a source of bleeding that is difficult to control. However, the enlargement obtained is very wide, and involves all sequential structures in the pathway of left ventricular ejection, i.e. subvalvular, valvular and supra-valvular areas.

Some authors have advocated the use of an aortic valve homograft as a technique of choice for aortic root enlargement (98-101). This procedure combines the concept of aorto-ventriculoplasty with aortic root replacement and coronary reimplantation. The size of homograft valve can be preoperatively determined (98).

We shall only mention two procedures which have been used as palliative measures in the case of a small aortic annulus and currently are seldom used because of their disadvantages:

- suturing the prosthesis in oblique supra-annular position results in little gain in the size of the prosthesis that can be implanted (102,103), and this oblique position can lead to dysfunction and thrombosis, furthermore, if a narrow annulus remains below the prosthesis, the operation does not achieve its objective.
- Installation of a composite graft between the apex of the left ventricle and the descending aorta is an attractive idea, however, many secondary complications - thrombosis and embolism - make this procedure hazardous and leaves it be reserved for specific cases.

Indications

Moderate enlargement of the aortic annulus achieved by posterior enlargement in our opinion appears to limit their application to adult patients or older children and to cases involving a small aortic annulus alone, without hypoplasia of the initial aorta and concomitant subvalvular stenosis. In these cases, whenever the diameter of the annulus is less than 20 or 21 mm, it should be enlarged towards the anterior mitral leaflet (91,92,104).

In growing children who have a normal aortic annulus, it is also possible to use posterior enlargement to install an adult size prosthesis (105). Nonetheless, in severe forms of congenital aortic stenosis involving the entire left ventricular outflow tract, only procedures of anterior enlargement resulting in an "aorto-ventriculoplasty" appear to be effective.

In this type of malformation, indeed, there is coexistent subvalvular tunnel stenosis, a narrow aortic annulus with valvular stenosis and a more or less marked degree of hypoplasia of the ascending aorta. A modified version of Konno's technique or root replacement with a homograft could then be used as required depending on the lesion (96,97,99,101,106).

Apico-aortic composite graft is no longer used as a temporary palliative measure in very young children.

Results

The results of aortic annulus enlargement appear to be satisfactory, although a truly large series has not been published yet, nor is there sufficiently long follow up information available (91,94). Procedures for posterior enlargement appear to involve operative risk similar to that of standard aortic valve replacement (89,91,92). Konno-type procedures carry a higher surgical risk: 20% in our own experience. Furthermore, the subsequent risks of disinsertion of the prosthesis and of bacterial endocarditis appear to worsen the clinical outcome. Long term results of homografts have been encouraging (100).

Regardless of the difficulties, these techniques may be perfected with experience and represent the only surgical treatment possible for management of severe forms of aortic stenosis in children and young adults.

References:

1. Di Matteo J, Vacheron A, Cachera JP, Heulin A, Lafont H. Pontage aorto-coronarien avec remplacement valvulaire aortique et commissurotomie mitrale. Ann Med lnt 1971;122:867
2. Dietrich EB. Technical considerations in combined valvular replacement and coronary artery bypass operations. Surg Gynec Obstet 1979;133:1015
3. Cachera JP, Vouhe PR, Loisance DY, Poulain H, Bloch G, Galey JJ. Protection hypothermique du myocarde. Application A la chirurgie combin6e vaivulaire et coronarienne. Serie de 43 cas. Ann Chir: Chir Thorac Cardiovasc 1979;33:571
4. Carlton LM. Local deep hypothermia for combined valvular and coronary heart disease. Ann Thorac Surg 1976;21:508
5. Luxereau PH, Heulin A., Verdier-Taillefer MH, et al. Les lesions coronaires des valvulopathies aortiques operees. Arch Mal Coeur 1979;72:1114
6. Anderson RP, Bonchek LI, Wood JA, Chapman RP, Starr A. Surgical management of coexisting coronary artery and valvular heart disease. Am J Surg 1974,128:282
7. MacManus 0, Grunkemeier G, Lambert L, Dietl CH, Starr A. Aortic valve replacement and aorto-coronary

bypass surgery. J Thorac Cardiovasc Surg 1978;75:865

8. Okies JE, Phillips SJ, Chaitman BR, Starr A. Technical consideration in multiple valve and coronary artery surgery. J Thorac Cardiovasc Surg 1974;67:762

9. Assad-Morel JL, Connolly DC, Brandeburgg RO, et al. Aorto-coronary artery saphenous vein bypass grafts isolated and combinated with others procedures. J Thorac Cardiovasc Surg 1975;69:841

10. Berndt TB, Hancock EW, Shumway NE, Harrison DC. Aortic valve replacement with and without coronary artery bypass surgery. Circulation 1974;50:967

11. Donzeau-Gouge P, Blondeau P, Enriquez O, et al. Calcified aortic stenosis and coronary disease. A propos of 115 surgically-treated cases. Arch Mal Coeur 1984;77:856

12. Cachera JP, Vouhe PR, Loisance DY, Poulain H, Galey JJ. La chirurgie combinee des lesions valvulaires et coronariennes. Coeur Med Int 1977;16:259

13. Lytle BW, Cosgrove DM, Gul CC, et al. Aortic valve replacement combined with myocardial revascularization. Late results and determinants of risk for 471 in hospital survivors. J Thorac Cardiovasc Surg 1988;95:402

14. HE GW, Hughes CV, McCaughan B, et al. Mitral valve replacement combined with coronary artery operation: determinants of early and late results. Ann Thorac Surg 1991;51:916

15. Cohn LH, Douper GS, Kinchla NM, Collins JJ. Decreased operative risk of surgical treatment of mitral regurgitation with or without coronary artery disease. J Am Coll Cardiol 1990;16:1575

16. Goor DA, Mohr R, Lavee J, Serraf A, Smolinsky A. Preservation of the posterior leaflet during mechanical valve replacement for ischemic mitral regurgitation and complete myocardial revascularization. J Thorac Cardiovasc Surg 1988;96:253

17. Cachera JP, Loisance DY, Vouhe PR, et al. Triple combined repair in the surgical management of ischemic heart failure. XXXth International Congress of the European Society of Cardiovascular Surgery. 1982;Abstract C6619

18 Akins CW, Buckley MJ, Daggett WM, Hilgenberg AD, Austen WG. Myocardial revascularization with combined aortic and mitral valve replacements. J Thorac Cardiovasc Surg 1985;90:272

19. Dor V, Mermet B, Kreitmann P, et al. Chirurgie valvulaire et coronaire associees. Problemes tactiques, techniques et resultats. Arch Mal Coeur 1981;74:1045

20. Kirklin JK, Naftel DC, Blackstone EH. Factors for mortality after primary combined valvular and coronary artery surgery. Circulation 1989;79 (suppl I):185

21. Loop FD, Phillips DF, Roy M, Taylor PC, Groves LK, Effler DB. Aortic valve replacement combined with myocardial revascularization. Circulation 1977;55:169

22. Miller DC, Stinson EB, Oyer PHE, Rossiter SJ, Reitz BA, Shumway NE. Surgical implications and results of combined aortic valve disease. Am J Cardiol 1979;43:494

23. Baudet M, Leguerrier A, Gandjbakhch I, Guiraudon G, Cabrol C. La chirurgie coronarienne associee aux remplacements valvulaires mitraux et aortiques. Rev Prat 1977;27:1775

24. Flemma RJ, Johnson WD, Lepley D, Auer JE, Tector AJ, Blitz J. Simultaneous valve replacement and aorta to coronary saphenous vein bypass. Ann Thorac Surg 1971;12:163

25. Merin G, Danielson GK, Wallace RB, Rutherford BD, Pluth JR. Combined one stage coronary artery and valvular surgery. A clinical evaluation. Circulation 1973;48:suppl III:173

26. Nottin R, Piwnica A, Carpentier A, et al. La chirurgie valvulaire avec revascularisation myocardique associee. Ann Chir Thorac Cardiovasc 1979;33:557

27. Oury JH, Quint RA, Angell WW, Wuerflein RD. Coronary artery vein bypass grafts in patients requiring valve replacement. Surgery 1972;72:1037

28. Loop FD, Favaloro RG, Shirey EK, Groves LK, Effler DB. Surgery for combined valvular and coronary heart disease. JAMA 1972;220:372

29. van Herwerden LA, Tjan D, Tijssen JG, Quaegebeur JM, Bos E. Determinants of survival after surgery for mitral valve regurgitation in patients with and without coronary artery disease. Eur J Cardiothorac Surg 1990;4:329

30. Bonow RO, Kent KM, Rosing DR, et al. Aortic valve replacement without myocardial revascularization in patients with combined aortic valvular and coronary artery disease. Circulation 1981;63:243

31. Heulin A, Joffe G, Audoin J, et al. Retrecissement aortique calcifie et atherosclerose coronarienne. Arch Mal Coeur 1973;66:1381

32. Kirklin JW, Kouchoukos NT. Editorial: aortic valve replacement without myocardial revascularization. Circulation 1981;63:252

33. Logeais Y, Rioux C, Leguerrier A, Laine P. Remplacement valvulaire aortique dans le retrecissement aortique caicifie. Coeur 1979;10:17

34. Cachera JP, Vouhe PR, Loisance DY, et al. Combined cardiac valve replacement and myocardial revascularization: operative risk and late results. 33rd Congress of the European Society for Cardiovascular Surgery. 1984;Abstract C 85

35. Richardson JV, Kouchoucos NT, Wright JO, Karp RB. Combined aortic valve replacement and myocardial

revascularization: results in 220 patients. Circulation 1979;59:75

36. Karp RB, Mills N, Edmunds LH Jr. Coronary artery bypass grafting in the presence of valvular disease. Circulation 1989;79 (suppl 1):1182

37. Tsai TP, Matloff JM, Chaux A, et al. Combined valve and coronary artery bypass procedures in septuagenarians and octogenarians: results in 120 patients. Ann Thorac Surg 1986;42:681

38. Bickerstaff L, Pairolero P, Hollier L, Melton J, van Pennen J, Cherry K. Thoracic aortic aneurysm: a population based study. Surgery 1982;92:1103

39. Acar J, Guyomard A, Baudouy PH et al. Les insuffisances aortiques par anevrysme dystrophique de l'aorte ascendante. Arch Mal Coeur 1979;72:596

40. Faivre G, Pesch C, Souris D, Cherrier F, Cure R, Neimann JL. La maladie annulo-ectasiante de l'aorte. Coeur Med Int 1980;XIX:177

41. Cooley DA, Ott DA, Frazier OH, Walker B. Surgical treatment of aneurysm of transverse aortic arch. Ann Thorac Surg 1981;32:260

42. Crawford ES, Crawford JL, Safi HJ, Coselli JS. Redo operations for recurrent aneurysmal disease of the ascending aorta and transverse aortic arch. Ann Thorac Surg 1985;40:439

43. Crawford ES, Svensson LG, Coselli, JS, Safi HJ, Hess KR. Surgical treatment of aneurysm and/or dissection of the ascending aorta, transverse aortic arch: factors influencing survival in 717 patients. J Thorac Cardiovasc Surg 1989;98:659

44. Culliford A, Ayvaliotis B, Shemin R, Colvin S, Isom W, Spencer F. Aneurysms of the ascending aorta and transverse arch. J Thorac Cardiovasc Surg 1982;83:703

45. Ergin A, O'Connor J, Guinto R, Griepp R. Experience with profound hypothermia and circulatory arrest in the treatment of aneurysm of the aortic arch. J Thorac Cardiovasc Surg 1982;82:649

46. Collins I, Schoen F, Mudge G, Collins J. Thrombosis associated with a porcine bioprosthesis and ascending aortic graft in a patient with Marfan syndrome. J Thorac Cardiovasc Surg 1983;85:5;794

47. DeBakey M, McCollum CH, Crawford ES, Morris G., Howell J, Noon G, Lawrie G. Dissection and dissecting aneurysm of the aorta. Surgery 1982;92:1118

48. Kouchoukos L, Karp R, Lell W. Replacement of ascending aorta and aortic valve with composite grafts. Results with 25 patients. Ann Thorac Surg 1977;24:2;140

49. Blondeau PH, d'Allaines C, Guilmet D, Soyer R, Grandi A, Dubost CH. Traitement chirurgical des anevrysmes de l'aorte ascendante avec insuffisance aortique majeure. 45 observations. Ann Chir Thorac Cardiovasc 1970;9:51

50. Bahnson HT, Nelson AR. Cystic media] necrosis as a cause of localized aortic aneurysm amenable to surgical treatment. Ann Surg 1956;144:519

51. Wheat M, Wilson M, Bartley TD. Successful replacement of an entire ascending aorta and aortic valve. JAMA 1964;188:717

52. Miller DC, Stinson E, Oyer P, et al. Concomitent resection of ascending aortic aneurysm and replacement of the aortic valve. J Thorac Cardiovasc Surg 1985;79:388

53. Najafi H. Acute aortic regurgitation secondary to aortic dissection. Surgical management without valve replacement. Ann Thorac Surg 1972;14:474

54. Egloff L, Rothlin M, Kugelmeister J, Senning A, Turina M. The ascending aortic aneurysm: replacement of repair? J Thorac Cardiovasc Surg 1982;83:117

55. Robicsek F. A new method to treat fusiform aneurysm of the ascending aorta associated with aortic valve disease. Ann Thorac Surg 1982;34:92

56. Carrel T, von Segesser L, Jenni R, et al. Dealing with dilated ascending aorta during aortic valve replacement: advantages of conservative surgical approach. Eur J Cardiothorac Surg 1991;5:137

57. Bentall H, de Bono AD. Technique for complete replacement of ascending aorta. Thorax 1968;23:338

58. Edward WS., Kerr AR. A safer technic for replacement of entire ascending aorta and aortic valve. J Thorac Cardiovasc Surg 1970;59:837

59. Singh MP, Bentall M. Complete replacement of ascending aorta and aortic valve for treatment of aortic aneurysm. J Thorac Cardiovasc Surg 1972;63:218

60. Crosby HK, Ashcraft W, Reed W. Surgery of proximal aorta in Marfan syndrome. J Thorac Cardiovasc Surg 1973;66:75

61. Tadawarthy SM, Castaneda W, Amplatz R, Edwards JE. Systolic collapse of an ascending aortic graft. Am J Roentgenol 1982;138:353

62. Kitamura S, Ohnishik, Nakano S, et al. Surgery for ascending aortic aneurysm with aortic regurgitation. Jap Circ J 1982;46:205

63. Koizumi S, Mohri H, Kagawa Y, Saji K, Haneda R. Surgical treatment of annulo-aortic ectasia: experience with 7 patients. Ann Thorac Surg 1978;25:425

64. Donaldson RM, Ross DN. Composite graft replacement for the treatment of aneurysm of the ascending aorta with aortic valvular disease. Circulation 1982;66:116

65. Houser S, Mijangos J, Sengupta A, Zaroff L, Weiner R, de Weese J. Management of fusiform ascending

aortic aneurysm. Ann Thorac Surg 1980;30:70

66. Mayer JE, Lindsay W, Wang Y, Jorgensen CR, Nicoloff D. Composite replacement of the aortic valve and ascending aorta. J Thorac Cardiovasc Surg 1978;75:816

67. Soots G, Stankowiak D, Warenbourg H. Les differentes modalites du geste de revascularisation coronaire dans le traitement de la maladie annuloectasiante de l'aorte ascendante. Ann Chir 1982;36:183

68. Cabrol C., Gandjbakhch I, Cham B. Anevrysmes de I'aorte ascendante: remplacement total avec reimplantation des arteres coronaires. Nouv Presse Med 1978;7:363

69. Cabrol C, Pavie A, Mesnildrey P, et al. Long-term results with total replacement of the ascending aorta and reimplantation of the coronary arteries. J Thorac Cardiovasc Surg 1986;91:17

70. Stellin 0, Bortolotti U, Faggian G, et al. Surgical treatment of mitral aortic incompetence and aneurysm of the ascending aorta in a child, with Marfan syndrome. Texas Heart Inst. J 1983;10:67

71. Crawford EF, Snider D. Treatment of aneurysm of the aortic arch. J Thorac Cardiovasc Surg 1983;85:227

72. McCready R, Pluth J. Surgical treatment of ascending aortic aneurysm associated with aortic valve insufficiency. Ann Thorac Surg 1979;28:307

73. Liddi Coat JE, Bekassy SM, DeBakey M. Ascending aortic aneurysm. Circulation 1975;52:202

74. Berckman M, Farkas E, Tabet J, Jeban C, Langlois J, Binet JP. Les anevrysmes de I'aorte ascendante avec infiltrations muccoides de la media et des sigmoides. Arch Mal Coeur 1979;72:831

75. Cachera JP, Domzeau Gouge G, Poulain H, Loisance DY, Bloch G, Galey JJ. Technique actuelle de reparation des dissections aortiques aigues. Chirurgie 1977;103:273

76. Soma Y, Kawada K, Kono N, et al. Clinical results of cardiopulmonary bypass with selective cerebral perfusion for aneurysm of the ascending aorta and aortic arch. J Thorac Cardiovasc Surg 1982;83:659

77. Cachera JP, Vouhe PR, Loisance DY, et al. Surgical management of acute aortic dissection involving the ascending aorta. J Thorac Cardiovasc Surg 1981;82:576

78. Bachet S, Gigou F, Laurian C, Bical 0, Guilmet D. 5 years clinical experience with G.R.F. biological glue in acute aortic dissection. J Thorac Cardiovasc Surg 1982;83:212

79. Diehl JT, Moon B, Leclerc Y, Wiesel RD, Salerno A, Goldman BS. Acute type A dissection of the aorta: surgical management with the sutureless intraluminal prosthesis. Ann Thorac Surg 1987;43:502

80. Dureau G, Villard J, George M, Delirm P, Froment JC, Clermont A. New surgical technique for the operative management of acute dissection of the ascending aorta. J Thorac Cardiovasc Surg 1978;76:385

81. Lemole F, Strong M, Spagna P, Karmilowitz P. Improved results for dissecting aneurysm: intraluminal sutureless prosthesis. J Thorac Cardiovasc Surg 1982;82:249

82. Carpentier A, Deloche A, Fabiani JN, et al. New surgical approach to aortic dissection: flow reversal and thrombo exclusion. J Thorac Cardiovasc Surg 1981;81:660

83. Mazzucotelli JP, Deleuze PH, Baufreton C, et al. Preservation of the aortic valve in acute aortic dissection: long-term echographic assessment and clinical outcome. Ann Thorac Surg 1993;55:1513

84. Randkivi PJ, Williams JD, Monro JL, Ross JK. Surgical treatment of the ascending aorta. Fourteen years' experience with 83 patients. J Thorac Cardiovasc Surg 1989;98:675

85. Heinemann M, Laas J, Karck M, Borst HG. Thoracic aortic aneurysms after acute type A aortic dissection: necessity for follow up. Ann Thorac Surg 1990;49:580

86. Hatcher CR. Aortic valve replacement: the problem of the small aortic annulus. Ann Thorac Surg 1976;22:400

87. Nicks K, Cartmill T, Bernstein L. Hypoplasia of aortic root: the problem of aortic valve replacement. Thorax 1970;25:339

88. Blanck PH, Pupello DF, Bessone LN, Harrison EE, Sbar S. Method of managing the small aortic annulus during valve replacement. Ann Thorac Surg 1976;22:356

89. Manouguian S, Epting S. Patch enlargement of the aortic valve ring by extending the aortic incision into the anterior mitral leaflet. J Thorac Cardiovasc Surg 1979;78:402

90. Najafi H, Ostermiller WE, Boolooki HJ. Narrow aortic root complicating aortic valve replacement. Arch Surg 1969;99:690

91. Nakano S, Matsuda H, Shimazaki Y, et al. An appraisal of patch enlargement of the small aortic annulus in 33 patients undergoing aortic valve replacement. Eur J Cardiothoracic Surg 1992;6:347

92. Bortolotti U, Mossuto E, Maraglino G, et al. Annular enlargement during aortic valve replacement: preliminary results with a simplified technique. J Card Surg 1992;7:235

93. Nunez L, Aguado MG, Pinto AG, Larrea JL. Enlargement of the aortic annulus by resecting the commissure between the left and non coronary cusp. Texas Heart Inst J 1977;10:301

94. Pugliese P, Bernabei M, Santi C, Pasoui A, Eufrate S. Posterior enlargement of the small aortic annulus during aortic valve replacement versus implantation of a small prosthesis. Ann Thorac Surg 1984;38:31

95. Piehler JM, Danielson GK, Pluth JR, et al. Enlargement of the aortic root or annulus with autogenous pericardial patch during aortic valve replacement. J Thorac Cardiovasc Surg 1983;86:350

96. Konno S, Imai Y, Ilda Y, Nakajima M, Tatsuno K. A new method for prosthetic valve replacement in congenital aortic stenosis associated with hypoplasia of the aortic valve ring. J Thorac Cardiovasc Surg

1975;70:909

97. Rastan H, Koncz J. Aorto ventriculoplasty. A new technique for the treatment of left ventricular outflow tract obstruction. J Thorac Cardiovasc Surg 1976;71:920

98. Moscucci M, Weinert L, Karp RB, Neumann A. Prediction of aortic annulus diameter by two-dimensional echocardiography. Application in the preoperative selection and preparation of homograft aortic valves. Circulation 1991;84(Suppl):III76

99. Konertz W, Hamann P, Hachenberg T, Schluter E, Scheld HH. Aortic annular enlargement with the use of a homograft valve. Thorac Cardiovasc Surg 1992;40:222

100. Bodnar E, Matsuki O, Parker R, Ross DN. Viable and nonviable aortic homografts in the subcoronary position: a comparative study. Ann Thorac Surg 1989;47:799

101. McKowen RL, Campbell DN, Woelfel GF, Wiggins JW Jr, Clarke DR. Extended aortic root replacement with aortic allografts. J Thorac Cardiovasc Surg 1987;93:366

102. Kinsley RH. The narrow aortic annulus. A technic for inserting a large prosthesis. Am Heart J 1977;93:759

103. Kinsley RH, Antunes MJ, McKibbin JK. Enlargement of the narrow aortic root and oblique insertion of a St Jude prosthesis. Br Heart J 1983;50:330

104. Bloch G, Cachera JP, Galey JJ, Poulain H, Vouhe PR. Le petit anneau aortique: un espoir de solution chirurgicale. Arch Mal Coeur 1978;71:558

105. Wittig J, McConnell D, Buckberg D, Mulder D. Aortic valve replacement in the young child. Ann Thorac Surg 1975;18:40

106. Fleming WH, Sarafian LB. Aortic valve replacement with concomitant aortoventriculoplasty in children and young adults. Long-term follow-up. Ann Thorac Surg 1987;43:575

Chapter 8.2

Mitral Valve Repair

Robert W. M. Frater MD

Mitral commissurotomy was the first consistently successful operation for acquired valvular heart disease. As this operation was developed, it was soon clear that there were heavily diseased stenotic cases that were not suitable for commissurotomy and that there were cases of mitral insufficiency for which an entirely different approach was needed. Indeed, bold and imaginative surgeons were devising extraordinary procedures for attempting to correct mitral and aortic insufficiency. With the advent of cardiopulmonary bypass, progress to the development of effective artificial heart valves was rapid. However, it became apparent that, for the mitral valve at any rate, there remained a gap in the surgical armoury between the operation of commissurotomy for mitral stenosis, with the pathology confined to fusion of the cusps, and mitral valve replacement (with imperfect devices) for more extensive pathology and for cases of insufficiency.

The initial approach to filling the gap between simple commissurotomy and replacement was to add tissue (1,2). Unfortunately, the tissue used, autogenous pericardium, proved unsuitable as a result of an excessive function-destroying healing process. The development of annuloplasty, which reduces the orifice to the dimensions of the existing cusp tissue rather than enlarging the cusps to cover a widened annulus, was a critical addition to the techniques for repair of mitral insufficiency (3). Strenuous efforts were also made to increase the scope of mitral valve surgery for stenosis (4). Despite all of this effort and even though artificial heart valves were admittedly imperfect, most cardiac surgeons continued to have at their disposal only two operations for mitral valve disease; commissurotomy for cases with pure cusp fusion and replacement for all the rest. Over the last 20 years, Alain Carpentier, Carlos Duran and others have changed this by persistent advocacy of new techniques for the extension of mitral valve repair (5-7).

This chapter describes the author's personal efforts to widen the scope of valvular repair and to evaluate its worth as objectively as possible.

MITRAL VALVE ANATOMY AND FUNCTION

An absolute prerequisite for mitral valve repair is an understanding of the anatomy and function of the valve and the cardiac structures related to it (8-10).

ANATOMY

The mitral valve is a continuous sleeve of tissue which is attached anteriorly to the subaortic curtain, and posteriorly is connected to the left atrium and ventricle by the atrioventricular membrane. The sleeve in turn is connected to the ventricular wall by the chordae tendineae.

Cardiac skeleton

The cardiac skeleton is a fibrous structure attached to the ostium of the left ventricle. A bar of fibrous tissue (the intervalvular trigone or the subaortic curtain) crosses the ostium and divides it unevenly into an inflow mitral portion and an outflow aortic portion. At the site of this division, the membrane is thickened into two distinct nodules, known as the left and right fibrous trigones. The three U-shaped cords of the aortic annulus are attached, at the base of the left coronary cusp, to the left fibrous trigone and, at the base of the right coronary cusp, to the right fibrous trigone. The depth of the intervalvular trigone is such that together with the trigones, it tilts the aortic orifice so that the plane of this orifice is always at an angle with the plane of the mitral orifice.

The atrioventricular membrane sweeps around the ventricular ostium posteriorly from the right and and left fibrous trigones. Close to the trigones, it is ribbon-like. Posteriorly, it is more cord-like and may have very little depth. It serves to connect the left ventricular ostium to the left atrial wall and the mitral valve. The ventricle thus has a definable fibrous membrane separating it from the left ostium and mitral cusps. This is often seen as a cul-de-sac under the posterior cusp of the mitral valve in the right anterior oblique projection of a ventriculogram. Anteriorly, the mitral valve and left atrium are attached to each trigone and the subaortic curtain.

Finally, the right fibrous trigone is the most substantial part of the skeleton, connecting the mitral, aortic, and tricuspid parts of the skeleton. Behind it, the artery to the atrioventricular node is located quite close to the mitral part of the atrioventricular membrane. The node itself is located toward the tricuspid side of the artery, also behind the right fibrous trigone.

The location of the skeleton is commonly discernible as a fine indentation at the junction of the atrium and posterior cusp. The right fibrous trigone is deep to a dimple in the atrial wall adjacent to the anterior cusp about a centimeter in front and to the right of the medial commissure.

The mitral orifice

The orifice of the mitral valve defined by the intervalvular trigone and the atrioventricular membrane is basically D shaped. The straight part of the D has a fixed width and gives attachment to the large semi-circular anterior cusp. The curved part of the D gives attachment to the posterior cusp and by virtue of its attachment to the atrium and ventricle is dynamic. The orifice is wide during diastolic flow and narrows for closure. This sphincteric action of the mitral orifice is crucial to both free diastolic flow and good apposition during systole. The average minimum annular systolic area is 5.2 cm^2, and the average maximum diastolic area is 7.1 cm^2, giving a systolic area reduction of the annulus of 26% (11). When the annulus is fixed in the end-systolic dimension a modest diastolic gradient can always be demonstrated.

The sphincter is sensitive to alterations in preload, afterload, and inotropy (12-14). Preload increases, i.e. volume infusions, result in a larger end-systolic size. Afterload increases have the same effect. Decreases in afterload result in a smaller end-systolic dimension. Increases in inotropy have the same effect (12).

The cusps

The cusp tissue is scalloped so that its free-edge length is much greater than the circumference of the atrioventricular orifice. A large deep anterior cusp swings from the subaortic curtain to form a curved line of closure with the generally tri-scalloped posterior cusp. The free edge of the posterior cusp is longer than that of the semicircular anterior cusp, but in closure the scallops meet each other as well as the anterior cusp. In fact it is the multi-scalloped nature of the posterior cusp that makes expansion of the mural annulus possible in diastole. Without scallops the free edge of the posterior cusp must limit the benefit to be obtained from annular expansion, and an unscalloped posterior cusp that opens widely can close only by developing folds and crimps. By contrast a scalloped posterior cusp, with a free edge much longer than the length of annulus to which it is attached, can respond to a lengthening of the muscular annulus by having its scallops separate from one another, and can ensure tight closure in systole by having them meet one another as well as the anterior cusp.

The result is the characteristic curved closure line and a closed orifice in which the anterior cusp is dominant. In the normal valve about 30% of the anterior cusp area is in contact with about 50% of the posterior cusp during systole. Even though the cusp tissue is formed into scallops and cusps there is no interruption of the continuity of the sleeve of tissue attached to the orifice. Even at the commissures there is a depth of tissue of at least 5mm.

The chordae and papillary muscles

There are three types of chordae tendineae defined by their attachment to the cusps: (i) Free edge chordae which support the whole length of the free edge of the valve. There are two watershed areas in the center of the anterior cusp and the center of the middle scallop of the posterior cusp which mark the separation of the cuspal attachments of chordae arising from the anterolateral papillary muscle on one side and the posteromedial papillary muscle on the other. (ii) Appositional area chordae attached away from the free edge, a few of which may arise directly from the posterior ventricular wall. These chordae mark the division between the part of the cusp that is in contact with its opposite member during systole and that which is not. They have also been called strut chordae, rough zone chordae, and second-order chordae (15). (iii) Commissural chordae, which differ from all other chordae in that they fan out from a single origin on the papillary muscle to insert into both the anterior and posterior cusps. These serve as the definitive marker of the commissures. There are several varieties of these chordae, well described by Victor et al. (16).

The three types of chordae may originate separately or together from the papillary muscles. Most often they originate in common chordae which then branch to end as one or other type of chorda. One absolute rule is that all chordae to the anterior cusp originate from the anterior parts of the anterolateral or posteromedial papillary muscles, and all chordae to the posterior cusp originate from the posterior parts of the respective papillary muscles (9).

Casual observation of the chordae tendineae reveals great variability in length between the free-edge insertion and the papillary muscle origin. Despite this apparent variability, the chordae follow three absolute rules: (i) Whatever the lengths of anterior and posterior cusp chordae, those lengths are such that they keep the opposing points of the two cusps exactly parallel to each other during systole and diastole; (ii) the chordae are always under some tension throughout systole and diastole. In systole the fact of tension is obvious. In diastole, as the posterior ventricular wall lengthens and the papillary muscles move away from the atrioventricular ring, the chordae are kept taut and the cusps are pulled down. This both opens the cusps and restrains them so that the anterior cusp, in particular, is prevented from moving out to the septum. (iii) In systole, the free edges are always kept below the plane of the atrioventricular orifice (8).

Papillary muscles

The papillary muscles vary anatomically from flat and sessile to tall and protuberant, and from single to multiheaded. A common arrangement has the appearance on the short axis echocardiogram of two U-shaped muscles facing each other with all the chordae to the anterior cusp originating from the anterior limbs of the"U's", the fan chordae on each side from the base of each "U", and the posterior chordae from the posterior limbs of each "U". Studies of length changes in papillary muscles during the cardiac cycle show the muscles actually elongating during the early part of systole (17), suggesting a use as shock absorbers (9).

Left ventricular-valvular interactions

During systole the following changes occur: (i) the posterior annulus shortens, bringing the semicircular base of the posterior cusp nearer to the anterior cusp, and (ii) the free wall shortens, bringing the attached papillary muscles closer to the annulus. During diastole the opposite changes occur; (i) the posterior annulus elongates, separating the scallops from one another and the anterior cusp, and enlarging the orifice, and (ii) the free wall elongates, keeping the chordae under tension as they pull the cusps open. In the absence of the annular- ventricular connection there is less shortening of the free wall in systole, enlargement of the left ventricular chamber, and a fall in stroke volume at any given end-diastolic volume (18).

Force, strength and structural correlations

Crimped collagen fibers run longitudinally in the chordae to the anterior cusp and then fan out on each side towards the base. The breaking strength of the cusp is greater in the direction of the collagen fibers than it is perpendicular to them. Figures for the breaking strength of anterior cusp tissue vary; in one study the breaking strength was 750 G/mm^2 in the direction of the collagen fibers and 400 G/mm^2 perpendicular to the collagen fiber direction. The strain maximum ($\Delta L/L_o$ where L_o is the original unloaded length) was similar for both orientations at 0.8. Others have measured the anterior cusp strength at 349-638 G/mm^2. Stresses in the anterior cusp have been calculated by finite element analysis to reach a maximum of 89 G/mm^2 which would provide a large safety margin.

The posterior cusp has significantly less collagen than the anterior cusp (the thickness of the posterior cusp fibrosa is 60% of that in the anterior cusp). In the finite element analysis model the stresses in the anterior cusp are tensile while those in the posterior cusp are compressive. The peak stresses calculated for the posterior cusp are only 21 G/mm^2 (19-24).

The breaking strength of marginal (free edge, first order) chordae has been measured at 310 G/mm^2. The stress in the anterior marginal chordae has been measured at 187 G/mm^2. Salisbury (25) measured the stress in the main chorda of a dog at 60 G. With other chordae cut, this rose to 100 G and with hypertension (produced by aortic constriction) to 200 G. In the finite element analysis model anterior marginal chordae peak stress has been calculated at 66 G/mm^2 and posterior marginal chordae peak stress at 2-4 G/mm^2.

It is clear from these data on structure, breaking strengths, measured and calculated stresses that (i) there is a reasonable margin of safety between strength and load under normal conditions, (ii) the load can increase considerably under special conditions, (iii) there is a clear correlation between the very different structures, strengths and expected stresses of the two cusps, and (iv) the posterior cusp does not have the structure or strength to tolerate the stresses experienced by the anterior cusp.

The circumstances which increase the stresses on the valve are increases in annular dimension, cuspal area, and chordal length, together with ruptures of chordae. Systolic stresses are normalized when the systolic annulus is small, the cusps have supportive contact with each other, and the free edges are completely supported by chordae.

MITRAL INSUFFICIENCY

Pathology

The characteristics of the pathologies that the surgeon must deal with (26-33) are summarized in Chapters 1.2, 4.1, 4.2, 4.3 and 8.3.

Pre- and intraoperative evaluation

While in the younger patient without symptoms or risk factors for coronary artery disease cardiac catheterization and angiography are not needed, patients will come to the surgeon having had these studies. Inspection of the first few frames of the left ventriculogram will often reveal the direction of the incompetent jet. If this travels along the posterior wall of the left atrium, anterior cusp prolapse is obviously the cause of the insufficiency and vice versa. Sometimes the prolapsing cusp itself is outlined and the excessive cusp area of the Barlow's syndrome cases may be seen.

Echocardiography is vital for proper evaluation, providing clear information on the dimensions and quality of the cusps and chordae, the dimensions, motion and contractility of the ventricular annulus and walls, and the quality and direction of the insufficient blood flow. The evaluation starts with preoperative echocardiography, but must be complemented with intraoperative studies, even though sometimes the quantity of insufficiency in significantly symptomatic patients may be greatly reduced with the unloading effect of good anesthesia. It is also vital for the surgeon to interpret the echocardiograms himself and then correlate that interpretation with direct evaluation of the valve in the open heart.

It is routine in our practice to measure the systolic and diastolic annular dimension and the length of the anterior cusp in a long axis view. Normally the anterior cusp length should not be less than the diastolic annular diameter (from the base of the anterior cusp to the junction of the posterior left ventricular base and the left atrium). Careful observation of the free edges of the anterior and posterior cusps in the long axis will identify prolapse of the free edge relative to the opposite cusp and to the plane of the annulus. In short axis views the particular posterior scallop or the side of the anterior cusp involved can often be identified by seeing a free edge moving in and out of the plane of the rest of the free edge of the valve. Color flow images in the short axis can also help define the location of the leaking portion and in the long axis the direction of the jet confirms the anterior or posterior location of prolapse.

In a difficult case epicardial echocardiography allows the most precise identification of the faulty part or parts of the valve. The probe is placed with its scanning plane to the left and parallel to the anterior descending coronary artery. When a good long axis image of the middle of the valve is seen the probe is slowly tilted to the left and right so as to identify the location and extent of prolapse or flail precisely.

For the surgeon, inspection of the valve is through the atrium and, for proper evaluation of the mechanisms of insufficiency, must be done segment by segment. There are six valvular segments. The anterior cusp has two of them, anterolateral and posteromedial, defined by the origin of the chordae from one or other papillary muscle. On each side of the central bare area are main chordae leading to their respective papillary muscles. Between the commissure and the main chordae are the paramedial chordae. The posterior cusp has multiple scallops, but the central or middle scallop can also be divided, like the anterior cusp, into an anterolateral and a posteromedial half because of the fact that the chorda of each half lead to separate papillary muscles. For each of these segments, the evaluation proceeds as follows:

Cusps: area; pliability (free edge, appositional, and non-appositional parts); restriction of mobility. The area of the cusps must be related to the dimension of the annulus. This is easily done with commercial sizers used for sizing annuloplasty rings, but may be done equally well with valve sizers. The anterior cusp is pulled forward with Wells or other right angle chordal retractors and the sizer is found that matches it precisely. The annulus is measured by finding which sizer fits through it most closely.

Pliability in the open heart, defined by two tests: (i) the "gravity test", in which normal cusps assume a position responsive to gravity; abnormal cusps assume a form or shape resistant to gravity, and (ii) the "bounce back" test; a cusp too stiff for good repair, when pushed on and indented with an instrument, immediately bounces back to its original shape on release of the pressure.

Chordae: length (short or long); integrity (intact or ruptured); consistency (thickened and immobile or normally thin and pliable). Gentle tension on the free edge of anterior and posterior cusps at points opposite each other will determine whether the crucial free-edge relationships have been altered and will determine whether the free edges rise above the plane of the atrioventricular ring. Gentleness is the key to this assessment, but in the paralysed heart it may be difficult to be sure about prolapse. The echo evaluation then becomes invaluable; if the anterior cusp was seen on echo before bypass not to prolapse, then this observation can be relied on even if there is an appearance of prolapse when the cusp edge is pulled on in the paralysed heart.

Annulus: size relative to anterior cusp area is evaluated as described above.

Quantitative overall assessment: the 50% rule; the surgeon should also assess what proportion of the valvular apparatus is grossly abnormal. If abnormalities of structure and function are present in more than 50% of a rheumatic valve the virtue of repair is very questionable (8). Although this may not apply with as much force with degenerative disease, it remains an important quality check for the surgeon.

Maneuvers available for repair of mitral insufficiency

The maneuvers used to repair mitral insufficiency (2,6,7,8,16,17) are described below. Methods used to repair mitral insufficiency caused by cusp pathology include the following: (i) excision or exclusion, the former popularized by Carpentier for the treatment of ruptured chordae and the latter first introduced by McGoon for the same purpose; (ii) cusp extension using additional material; and (iii) cusp and chordal replacement, which was first used by us in the 1960s.

Originally, we used autogenous pericardium for this, but found it to be unsatisfactory because of an excessive fibrosis in healing which led to contracture and complete loss of flexibility and function. Aldehyde tanned xenograft tissue does not shrink but does thicken and lose flexibility so that it is not suitable as a cusp substitute. Aldehyde tanning of autogenous tissue has been proposed as a satisfactory alternative but it has been shown that more than brief (i.e. 10-15 min.) aldehyde tanning results in similar behavior of tanned autogenous and tanned xenograft tissue (34). Alternatively, capping of residual aldehydes on tanned xenograft tissue produces a material suitable for cusp addition and substitution. Homograft tissues have begun to be used for partial valve tissue replacements (35).

Methods used to repair mitral insufficiency caused by chordal pathology include the following: (i) chordal shortening, which was introduced by Carpentier (6), (ii) chordal replacement, which was done experimentally very early in the history of open-heart surgery and which we used back in the 1960s and subsequently, reintroduced more recently (36-40), (iii) transposition of chordae (41), and (iv) section of shrunken appositional chordae restricting posterior cusp mobility, popularized by Carpentier and his disciples (Fig. 8.2-1) (6).

Finally, annuloplasty is the method used to reduce the size of the annulus to the size of the available cusps (3,5,42). Whatever the method used, it is basically the mural muscular part of the mitral orifice that is being reduced either completely or partially.

Cusp excision

The excision of flail cusps for chordal rupture works well for rupture of segments of the posterior cusps because there is invariably an elongation of the mural annulus, which must be shortened in any case. Anterior cusp excision, even when restricted to a small proportion of the cusp, inevitably shortens the free edge so that the crucial semicircular shape of the anterior cusp that is essential for proper apposition with the posterior cusp is lost. Shortening of the mural annulus does not easily bring the posterior cusp to meet this shortened, straightened anterior cusp edge, and this is not compensated for by any attempts to shorten the distance between the trigones at the base

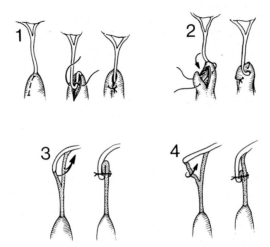

Figure 8.2-1: Shortening of elongated chordae. (1) Carpentier technique for chordal shortening. (2) Duran method. (3) Cusp level shortening used in some rheumatic cases. (4) Disproportionate elongation of anterior cusp free-edge chordae and method of correction.

of the anterior cusp, because not only will this not elongate the anterior free edge, it will distort the aortic root and the aortic valve. However, when Barlow's syndrome is present there is often excess tissue which allows some anterior cusp excision without loss of the curved shape. In fact Carpentier and Mihaileanu believe that the occurrence of systolic anterior motion of the anterior cusp that has been seen after mitral valve repair incorporating the rigid Carpentier annuloplasty ring is due to excessive size of the posterior cusp in cases of Barlow's syndrome and is effectively treated by cusp excision at the base of the cusp, reducing its depth from the annulus to the free edge. It is the fashion to excise rectangular rather than triangular segments of flail posterior cusp tissue, but, in this author's experience, virtually all excisions of posterior cusp tissue have the effect of rendering the posterior cusp less mobile. This is because the free edge is inevitably shortened and becomes equal to or less than the annulus in length. So long as the anterior cusp has a normal area and a curved free edge it can still make excellent contact with a still pliable but less mobile than normal posterior cusp.

Sliding cusp plasty

The operation of sliding plasty of the posterior cusp introduced by Carpentier may have the effect of lessening the consequences described above of posterior cusp excision (43,44). After excision of a flail segment the adjacent remaining posterior cusp tissue is detached from the atrioventricular membrane to each side of the excised portion. Uneven simple stitches are then placed close together on the cusp tissue and further apart on the atrioventricular membrane so that the excised edges come together in the middle of the gap produced in the annulus by the rectangular ("quadrantic") excision.

Chordal shortening

Chordal shortening as practised by Carpentier and Lessana and others involves the folding over and securing of an elongated chorda into a longitudinal trench cut in the papillary muscle (Fig. 8.2-1) (26,45). A transverse incision with a folding over of the apex of the papillary muscle and its attached elongated chorda down into the bottom of this incision is used by Duran (Fig. 8.2-1) (42). We have used both of these techniques and found both to work. We judge the degree of folding needed by first establishing the difference between the free edges with the chordae under gentle tension.

Another technique that we have used and have found useful with somewhat thickened rheumatic chordae is to fold them up behind the free edge of the cusp to shorten them (32,46). The differential elongation of free-edge chordae described earlier may be overcome by suturing the cusp free edge down to the chorda (Fig. 8.2-1). Groups of chordae may be shortened by shortening the papillary muscles. This can be done by cutting a wedge from the papillary muscle and suturing closed the resultant gap. For the elongated, scarred muscle a sliding plasty is effective.

Although chordal shortening can be very effective, variations in papillary muscle anatomy can make it difficult, while chordal pathology may produce chordae that are too thick to be folded comfortably or too attenuated to be shortened with safety.

Chordal transposition

In this procedure posterior chordae of normal length are moved with a piece of cusp across and sutured to the opposing anterior cusp. When we used this years ago, we had a dilated annulus and a dilated orifice, and rather than reducing the annulus size, we added tissue (8). Posterior-to-anterior chordal transposition has been effectively combined with annuloplasty by Carpentier and Lessana (26,41). The defect in the posterior cusp must then be repaired. The conditions for this procedure are (i) the posterior cusp must be normal opposite the point of anterior cusp pathology, and (ii) if a part of the normal posterior cusp is to be sacrificed there must not be any abnormality requiring further excision in the remainder of the posterior cusp.

Chordal replacement

This was among the earliest maneuvers used in mitral valve repair (47,48). Our initial experience was with autogenous pericardium (49). Later we used aldehyde tanned xenograft pericardium, having shown experimentally that it neither shortened nor elongated. Although the experience was successful the fact that the new chordae thickened and stiffened made the technique unsuitable for multiple chordal replacement. Further experiments with extruded polytetrafluorethylene sutures (GoreTex) in which there were internodal spaces, giving hope that fibrous tissue would cover the surface, turned out to exceed expectations; the fibrocyte covering did indeed occur, and was followed by a monolayer of host endothelial cells. The resultant fibrosa and intima not only duplicated the structure of a natural chorda, but the growth of the new chorda proceeded only as far as it needed to achieve the object. The progressive function-destroying scarring that was seen with other materials did not occur (50).

The proper length of a new chorda is determined using two principles; (i) that the chordae are always under tension, and (ii) that opposing free anterior and posterior cusp edges are parallel throughout the cycle. Presuming the chorda opposite a ruptured

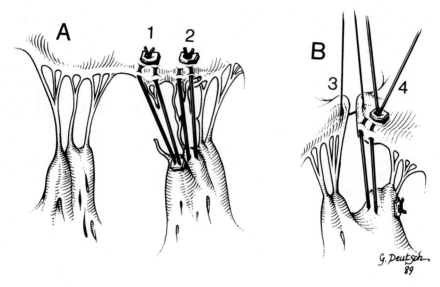

Figure 8.2-2: Panel A: Replacement of anterior rupture elongation. (1) Replacement of ruptured main chorda to the medial side of the anterior cusp. Extruded polytetraflourethylene suture is tied at the papillary level on a pledget. At the cusp, the suture has been passed through the thickened free edge and tied over a piece of autologous pericardium; (2) attenuated, elongated, paramedial chordae have been judged too thin for shortening. Furthermore, the papillary muscle is sessile. Another pair of new chordae function for these. An alternative papillary technique with a pledget on the side only is used. Panel B: Length is adjusted so that the opposing free edges are parallel with the chordae under tension. A temporary suture (3) is pulled to keep the chordae taut while the chordae are tied (4).

chorda is found to be of normal length, it is placed under mild tension by retraction of the free edge of the cusp. The new chordae are fastened to the papillary muscle and sutured to the free edge of the cusp under mild tension to a length that ensures that the edges of the anterior and posterior cusps meet at the same level (Fig. 8.2-2).

This technique of chordal replacement has now been widely adopted in many centers around the world and the indications have been extended beyond the original indication of replacement of ruptured chordae. Chordal replacement is now used for elongated as well as ruptured chordae (especially when the anatomy of the papillary muscles or the pathology of the chordae make shortening or transposition techniques difficult or unwise), to replace chordae that have been injured in decalcification or removal of fibrous scar during surgery for rheumatic stenosis, and for support of flail posterior scallops, reducing the amount of excision needed and thus avoiding the need for excessive loss of the posterior cusp or an uncomfortably tight annuloplasty. As many as 14 new chordae are used in one case. Different users develop their own variations on the technique (38,40,51,52).

Subannular calcification

This may be removed surgically. The endothelium is opened over the calcium where the cusp meets it on one side and the atrium meets on the other. Using blunt and sharp dissection the calcium is separated from the base of the ventricle. Once the calcium is out, the atrial wall, ventricular base and base of the mitral posterior cusp must be joined together again (43). Whatever additional maneuvers are needed to correct the insufficiency are then performed. Since this condition occurs in the elderly, it is often easier and safer to insert a stented bioprosthesis within the calcium rather than attempt the undoubtedly difficult and complex repair.

Annuloplasty

The goal of mitral annuloplasty is to fix the systolic dimension at a size that will be closed by the area of available cusp tissue. This can be done with relatively rigid (Carpentier) or more flexible rings (Duran, Puig-Messana, Wells et al.) (53,54). However, the same effect is achieved by a mural annulus shortening stitch (MASS), criss-crossing through the atrioventricular membrane, taking in 1 mm of the cusps and 2 mm of the atrium, starting at the left fibrous trigone and ending at the right, with the actual shortening being done with an obturator in the orifice. The size of the obturator is determined by the size of the anterior cusp. Reduction of the annulus dimension to the size of the anterior cusp guarantees that the anterior cusp will have an adequate area of contact with the posterior cusp. It is also possible to use a strip of synthetic material or short tanned autogenous or regularly tanned xenograft tissue to reduce the annulus (55-57). The length is the length of the free edge of the anterior cusp. We cut xenograft pericardium to the shape of the free edge of the anterior cusp and then suture it to the atrioventricular membrane.

When a rigid ring is used, annular contraction is inevitably abolished. Some annular contraction is demonstrable in the other forms of annuloplasty, suggesting some potential benefit in valve closure and possibly better ventricular function (58,59). It is also possible that the occasional occurrence of systolic anterior motion of the anterior cusp, while ascribed to excessive posterior cusp size, is also influenced by a rigid bar attached to the base of the anterior cusp (60,61). Certainly the phenomenon does not occur with the pliable mural annular shortening techniques. A major difference between the techniques that use either the mural annulus shortening suture or one or other form of pericardial annuloplasty, is the absence of hemolysis that results when residual jets of insufficiency impact on the fabric of synthetic rings (62).

When the atrioventricular junction is inspected in the long axis echocardiogram after annuloplasty, the same appearance is seen in all cases whether a ring, a mural annulus shortening suture or a pericardial annuloplasty has been used; the posterior annulus is bent forward towards the base of the aorta, thereby bringing the curved posterior annulus and its attached cusp in contact with the semicircular anterior cusp.

Not only do the various types of annuloplasty appear the same on echocardiography, they also all produce some obstruction to forward flow. The degree of obstruction depends on how much the orifice is reduced and how pliable the cusps are. The area of 25 mm and 23 mm sizers and an 18 Hegar dilator are 4.9 cm^2, 4.2 cm^2 and 2.5 cm^2, respectively. The effective orifice areas of valves after the annulus has been tightened to these dimensions are inevitably less than these figures. When the tissues are stiff (i.e. rheumatic) it is unwise to use less than a 25 mm circular obturator. However, with the normal pliable cusps found in cases of ischemic mitral insufficiency it is possible to tighten down the annulus around an 18 Hegar dilator without excessive obstruction.

Note that an orifice of 4 cm^2 is only 56% of the normal average adult diastolic dimension; some mitral obstruction is inevitably produced by fixing the annulus in a systolic position. By comparison the geometric orifice areas (which of course are always larger than the hemodynamically determined effective orifice areas) of 25 mm mounting size artificial mitral valves, range from less than 2.5 cm^2 to slightly over 3.0 cm^2.

Repair for endocarditis

This is feasible when the following conditions are met: (i) the infection is localized to less than half of the valve, (ii) the grossly visible infection can all be removed, (iii) the margins of the residual valve tissue are not weakened by the inflammatory response, and (iv) the surgeon has material available for substitution of the removed tissue. The fact that there may still be residual live organisms in the field after all the above conditions are met is not important; endocarditis in the absence of vegetations is generally cured by antibiotics and the same question is invariably raised when a prosthetic replacement is performed (35,63,64).

MITRAL STENOSIS

Mechanisms of mitral stenosis

Rheumatic pathology produces obstruction of flow in a number of ways (Fig. 8.2-3).

Reduction of orifice at the free-edge level

In essentially all cases of rheumatic disease, the separate definition of the posterior cusp scallops is lost. This occurs even without fusion between the anterior and posterior cusps and is always evident after successful commissurotomy. In addition there appears to be, in some cases, a further shortening of the length of the free edge, as though a purse string suture running through it had been tightened (Fig. 8.2-3C).

Cusp fusion

This occurs between the chordally supported parts of the opposing cusps, leaving only the central bare areas open (Fig. 8.2-3B).

Chordal fusion

Chordal fusion occurs between anterior and posterior cusp chordae (Fig. 8.2-3B).

Chordal shortening and thickening

In patients with this pathology, cusp motion is inevitably restricted by both the reduced arc through which the chordae can move and by their inability to flex at their papillary muscle attachment.

Cusp fibrosis and calcification producing loss of pliability

Cusp fibrosis largely produces thickening of the appositional parts of the cusps. An anterior cusp afflicted in this way will hold its bowed systolic form against the influence

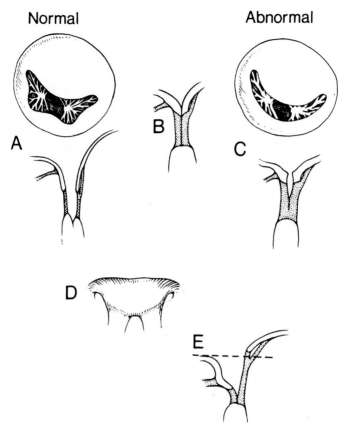

Normal   Abnormal

Figure 8.2-3: Mechanisms of stenosis. (A) Normal valve. Posterior scallops are defined. Chordae and cusps are thin and pliable. (B) Cusps and chordae are thickened, stiffened and fused. (C) Separation of fused cups and chordae does not restore the orifice to normal because of fusion of the posterior scallops. (D) Anterior chordal fusion. (E) Posterior cusp restrained by third order chorda. Elongation of anterior cusp chordae.

of gravity (Fig. 8.2-4). Calcification occurs most prominently at the commissures. It may be on the cusps with a definable plane of dissection or within their substance. Fibrous thickening of the cusps and chordae may also have a definable plane of dissection, making it possible to separate it from the original underlying valve.

Fusion of adjacent anterior cusp chordae

This type of fusion confines flow to the central space between the papillary muscles (Fig. 8.2-3D).

Methods for relief of stenosis

Separation of fusion

In the classic case of pure mitral stenosis with pliable cusps and unfused pliable

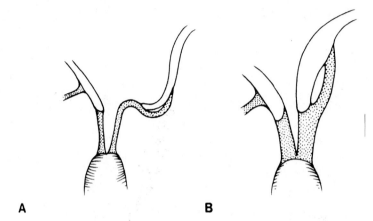

Figure 8.2-4: Cusp stiffness. (A) Gravity determines the position of the cusp. (B) Tissue stiffness causes the cusp to resist gravity.

chordae, separation of fused cusps is all that is needed, but in cases with more extensive pathology, which might ordinarily be considered for replacement, the essential point is that pliable tissue must be reached, so that despite the degree of stiffness that remains in the anterior cusp, it will hang from good hinges and will be able to swing open and closed with minimal restriction. To achieve this, it is necessary to go beyond the fan chordae at each commissure and down into the papillary muscles. Thickened fan chordae can be split. If this is not possible, the cut extends out beyond the central branch (Fig. 8.2-5).

Thin pliable tissue is almost always reached by this maneuver. Similarly, the papillary muscles almost always remain muscular and, therefore, pliable, so that splitting them compensates for the stiffness and limited arc of short, thick chordae (Fig. 8.2-5B).

Decalcification and thinning of cusps and chordae

Surface calcific nodules can frequently be removed by incising endothelium at the base of the nodule and finding a plane of dissection. The cups are commonly remarkably pliable under such nodules. Calcification within the cusp, of course, is not treatable without cusp destruction. Fibrous thickening and, in particular, the build-up of scar within the appositional area can be shaved off until the cusps and chordae no longer maintain their form in resistance to gravity. A plane may be found between fibrous thickening and quite thin and pliable cusps (Fig. 8.2-5B).

Fenestration of fused anterior chordae

Quadrangles of tissue approximately 2 mm wide are excised between the papillary muscle and the cusp edge, leaving chordae that are themselves 2 mm wide. If two such openings with an average length of 4 mm are made on each side, the potential gain in flow area would be 0.32 cm^2. This is, obviously, a modest return for a significant amount of quite delicate work, and unless the chordae and cusps were rendered pliable at the same time a benefit might not be realized.

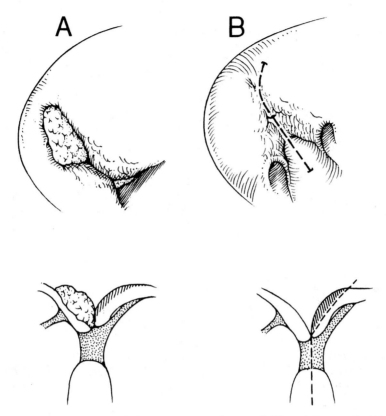

Figure 8.2-5: Mitral valve plasty. (A) Anterior commissure calcific nodule, cusp fusion, chordal fusion, cusp thickening, chordal thickening and shortening. (B) Calcium removed. Incision between the cusps through fused chordae into the papillary muscle. Fenestration of fused anterior chordae. Thinning of the cusp.

MITRAL STENOSIS AND INSUFFICIENCY

In many of the cases at issue in this presentation, namely those that might ordinarily be treated by replacement, there is a combination of stenosis and insufficiency. Treatment of the insufficiency involves shortening of chordae and/or adjusting the relative areas of the cusps and the systolic orifice. In the early days, we added tissue in the form of autogenous pericardium, but pliability was lost in the healing process (1). Because of the thickening and stiffening seen so commonly in implanted tanned xenograft pericardium, it is clearly not suitable for use as the pliable appositional part of mitral cusps. We have, however, used it selectively to advance the base of the mitral anterior cusp or to patch a hole in the base of the anterior cusp, provided the appositional parts of the valve have retained appropriate pliability.

Tanned autogenous pericardium has been advocated as suitable (65) but our experimental work indicates that the tanning period must be short (i.e. 10-13 min..) if the material is not to behave in the same way as tanned xenograft pericardium (34). The latter material has significantly improved biocompatibility when the residual aldehydes, normally present in partly bound form in the tissue, are chemically capped. The tendency to calcification is dramatically reduced and spontaneous host coverage by endothelium occurs. This material has worked well as a valve substitute in weanling sheep (66). Homograft valve material is also potentially useful.

The possibility of adding tissue in these patients is important because even though there is evidence of some annular enlargement, the latitude available to the surgeon for reducing the area of the systolic orifice is small. Even when the anterior cusp has enough depth to form a semicircular line of closure in systole, annular reduction in the presence of stiff tissues very easily produces competence at the expense of unacceptable obstruction. Cutting posterior and anterior second order chordae has been advocated as useful in improving cusp pliability but has been disappointing in our experience.

In general, mixed stenosis and insufficiency is a mark of advanced rheumatic pathology. The implication is that the process has led to shrinkage of tissue. This not only makes the initial repair difficult, it presages the progression of pathology leading to the undoing of the repairs.

INTRAOPERATIVE TESTING

The testing of insufficiency is a critical step in all cases. There are many ways of doing this. It is convenient to do the testing in the arrested heart. If the aortic valve is incompetent antegrade cardioplegic injection will fill the ventricle appropriately. Even with a competent valve, digital distortion of the aortic root may achieve the same purpose. Otherwise, forcible injection of fluid into the ventricular cavity (either through the orifice, the ventricular apex, or the aorta and aortic valve), achieves the same purpose.

When the injection is made with a bulb syringe through the orifice, if the valve is competent the left ventricle swells visibly and stays that way, collapsing only when the anterior cusp is pushed open with a large blunt right angle clamp. If the valve is competent with no more than small, circumscribed jets of insufficiency, then that valve will be competent when the heart is beating. Care has to be taken not to distort the skeletal framework of the heart by excessive retraction during testing. Distortion may be needed to see the valve but the test may then show significant regurgitation. However, if the valve will not close with forcible fluid injection it is better to accept that there is something wrong with the valve rather than the testing system.

Any testing system must avoid the risk of pumping air into the coronary arteries, and there must be a way of clearing air from the ascending aorta and the ventricular cavity before applying pressure to the ventricular cavity. We fill the heart with fluid and suck gently on the ascending aorta cardioplegia line and jiggle the ventricle and aorta until bubbles stop coming through the line, before making the ventricular injection.

After coming off bypass the valve is evaluated with 2-D echocardiography. As soon as the heart is producing a satisfactory output and systemic pressure the echo is used to evaluate residual insufficiency, the state of the anatomy (i.e. the restoration of parallel coapting anterior and posterior free edges on a plane well to the ventricular side of the atrioventricular plane), and the absence of systolic anterior motion. It is appropriate to measure left atrial and left ventricular pressures and cardiac outputs in order to determine the degree of obstruction as well as incompetence. Good myocardial protection must have been achieved if the cardiac output is to be high enough to evaluate the result properly. Either too much incompetence (more than trivial to mild) or too much stenosis (valve area less than 1.4 cm^2) is an indication to go back on bypass and correct the disorder or replace the valve.

These initial evaluations, whether intra- or postoperative, are of great importance to the later assessment of the course of the patient. Baseline observations make subsequent observations all the more valuable.

Without these measurements, no quality control of the surgeon's performance is possible. Such quality control is an essential part of this branch of cardiac surgery. Nothing less than this is acceptable for evaluation of the immediate mechanical results of the operations. Comparison with the preoperative observations, and the intraoperative descriptions of pathology and the maneuvers used to correct them, will then allow the establishment of the limits and potential benefits of reparative surgery in that surgeon's hands.

CLINICAL MATERIAL AND RESULTS

During the last 15 years, since restarting an active program of mitral valve repair, 712 patients have had mitral valve surgery. Not included are patients with congenital atrioventricular defects who underwent primary mitral and tricuspid valve repairs. A small number of patients with aortic valve disease and secondary dilatation of the atrioventricular orifice were excluded. In this group a mitral annuloplasty was performed when there was a failure of immediate resolution of the mitral incompetence after aortic valve replacement. However, patients with failed primary repairs of atrioventricular defects are included, as are patients who received annuloplasty alone either for rheumatic heart disease or myocardial ischemic mitral insufficiency. Also included are patients who received coronary artery bypass grafts, patients operated on as emergencies, all patients with class IV disability, patients who had tricuspid valve surgery, patients with aortic valve disease who had primary pathology of the mitral valve, and patients with previous mitral valve surgery.

There were, then, 361 repairs, 273 replacements and 78 re-replacements. Of the 361 repairs there were 90 simple commissurotomies, leaving 271 patients with complex repairs for whom replacement would have been done by surgeons not experienced or trained in valve repair.

Among the repairs, the diagnoses were: 132 rheumatic cases, 57 degenerative cases, 43 ischemic cases, 25 infective cases, and 14 congenital cases. Since these patients cover a wide span of years it is important to recognize that over the last five years over 90% of patients with degenerative or ischemic disease have had repairs while over 90% of patients with rheumatic disease have had replacements. The mean age for degenerative patients was 59 years, the oldest being 81 years. The rheumatic patients had the same mean age with the oldest rheumatic patient also being 81. For rheumatic disease advanced age automatically implies long-standing pathology and since rheumatic pathology is progressive, this implies also that the patients are very different from the rheumatic patients seen in Third World countries, whose mean age is 20-30 years younger.

Thirty-three percent of patients were in class IV, 62% in class III and 5% in class II of the New York Heart Association classification. Coronary artery surgery was performed in 25% of cases and tricuspid surgery in 15%.

Mortality

The hospital mortality for 361 valve repairs was 2.2%. The mortality was virtually confined to patients with severe acute coronary disease. The mortality for simple commissurotomy or dominant non-ischemic mitral insufficiency has been zero in more than 250 cases. The mitral valve replacement mortality is 4%, but includes cases in which repair was avoided because of a judgement that the shortest possible operation was needed because of the general condition of the patient. Part of the difference is related to the maintenance of a pliable annulus and the annular papillary connection, but it must be emphasized that the deterioration formerly accepted as normal after mitral valve replacement for mitral insufficiency can no longer, by itself, be invoked as a reason for performing repair rather than replacement, since for the last 11 years, at least the posterior chordae have been preserved in all our cases of mitral valve replacement, and this deterioration has become minimal or none at all. Other recent reports of mortality for repair and replacement have presented similar data to ours.

Clinical results

These must be considered under the headings of hemodynamic performance, thromboembolism, endocarditis, hemolysis and reoperation, and comparison with other techniques.

Hemodynamic performance

In a previous publication we reported the results of 76 patients in whom very careful perioperative hemodynamic measurements were made. Obstruction to forward flow was expressed as an effective orifice area obtained from intraoperative hemodynamic measurements, as a planimetric orifice measurement in the echocardiographic short-axis view of the open mitral valve, and as a measurement obtained by half-time pressure Doppler methods. Correction of mitral insufficiency was judged by the presence and size of a V wave in the simultaneously obtained left atrial and ventricular pressures, by intraoperative contrast echocardiography, by echocardiographic observation of changes in cusp motion and Doppler-detectable insufficiency, by echocardiographic observation of the changes in left atrial and ventricular systolic and diastolic dimensions that occur with correction of mitral insufficiency and, of course, by auscultation. Clinically "good"

Table 8.2-I: Size of hole at free-edge level.

Obturator size Diameter (mm)	Geometric Area (cm^2)	Effective Orifice Area (cm^2)	Patients
18	2.54	1.76	5
22	3.8	1.35	1
23	4.1	1.62	2
25	4.9	1.6	2
2 (Fingers)	4.0	1.54	2

results are judged in the conventional manner by improvement in exercise capacity and by auscultatory evidence of the presence or absence of stenosis and insufficiency.

Thirty-three stenosis and stenosis-and-insufficiency patients with transvalvular flows of more than 100 ml/second had an average effective orifice area of 1.8 cm^2 (1.3 cm^2 to 2.1 cm^2), while thirty-four pure insufficiency patients had an average effective orifice area of 2.8 cm^2.

Among patients with flows of more than 100 ml/second, there were five in whom different sets of cardiac outputs were obtained with markedly different rates of transvalvular flow. In every case, at the higher flows the orifice areas were proportionally higher than they were at lower flows. The early two-dimensional echocardiographic data also show a marked difference between 35 patients with stenosis and insufficiency and 25 with pure insufficiency with average values of 1.8 cm^2 and 3 cm^2, respectively.

In seeking an explanation for the difference between stenosis and insufficiency patients and the failure to achieve normal hemodynamic function, there are several possibilities to discuss. These include the orifice size at the free-edge level, the orifice size at the atrioventricular level, and the degree of stiffness of the valve tissues.

There is no doubt that the pathology of rheumatic disease produces a shortening of the free edge. At the completion of a simple commissurotomy in which the chordae are normal and the cusps only somewhat thickened, it is always evident that the size of the orifice at the free-edge level is less than that at the ring. A major reason for this is the invariable loss of the capacity of the scallops to separate in diastole, because of the fusion of the commissures between them, that is routinely present in rheumatic cusps. The implication is that the benefit to forward flow provided by diastolic dilatation of the ring is lost and that there will be some measurable reduction of the orifice. For the rheumatic stenotic cases under discussion, invariably there are also changes in the consistency of cusps and chordae in addition to fusion, so that whatever the size of the orifice obtained by separation of fused structures, there is the potential for a significant extra interference with flow as a result of stiffness of the tissues.

In Table 8.2-I, the effective orifice areas obtained by hemodynamic measurements in 12 patients are compared with the size of the orifice measured by an obturator at the free-edge level at surgery. The hemodynamic area is invariably less than the area measured by the obturator, and the areas in general do not correlate well with the varying areas of the different-sized obturators. The explanation for this must be related to cusp and chordal stiffness.

Fixing the diastolic dimension at an end-systolic size by annuloplasty also produces some orifice obstruction. A 25 mm obturator (area 4 cm^2) was used to control the size of annulus reduction in four patients with stenosis and in 13 with insufficiency. All had effective orifice areas less than 4 cm^2, presumably related to fixing the diastolic atrioventricular size at a less than normal systolic level, but whereas the average area for the stenosis cases was 1.6 cm^2, the average for the insufficiency cases was 3 cm^2. Tissue stiffness presumably accounts for this difference.

Alternatively, when only stenosis cases were examined, eight patients who had annuloplasty in addition to other procedures had a mean effective orifice area of 1.46 cm^2, while 27 without had a mean area of 1.9 cm^2, suggesting that the addition of annuloplasty in cases of stenosis produced an additional measure of obstruction.

Most other studies have relied on echocardiographic methods, with pressure-half time being used most often. The continuity equation produces more homogeneous results in the analysis of mitral valve repair, and also results that give higher areas than the pressure half-time method, which has also been criticized as less accurate (67). Nevertheless the results are on a par with those we reported and it is possible from this data to draw general conclusions.

Pure tight mitral stenosis with pliable cusps and chordae and no calcification or insufficiency

Relief of obstruction is uniformly good, and this is true for good balloon commissurotomy, good closed surgical commissurotomy and good open commissurotomy (68-73). However, significant mitral insufficiency occurs in up to 8% of cases of balloon commissurotomy, and a residual atrial septal defect in 1% to 3% (28,29,74) (see also Chapter 7.2). Closed mitral commissurotomy has very similar results; inadvertent cusp tears leading to severe insufficiency were essentially the same as are now seen with balloon commissurotomy (30). An experienced surgeon had a substantial degree of control and would accept a lesser area in a particular case in order to avoid a likely injury but so also does the complication rate fall with the balloon technique as experience is gained.

The use of transesophageal echocardiography during balloon commissurotomy will provide the kind of sensitive control that surgeons used in determining how much to dilate (75). It is also interesting that both the area achieved and the rate of significant insufficiency with the Inoue balloon are less than with the double balloon (28). However, this discussion is irrelevant to the modern era. Balloon commissurotomy has displaced (or will very soon displace) closed commissurotomy as the primary treatment, even in less developed countries. There will be no experienced surgeons to do the closed operation. For the pregnant patient, using echocardiography for control, there is no doubt that balloon commissurotomy will be the best technique (76).

Mitral stenosis with undesirable features

These features include thick cusp edges, thick and/or short chordae, short anterior cusps, some calcification, with or without mild insufficiency. Surgeons learned 25 years ago that in the best hands these features led to poorer initial results, especially with closed commissurotomy. The preceding discussion emphasized the pathology determined imperfections of commissurotomy in "ideal valves". With less than ideal pathology the ability to correct the hemodynamic abnormality is inevitably worse. Balloon commissurotomy certainly does quite poorly in cases with these features (28,68,77).

Open commissurotomy, better described in these kinds of cases as open mitral plasty, unquestionably allows some patients to do well who will not do well with closed forms of commissurotomy. This is mostly related to the ability to achieve mobility by incising some commissures in which the chordae have fused into a solid sheet and, in particular, by dividing unscarred still muscular papillary muscles, as well as the ability to detect and repair, at the table, insufficiency that would otherwise mar the postoperative result.

Nevertheless the correlation between advanced pathology and less perfect results is clear (71,73,78). There is no doubt that current efforts to extend balloon commissurotomy to mitral stenosis patients with more and more advanced disease are egregiously wrong. A significant number of patients will have either no improvement in hemodynamics or some improvement with the unfortunate addition of increased insufficiency (77).

Thromboembolism

Since all of the cases considered would, in some surgeons' hands, have been replaced, it is appropriate to compare the results of valve repair with those of valve replacement. For comparisons between valve repair and replacement to be valid, we contend that the cases must be contemporaneous and from the same institution, that all patients must be followed at least annually by direct contact; and that during this contact all patients must receive the same detailed questionnaire designed to assess their symptomatic status and to determine, as precisely as possible, the occurrence of transient ischemic attacks and other embolic episodes. This questionnaire has been published before and its deficiencies have been objectively criticized (79).

Major embolic episodes are defined as strokes, especially those that leave residua, or produce symptoms for at least five days. Minor episodes are characteristically episodic; they should be clearly defined and, of course, transient. There are obvious difficulties in these definitions; patients with migraine equivalents, Meniere's syndrome, and previous strokes are commonly quite difficult to analyze. We have chosen to regard scintillation scotomata as evidence of emboli, but there are many patients in whom events occur that we classify as "possible". In this discussion we shall exclude the "possible" episodes from analysis and look only at those with major and minor episodes.

Because we are taking cohorts of patients followed for 14 to 18 years, we have only 39 of the valvuloplasty patients to be compared with 29 patients with Starr ball valve replacements and 59 with bioprosthetic replacements. The percentage of patients with atrial fibrillation is the same for all three groups. Ninety percent of the mechanical valve recipients, 47% of the bioprosthetic recipients, but only 21% of those who had valvuloplasties were anticoagulated. At 14 years, 48% of the mechanical valve recipients, 70% of those with bioprostheses, and 85% of those with plasties were free of emboli. These differences were significant.

Given the inevitably subjective nature of estimation of thromboembolic rates, these rates are slightly higher but not far different from follow up studies of similar duration for porcine and ball valve series of similar duration (80,81). There are no data of comparable duration for modern pyrolytic carbon bileaflet valves, but it is likely that their incidence will be lower and closer to rates for bioprosthetic valves. The very real advantage of the absence of an absolute obligation to use anticoagulants will, of course, persist for both repair and bioprosthetic cases and it would appear that there is a persistent lower risk of thromboembolism for valve repair.

Durability

The durability of valve repair is dominated by the pathology of the valve operated on. If tissue substitution is used the durability of the materials and their interaction with the host also become important.

There is a clear difference between patients with rheumatic and degenerative pathology. Although there are cases in which further chordal ruptures occur after repair of degenerative disease the overall durability of repairs of degenerative disease appears to equal that of mechanical valves in comparative studies. Patients who have had repairs of degenerative disease are, of course, selected; it is the simpler pathology that is most often repaired (70% of cases involve prolapse or flail of one or less than one scallop). Very often the remaining valve in these cases appears relatively normal. There is no data that attempts to quantitate repair durability with the proportion of remaining tissue that appears to be pathologic. There are no randomized studies.

With rheumatic disease there are very long (15-25 years) symptom-free survivals for commissurotomy performed under ideal circumstances. Even these cases, however, show evidence of an inexorable progression of pathology and we have alluded to the certainty of the continuation of the fibrotic process in rheumatic valves. Modern studies using repeated echocardiographic follow up examinations are rapidly producing data on this process. Within the first year after successful balloon dilatation of ideal cases of pliable pure mitral stenosis there is a detectable narrowing of the orifice originally attained in 10% of cases, and an increase in regurgitation in as many as 8% (28,74,82). Nevertheless, the rate of this progression when the pathology is less advanced may be quite slow.

Between 1975 and 1980 we performed repair for rheumatic disease in 41 cases. The maneuvers included the shaving and decalcification of cusps, fenestration, shaving, shortening and replacement of chordae, division of papillary muscles and annuloplasty. However, although these were not simple commissurotomies, the greater part of each valve was still thin and pliable and the end result in each case was very close to the end result of commissurotomy in an ideal case of mitral stenosis. At 10 years patient survival was 88% and at 15 years 75%. Valve survival was 83% at 10 years and 70% at 15 years. These results are remarkably similar to long term analysis of open and closed commissurotomy for pure mitral stenosis in Padua, Italy and Birmingham, Alabama (71,72).

When the pathology is less than ideal the results are distinctly less good. Although skilful surgeons can achieve satisfactory early results in combined stenosis and insufficiency (70), the progressive valve failure rate in these cases appears to be such that in the industrial western world, where the patients are older and follow up easier, the patient with rheumatic valvular disease with less than ideal pathology may do better with valve replacement (83,84). If the 50% rule and the gravity response of the cusps are observed and used to judge whether to repair rheumatic valve disease, the incidence of early and late treatment failure will be reduced.

The use of balloon dilatation with advanced pathology is indefensible in this author's opinion. A recently published two year survival rate in patients with calcification (35% Grade 1, 48% Grade 2, 11% Grade 3 and 6% Grade 4) of only 80% is totally unacceptable (77).

Pure rheumatic insufficiency is essentially a disease of young patients in the Third World and the least common rheumatic valvular disease. Despite what would seem a more desirable pathology the association of anterior chordal elongation and tissue stiffness makes good repair more difficult to achieve than with degenerative disease, and some published results have been poor. Even with pure insufficiency, echocardiographic follow up documents significant continued progression of pathology (85). If the surgeon can achieve a valve that is equivalent to the end result of commissurotomy in an ideal case, then it is reasonable to hope for a desirable long term result. Evidence of tissue stiffness that was discussed earlier in this chapter should preclude the performance of repair.

For the young Third World patient, and particularly the young female of child bearing age, the inevitability of reoperation is a quite reasonable alternative to the hazards of anticoagulation in pregnancy and the commonly accelerated calcification of current xenograft bioprostheses. New designs and anticalcification treatments may change this. At present the dilemma of poor results of repair and unsatisfactory choice of devices persists (86).

Chordal replacement

EPTFE chordae have been implanted in patients for up to nine years. Thus far late rupture has not been reported and the few that have been seen late have shown an appropriate and apparently stable tissue covering. The technique is being increasingly reported and results continue to be encouraging (51,52).

Annuloplasty without synthetic rings

The results of these various and increasingly performed methods of bringing the anterior and posterior cusps closer to each other are good. In 120 of our patients receiving the mural annulus shortening suture and followed for five to 16 years, there was one dehiscence of the suture and two that needed early reoperation for tightening or retying the suture. There were no other failures of the repair related to the annuloplasty. Hemolysis did not occur in any case.

Cusp extension with biologic tissue

There is reasonable satisfaction with tanned autogenous pericardium, although the warning not to exceed a brief (10 minute) tanning period is probably important. Conventional tanned xenograft pericardium should not be used in the free edge of the valve because of its tendency to stiffen, but has had successful use in extending the base of cusps so that the pliable natural cusp tissue makes a better apposition.

LEARNING REPAIR

Learning to perform mitral valve repair presents many difficulties. The first of these is that it is much easier and demands less from the surgeon to take a competent and mildly stenotic valve from a shelf than to create one from diseased tissue at the operating table. Failure of an artificial device can be laid at the manufacturer's door. Failure of a repair will be seen as a failure of either surgical technique or surgical judgement. Secondly, the surgeon practising in a modern industrial state, embarking on the task of learning mitral valve repair, is faced with the obvious problems that learning is directly linked to experience, that the volume of mitral valve surgery is generally too low to provide optimal experience, and that failures along the way are likely to cause voluntary or involuntary termination of the venture.

There have in recent years been numerous courses on valve repair. These are unquestionably useful but, on returning home, the surgeon is still faced with the problems described above. The necessary ingredients for success are:

(i) Meticulous cardioplegic myocardial protection. We believe that continuous retrograde warm blood cardioplegia combined with removal of air from the aorta before fluid testing of competence produces excellent results but other surgeons will prefer intermittent cold cardioplegia. Whatever the method of protection it must allow the surgeon to spend time on a repair, to decide that it has failed and to proceed to valve replacement with no more risk than proceeding immediately to replacement.

(ii) A careful analysis of the preoperative echo by the surgeon with specific attention paid to the length, pliability and thickness of cusps and chordae, the presence of prolapse or flail, and the annular dimension in systole and diastole.

(iii) A repeat of this analysis in the operating room using transesophageal, and if necessary, epicardial echocardiography.

(iv) A comparison of the echocardiographic appearance with the valvular pathology systematically analyzed segment by segment for cusps, chordae and annulus.

(v) Post repair testing using fluid under pressure in the ventricle.

(vi) Confirmation of the result with good transesophageal echo and, in cases of rheumatic disease, the measurement of cardiac outputs and transvalvular gradients.

References

1. Frater RWM, Berghuis J, Brown AL, Ellis FH, Jr. Autogenous pericardium for posterior mitral leaflet replacement. Surgery 1963;84:260-269
2. Bailey CP, Zimmerman J, Hirose T, Folk FS. Reconstruction of the mitral valve with autologous tissue. Ann Thorac Surg 1970;9:103-110
3. Wooler GH, Nixon GPF, Grimshaw VA, Watson DA. Experience with repair of the mitral valve in mitral incompetence. Thorax 1962;17:49-54
4. Bailey CP, Zimmerman J, Likott W. The complete relief of mitral stenosis: ten years in progress toward this goal. Dis Chest 1960;37:1-12
5. Carpentier A. La valvuloplastie reconstitutive. Une nouvelle technique de valvuloplastie mitrale. Presse Med 1969;77:251-253
6. Manhas DR, Ritterhause HA, Hessel EA, Merendino KA. Reconstructive surgery for the treatment of mitral incompetence. J Thorac Cardiovasc Surg1978;62:781-787
7. Duran CG, Pomar JL, Revuelta JM, Gallo I, Poveda J, Ochoteco A, Ubago JL. Conservative operation for mitral insufficiency. J Thorac Cardiovasc Surg 1980;79:326-337
8. Frater RWM. Anatomical rules for the plastic repair of the mitral valve. Thorax 1964;19:458-464
9. Frater RWM. Functional anatomy of the mitral valve. In: Ionescu M. Cohn L (eds). Mitral valve disease. Diagnosis and treatment. London, Butterworths, 1985:123-134
10. McAlpine WA. Heart and coronary arteries. Berlin, Springer-Verlag, 1975
11. Ormiston JA, Shah PM, Tei C, Wong M. Size and motion of the mitral annulus in man. Circulation 1981;64:113
12. Yellin EL, Yoran C, Sonnenblick EH, et al. Dynamic changes in the canine mitral regurgitant orifice during ventricular ejection. Circ Res 1979;45:667-683
13. Yoran C, Yellin EL, Becker RM, et al. Mechanism for reduction of mitral regurgitation with vasodilator therapy. Am J Cardiol 1979;43:773-777
14. Yoran C, Yellin EL, Becker RM, et al. Dynamic aspects of mitral regurgitation: effects of ventricular volume, pressure and contractility on the effective regurgitant area. Circulation 1979;60:170
15. Lam JHC, Ranganathan W, Wigle ED, Silver MD. Morphology of the human mitral valve: J chordae tendineae: a new classification. Circulation 1970;41:449
16. Victor S, Nayak VM. Definition and function of commissures, slits and scallops of the mitral valve: analysis in 100 hearts. Asia Pacific J Thorac Cardiovasc Surg 1994;3:10-16

17. Hagl S, Heimisch W, Meisner H, Mendler N, Sebening F. In situ function of the papillary muscles in the canine left ventricle. In: Duran C, Angell W, Johnson A, Oury J (eds). Recent progress in mitral valve disease. 1984:397-409
18. Gams E, Schad H, Heimisch W, Hagl S, Mendler N, Sebening S. Importance of the left ventricular subvalvular apparatus for cardiac performance. J Heart Valve Dis 1993;2:642-645
19. Kunzelman KkS, Cochran RP, Murphree SS, Steves Ring W, Verrier ER, Eberhart RC. Differential collagen distribution in the mitral valve and its influence on biomechanical behaviour. J Heart Valve Dis 1993;2:236-244
20. Kunzelman KS, Cochrane RP. Stress/strain characteristics of porcine mitral tissue: parallel versus perpendicular collagen orientation. J Cardiac Surg 1992;7:71-78
21. Liao K, Frater RWM, Stevenson-Smith W, Nikolic SD, Macaluso F, Yellin EL. Two dimensional mechanical and ultrastructural correlates of bovine pericardium for prosthetic valves. ASAIO Transactions 1991;37:M349-M351
22. Kunzelman KS, Cochran NM, Chuong C, Steves Ring W, Verrier ED, Eberhart RD. Finite element analysis of the mitral valve. J Heart Valve Dis 1993;2:236-340
23. Clark RE. Stress/strain characteristics of fresh and frozen human aortic and mitral leaflets and chordae tendineae. J Thorac Cardioivasc Surg 1973;66:202-208
24. Lim KO, Banghner DR: Scanning electron microscopical study of human mitral valve chordae tendineae. Arch Pathol Lab Med 1977;101:236-246
25. Salisbury PF, Cross CE, Weben PA. Chordae tendineae tension. AM J Physiol 1963;205:285-392
26. Carpentier A. Cardiac valve surgery - the "French Correction". J Thorac Cardiovasc Surg 1983;86:323-337
27. Frater RWM, Cornelissen P, Sisto D. Mechanisms of ischemic mitral insufficiency and their surgical correction. In: Vetter HO, Hetzer R, Schmutzler H (eds). Ischemic mitral incompetence. 1991:117-130
28. Rothlisberger C, Essop IM, Skudicky D, Skoularigis J, Wisenbaugh T, Sareli P. Results of percutaneous balloon mitral valvotomy in young adults. Am J Cardiol 1993;72:73-77
29. Hermann HC, Lima JAC, Feldman T, Chrisholm R, Isner J, O'Neill W, Ramaswamy K. Mechanisms and outcome of severe mitral regurgitation after Inoue balloon valvuluplasty. J Am Coll Cardiol 1993;22:783-789
30. Frater RWM. Traumatic mitral incompetence. J Thor Cardiovasc Surg 1967;53:312-321
31. Frater RWM, Ellis FH. The anatomy of the canine mitral valve: with notes on function and comparisons with other mammalian mitral valves. J Surg Res 1961;1:171
32. Frater RWM. Mitral valvuloplasty. In: Current Surgery of the Heart. Roberts AJ, Conti CR (eds). Lippincott, Philadelphia. 1987:62-67
33. Klues HG, Proschan MA, Dollar AL, Spirito P, Roberts WC, Maron BJ. Echocardiographic assessment of mitral valve size in obstructive hypertrophic cardiomyopathy. Anatomic validation from mitral valve specimen. Circulation 1993;88:548-555
34. Liao KJ, Frater RWM, Chang TH, LaPietra A, Ciuffo G, Seifter E. Time dependent effect of glutaraldehyde on the tendency to calcify of both autografts and xenografts. Ann Thoracic Surg 1995;60(Suppl):S343-S347
35. Dossche K, Vaverman H, Wellens F. Partial mitral valve replacement with a mitral homograft in subacute endocarditis. Thorac Cardiovasc Surg 1994;42:199-258
36. Frater RWM, Gabbay S, Shore D, Strom J. Reproducible replacement of elongated or ruptured mitral valve chordae. Ann Thorac Surg 1983;35:14-28
37. Vetter HO, Burack JH, kFactor SM, Frater RWM. Replacement of chordae tendineae of the mitral valve using the new expanded PTFE suture in sheep. In: Bodnar E, Yacoub M (eds). Biologic and bioprosthetic valves. New York, Pergamon Press, 1986:772-784
38. David TE, Bos J, Rakowski M. Mitral valve repair by replacement of chordae tendineae with polytetrafluorethylene sutures. J Thorac Cardiovasc Surg 1995;101:495-501
39. Revuelta JM, Garcia-Rinaldi R, Gaite L. Generation of chordae tendineae with polytetrafluorethylene stents. Results of mitral valve chordal replacement in sheep. J Thorac Cardiovasc Surg 1989;97:98-103
40. Zussa C. Artificial chordae in mitral valve surgery. R G Landes, Austin, TX, 1994:159
41. Lessana A, Romano M, Lutfalla G. Treatment of ruptured or elongated anterior mitral valve chordae by partial transposition of the posterior leaflet: experience with 29 patients Ann Thorac Surg 1988;45:404-408
42. Duran CMG, Ubago JL. Clinical and hemodynamic performance of a totally flexible prosthetic ring for atrioventricular reconstruction. Ann Thorac Surg 1976;22:458
43. Deloche A, Jebara VA, Rellamel JYM, Carpentier A. Valve repair with Carpentier techniques. The second decade. J Thorac Cardiovasc Surg 1990;99:990-1002
44. Perier P, Clausmizer B, Mistanz K, Carpentier A. "Sliding Leaflet" technique for repair of the mitral valve: early results. Ann Thorac Surg 1994;57:383-386
45. Lessana A, Herreman F, Boffety C, et al. Hemodynamic and cineangiographic study before and after mitral valvuloplasty. Circulation 1981;11:195
46. Kumar AS, Bhan A, Kumar RV, Shrivastava S, Sood AK, Gopinath N: Cusp- level chordal shortening for

rheumatic mitral regurgitation. Texas Heart Inst J 1992;19:47-50

47. Marchand P, Barlow JB, DuPlessis LIA, Webter I. Mitral regurgitation with rupture of normal chordae tendineae. Brit Heart J 1966;28:746-758
48. January LE, Fisher JM, Ehrenhaft J. Mitral insufficiency resulting from rupture of normal chordae tendineae. Circulation 1962;26:1329-1333
49. Frater RWM, Berghuis J, Brown AL, Ellis FH Jr. The experimental and clinical use of autogenous pericardium for the replacement and extension of mitral and tricuspid cusps and chordae. J Cardiovasc Surg 1965;6:214-228
50. Frater RWM, Vetter HO, Zussa C, Dahm M. Chordal replacement in mitral valve repair. Circulation 1990;82(Supp IV):IV-125-IV-130
51. Eishi K, Kawazoe K, Sasaka Y, Kosakai Y, Kitoh Y, Kawashima Y. Comparison of repair techniques for mitral valve prolapse. J Heart Valve Dis 1994;3:432-438
52. Lawnie U, Eckhoidt G, Brown A, VanCleve G, Earle N, Pak M. Resection v PTFE chordal replacement for repair of mitral insufficiency. J Am Coll Cardiol 1995:396A
53. Duran CMG, Pomar JI, Cucchiara G. A flexible ring for atrioventricular heart valve reconstruction. J Thorac Cardiovasc Surg 1978;19:417-420
54. Gorton ME, Piehler JM, Killen DA. Mitral repair using a flexible and adjustable annuloplasty ring. Ann Thorac Surg 1993;55:860-863
55. Pellegrini A, Quaini E, Colombo T, Laufranchi M, Russo C, Vitali E. Posterior annuloplasty in the surgical treatment of mitral insufficiency. J Heart Valve Dis 1993;2:633- 638
56. Salati M, Scrofani R, Santoli C. Annular remodelling with pericardial reinforcement: surgical technique and early results. J Heart Valve Dis 1993;2:639-641
57. Salvador I, Rocco F, Ius P. The pericardium reinforced suture annuloplasty. Another tool for mitral annulus repair? J Card Surg 1993;8:79-84
58. Van Rijk-Zwikker GL, Mast F, Schipperlyn JJ, Huysmans HA, Bruschke AVG. Comparison of rigid and flexible rings for annuloplasty of the porcine mitral valve. Circulation 1990;82(Supp IV):58-64
59. David TE. Effect of mitral annuloplasty ring on left ventricular function. Thorac Cardiovasc Surg 1989;1:144-148
60. Lee KS, Stewart WJ, Lever HM. Mechanism of outflow tract obstruction causing failed mitral valve repair: anterior displacement of leaflet cooptation. Circulation 1992;86(Supp I):I-496
61. Kreinckl MS, Schiavone WA, Lever RM. Systolic anterior motion of the mitral valve after Carpentier ring valvuloplasty for mitral valve prolapse. Am J Cardiol 1986;57:408-412
62. Wilson JH, Rath R, Glaser R. Severe hemolysis after incomplete mitral valve repair. Ann Thorac Surg 1990;50:136-137
63. Gammage MD, Littler WA, Abrams LI. Conservative surgery of the mitral valve in bacterial endocarditis. Thorax 1984;39:868-871
64. Dreyfus G, Serraf A, Jebara VA, Chauvand S, Chacques JC, Carpentier A. Valve repair in acute endocarditis. Ann Thorac Surg 1990;49:706-713
65. Chauvand S, Jebara V, Chacques JC, Carpentier A. Valve extension with glutaraldehyde-preserved autologous pericardium. Results in mitral valve repair. J Thorac Cardiovasc Surg 1991;102:171-178
66. Frater RWM, Liao KJ, Seifter E. Stentless chordally supported mitral bioprosthetic valve. In: New horizons and the future of heart valve bioprostheses. Gabbay S, Frater RWM (eds). Silent Partners, Austin. 1994:103-122
67. Acar J. Editorial: Open mitral commissurotomy or percutaneous mitral commissurotomy. J Heart Valve Dis 1994;3:133-135
68. Eguaras MG, Garcia Jimenez MA, Colleja F, Roman M, Casares J, Fresnella F, Concha M. Early open commissurotomy: long-term results. J Thorac Cardiovasc Surg. 1993;106:421-426
69. Antunes MJ, Nascimento J, Andrade CM, Fernandes LIE. Open mitral commissurotomy: a better procedure. J Heart Valve Dis 1994;3:88-89
70. Kumar AS, Pantula N Rao. Mitral valve reconstruction: intermediate term results in rheumatic mitral regurgitation. J Heart Valve Dis 1994;3:161-164
71. Scalia D, Rizzoli G, Campanile F, et al. Long-term results of mitral commissurotomy. J Thorac Cardiovasc Surg 1993;105:633-642
72. Hickey MS, Blackstone EH, Kirklin JW, Dean LS. Outcome probabilities and life history after surgical mitral commissurotomy implications for balloon commissurotomy. J Am Coll Cardiol 1991;17:29-42
73. Cohen JM, Glower DD, Harrison JK, et al. Comparison of balloon valvuloplasty with operative treatment for mitral stenosis. Ann Thorac Surg 1993;56:1254-1263
74. Ribeiro PA, Fawzy ME, Minish L, Swad M, Dunn BE, Arafah MR, Duran CGM. Mitral restenosis and mitral regurgitation 1 year after Inoue mitral balloon valvotomy in a population of patients with pliable mitral valve stenosis. Am Heart J 1993;126:136- 140
75. Goldstein SA, Campbell A, Mintz GS, Richard A, Leon M, Lindsay J. Feasibility of on-line transesophageal echocardiography during balloon mitral valvotomy. Experience with 93 patients. J Heart Valve Dis

1994;3:131-148

76. Ribeiro PA, Al Zaibag M. Mitral balloon valvotomy in pregnancy. J Heart Valve Dis 1992;1:206-208

77. Tuzcu EM, Block PC, Griffin B, Dinsmore R, Newell JB, Palacios IF. Percutaneous mitral balloon valvotomy in patients with calcific mitral stenosis: immediate and long-term outcome. J Am Coll Cardiol 1994;23:1604-1609

78. Okamura K, Alsumi N, Terada Y, et al. A reconsideration of surgery for mitral stenosis based on the extent of valvular distention shown by two dimensional echocardiography preoperatively. Thorac Cardiovasc Surg 1993;41:167-172

79. Bodnar E, Horstkotte D. Potential flaws in the assessment of minor cerebrovascular events after heart valve replacement. J Heart Valve Dis 1993;2:287-290

80. Jamieson WRE, Gallucci V, Thiene G, et al. Porcine valves. In: Bodnar E, Frater RWM (eds). Replacement cardiac valves. New York, Pergamon Press 1991:229- 275

81. Fanin JI, Moreno-Cabral CE, Miller C. Caged-ball valves. In: Bodnar E, Frater RWM (eds). Replacement cardiac valves. New York, Pergamon Press 1991:149-186

82. Woroszylska M, Ruzyllo W, Konka M, et al. Long term follow up after percutaneous commissurotomy with the Inoue Balloon - incidence of restenosis. J Heart Valve Dis 1994;3:594-601

83. Gross EA, Galloway AC, LeBoutillier M, et al. Anterior leaflet procedures during mitral valve repair do not adversely influence long-term outcome. J Am Coll Cardiol 1995;25:134-136

84. Lessana A, Carbone C, Romano M. Mitral valve repair: result and decision making process in reconstruction report of 275 cases. J Thorac Cardiovasc Surg 1990;99:622-630

85. Skoularigis J, Sinovich V, Sareli P. Echocardiographic assessment of 148 young surviving patients with mitral valve repair for rheumatic mitral regurgitation: long term observations. J Am Coll Cardiol 1995;special issue:63A

86. Gometza B, Kumar N, Prabhakar G, Gallo R, Kandeel M, Duran CMG. The challenge of valve surgery in a developing population. J Heart Valve Dis 1993;2:194-199

Chapter 8.3

Reconstructive Surgery of the Mitral Valve

Christophe Acar, Alain Deloche

In the past few years reconstructive surgery of the mitral valve has experienced a growing popularity. It is now clearly established that restoration of a normal valve function is preferable to replacement with a device, whether bioprosthetic or mechanical. In 1968, Carpentier proposed a functional approach to the mitral valve reconstructive surgery and introduced the concept of prosthetic ring annuloplasty that transformed this operative procedure into a reliable and reproducible technique (1,2). The guidelines set at that time have not changed since despite the modifications and the introduction of new methods.

In this chapter we will review mitral valve repair according to Carpentier's techniques.

FUNCTIONAL CLASSIFICATION

Reconstruction of the mitral valve requires a perfect understanding of the functional abnormalities responsible for the regurgitation. The functional classification described below is the guiding line for the operation.

Pre-operative echocardiographic analysis as well as intra-operative inspection of the valve allow classification of any mitral insufficiency into three groups according to the amplitude of the leaflet motion (Fig. 8.3-1):

Type I: leaflet motion is normal. Regurgitation results, as a rule, from insufficient coaptation of the free margins due to dilatation of the annulus.

Type II: leaflet prolapse. Leaflet motion is increased in such a way that its free margin overrides the plane of the mitral annulus during systole.

Type III: restricted leaflet motion. Regurgitation results from insufficient systolic closure of the leaflets. Diastolic opening of the valve may also be affected resulting in a certain degree of stenosis.

The different types of functional abnormalities can coexist, and one may observe a prolapse of the anterior leaflet associated with a restricted posterior leaflet (anterior type I and posterior type III).

As seen from this classification prolapse is a functional abnormality and not a lesion. It should be distinguished from valvular billowing of both leaflets, the free margin of which do not override the plane of the annulus during systole (Fig. 8.3-2) (3,4). Valvular billowing or Barlow's disease do not necessarily imply valvular dysfunction although it may become complicated by prolapse and regurgitation whenever chordae become elongated or ruptured or both.

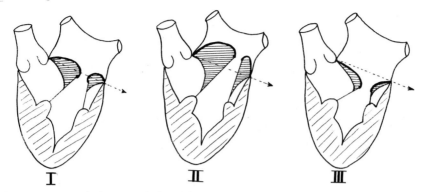

Figure 8.3-1: Carpentier's functional classification of valvular disease. Type I: normal leaflet motion. Type II: leaflet prolapse. Type III: restricted leaflet motion.

The valvular lesions responsible for functional abnormalities are recognized during the operation. However, pre-operative echocardiography (transthoracic or transoesophageal) can sometimes identify the mechanism of mitral regurgitation. Table 8.3-I shows the valvular lesions encountered in mitral valve insufficiency and their functional significance. A unique lesion is a rarity. As a rule, several lesions are involved in a functional abnormality: ruptured chordae are very frequently associated with elongated chordae and chordal fusion is almost always accompanied by commissural fusion. One should keep in mind this polymorphism, each lesion requiring a specific technique and each dysfunction requiring to be corrected.

PATHOMORPHOLOGY

While functional classification serves as a guideline in valve reconstruction, the etiologic diagnosis has a prognostic value. In addition, each pathology has specific pathological features. Figure 8.3-3 illustrates the mechanisms of regurgitation in relation to the most frequent etiologies.

Table 8.3-I: Distribution of functional types and valvular lesions.

FUNCTIONAL TYPE	VALVULAR LESIONS
Type I	Annular dilatation Leaflet perforation
Type II	Chordal rupture Chordal elongation Papillary muscle rupture Papillary muscle elongation
Type III	Commissural fusion Leaflet thickening Chordal fusion Chordal thickening Excess traction on chordae

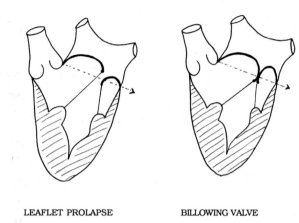

LEAFLET PROLAPSE   BILLOWING VALVE

Figure 8.3-2: Nosologic definition of leaflet prolapse and billowing valve.

Degenerative diseases

Degenerative diseases of the mitral valve have emerged as the most frequent cause of acquired mitral insufficiency in the industrialized countries (5). This disease is characterized by a tendency towards mitral valvular prolapse. Degenerative mitral regurgitation refers to two separate pathologic entities: Barlow's disease and fibro-elastic deficiency (6). The distinction between these diseases is based on age at onset, clinical course and, most notably, the macroscopic aspect of the leaflet tissue.

Barlow's disease appears early in life, often before the age of 50, with a long history of mitral click or systolic murmur. Macroscopically the valve is thick with yellowish leaflets. Excess valvular tissue can be considerable, producing an undulating pattern at the free edges of the leaflets. The chordae are thickened, elongated, and may be ruptured. The papillary muscles may also be elongated. The annulus is dilated and frequently calcified. Calcification may invade the adjacent muscular wall and the attachment of the posterior leaflet papillary muscles (see also Chapter 4.3)

Fibro-elastic deficiency appears mostly in elderly patients beyond the age of 65 and is probably a manifestation of the tissue aging (6). The time course of the disease is shorter, limited to few years. The macroscopic features of the valve differs from Barlow's disease. The leaflets contain no excess tissue, the chordae are elongated, thin and frail, and often ruptured. The annulus is dilated without calcification. Marfan's disease with mitral insufficiency resembles a fibro-elastic deficiency with excess tissue and no myxoid degeneration.

In some instances the distinction between a form fruste of Barlow's disease and fibro-elastic deficiency may be difficult (5). The prolapsed portion presents sometimes a myxoid aspect with excess tissue resembling a Barlow's disease. These lesions are secondary to the jet of regurgitation.

Rheumatic heart disease

Rheumatic disease affects the mitral valve in an inflammatory or fibro-rectractive manner or both. Fibrosis is a slowly evolving process with considerable individual variation. It involves both leaflets and chordae, and eventually leads to valvular

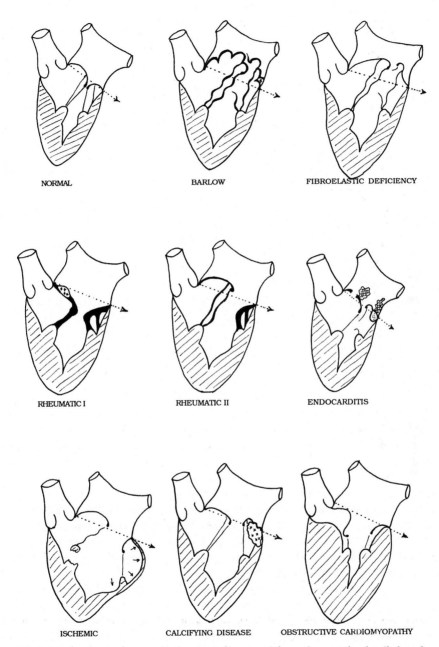

Figure 8.3-3: Mechanisms of regurgitation according to etiology. See text for detailed explanation.

calcification. Shrinkage of leaflet tissue is a prime feature. The chordae are frequently shortened and fused. These lesions typically result in a type III mitral insufficiency with restricted leaflet motion (Fig. 8.3-3). A certain degree of mitral stenosis is always present. The mechanism of stenosis includes commissural fusion and leaflet rigidity resulting in inadequate opening. The annulus is normal or moderately dilated.

In children pure mitral insufficiency (MI) of rheumatic origin may be encountered (Fig. 8.3-3). The typical lesion is anterior leaflet prolapse due to chordal elongation with restricted motion of the posterior leaflet. The annulus may be considerably dilated in this case.

Endocarditis

Lesions resulting from acute endocarditis of the mitral valve include: abscess, perforation, vegetation and chordal rupture (Fig. 8.3-3).

The valvular abscess is characterized by a mass protruding underneath the endocardium of the leaflets surrounded by a halo of infiltration. Abscesses are usually located inside the leaflet tissue (more frequently the anterior leaflet) and may extend to the annulus. Perforation is the natural evolution of an abscess. When the infection involves the leaflet margin or the chordae, prolapse may result from chordal ruptures. Vegetations attest to the acute nature of an endocarditis and are made up of bacteria and altered polynucleated cells embedded within fibrin deposits. The vegetations may be mobile or adherent, pedicled or consist of fine endocardial granulations. In the acute phase of endocarditis, annular dilatation is minimal when present.

Certain lesions may be indicative of a remote episode of endocarditis: leaflet perforation, isolated chordal rupture especially when associated with tissue loss and calcified remains of vegetations.

Ischemic heart disease

Ischemic heart disease may give rise to MI of three different functional types (7).

In type I with normal leaflet motion, the insufficiency results from an isolated dilatation of the annulus.

In type II, leaflet prolapse results from a papillary muscle rupture which usually involves the postero-medial papillary muscle because of the precarious arterial supply at this level. Indeed the vascularization is selectively furnished by distal branches of the circumflex or the right coronary artery. Rupture may be limited to a single bundle of the papillary muscle. The consequence is a prolapse of the corresponding commissural area and the adjacent leaflets. With time, the necrotic papillary muscle will become fibrotic. A necrotic papillary muscle, once fibrotic, may account for ischemic MI by producing commissural prolapse from an elongated papillary muscle or by restricting valvular motion from a shortened papillary muscle.

In type III, restricted leaflet motion with restricted closure during systole is due to a segmental dyskinesia or aneurysm of the left ventricle. In this case, the distance separating the papillary muscle from the plane of the annulus is increased during systole by the dyskinetic motion. Consequently, impaired valve closure will result from excess traction applied to the chordae.

Some authors have proposed papillary muscle dysfunction as the cause of ischemic mitral insufficiency, but this concept is not supported by any laboratory study (7). The sole absence of papillary muscle contraction cannot explain the onset of ischemic mitral insufficiency.

Association of coronary lesions with a degenerative disease of the mitral valve is not a rare finding. Therefore, the diagnosis of MI of ischemic origin implies the presence of specific lesions (rupture or fibrosis of a papillary muscle, dyskinesia of the base of the left ventricle).

Calcifying disease of the mitral annulus

Calcification of the annulus results from a degenerative process involving the base of the mitral leaflets. The calcifications are commonly located at the posterior portion of the annulus including the insertion of the corresponding leaflet (8). The process may be extended to the entire annulus and spread towards the base of the left ventricle. The mechanism of MI in this circumstance is twofold: loss of contraction of the annulus, as it becomes fixed in diastole by calcifications, and restricted motion of the posterior leaflet. This restriction is due to invasion of the leaflet or its chordae by the calcifying process. In addition, the calcifying disease of the annulus is frequently associated with a degenerative lesions of the leaflets and the chordae (5).

Trauma

Mitral insufficiency secondary to blunt or penetrating trauma is rare. Chordal rupture is the most frequently encountered lesion (9). A common cause of traumatic MI is percutaneous balloon dilation (10,11). For the surgeon, this etiology is characterized by a combination of traumatic and rheumatic lesions. Most often the lesions consist of a leaflet tear in a paracommissural area. Rarely the tear involves the mid-part of a leaflet. In addition, rupture of papillary muscle may be observed. The predisposing factors to this kind of injury are a very tight mitral stenosis with fibrous commissural nodules and a narrow mitral annulus.

Cardiomyopathy

In obstructive cardiomyopathy, MI is usually of secondary importance regarding left ventricular outflow tract obstruction. Regurgitation results from systolic anterior motion of the anterior leaflet. A jet lesion at this level with a pseudomyxoid component is a frequent finding. Also, the mitral valve is displaced such that the anterior leaflet protrudes into the outflow tract of the left ventricle.

In dilated cardiomyopathy mitral insufficiency is a consequence of annular dilation.

Endomyocardial fibrosis

Mitral insufficiency results from invasion of the posterior leaflet and its chordae by the fibrotic process. The posterior leaflet becomes fixed in the opening position by the fibrosis (12).

In Libman-Sacks endocarditis the lesions resemble those observed in rheumatic valve disease.

SURGICAL TECHNIQUE

Following a median sternotomy extra-corporeal circulation is established between the venae cavae and the ascending aorta. Myocardial protection is achieved using intermittent anterograde cold cardioplegia.

The mitral valve is approached via a standard left atriotomy parallel to the interatrial sulcus. Carpentier's retractor is positioned for optimal exposure.

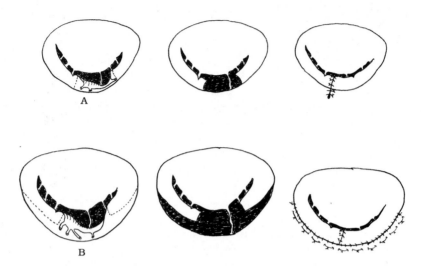

Figure 8.3-4: Correction of a prolapsed posterior leaflet. A: No excess tissue, quadrangular resection with annular plication. B: Excess tissue, quadrangular resection with sliding plasty using compression sutures on the annulus.

Valve analysis

The entire valvular apparatus must be carefully examined in order to assess the feasibility of reconstructive surgery and to plan the operative technique (4).

The left atrium is first examined for jet lesions which indicate a prolapse of the opposing leaflet. The valvular apparatus is then mobilized as an entire unit with a nerve hook in order to assess tissue flexibility and to identify leaflet prolapse or restriction. The extent of prolapse can be determined by applying traction to the free edge of the suspected leaflet segment and then comparing it to a non-prolapsed segment (reference point) (4), usually the anterior paracommissural scallop of the posterior leaflet.

Correction of posterior leaflet prolapse: the quadrangular resection

A prolapse of the posterior leaflet, resulting from chordal rupture or elongation, is treated by a quadrangular resection of the prolapsed area. Stay sutures are placed around the normal chordae adjacent to the prolapsed area. An incision in the prolapsed posterior leaflet is made perpendicular to the free edge towards the annulus and then parallel to is. A quadrangular portion of leaflet is excised. Valvular continuity is restored by annular plication and direct suture of the leaflet remnants (Fig. 8.3-4) (4).

In cases of excess posterior leaflet tissue, as in Barlow's disease, the height of the posterior leaflet must be reduced in order to avoid a SAM (systolic anterior motion) (13). This is achieved, following quadrangular resection, by the sliding leaflet technique. The posterior leaflet is detached from the annulus and a triangle of tissue is resected at the base of each leaflet remnant. Compression sutures are then placed in the annulus allowing reattachment of the leaflet remnants (Fig. 8.3-4). In all cases a prosthetic annuloplasty ring must be inserted to reinforce the repair (13).

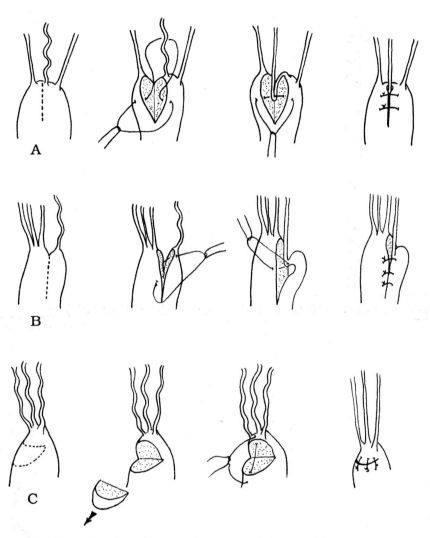

Figure 8.3-5: Correction of a prolapsed anterior leaflet due to chordal elongation. A: Chordal shortening by embedding into the papillary muscle. B: Chordal shortening by sliding plasty. C: Papillary muscle shortening.

Correction of anterior leaflet prolapse

Several techniques are available depending on the lesions (Fig. 8.3-5 and 6):

Chordal shortening by embedding into the papillary muscle

Elongated chordae of the anterior leaflet is a frequent finding in MI. The abnormality can be corrected by the technique of burying of the excess of chordae into the papillary muscle (4). A trench is made into the corresponding papillary muscle. The elongated chorda is then invaginated within the trench (Fig. 8.3-5). The degree of shortening is greater as the trench is placed closer to the papillary muscle base.

Chordal shortening by sliding plasty of the papillary muscle

This technique is best suited for moderate chordal elongations. The portion of the papillary muscle supporting the elongated chordae is split longitudinally and sutured at a lower level towards its base (Fig. 8.3-5) (4).

Papillary muscle shortening

Papillary muscle elongation or chordal elongation involving the entire population of chordae may be corrected using papillary muscle shortening (Fig. 8.3-5). The technique consists of resecting a wedge of papillary muscle at its base. The defect is closed by direct suture resulting in reduction of the height of the papillary muscle.

Chordal transposition

Chordal transposition is the technique of choice in case of chordal rupture of the anterior leaflet. If the number of chordae involved is limited, a single secondary chordae is detached from its insertion on the valve and sutured to the free margin of the leaflet (4). If rupture involves multiple chordae or if no secondary chordae are available, the opposite segment of posterior leaflet including its chordae may be employed (Fig. 8.3-6) (4). This segment is disinserted from the annulus and reattached to the free margin of the anterior leaflet at the site of prolapse. The papillary muscle corresponding to the transposed chordae is mobilised and the defect created in the posterior leaflet is closed by direct suture.

Correction of commissural prolapse

Correction of commissural prolapse may require different techniques according to the lesion. Elongation of the commissural chordae can be treated by burying the extra length into the papillary muscle; chordal rupture requires quadrangular resection of the commissure and sliding plasty of the paracommissural scallop of the posterior leaflet.

Finally, a ruptured papillary muscle, when fibrotic can be reattached to the remnant papillary muscle directly or to the ventricular wall.

Correction of restricted leaflet motion

Commissurotomy

Locating the commissural zone in the presence of gross valvular alteration due to rheumatic disease may be difficult. Traction on the edge of the anterior leaflet may be helpful to identify the commissural groove. The commissure is incised while leaving intact three millimeter of valvular tissue as in the normal anatomy. The underlying chordae and papillary muscle are then incised accordingly.

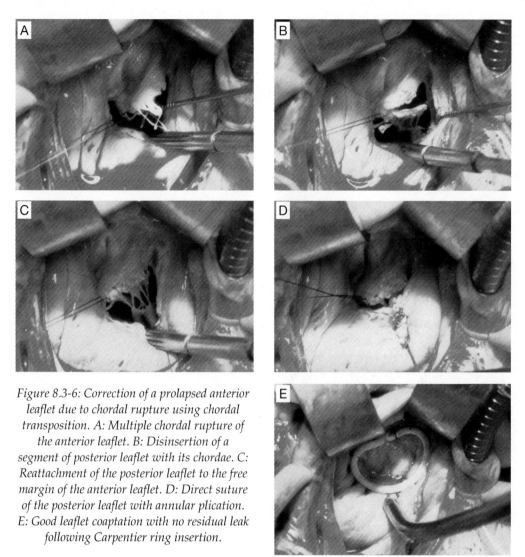

Figure 8.3-6: Correction of a prolapsed anterior leaflet due to chordal rupture using chordal transposition. A: Multiple chordal rupture of the anterior leaflet. B: Disinsertion of a segment of posterior leaflet with its chordae. C: Reattachment of the posterior leaflet to the free margin of the anterior leaflet. D: Direct suture of the posterior leaflet with annular plication. E: Good leaflet coaptation with no residual leak following Carpentier ring insertion.

Resection of secondary chordae

Restriction of the posterior leaflet often results from thickened and shortened secondary chordae. Removal of these chordae may restore leaflet mobility (4).

Chordal fenestration

Fused chordae may create a sub-valvular obstruction which can be corrected by triangular resection of the fibrotic tissue (4).

Pericardial patch enlargement

Total fixation of the posterior leaflet may be corrected by using a pericardial patch

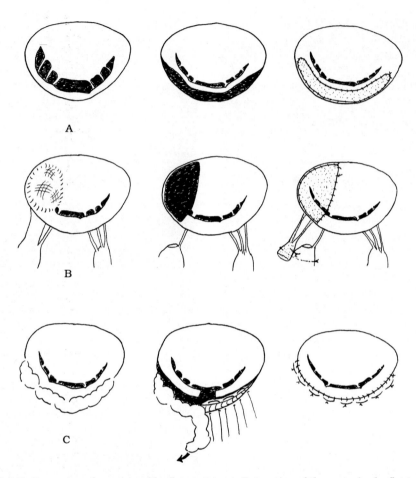

Figure 8.3-7: Correction of a restricted leaflet motion. A: Retraction of the posterior leaflet treated by enlargement with a pericardial patch. B: Calcification of a commissural area: partial valvular replacement using a segment of a cryopreserved mitral homograft. C: Calcifying disease of the mitral annulus: decalcification and reconstruction of the annulus with contraction suture.

(Fig. 8.3-7). The posterior leaflet is detached from the mitral annulus from one commissure to the other and the secondary chordae are removed. The leaflet tissue is reconstructed using an autologous glutaraldehyde treated pericardial patch, inserted between the posterior leaflet and the annulus.

Decalcification

A localized calcified nodule embedded in a leaflet can be excised and the tissue defect replaced by a pericardial patch. If the calcification has invaded both leaflets and their chordae, particularly at the commissural level, the entire diseased segment may be excised en bloc and replaced by a segment of cryopreserved homograft including its chordae (personal technique) (14)). Implantation is performed by suturing the

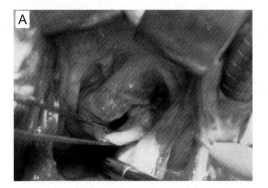

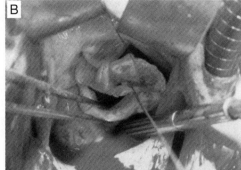

Figure 8.3-8: Partial replacement of the mitral valve using a portion of cryopreserved mitral homograft. A: Large calcification on the anterior commissure. B: Resection of the calcified leaflet tissue with chordae. C: Replacement of the commissure using the corresponding segment of a cryopreserved homograft (personal technique (14)).

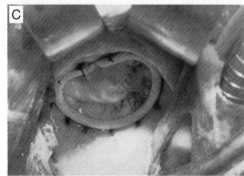

homograft papillary muscle to the corresponding papillary muscle of the recipient (Fig. 8.3-7,8).

In case of calcification of the annulus, decalcification may be achieved by detachment of the leaflet followed by en bloc excision of the calcific deposits (Fig. 8.3-7) (8). Annular reconstruction is performed using mattress sutures to approximate the ventricular and the atrial myocardium. The posterior leaflet is then reattached and the suture line is reinforced by a prosthetic ring.

Treatment of the infected lesions

The first step of mitral valve surgery in the acute phase of endocarditis is a complete resection of all infected tissues. This includes debridement of valvular abscesses with the surrounding tissue and removal of vegetations and ruptured chordae. Reconstruction of the valvular defects will be performed as a second step employing various techniques: pericardial patch reconstruction, chordal transposition, direct valvular suture or leaflet sliding plasty. The use of a portion of cryopreserved mitral homograft will permit to widen the possibilities for valvular repair during the acute phase of endocarditis (14).

Carpentier prosthetic ring annuloplasty

Annuloplasty is a fundamental step of valvular reconstruction (2). It is used in combination with the previously described techniques and shall not be considered as an alternative procedure. The basic concept is remodelling rather than narrowing of the mitral annulus.

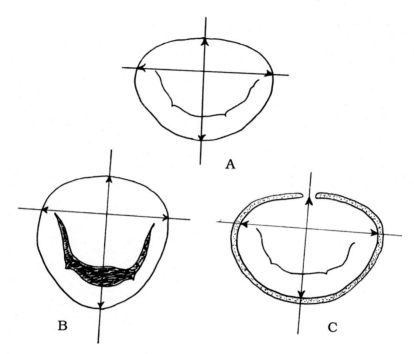

Figure 8.3-9: The concept of Carpentier remodelling annuloplasty. A: Normal mitral valve orifice in systole: the transverse diameter is greater than the anteroposterior diameter. B: Mitral valve incompetence: the annulus is selectively dilated in its posterior portion resulting in an inversion of the diameters ratio (anteroposterior>transverse). C: Remodelling Carpentier ring annuloplasty restores the physiologic ratio.

Dilatation of the mitral annulus is a common finding in MI. The dilatating process is not homogeneous and affects preferentially the posterior portion of the annulus. Remodelling annuloplasty, according to Carpentier, consists in restoring both the size and the shape of the annulus (anteroposterior diameter less than the transverse diameter) by reducing selectively the dilated areas (Fig. 8.3-9) (1-2). Carpentier's ring is a semi-rigid structure open at its anterior portion in contact with the aortic valve. Its implantation is indicated in the case of annular dilatation or for reinforcement following posterior leaflet reconstruction.

Consequently, the annuloplasty ring is employed in the majority of mitral valve reconstructions. In some rare occasions, however, the ring may not be mandatory such as in rheumatic mitral valve disease with predominant stenosis or selected cases of acute endocarditis or congenital malformations.

Intra operative assessment of the repair

The surgeon has two methods to evaluate the repair during surgery: injection of saline into the ventricular cavity and transesophageal Doppler echocardiography. With the heart open the surgeon may assess the quality of the repair according to the aspect of the line of closure of the leaflets. A "smiling" mitral valve with a symmetrical line parallel to the posterior leaflet attachment indicates a satisfactory result even in the presence of a tiny leak due to irregularity of the coaptation surfaces. The advantage of using a remodelling annuloplasty ring as opposed to deformable rings is that the symmetrical closure line, which proves the good coaptation of the leaflets, remains after the heart has resumed its contractility.

Using the remodelling annuloplasty and the Carpentier's techniques makes intraoperative transesophagal echocardiography less important. This technique has the disadvantage that it is to be used after closing the left atrium and discontinuing bypass. However, transesophageal echo is useful during the learning period of the surgeon or for complex cases in order to verify leaflet motion, absence of leak and free left ventricular outflow tract.

RESULTS

Since August 1968, date of the first reconstructive mitral surgery using a Carpentier prosthetic ring, more than 7,000 mitral valve repairs have been performed at the Hospital Broussais in Paris. With the advent of new techniques, the indications of mitral valvuloplasty which were initially restricted to some cases of rheumatic and degenerative valves have broadened to other cases and other etiologies.

Long term assessment of the clinical results must be analyzed taking into consideration the heterogeneity of the patient population and the diversity of surgical techniques.

Operative mortality

Operative death was 4.2% during the first decade (69-78) (6) but it has progressively declined to 1.3% by 1990 (15). Paradoxically, the decrease in mortality has occurred despite extension of the indications to high risk groups such as elderly patients, acute endocarditis and ischemic heart disease. The reduction in mortality is likely related to the general improvement of cardiac surgical results due to the advancements in myocardial protection and postoperative care.

Long term results

It appears that mitral valve repair offers superior long term results in terms of mortality, thromboembolic events and risk of reoperation when compared to replacement with mechanical or bioprosthetic valves (17).

Long term results have been evaluated on a series of 206 patients operated consecutively before 1979 and followed up during a period of two to 17 years (mean 13.2 years) (15). The actuarial curve shows a survival rate of 81% at 10 years and 72% at 15 years. If only valve related deaths are taken into account, the survival rate is 85% at 15 years. At 15 years, 94% are free of thromboembolic complications (linearized rate: 0.4% per patient-year), 97% of the patients are free of endocarditis and 96% have not had any episodes of anticoagulant related hemorrhage. In addition 87% of the patients have not been reoperated at 15 years (linearized rate of reoperation: 1% per patient-year). These data have been confirmed by other comparable series (18).

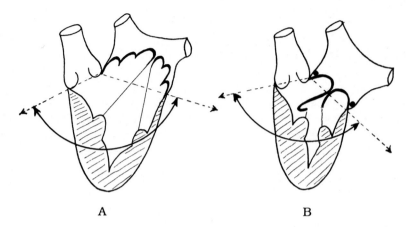

Figure 8.3-10: Mechanism of SAM after mitral valve repair. A: Degenerative mitral insufficiency with excess tissue and annular dilatation. B: Reduction of the aorto-mitral angle following annuloplasty, residual excess leaflet tissue is obstructing the outflow tract.

The presence of a mild residual insufficiency can be recognized by postoperative echo Doppler studies in one out of three cases (18).

Early reoperation within the first two years is usually due to technical errors such as residual prolapse, mitral stenosis (narrow mitral ring associated with a rigid valve), secondary annular dilation (when no prosthetic ring was placed), pericardial patch or valvular suture line dehiscence and, rarely, prosthetic ring dehiscence. Triangular resection of the anterior leaflet, which is no longer practised, has been a frequent cause of early reoperations (19). Late reoperations are generally unrelated to surgical technique. Most often the cause is mitral stenosis or leaflet retraction which attest to the progression of the rheumatic process. Rarely, a recurrent valvular prolapse may be observed as a result of chordal rupture occasionally due to endocarditis. It should be noted that the development of a mild aortic regurgitation may occasionally be observed (18).

Left ventricular outflow tract obstruction after mitral valve reconstruction

Obstruction of the left ventricular outflow tract may occur following reconstructive mitral valve surgery (20). This complication may be suspected intraoperatively by a hemodynamic failure shortly after the discontinuation of bypass or later in the postoperative period by a systolic murmur. Diagnosis is confirmed by echo Doppler study which demonstrates systolic anterior motion (SAM) of the anterior leaflet accompanied by a ventriculo-aortic pressure gradient.

The cause of SAM after valve repair is the interplay of two phenomena: narrowing of the aorto-mitral angle and excess valvular tissue (Fig. 8.3-10). Any intervention on the mitral valve that reduces the annular diameter will decrease the angle between the mitral valve and the aortic valve plane thereby positioning the mitral valve closer to the septum. The second mechanism responsible for SAM is the excess valvular tissue as observed in Barlow's disease. In this case, the redundant posterior leaflet displaces the anterior leaflet into the outflow tract during systole. The protruding anterior leaflet is then forced against the interventricular septum by the high velocity blood stream and, as a result, obstructs ventricular ejection.

EVENT-FREE SURVIVAL

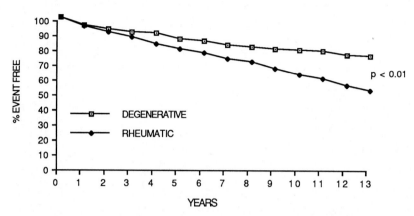

Figure 8.3-11: Cumulative freedom from valve related mortality and morbidity after mitral valve repair. Comparison of rheumatic and degenerative diseases.

The prognosis of reconstruction-related SAM is favorable and the phenomenon tends to disappear under fluid administration and vasodilator therapy. In order to eliminate the risk of SAM in patients presenting an important amount of excess of tissue, a specific technique has been developed to reduce the excess tissue of the valve leaflet (13). No case of SAM has been reported since the development of this technique (21).

Results according to etiology

In *degenerative and in rheumatic valvular disease* the long term results vary according to the progress of the underlying disease (Fig. 8.3-11) (15,18). In degenerative diseases the results of mitral valve repair remain stable: at 15 years 93% of the patients are free of reoperation. In rheumatic valvular disease the results slightly deteriorate with time with 76% of the valvular patients free of reoperation at 15 years.

Acute endocarditis: In a series of 35 patients having undergone a mitral valve repair during the acute phase of endocarditis, operative mortality was 5.7% (22). Additional repair had to be performed at the 9th postoperative day in a patient developing dehiscence of a pericardial patch. After a mean follow up of two years no recurrence of endocarditis has been noted. One patient in the series was reoperated after one year for stenosis. Follow up Doppler echocardiography demonstrates in all cases a competent valve or a minimal residual leak.

Calcifying disease of the annulus: Forty-one patients have undergone annular decalcification associated with a valve repair with a 3-year follow-up (operative mortality 5%) (23). One death occurred during the observation period while three patients have undergone reoperation. Echocardiography confirmed good functional results in all other patients without stenosis or significant residual leak.

Endomyocardial fibrosis: Nine patients with a severe fibrosis related MI were followed for a mean period of 18 months (24). One patient has been reoperated within a year while the others had excellent long term outcomes.

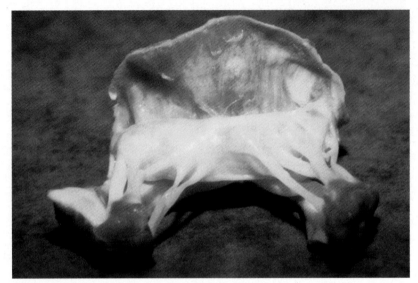

Figures 8.3-12: Operative specimen of a mitral valve obtained 18 months after insertion of an autologous pericardial patch: note the unshrunken pericardial tissue without calcification.

Results according to operative technique

Pericardial patch: The performance of the autologous pericardial patch, fixed in glutaraldehyde, has been studied in a series of 64 patients followed over a three year period (25). Repeat echocardiographic studies have revealed unshrunken pericardial tissue with normal compliance and without evidence of calcification. These satisfactory results have also been noted in children. The occasional reoperation has verified well preserved pericardial patches free of significant deterioration (Fig. 8.3-12).

Chordal transposition: 44 cases of transposition of chordae on the anterior leaflet were followed during a 3-year period (26). In half of the cases, transposition involved secondary chordae of the anterior leaflet which were sutured to the free margin and, in the other half, chordae of the posterior leaflet were transposed to the anterior leaflet. No recurrence of prolapse was observed. Two patients were reoperated at 6 months whereas the others had a stable result.

Commissural prolapse: The commissural area is a hinge the integrity of which is mandatory for normal opening and closure of the valve. The etiologies of the commissural prolapse are by order of frequency: degenerative valvular disease, endocarditis and papillary muscle necrosis (ruptured or elongated).

Analysis of a series of 97 patients presenting with commissural prolapse, followed over a five year period showed that Carpentier's techniques of reconstruction offer the same quality results as for the other sites of valvular prolapse (27). No recurrence of prolapse was observed. Two patients required reoperation at six months whereas the others maintained a satisfactory result.

Results according to age

Mitral repair in children: Long term results of mitral valve repair using Carpentier's

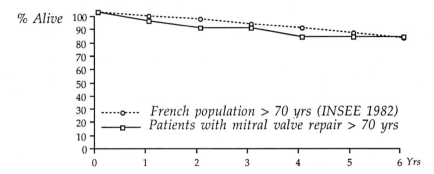

Figure 8.3-13: Actuarial survival of patients over 70 years of age with mitral valve repair versus normal population of the same age group.

techniques have been assessed in 89 children aged two to 12 years with acquired, mainly rheumatic, type II MI (28). At 10 years, 90% of the patients were alive and 78% were free of reoperation with 98% of patients being free from thromboembolic events.

Mitral repair in the elderly: Mitral valve reconstruction was performed in 79 patients over 70 years of age (29). In 90%, the etiology of MI was degenerative disease with a valvular prolapse. Operative mortality (3.8%) was not significantly different from that of younger cohorts. Conversely, postoperative complications have occurred frequently; these complications were related to the medical history of the patients such as renal or respiratory insufficiency, neurologic disorders and infections. Interestingly, the actuarial survival curve was identical to that of a normal population of the same age group (Fig. 8.3-13). Repeat echocardiography demonstrated stable results in all cases during a two-year follow up period.

INDICATIONS

Optimal timing for surgery

Because of the excellent early and late results, the indication for mitral reconstructive surgery has been extended during the recent years. Any significant MI should be considered for surgical repair.

The onset of atrial fibrillation or the appearance of echocardiographic signs of left ventricular dysfunction calls for early surgical intervention: surgery must be considered in patients with the cardiothoracic ratio > 0.56, ejection fraction < 0.55 and left ventricular end-diastolic diameter (LVEDD) > 65 mm (30). Mitral valve repair may permit return of sinus rhythm thereby obviating the need for anticoagulation and the attendant complications. It may also restore a normal left ventricular function.

The date of the operation will obviously be influenced by the feasibility of valve repair.

Indications according to age

Mitral valve repair must be considered as the procedure of choice in children where the mandatory anticoagulation therapy after replacement with a mechanical prosthesis or the high rate of early calcification of a bioprosthesis remain problematic. On the other hand, in elderly patients (over 70 years of age) mitral valve repair remains also the preferred surgical treatment whenever technically feasible (27). Indeed, this technique carries a lower operative mortality than mitral valve replacement in this age group and offers excellent midterm results.

In the other age groups, the indication for valve repair depends mainly on the anatomy of the mitral valve.

Feasibility

The majority of cases of mitral insufficiency can be corrected by this system of reconstructive valve surgery. However, the feasibility of the repair depends partly on the etiology of the valvulopathy and partly upon the experience of the surgeon. The great majority of degenerative or ischemic mitral insufficiencies are amenable to reconstruction.

In rheumatic heart disease valve repair is possible only in 70% of cases using the conventional techniques; calcification and extensive fibrosis are the main obstacles to valve reconstruction. At the acute phase of mitral endocarditis the possibility of repair depends on the extent of valvular mutilation and also approximates 70% of cases. With the introduction of new methods (decalcification, leaflet substitution with a pericardial patch or partial replacement with a homograft) the feasibility of the repair has been extended to many complex cases of rheumatic heart disease and endocarditis.

The presence of massive annular calcification constitutes a technical challenge in any mitral valve surgical procedure. Valvular replacement carries a high risk of mitral annular rupture or early prosthetic dehiscence. In contrast, valve reconstruction after annular decalcification is free of these complications and should be the preferred procedure. Nevertheless, valve repair is not possible when calcifications are either transmural or invade the left ventricular wall.

Indications at the acute phase of endocarditis

Replacement with a mechanical prosthesis during the acute phase of mitral endocarditis carries a high risk of recurrent infection with prosthetic dehiscence. This complication frequently leads to death or multiple reoperations. Valve reconstruction has the advantage of introducing minimal foreign material in the septic environment. For details of surgical indications see Chapter 6.3.

Poor left ventricular function

In the presence of severe ventricular contractile impairment associated with MI, mitral valve repair that preserves the integrity of the subvalvular apparatus, the role of which in left ventricular function has been well demonstrated, is probably the best surgical alternative. However in the case of severe regurgitation an ejection fraction below 20% implies a major systolic impairment. In these cases, the correction of the MI, which serves as a safety vent, carries a prohibitive surgical risk. Cardiac transplantation then remains the procedure of choice (30).

References

1. Carpentier A. La valvuloplastie reconstitutive. Une nouvelle technique de valvuloplastie mitrale. Press Med 1969;77:251-253
2. Carpentier A, Deloche A, Dauptain J, et al. A new reconstructive operation for correction of mitral and tricuspid insufficiency. J Thorac Cardiovasc Surg 1971:61:1-13
3. Carpentier A, Relland J, Deloche A, et al. Conservative management of the prolapsed mitral valve. Ann Thorac Surg 1978;26:294-302
4. Carpentier A. Cardiac valve surgery - The "French correction". J Thorac Cardiovasc Surg 1983;86:323-337
5. Luxereau P, Dorent R, De Gevigney G, Bruneval P, Chomette G, Delahaye G. Aetiology of surgically treated mitral regurgitation. Eur Heart J 1991;12 (Suppl B):B2-B4
6. Carpentier A, Chauvaud S, Fabiani JN, et al. Reconstructive surgery of mitral valve incompetence. Ten year appraisal. J Thorac Cardiovasc Surg 1980;79:338-348
7. Carpentier A, Loulmet D, Deloche A, Perier P. Surgical anatomy and management of ischemic mitral valve incompetence. Circulation 1987;76(Pt2):IV446
8. Carpentier A. Mitral valve repair in calcified mitral valve annulus. Le Club Mitrale Newsletter 1989;I:6-8
9. Jebara V, Acar C, Deloche A, Couetil JP, Dreyfus G, Fabiani JN, Carpentier A. Mitral valve repair for traumatic mitral valve incompetence. Eur Heart J 1989;101:277
10. Acar C, Deloche A, Tibi PR, et al. Operative findings after percutaneous mitral dilation. Ann Thorac Surg 1990;49:959-963
11. Acar C, Jebara V, Grare P, et al. Traumatic mitral insufficiency following percutaneous mitral dilation: mechanisms and surgical implications. Eur J Cardiothorac Surg 1992;6:660-664
12. Dubost C, Maurice P, Gerbaux A et. The surgical treatment of constrictive fibrous endocarditis. Ann Surg 1976;184:303-307
13. Carpentier A. The SAM Issue. Le Club Mitrale. Newsletter 1989;I:5
14. Acar C, Deloche A, Forge A, et al. A new surgical approach in acute mitral valve endocarditis: partial and total replacement using a mitral homograft. Circulation 1994;90:I-310
15. Deloche A, Jebara V, Relland J, et al. Valve repair with Carpentier techniques: the second decade. J Thorac Cardiovasc Surg 1990;99:990-1002
16. Mihaileanu S, El Asmar B, Acar C, et al. Intraoperative transesophageal echocardiography after mitral repair-specific conditions and pitfalls. Eur Heart J 1991;12 (Suppl B):26-29
17. Pèrier P, Deloche A, Chauvaud S, et al. Comparative evaluation of mitral valve repair and replacement with Starr, Björk and porcine valve prostheses. Circulation 1984;70:I-187-192
18. Michel PL, Iung B, Blanchard B, Luxereau P, Dorent R, Acar J. Long term results of mitral valve repair for non-ischaemic mitral regurgitation. Eur Heart J 1991;12 (Suppl B):B39-B43
19. Chauvaud S, Deleuze P, Perier P, Carpentier A. Failure in reconstitutive mitral valve surgery. Circulation 1986;74:II-393
20. Mihaileanu S, Marino JP, Chauvaud S, et al. Left ventricular outflow obstruction after mitral valve repair (Carpentier's technique): proposed mechanisms of disease. Circulation 1988;78:I-78-84
21. Jebara V, Mihaileanu S, Acar C, et al. Left ventricular outflow tract obstruction after mitral valve repair. Results of the sliding leaflet technique. Circulation 1993;88:II 30-34
22. Fuzellier JF, Acar C, Jebara V, et al. Plasties mitrales au cours de la phase aigue de l'endocarditis. Arch Mal Coeur 1993;86:197-201
23. Fuzellier JF. Maladie calcifiante de l'anneau mitral: anatomopathologie et chirurgie reconstructrice. These pour le Doctorat en Medecine, Paris 1993
24. Sousa-Uva M, Jebara V, Acar C, et al. Mitral valve repair in patients with endomyocardial fibrosis. Ann Thorac Surg 1992;54:89-92
25. Chauvaud S, Jebara J, Chachques JC, et al. Valve extension with glutaraldehyde preserved autologous pericardium: results in mitral valve repair. J Thorac Surg 1991;102:171-178
26. Sousa-Uva M. Transposition of chordae in mitral valve repair: mid term results. Circulation 1993;88:35-38
27. Radermecker M, Pellerin M, Acar C, et al. Mitral valve repair of commissural prolapse. Ann Thorac Surg (in press)
28. Chauvaud S, Perier P, Touati G, et al. Long term results of valve repair in children with acquired mitral valve incompetence. Circulation 1986;74:I-104-109
29. Jebara V, Dervanian P, Acar C, et al. Mitral valve repair using Carpentier techniques in patients more than 70 years old: early and late results. Circulation 1992;86:II 53-59
30. Acar J, Michel SL, Luxereau P, Dervanian, Cormier B. Indication for surgery in mitral regurgitation. Eur Heart J 1991;12 (Suppl B):B52-54

Chapter 8.4

Surgical Commissurotomy of the Mitral Valve

Philippe Grare, Alain Deloche

Closed mitral commissurotomy (CMC) was historically the first surgical treatment for mitral stenosis. The first successful operation was performed in 1925 by Souttar (1), but gave rise to harsh criticism at that time. Three decades later, the procedure was made popular by Harken (2), Bailey (3) and Baker (4) and was used extensively in the fifties and sixties. The ideal indication was a tight, pure, and non-calcified stenosis in a patient in sinus rhythm.

Later, with the development of extra-corporeal circulation (ECC), open mitral commissurotomy (OMC) evolved. This new technique allowed direct inspection and treatment of the valve and its subvalvular apparatus, and gradually replaced the closed technique.

In 1984 the introduction of percutaneous mitral dilatation once again modified the therapeutic strategy of treating mitral stenosis, decreasing the need for surgical commissurotomies. Although less invasive, percutaneous mitral dilatation does have its limitations, which may include cost, lack of expertise or advanced mitral stenosis. Consequently, there still remains an important role for surgical commissurotomy in the management of mitral stenosis.

CLOSED MITRAL COMMISSUROTOMY

Technique

Through a left thoracotomy the left atrial appendage is approached. Dilatation is performed blindly. The initial attempt is made with the surgeon's finger (Fig. 8.4-1) followed by, if unsuccessful, using a mechanical dilator through the left appendage (Dubost's dilator), or via the left ventricular apex (Tubb's dilator) (Fig. 8.4-2). Occasionally, the left appendage can be exposed via a right thoracotomy or a median sternotomy.

Immediate results

Operative mortality for closed commissurotomy has been reported to be 2%-3% in most series (5-8). In a series of over 1,000 patients at the Broussais hospital, the hospital mortality was less than 1%, the predominant cause of operative mortality being refractory heart failure.

Postoperative complications

The major complications include mitral insufficiency and thromboembolic events.

846

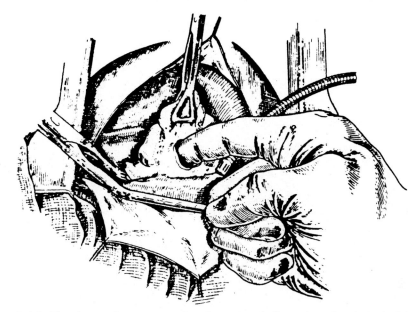

Figure 8.4-1: Closed commissurotomy using the surgeon's finger introduced via the left atrial appendage.

Mitral insufficiency

Mitral insufficiency has been clinically detected in 10%-23% of patients undergoing CMC (8-11). However, severe mitral insufficiency requiring urgent valvular replacement was rare (0.4%) (8,12).

The diagnosis of mitral insufficiency and its severity following CMC may be difficult. Mitral insufficiency is usually recognized by the surgeon using finger palpation of the mitral orifice immediately following dilatation. The precision of this evaluation is dependent on the hemodynamic status, (cardiac output, arterial pressure). A certain number of significant mitral insufficiencies have probably been under-estimated (11). Today the method of choice for diagnosis and quantification of mitral insufficiency during surgery is Doppler echocardiography.

Early thromboembolic events

Most series have reported an incidence of 2.5% (13-15). The risk of thromboembolic complications was lower in patients submitted to a prolonged period of anticoagulation therapy prior to CMC. For this reason, the existence of preoperative atrial fibrillation (which was an indication for anticoagulation) was not associated with a higher rate of thromboembolic complications (8,9). Intraoperative discovery of a left atrial thrombus is considered by some as a contra-indication to completing the closed commissurotomy (16).

Functional results and changes in mitral valve area

All study groups have reported good clinical results, with immediate relief of

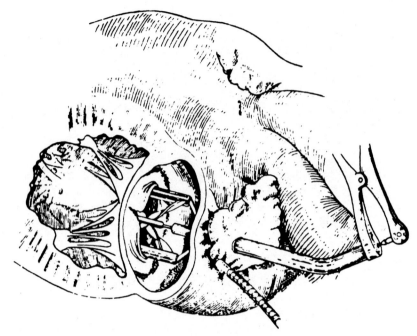

Figure 8.4-2: Closed commissurotomy using a mechanical dilator.

symptoms, in patients who were mostly in NYHA class III or IV prior to CMC (8,17). Nevertheless, a quantitative evaluation in terms of valve surface area has rarely been available. The results of dilatation were assessed by the surgeon's finger during the operation, and a satisfactory result was reported in 98% of cases (8).

Recent echocardiographic and catheter studies have reported pre- and postoperative measurements of the valve surface area. The results, in highly selected patients (free of calcification) showed an increase of 70% to 170% in valve surface area. Doppler-echocardiography studies (10) have reported a mean valve surface area of 0.79 cm^2 which increased to 2.2 cm^2. In other series, hemodynamic assessment of the valve surface area showed an increase from 1.0 cm^2 to 1.8 cm^2 and from 0.82 cm^2 to 1.4 cm^2 following CMC (18,19).

Long term results

Survival rate and functional results

Actuarial survival rates of 75%, 58% and 38% have been found at 10, 20 and 28 years, respectively (20). The long term causes of death were heart failure and cerebro-vascular accidents. The initial functional improvement remained stable, with 86% of patients in NYHA classes I or II at 15 years (8).

Reoperation

Recurrence of symptoms implies restenosis, underlining the importance of regular clinical and echocardiographic follow up. Opinions vary as to the incidence of restenosis following closed mitral commissurotomy, but the rate of restenosis clearly increases as survival reaches 20-30 years (8,20,21). The rate of occurrence of restenosis has been found to vary from 4.2 to 11.4 per 100 patient-year between the fifth and fifteenth years of follow up. Rates of reoperation of 18% at 10 years and 32% at 25 years have been reported (6,22).

Restenosis is a consequence either of a fibrotic process or a commissural fusion. In many patients both lesions are associated (23).

Restenosis raises the problem of which surgical technique should be used for the second procedure. A second closed commissurotomy is occasionally possible with a relatively high mortality (6.7% to 9.5%) (8,9,11,20). An open heart operation such as open commissurotomy or valvular replacement should be favored in cases of advanced lesions (6,8,9,20,24). Mitral balloon valvuloplasty for restenosis following surgical commissurotomy has also been employed with success (25,26).

OPEN MITRAL COMMISSUROTOMY

Technique

Following a median sternotomy, institution of cardiopulmonary bypass and cardioplegic arrest, the left atrium is opened. The commissures are incised, and the fused chordae as well as the papillary muscles are split in order to remove the subvalvular obstruction.

Immediate results

Operative mortality

Most series have reported an operative mortality of approximately 1% (27,30,33). The main causes of death are myocardial failure, thromboembolic events and infection.

Postoperative complications

Moderate mitral insufficiency has been noted in less than 7% of cases (19). Significant mitral insufficiency requiring an early reintervention is rare (2%-3%) (27,28), as is the incidence of thromboembolic events (1%-2%) (27,29). In 1%-13% of cases an atrial thrombus is discovered intraoperatively and removed (27,30).

Functional results and changes in mitral valve area

The immediate functional results are excellent (27,30,31); in one study 53% of the patients were in NYHA class I or II and 47% in class III or IV before the intervention, after the operation 86% were in class I or II and 14% in class III or IV (31). Unfortunately, changes in valve surface area are rarely reported. According to Nakano (31), it increased from 0.75 cm^2 to 2.2 cm^2 postoperatively. More recently a prospective hemodynamic study has shown an increase from 0.84 cm^2 to 2.14 cm^2 (19). In selected cases, with pliable valves, surgery could obtain a valve area greater than 2.5 cm^2 (32).

Long term results

Survival rate and functional results

The cardiac causes of late mortality include thromboembolic accidents, sudden death, and congestive heart failure (27,30,31).

Actuarial survival rates of 89% and 75% have been found at 15 and 18 years, respectively (30,31). Functional results remain stable; at 10 years 92% of patients are in NYHA class I or II. Late thromboembolic accidents are rare. In Nakano's series (31) an incidence of 0.14% per patient-year was found (31).

Reoperation

The main cause of reoperation is the development of mitral insufficiency rather than restenosis (31,33), reported as the cause of 88% of reoperations (31).

CONCLUSION

The respective merits of the two techniques of commissurotomy have been largely debated (9,20,29). Some surgeons have abandoned closed commissurotomy altogether in favor of the open version as it provides more precise correction of the lesions. In fact, open commissurotomy allows satisfactory opening of both commissures whereas closed commissurotomy usually relieves the anterior commissure only (34). A recent randomized study comparing the two techniques showed the postoperative valve surface area to be superior with open commissurotomy (19).

Today, the debate between the closed and the open commissurotomy is outdated due to the tremendous progress achieved both in interventional cardiology and in mitral valve reconstructive surgery. At the present time a surgical commissurotomy should be performed only if a balloon dilatation is contra-indicated. In such a case an open commissurotomy should be performed, taking advantage of the techniques of mitral reconstructive surgery such as localized calcification removal, posterior leaflet mobilization with a pericardial patch, and remodelling annuloplasty with a prosthetic ring.

However, in developing countries, socio-economic restraints often influence the therapeutic strategy for treating mitral stenosis. In this scenario closed commissurotomy is the less expensive and provides a reliable surgical intervention for mitral stenosis (18,35,36). Also, in pregnant women with critical mitral stenosis, closed commissurotomy (37) and, at the present time, percutaneous mitral commissurotomy (38) provide an important alternative for the treatment of these high risk patients.

References

1. Souttar HS. The surgical treatment of mitral stenosis. Br Med J 1925;2:603-606
2. Harken DE, Ellis LB, Ware PF, Norman LR. The surgical treatment of mitral stenosis. N Engl J Med 1948;239:801-808
3. Bailey CP. The surgical treatment of mitral stenosis (mitral commissurotomy). Dis Chest 1949;15:377-384
4. Baker C, Brock RC, Campbell M. Valvotomy for mitral stenosis. Br Med J 1950;2:46-65
5. Ellis IB, Singh JB, Morales DD, Harken DE. Fifteen-to-twenty year study of thousand patients undergoing closed mitral valouloplerty. Circulation 1973;48:357-369
6. Salemo TA, Neilson DR, Chamette EJP, Lynn RB. A 25 year experience with the closed method of

treatment in 139 patients with mitral stenosis. Ann Thorac Surg 1980;31:300-304

7. Commerford PJ, Hastie T, Beck W. Closed mitral valvotomy: actuarial analysis of results in 654 patients over 12 years and analysis of preoperative predictors of long-term survival. Ann Thorac Surg 1982;33:473-479
8. Stanley J, Bashi VV, Muralidharan S, et al. Closed mitral valvotomy: early results and long-term follow-up of 3724 consecutive patients. Circulation 1983;68:891-896
9. Molajo AO, Bennett DH, Bray CL, et al. Actuarial analysis of late results after closed mitral valvotomy. Ann Thorac Surg 1988;45:364-369
10. Arora R, Nair M, Karla GS, et al. Immediate and long-term results of balloon and surgical closed mitral valvotomy: a randomized comparative study. Am Heart J 1993;125:1091-1094
11. Spencer FC. Results in closed mitral valvotomy. Ann Thorac Surg 1988;45:355
12. Otto TJ. Surgical treatment of mitral stenosis. Thorax 1964;19:541-547
13. Belcher JR, Somerville W. Systemic embolism and left auricular thrombosis in relation to mitral valvotomy. Br Med J 1955;2:1000-1003
14. Bakoulas G, Mullar K. Mitral valvulotomy and embolism. Thorax 1966;21:43-46
15. Hoeksema TD, Wallace RB, Kirklin JW. Closed mitral commissurotomy: recent results in 291 cases. Am J Cardiol 1966;17:825-829
16. D'allaines Cl, Blondeau Ph, Dubost Ch, et al. La commissurotomie mitrale a coeur fermie. Vingt ans apres. Arch Mal Coeur 1977;11:1145-1153
17. Lainee R, Acar J, Joly F, Carlotti J. Resultats eloignes de la commissurotomie mitrale. Arch Mal Coeur 1963;56:1326-1345
18. Turi ZG, Reyes VP, Raju BS, et al. Percutaneous balloon versus surgical closed commissurotomy for mitral stenosis. A prospective randomized trial. Circulation 1991;83:1179-1185
19. Ben Farhat M, Bousssadia H, Gandjbakhch I, et al. Closed versus open mitral commissurotomy in pure non-calcific mitral stenosis: hemodynamic studies before and after operation. J Thorac Cardiovasc Surg 1990;99:639-644
20. Nakano S, Kawashima Y, Hiros H, et al. Reoperation-free survival after closed mitral commissurotomy. J Cardiovasc Surg 1986;27:103-107
21. Hickey MSJ, Blackstone EH, Kirklin JW, et al. Outcome probabilities and life history after surgical mitral commissurotomy implications for balloon commissurotomy. J Am Coll Cardiol 1991;17:29-42
22. Rutledge R, Mc Intosh CL, Morrow AG, et al. Mitral valve replacement after closed mitral commissurotomy. Circulation 1982;66:I-162-I-166
23. Degeorge JM, Joly F, Acar J, Lainee R. Les retrecissements mitraux recidivants. Sem Hop Paris 1965;53:3117-3130
24. Peper WA, Lytle BW, Cosgrove DM, et al. Repeat mitral commissurotomy: long-term results. Circulation 1987;76:Suppl III-97-III-101
25. Rediker DE, Block PC, Abaseal VM, et al. Mitral balloon valvuloplasty for mitral restenosis after surgical commissurotomy. J Am Coll Cardiol 1988:11:252-256
26. Vahanian A, Michel PL, Cormier B, et al. Mid-term results of mitral balloon valvulotomy for restenosis after surgical commissurotomy (Abstract). Circulation 1990;82(Suppl III):80
27. Halseth WL, Elliott DP, Walker EL, et al. Open mitral commissurotomy. A modern re-evaluation. J Thorac Cardiovasc Surg 1980;80:842-848
28. Mullin MJ, Engelman RM, Isom OW, et al. Experience with open mitral commissurotomy in 100 consecutive patients. Surgery 1974;76:974-982
29. Housman LB, Bonchek L, Lambert L, et al. Prognosis of patients after open mitral commissurotomy. J Thorac Cardiovasc Surg 1977;73:742-745
30. Herrera JM, Vega JL, Berual JM, et al. Open mitral commissurotomy: fourteen- to-eighteen-year follow-up clinical study. Ann Thorac Surg 1993;55:641-645
31. Nakano S, Kawashima Y, Hirose H, et al. Reconsiderations of indications for open mitral commissurotomy based on pathologic features of the stenosed mitral valve. J Thorac Cardiovasc Surg 1987;94:336-342
32. Antunes MJ, Nascimento J, Andriade CM, Fernandes LE. Open mitral commissurotomy: a better procedure? J Heart Valve Dis 1994;3:88-92
33. Antunes MJ. Mitral valve repair. Verlag R. S. Schulz, Kempfenhausen, 1989:55-62
34. De Vernejoul F, Cabrol C, Cabrol A, et al. Commissurotomie mitrale a coeur ouvert. Arch Mal Coeur 1979;72:606-614
35. Rihal CS, Schaff HV, Frye RL, et al. Long-term follow-up of patients undergoing closed transventricular mitral commissurotomy: a useful surrogate for percutaneous balloon mitral valvuloplasty? J Am Coll Cardiol 1992;20:781-786
36. Enriquez-Sarano M, Louvard Y, Darmon D, et al. Faut-il encore faire des commissurotomies mitrales a coeur ferme? Arch Mal Coeur 1984;7:782-790

37. Vosloo S, Reichart B. The feasibility of closed mitral valvotomy in pregnancy. J Thorac Cardiovasc Surg 1987;93:675-679
38. Iung B, Cormier B, Elias J, et al. La commissurotomie mitrale percutanee durant la grossesse. Arch Mal Coeur 1993;86:995-999

Chapter 8.5

Reconstructive Surgery of the Aortic Valve

Christophe Acar, Victor Jebara

The first surgical attempts to treat aortic insufficiency were performed using reconstructive techniques on the aortic valve (1-4). Over the past 25 years, progressive development of various types of mechanical and biologic prostheses have offered a relatively simple and efficient solution to treat patients with acquired disease of the aortic valve. This explains the lack of interest and the limited development of the techniques of aortic valve repair during this period. However, valve related complications observed after aortic valve replacement and the absence of an "ideal" prosthetic valve have led in recent years to a resurgence in interest in the use of aortic valve reconstructive techniques in a selected group of patients.

PATHOPHYSIOLOGY

Misunderstanding of the exact physiopathology of aortic insufficiency has remained a significant drawback for valve repair. Schematically, the competence of the aortic valve depends on the integrity of its two components, the annulus and the aortic cusps. The normal aortic valve can be considered as a cylinder comprising three identical semilunar leaflets. By definition, the length of the free margin of each cusp is equal to two radii (i.e. diameter) of the aortic annulus at the level of the sinotubular junction (Fig. 8.5-1).

Based on these criteria, four types of aortic insufficiency can be identified (Fig. 8.5-1): Type I: Annular dilatation, where due to the dilatation process of the aortic root, the length of the free margin of the cusps has become not long enough for the diameter of the annulus. Type II: Cusp prolapse, where the cusps are displaced towards the ventricle in diastole, preventing coaptation due to pathologic excess tissue along the free edges of the cusps making them too long for the annular diameter. Type III: Cusp retraction, where shrinkage of the cusp tissue results in a lack of coaptation in diastole with the cusp free edge being too short for the annular diameter. Type IV: Cusp perforation, where the sizes of both the annulus and the cusps are normal, and the regurgitation is secondary to a localized lesion (perforation/tear) involving one or more cusps.

The different etiologies of aortic valve disease are tightly correlated with the functional classification. Degenerative aortic insufficiency, as well as insufficiency secondary to a bicuspid valve, are associated with type I and/or II. Type III is almost exclusively encountered in rheumatic aortic insufficiency, while type IV is the consequence of bacterial endocarditis.

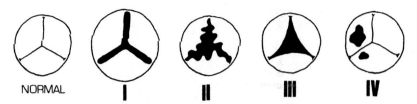

Figure 8.5-1: Functional classification of aortic insufficiency. Normal valve - Cusp free edge = annulus diameter. Type 1: Annular dilatation - Cusp free edge < annulus diameter. Type II: Cusp prolapse - Cusp free edge > annulus diameter. Type III: Cusp retraction - Cusp free edge < annulus diameter. Type IV: Cusp perforation - Cusp free edge = annulus diameter.

SURGICAL TECHNIQUES

Commissurotomy

Incision of the fused commissures can improve valve motion. Resection of the fibrotic tissue involving the inter-leaflet triangle is frequently necessary (5,6) (Fig. 8.5-2A).

Cusp shaving

Thickening and fibrosis at the level of the free edge of the cusps is frequently encountered. This is treated by tangential excision of the fibrotic tissue from both the aortic and ventricular aspects, allowing increased mobility and unrolling of the cusps. This maneuver leads to a slight increase in the depth of the cusp, with a larger surface of coaptation of the adjacent cusps (5,6) (Fig. 8.5-2B).

Treatment of leaflet prolapse

Various techniques have been described to treat patients with cusp prolapse of the aortic valve (Fig. 8.5-3). The first in time was cusp plication at the level of the commissure (6,7). This technique was originally described to treat aortic regurgitation in Pezzy and Laubry syndrome, which is associated with aortic insufficiency due to prolapse of the right coronary cusp and ventricular septal defect (8,9). Carpentier developed triangular resection and direct reconstruction of the cusp to treat cusp prolapse (5). The extent of resection is adjusted in order to obtain an identical length of the free edges of the three cusps. Cosgrove proposed the use of this technique in aortic insufficiency due to bicuspid aortic valves (10). In this case the resection is performed on the prolapsed cusp at the level of the raphe when present in order to reconstruct two aortic cusps whose free margins are equal.

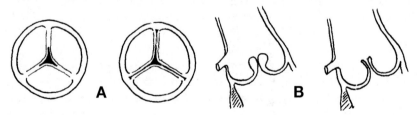

Figure 8.5-2: Correction of restricted leaflet motion. A: Commissurotomy. B: Cusp shaving.

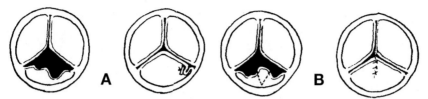

Figure 8.5-3: Correction of leaflet prolapse. A: Cusp resuspension (Duran). B: Triangular resection (Carpentier).

Surgical annuloplasty

Sub-commissural annuloplasty

This technique was first described by Cabrol in 1966 and consists of plication of the aortic commissures using an inverted suture with Teflon pledgets placed on the ventricular aspect (11) (Fig. 8.5-4A). The rationale of this technique is based on the hypothesis that annular dilatation preferentially involves the commissural areas where fibrous tissue becomes scarce. Plication of these areas remodels the annulus to a normal size.

Continuous circular annuloplasty

Described by Carpentier, this technique consists of performing two continuous circular suture lines passing alternatively from the ventricular to the aortic aspect of the aortic annulus (5). This technique not only reduces the size of the aortic annulus but also prevents further dilatation (Fig. 8.5-4B).

Supra-aortic crest enhancement

The role of the sinuses of Valsalva in the function of the aortic valve has been well documented. It has been shown that circular flow patterns occur at the superior edge of the sinus of Valsalva and that these patterns persist throughout the period of valve closure (12). It has also been demonstrated that the intensity of these circular flow

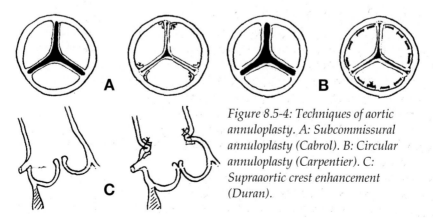

Figure 8.5-4: Techniques of aortic annuloplasty. A: Subcommissural annuloplasty (Cabrol). B: Circular annuloplasty (Carpentier). C: Supraaortic crest enhancement (Duran).

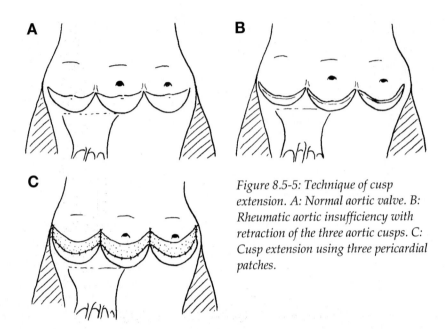

Figure 8.5-5: Technique of cusp
extension. A: Normal aortic valve. B:
Rheumatic aortic insufficiency with
retraction of the three aortic cusps. C:
Cusp extension using three pericardial
patches.

patterns is directly proportional to the degree of pre-eminence of the aortic crest and
affects the rapidity of the closure of the aortic valve. Duran provided experimental
confirmation of this hypothesis (13). He then advocated the enhancement of the supra-
aortic crest using a continuous circumferential mattress suture constructed at the
superior edge of the sinuses of Valsalva (6) (Fig. 8.5-4C).

Closure of cusp perforation

Cusp perforation secondary to bacterial endocarditis can be closed using a patch of
autologous pericardium. In the case of active infection, all necrotic tissue likely to be
contaminated must be previously removed.

Cusp extension using extravalvular material

Cusp extension was first described by Senning in 1960 using autologous fascia lata
(14). Since then the technique has evolved both in relation to the shape of the patch and
to the material used (Fig. 8.5-5). In 1986 Batista advocated the use of a single
glutaraldehyde-treated bovine pericardial patch to enlarge the aortic cusps (15). Almost
simultaneously, Yacoub and Al Fagih modified the technique by using three separate
patches of bovine pericardium to enlarge each of the aortic cusps (16,17). Duran then
proposed a similar technique using autologous pericardium treated briefly with
immersion in glutaraldehyde (18). The pericardium was tailored in three pieces (18) or
trimmed as a singular patch.

Recently, we described a standardized technique of cusp extension using autologous
pericardium (19). This technique can be applied in patients with type III aortic
insufficiency with cusp retraction. The valve should still be pliable and free of

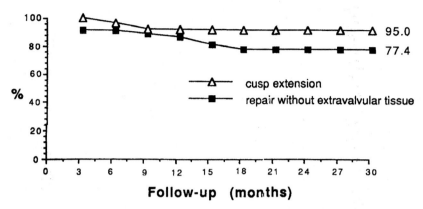

Figure 8.5-6: Actuarial freedom from reoperation following aortic valve repair with and without addition of extravalvular tissue (from Duran et al. (18)).

calcification. The free edge of the cusps when fibrotic is excised. Routine enlargement of the three aortic cusps are performed in order to obtain a large surface of coaptation (Fig. 8.5-5). The autologous pericardium is previously treated for 10 minutes in glutaraldehyde. Three rectangular patches are tailored, their width being equal to the diameter of the annulus measured with a valve sizer, and the height is approximately eight millimeter. Each patch is sutured to the free edge of the cusp and the commissures are reconstructed by fixing the vertical portion of the patch directly to the aortic wall). This results in a vertical shift in the commissures and restoration in excess of the surface of coaptation during diastole (Fig. 8.5-5 (19).

RESULTS

There are few reports in the literature describing the long term results of aortic valve repair for acquired valve disease. In a series from Bessou et al. reviewing the results of 95 patients who underwent aortic valve repair for aortic insufficiency over an 11-year period since 1971, 75% of the cases had associated mitral insufficiency (20). Operative mortality was 3.3%. Reoperation was required in 15% of the cases at three years due to significant residual aortic insufficiency. No embolic complications have been observed.

In a series from Duran, hospital mortality was 1.8% and actuarial survival of 50 patients operated between 1974 and 1986 was 86% at 13 years, with only four patients requiring reoperation for aortic insufficiency (7). More recently, Duran and associates reviewed 107 patients and concluded that cusp extension techniques using pericardium were superior to aortic valve repair without addition of extravalvular tissue (18). Reoperation rates were lower (94% versus 77% free from reoperation at 30 months, respectively) (Fig. 8.5-6). Furthermore, immediate and late echocardiographic follow up showed better results in the case of cusp extension. The majority of patients were free from anticoagulation therapy and thromboembolic events did not occur.

Poor clinical experience with fascia lata introduced by Senning showed that extravalvular material should be pre-treated before its insertion in the aortic root. On the other hand results of the use of bovine pericardium treated with glutaraldehyde seem interesting. Yacoub reported on 135 patients treated with this technique followed up to seven years: early rupture (three months) occurred in six cases and only four patients developed tissue failure. Similarly, Al Fagih reported on 20 patients followed up to two years with no complications (17). Following basic experimental studies, Chachques offered an attractive solution to the problem of the use of autologous pericardium in routine cardiac surgery by showing that adequate fixation of this material could be obtained by a brief immersion (10 minutes) in glutaraldehyde (21).

In our experience, 21 patients underwent aortic valve repair using cusp extension with glutaraldehyde treated autologous pericardium for rheumatic aortic regurgitation (19). All patients underwent a standardized technique of valve repair with cusp extension using three rectangular patches of autologous pericardium sutured to the free edge of the aortic cusp and the aortic wall adjacent to the commissures (19). The size of the patches was adapted according to that of the aortic annulus measured with a valve sizer at the level of the sinotubular junction. This allowed the adjustment of the tension exerted on the free edge of the cusp with great precision and the restoration of a large (greater than necessary) surface of coaptation so as to compensate for any geometrical asymmetry. Echocardiographic studies in most patients showed correction of the aortic regurgitation both intraoperatively and after a follow up of up to three years. Doppler studies demonstrated the absence of transvalvular gradients that could have been induced by the addition of extravalvular tissues; a prerequisite being that the remaining cusp tissue was pliable.

INDICATIONS

Aortic valve repair for acquired valve disease is still under investigation and its indication should remain restricted to selected cases. The expected results should always be balanced against those of aortic valve replacement using various types of prosthesis. The indications for aortic valve repair might be extended in the future according to the long term results of the cusp extension technique using autologous pericardium.

At the present time, aortic valve repair using cusp extension with autologous pericardium should be the preferred treatment in case of rheumatic aortic insufficiency in children; indeed valve replacement in this age group remains a dramatic problem because of the rapid calcification of bioprostheses and the difficulty with anticoagulation therapy in the case of mechanical prostheses. Moreover, small size homografts are rare and constitute a limiting factor to this technique. Valve repair for rheumatic aortic insufficiency may also be considered in young patients in whom anticoagulant therapy is contraindicated (22). The Ross procedure (pulmonary autograft) also appears to be a viable alternative (see Chapter 9.2).

References
1. Taylor WJ, Thrower WB, Black H, Harken DE. The surgical correction of aortic insufficiency by circumclusion. J Thorac Cardiovasc Surg 1958;35:192-205
2. Murphy JP. The surgical correction of syphilitic aortic insufficiency. J Thorac Cardiovasc Surg 1960;40:524-528
3. Starzl TE, Cruzat EP, Walker FB, Lewis FJ. A technique for bicuspidization of the aortic valve. J Thorac Cardiovasc Surg 1959;262-270
4. Hurwitt ES, Hoffert PW, Rosenblatt A. Plication of the aortic ring in the correction of aortic insufficiency. J Thorac Cardiovasc Surg 1960;39:654-662
5. Carpentier A. Cardiac valve surgery - the "French correction". J Thorac Cardiovasc Surg 1983;86:323-337
6. Duran CMG, Alonso J, Gaite L, et al. Long term results of conservative repair of the rheumatic aortic valve

insufficiency. Eur J Cardiothorac Surg 1988;2:217-223
7. Duran CMG. Reconstitutive techniques for rheumatic aortic valve disease. J Cardiac Surg 1988;3:23-28
8. Spencer FC, Doyle EF, Danilowicz DA, Bahnson HT, Weldon CS. Long term evaluation of aortic valvuloplasty for aortic insufficiency and ventricular septal defect. J Thorac Cardiovasc Surg 1973;65:15-31
9 Trusler GA, Moes CAF, Kidd BSL. Repair of ventricular septal defect with aortic insufficiency. J Thorac Cardiovasc Surg 1973;66:394-403
10. Cosgrove DM, Rosenkranz ER, Hendren WG, Bartlett JC, Stewart WJ. Valvuloplasty for aortic insufficiency. J Thorac Cardiovasc Surg 1991;102:571-577
11. Cabrol C, Guiraudon G, Bertrand M. Le traitement de l'insuffisance aortique par l'annuloplastie aortique. Arch Mal Coeur 1966;59:1305-1312
12. Belhouse BJ, Belhouse FH, Reid KG. Fluid mechanics of the aortic root with application to coronary flow. Nature 1968;219:1059-1061
13. Duran CG, Balasundaram S, Wilson N, Bianchi S, Eid Fawzy M. Study on the haemodynamic importance of the supraaortic ridge and its implications in aortic valve reconstruction. In: Bodnar E (ed). Surgery for Heart Valve Disease. London, ICR Publishers, 1990:389-401
14. Senning A. Facia lata replacement of aortic valves. J Thorac Cardiovasc Surg 1967;54:465-470
15. Batista RJV, Dobrianskij A, Comazzi M, et al. Clinical experience with stentless pericardial monopatch for aortic valve replacement. J Thorac Cardiovasc Surg 1987;93:19-26
16. Yacoub M, Khaghani A, Dhalla N, et al. Aortic valve replacement using unstented dura or calf pericardium: early and medium term results. In: Bodnar E, Yacoub M (eds). Biologic and Bioprosthetic Valves. New York, Yorke Medical Books, 1986:684-690
17. Al Fagih MR, AI Kasab SM, Ashmeg A. Aortic valve repair using bovine pericardium for cusp extension. J Cardiovasc Surg 1988;96:760-764
18. Duran C, Kumar N, Gometza B, AI Halees Z. Indications and limitations of aortic valve reconstruction. Ann Thorac Surg 1991;52:447-454
19 Acar C, Brizard C, Berrebi A et al. A standardized technique of aortic valve repair using cusp extension with autologous pericardium for rheumatic aortic insufficiency. Ann Thorac Surg 1996;(in press)
20. Bessou JP, Carpentier A. Valvuloplasties dans les insuffisances aortiques. Information Cardiol 1993;7:645-649
21. Chachques JC, Vasseur B, Perrier P, Balansa J, Chauvaud S, Carpentier A. A rapid method to stabilize biological materials for cardiovascular surgery. Ann NY Acad Sci 1988;529:184-186
22. Duran C, Gometza B, Al Halees Z. J Heart Valve Dis 1994; 3:439-444

Chapter 8.6

Reconstructive Surgery of the Tricuspid Valve

Philippe Grare MD, Alain Deloche MD

The surgical indications and therapeutics of tricuspid valve disease are closely related to their etiologies. Functional tricuspid valve insufficiency constitutes the most frequent cause of tricuspid valve disease and is therefore discussed first. Organic rheumatic tricuspid insufficiency is present in only a small group which will be discussed in the same section. Infective tricuspid insufficiency, less frequent and with different therapeutic strategies, will also be discussed. Finally, degenerative, ischemic and traumatic tricuspid valve diseases, which are the least frequently encountered etiologies, will be briefly overviewed. Whatever the etiology, the main objective of the surgical treatment is to preserve tricuspid valve function with conservative surgical techniques.

FUNCTIONAL AND ORGANIC RHEUMATIC TRICUSPID VALVE INSUFFICIENCY

Annuloplasty

In 1965, Kay (1) was the first author to apply a reconstructive surgical technique for tricuspid valve insufficiency. The operation he advocated consisted of the creation of a bicuspid valve, excluding the posterior leaflet, resulting in shortening of the annular circumference (Fig. 8.6-1).

Other surgical strategies were then developed; De Vega in 1972 (2) proposed an annuloplasty technique using a double purse-string to narrow the tricuspid annulus corresponding to the anterior and posterior leaflets (Fig. 8.6-2). The septal part of the annulus was not involved in the repair in order to avoid a complete atrio-ventricular (AV) block due to perioperative AV conduction pathway injury. This technique is simple and still remains popular and widely used. In 1972 a similar technique was described by Cabrol (3) in France.

Carpentier presented a remodeling semi-rigid prosthetic tricuspid ring annuloplasty to reconstruct native tricuspid valve geometry and selectively reduce the pathologic dilatation of the posterior and anterior parts of the tricuspid annulus in 1974 (4) (Fig. 8.6-3). Duran introduced a flexible prosthetic ring in 1975 (5). The objective of this prosthesis is to allow physiologic motion of the tricuspid annulus during the cardiac cycle.

All these surgical procedures are performed under cardiopulmonary bypass. The surgeon then proceeds to the analysis and correction of left heart valvular pathologies. The tricuspid valve is inspected and can be repaired after aortic unclamping in order to decrease global myocardial ischemia. Based on a systematic perioperative tricuspid valve analysis, numerous reconstructive techniques can be performed on the leaflet, subvalvular apparatus, or commissures; they are the applications of the well known mitral valve reconstructive surgery.

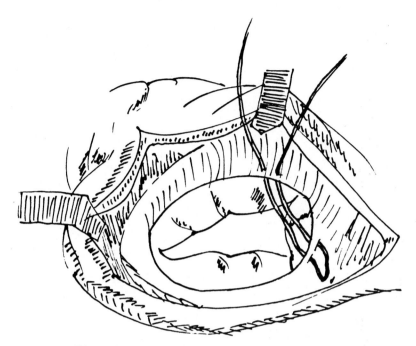

Figure 8.6-1: Kay technique of tricuspid annuloplasty.

Surgical indications

The surgical treatment of functional tricuspid valve insufficiency secondary to left sided valvular pathologies resulting from increased pulmonary artery pressure and right ventricular dilatation is relatively frequent (20% to 30% based on different clinical studies). The main objective of the treatment should be preservation of the native valve.

The avoidance of any correction of functional tricuspid valve insufficiency (FTVI) during left heart valvular surgery had been proposed in the past (6,7). The occurrence of progressive postoperative right heart failure secondary to massive FTVI after mitral and aortic valve surgery changed this therapeutic concept. Although there is a consensus to surgically treat any massive FTVI, the operative correction of moderate FTVI remains to some extent controversial. Some authors advise early repair of moderate FTVI (8). An argument in favor of early correction is the unpredictable decrease of pulmonary hypertension postoperatively (9). Moreover, recent studies have shown good results of tricuspid valvuloplasty whatever the surgical technique used. These results are in favor of a more widespread use of this type of operation. This therapeutic strategy helps optimize the postoperative clinical outcome and can give better long term results.

The surgical correction of organic tricuspid valve stenosis and insufficiency is widely accepted, and only mild cases may be controversial (10,11). Even if there is a consensus concerning the surgical treatment of organic tricuspid valve disease, many options exist and vary among surgical teams. It is important to remember that tricuspid valvuloplasty can be performed in 93% of cases (10).

Chronologically, the first surgical treatment to be proposed was tricuspid valve replacement (TVR). At present, it is used only when valvuloplasty is technically

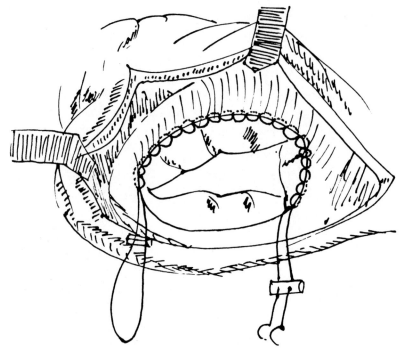

Figure 8.6-2: De Vega technique of tricuspid annuloplasty.

impossible. Mechanical prostheses were initially used, but were abandoned owing to major clinical drawbacks (12,13), including:

- increased risk of thrombosis (whatever the type of prosthesis chosen);
- inappropriate hemodynamics (>5 mmHg gradient postoperatively);
- prosthetic mitral ball valve encrustation into the wall of the right ventricle.

Presently, bioprostheses are the preferred alternatives. Their hemodynamic performance is better and they are associated with very low rates of thrombotic events. However TVR presents an increased risk of postoperative complete AV block because of the need to place sutures circumferentially around the tricuspid annulus.

Results

Comparison among different surgical series remains difficult to summarize. The evaluation of clinical outcome is global and takes into account each step of the treatment. Moreover preoperative or postoperative grading of the tricuspid valve insufficiency (TVI), and thus the evaluation of the surgical results is often incomplete owing to the specific limits of the various techniques used for diagnosis (clinical data, angiogram, cardiac catheterization, and perioperative digital evaluation of tricuspid valve regurgitation).

Doppler echocardiography (including intraoperative use) is of growing importance in the diagnosis of TVI (10-17) although it has not been widely used in the previous reports.

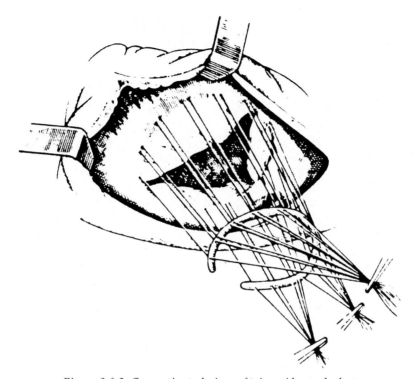

Figure 8.6-3: Carpentier technique of tricuspid annuloplasty.

Echocardiography also has its technical limits and can determine organic TV disease in only approximately 42% of cases (10).

Tricuspid valvuloplasty series have recently been evaluated and have demonstrated appropriate results overall (9,11,18-21). The operative mortality of multiple valve surgery depends on the extent of the procedure itself and on the patient's preoperative clinical status. The main predictive factors are preoperative left ventricular ejection fraction, patient age, functional NYHA class, the chronicity of left heart failure, pulmonary hypertension and the number of surgical maneuvers performed (11).

Operative mortality ranges from 5% to 31% in clinical series, this wide variation in results may be explained by inadequate myocardial protection techniques in earlier studies. Recent publications have demonstrated lower mortality rates from 5% to 16% (10,18-22). The main causes of death are congestive heart failure, acute myocardial infarction, malignant arrhythmias, gastrointestinal bleeding, infection and central nervous system complications.

As for hemodynamic results, Duran (11) found a mean postoperative gradient of 3 mmHg in 38% of all cases; this condition was more frequently encountered in organic (44%) than in functional TVI (31%). Postoperative TVI was noted in 30% of the patients (angiographic grade II - III) predominantly documented in organic (41%) rather than in functional TVI (18%).

Haerten (23), using the De Vega tricuspid annuloplasty, reported a moderate 2-7 mmHg postoperative gradient in 50% of his cases. The TVI was unchanged or increased in 41% of the patients.

Hanania (18) noted a small postoperative gradient (<3 mmHg) in 36% of cases after Carpentier tricuspid annuloplasty. Mild or severe postoperative TVI were respectively identified in 44% and 4% of patients. TVI was completely cured in 52% of cases.

Lambertz (9) showed a 4 mmHg postoperative right atrioventricular gradient in 33% of patients after Carpentier tricuspid annuloplasty. Postoperative TVI persisted in 31% of patients, was mild to moderate in 27% and severe in 4%. Relland (24), did not find any residual TVI after Carpentier annuloplasty in a group of 30 patients (15 functional, 15 organic); the mean postoperative gradient was 1.5 mmHg.

The global experience with various types of tricuspid valvuloplasty techniques demonstrates that approximately two third of patients do not demonstrate any or mild postoperative TVI, one third have moderate residual TVI, and finally approximately 4% of patients present with severe TVI after reconstructive surgery. Small postoperative gradients are documented postoperatively (<5 mmHg) whatever the technique used. The recurrence of TVI after a tricuspid valvuloplasty is rare, most authors relating this problem to failure of the associated mitral or aortic surgery which causes an elevated postoperative pulmonary artery pressure (14).

Reoperations for isolated failure of tricuspid valve repair are infrequent (25), and Carpentier (12) reported that tricuspid valve insufficiency was never implicated as a cause of reoperation in cases of combined mitral and tricuspid valve surgical procedures.

Even if reoperation for isolated recurrent TVI is a rare condition, results have been deceptive (9,14,15,25), in terms of mortality, morbidity and functional benefit, particularly in cases with poor right ventricular function.

In conclusion, late postoperative TVI after left sided heart valve surgery can be reduced by early treatment of mitral lesions and precise evaluation of TVI in combination with an adequate tricuspid valvuloplasty (26). Echocardiography in these circumstances constitutes an excellent diagnostic tool.

SURGICAL TREATMENT OF TRICUSPID VALVE ENDOCARDITIS

An increasing indication for tricuspid valve (TV) surgical intervention is infective endocarditis, which has become more widespread because of the rising incidence of intravenous drug abuse. Other causes of TV infections include pacemaker lead infections or intravenous catheter sepsis. Endocarditis complicating congenital heart diseases will not be discussed in this chapter.

The most frequently encountered infective micro-organism is *Staphylococcus aureus*. TV endocarditis is sometimes associated with mitral and aortic valvular infections (27).

Intravenous antibiotics should be started systematically according to the specific infecting micro-organism and should permit control of the septic process. However, surgical treatment is necessary in the presence of continued sepsis, moderate or severe right heart failure (secondary to septic valvular destruction) and multiple pulmonary septic emboli.

Several surgical alternatives can be considered:

- Tricuspid valvuloplasty is often successful and not associated with a late recurrence of infection (28,29). The surgical techniques involved may be vegetation resection, TV

leaflet pericardial patch and all other principles of mitral valve repair. Usually there is no tricuspid ring dilatation which does not dictate any TV annuloplasty.
- In 1971 Arbulu recommended tricuspid valvectomy to remove the infected focus, and avoid early or late re-infection in cases of intravenous drug addiction (30,31).
- Lastly, some authors have directly advocated tricuspid valve replacement (TVR) (27) with clinical results comparable to tricuspid valvectomy.

In summary, reconstructive TV surgery should be systematically attempted, particularly if the infection is localized (32). Tricuspid valve repair avoids foreign material use and improves the hemodynamic status. When tricuspid valvuloplasty is impossible the surgeon should consider valvectomy or TVR. Tricuspid valvectomy is usually well tolerated in patients with normal preoperative right ventricular function (28). However, right heart failure has been found in one third of patients (27). Moreover, TV excision does not eliminate the risk of left-sided endocarditis.

The disadvantages of tricuspid valvectomy are therefore hemodynamic, leading to right ventricular failure, while TV replacement may increase the risk of re-infection. Stern (27) does not suggest TVR as a risk factor for late endocarditis, since the main prognostic factor is the recurrence of drug addiction itself.

Finally, TVR with a mitral homograft has recently been suggested by Pomar (33). This procedure could be an interesting compromise when reconstructive surgery of the TV it is not possible.

In the case of combined mitral and tricuspid endocarditis a recent publication (34) reported the use of double mitral homografts in the tricuspid and mitral positions, avoiding the use of bioprostheses and preserving long term right ventricular function. However, these results have yet to be confirmed.

TRAUMATIC TRICUSPID INSUFFICIENCY

The incidence of traumatic tricuspid insufficiency is low but may be underestimated (35). This fact could be explained by diagnostic difficulties. Usually the tricuspid insufficiency is mild to moderate and clinically well tolerated. Also, serious multi-organ injuries are treated in priority in the acute phase of a major trauma. Nevertheless tricuspid valve insufficiency is sometimes massive and constitutes an indication for surgery, which should be performed early to avoid severe right ventricular failure. Tricuspid valve repair has rarely been attempted and TVR is usually done. However, well trained surgical teams with elective valve repair techniques have been able to successfully complete tricuspid valvuloplasties (35).

References
1. Kay JH, Maselli-Campagna G, Tsuji HK. Surgical treatment of tricuspid insufficiency. Ann Surg 1965;162:53-58
2. De Vega N. La annuloplastia selectiva, regulable y permanente. Rev Esp Cardiol 1972;25:555-560
3. Cabrol C. Annuloplastie valvulaire: un nouveau procede. Nouv Press Med 1972;1:1366
4. Carpentier A, Deloche A, Hanania G. Surgical management of acquired tricuspid valve disease. J Thorac Cardiovasc Surg 1974;67:53-65
5. Duran CG, Cucchiara G, Ubago JP. A new flexible ring for atrio-ventricular annuloplasty. In: Proceedings of the annual meeting of the Society of Thoracic and Cardiovascular Surgeons of Great Britain and Ireland. Glasgow, Scotland 1975
6. Ben-Ismail M, Richard C, Kamoun M. Evolution de l'insuffisance tricuspidienne corrigee ou non apres

reparation par protheses des valulopathies mitrales ou mitro-aortiques. Arch Mal Coeur, 70eme annee, 1977;5:461-468

7. Braunwald MS, Ross J, Morrow AG. Conservative management of tricuspid regurgitation in patients undergoing mitral valve re placement. Circulation 1967;35(Suppl 1):63
8. Lambertz H, Flachskampf FA, Minale C. Tricuspid regurgitation in patients with mitral valve disease. Who needs tricuspid repair? Circulation 1988;78(Suppl II):210
9. Lambertz H, Minale C. Long term follow up after Carpentier tricuspid valvuloplasty. Am Heart J ;117:615-622
10. Prabhakar G, Kumar N, Gometza N. Surgery for organic rheumatic disease of the tricuspid valve. J Heart Valve Dis 1993;2:561- 566
11. Duran C, Pomar J, Colman T. Is tricuspid valve repair necessary? J Thorac Cardiovasc Surg 1980;80:849-860
12. Kratz JM, Crawford FA, Stroud MR. Trends and results in tricuspid valve surgery. Chest 1985;88:837-840
13. Ben-Ismail M, Curran Y, Bousnina A. Devenir au long cours des protheses en position tricuspide. Arch Mal Coeur 1981;74:1035- 1044
14. Groves PH, Hall RJC. Late tricuspid regurgitation following mitral valve surgery. J Heart Valve Dis 1992;1:80-86
15. De Simone R, Lange R, Tanzeem A. Adjustable tricuspid valve annuloplasty assisted by intraoperative transesophageal color Doppler echocardiography. Am J Cardiol 1993;71:926-931
16. Chopra HK, Nanda NC, Pohoey Fan. Can two-dimensional echocardiography and Doppler color flow mapping identify the need for tricuspid valve repair? J Am Coll Cardiol 1989;14:1266-1274
17. Wong M, Matsumura M, Kutsuzawa S. The value of Doppler echocardiography in the treatment of tricuspid regurgitation in patients with mitral valve replacement. J Thorac Cardiovasc Surg 1990;99:1003-1010
18. Hanania G, Sellier PH, Deloche A. Resultats a moyen terme de l'annuloplastie tricuspide reconstitutive de Carpentier. Arch Mal Coeur, 1974;67:895-909
19. Chidambaram M, Sultan A, Abdulali. Long-term results of De Vega tricuspid annuloplasty. Ann Thorac Surg 1987;43:185-188
20. Nakano S, Kawashima Y, Hirose H. Evaluation of long-term results of bicuspidalization annuloplasty for functional tricuspid regurgitation. J Thorac Cardiovasc Surg 1988;95:340-345
21. Kay GL, Morita S, Mendez M. Tricuspid regurgitation as sociated with mitral valve disease: repair and replacement. Ann Thorac Surg 1989;48:593-595
22. Carpentier A, Chauvaud S, Fabiani JN. Reconstructive surgery of mitral valve incompetence. J Thorac Cardiovasc Surg 1980;79:338- 348
23. Haerten K, Seipel L, Loogen F. Hemodynamic studies after De Vega's tricuspid annuloplasty. Cardiovasc Surg, Circulation 1978;58:28- 33
24. Relland in discussion of Duran C, Pomar J, Colman T. Is tricuspide valve repair necessary? J Thorac Cardiovasc Surg 1980;80:849- 860
25. Donzeau-Gouge P, Villard A, Olivier M. Reintervention tricuspidienne dans la chirurgie des valvulopathies rhumatismales. Arch Mal Coeur, 1984;77:255-261
26. Deloche A. Chirurgie des valvulopathies tricuspidiennes ac quises. Chirurgie due coeur droit. Actutalites de Chirurgie Cardiovasculaire de l'Hopital Broussais. Masson, 1980:15-28
27. Stern HJ, Sisto DA, Strom JA. Immediate tricuspid valve replacement for endocarditis. J Thorac Cardiovasc Surg 1986;91:163-167
28. Yee ES, Khonsari S. Right-sided infective endocarditis: valvuloplasty, valvectomy or replacement? J Cardiovasc Surg, 1989;30:744- 748
29. Allen MD, Slachman F, Craig Eddy A. Tricuspid valve repair for tricuspid valve endocarditis: tricuspid valve "recycling". Ann Thorac Surg 1991;51:593-598
30. Arbulu A, Holmes RJ, Asfaw I. Tricuspid valvectomy without replacement. J Thorac Cardiovasc Surg 1991;102:917-922
31. Arbulu A, Holmes RJ, Asfaw I. Surgical treatment of intractable right-sided infective endocarditis in drug addicts: 25 years experience. J Heart Valve Dis 1993;2:129-137
32. Carrel T, Schaffner A, Vogt P. Endocarditis in intravenous drug addicts and HIV infected patients: possibilities and limitations of surgical treatment. J Heart Valve Dis 1993;2:140-147
33. Pomar JL, Carlos-A Mestres. Tricuspid valve replacement using a mitral homograft. Surgical technique and initial results. J Heart Valve Dis 1993;2:125-128
34. Acar C, Iung B, Cormier B, et al. Double mitral homograft for recurrent bacterial endocarditis of the mitral and tricuspid valves. J Heart Valve Dis 1994;3:470-472
35. Gayet C, Pierre B, Delahaye JP. Traumatic tricuspid insuf ficiency: an underdiagnosed disease. Chest 1987;92:429-432

Chapter 8.7

Reoperations on Cardiac Valves

Manuel J. Antunes

Since the first heart valve replacement in 1960, more than a million valve prostheses have been implanted throughout the world in patients affected by all forms of valve disease (1). However, all types of prostheses have complications which result in significant morbidity and mortality. On the one hand, bioprostheses are subjected to structural failure and calcification, which are accelerated in young patients and during pregnancy. On the other hand, mechanical prostheses are prone to thromboembolic phenomena, especially in patients who are non-compliant with medical therapy, including anticoagulation. The incidence of these complications is usually time-related. Finally, in recent years there has been a renewed enthusiasm for the use of homografts, especially in cryopreserved form. Also, the use of unstented heterografts is attracting the interest of many surgeons. Although the long term intrinsic durability of these valves may be enhanced, technical aspects of implantation may still determine the need for substitution at a later stage.

Valve replacement thus only exchanges one disease for another and reoperations have become more frequent as the number of patients who have been subjected to valve surgery increases (2). Besides, as the incidence of complications following valve re-replacement increases in an exponential manner, multiple reoperations become a significant feature in all large series (3).

DEFINITION AND INCIDENCE

In the majority of reports on valvular reoperation published in the past, the authors have used definitions varying from the very restrictive, including only isolated replacement of a prosthesis or a bioprosthesis in either the mitral or the aortic position (4,5), to the very wide, including repeat operation on any patient who has had a previous intrapericardial procedure, such as coronary artery surgery and other non-valvular open heart operations, closed mitral commissurotomy, pericardiectomy, and even pericardial poudrage (6).

Although a previous invasion of the pericardium is one of the factors which influence the technique of reoperation and the results thereof, we believe that the definition should be restricted to procedures primarily directed at one or more cardiac valves, subsequent to an initial open heart procedure involving a valve in the same anatomic position. In our view, the most important factor affecting the results is the condition of the annulus after removal of the previous prosthesis. Hence patients who have had a previous valvuloplasty should be included and considered as a reference group.

This definition conforms with the recently adopted guidelines for reporting morbidity and mortality after cardiac valve operations, which define reoperation as "any operation that repairs, alters or replaces a previously placed prosthesis or repaired valve" (7). Other cardiac procedures performed during valvular reoperation, such as myocardial revascularization, influence the results significantly. These should, therefore, be differentiated from those of isolated valve procedures.

In our past experience (4,5,8), reoperations constituted 16.1% of 4,956 valve procedures performed over a 12-year period beginning in 1974. Equivalent figures have generally not been reported from other centers, but the incidence of reoperation is mentioned in most series dealing with the late follow up of patients subjected to all kinds of valve surgery. Hence reoperation may be required at a rate of 2%-24% per patient year after replacement with a bioprosthesis, depending on the age of the patients (9,10). Even in the groups where the initial incidence is lower, the hazard function curves demonstrate a marked increment in the rate of reoperation 8-12 years after valve replacement (11).

In contrast, there is a far greater homogeneity in the reported incidence of reoperation after mechanical valve replacement, varying between 2% and 4% per patient year, but resulting from a wide array of complications, of variable importance in different populations (12,13). In this case, the incidence of reoperation appears to be greater in the first year after valve replacement because of the prevalence of early prosthetic valve endocarditis and of bland periprosthetic leakage. Five years after mechanical valve replacement, the freedom from reoperation is identical to that observed after replacement with a bioprosthesis, at around 90%, but after 10 years about 80% of the patients remain free from this complication, as compared to 70% of those with bioprostheses (14).

CAUSES AND INDICATIONS

The major causes of reoperation are structural dysfunction or deterioration, including native valve dysfunction following a previous valvuloplasty, prosthetic valve endocarditis, bland periprosthetic leakage and thrombosis and thromboembolism. Less frequent causes include hemolysis, tissue overgrowth and other causes of non-structural failure, and patient-valve mismatch.

With the exception of structural failure, each category may be related to either valve or patient factors, or may result from technical errors during implantation of the prosthesis or performance of the valvuloplasty (15).

Structural dysfunction

Structural dysfunction may be defined as "any change in valve function resulting from an intrinsic abnormality causing stenosis or regurgitation" (7), which includes biodegradation of tissue valves, mechanical valve failure, and functional deterioration of reconstructed valves.

Bioprostheses

Degeneration and/or calcification of bioprostheses is likely to become the most frequent cause of reoperation because most tissue valves will eventually require

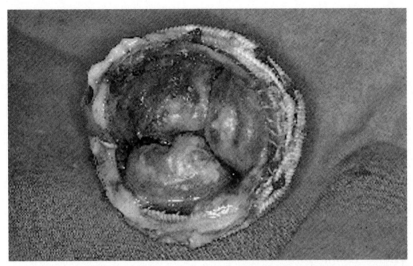

Figure 8.7-1: Degenerated porcine bioprosthesis explanted three years after implantation in a 14-year old patient. Note the egg-shell calcification of all three cusps.

replacement if the patients survive long enough; degeneration is clearly a time-related phenomenon (16). The incidence of this complication is related to several patient and valve-related factors. In general, the age of the population is the most influential (Fig. 8.7-1). The rate of failure of porcine bioprostheses may exceed 20% per patient year in patients less than 20 years of age (actuarial freedom from structural failure, 19% at five years) (9). However, it averages 2%-4% per patient year in patients older than 30 years, in whom the freedom from reoperation is 85%-90% at five years and 70%-75% at 10 years, but probably less than 40% at 15 years (17). For patients over the age of 70 years, primary tissue failure occurs at a rate of 0.2% per patient year (18).

The durability of these prostheses also varies with the position (lower in mitral than in aortic prostheses), type (lower in pericardial than in porcine) and make (design and quality of manufacture). Certain types and models of tissue valve were associated with earlier failure and some were removed from the market for this reason (19). One of the most illustrative cases was the Ionescu-Shiley bovine pericardial prosthesis, which was used for more than a decade, until very recently.

Reoperation for failure of a bioprosthesis is indicated, irrespective of the patient's symptomatic status, as soon as the signs of valve dysfunction occur, especially when there is regurgitation, which is usually a sign of eminent disintegration (20). The common belief that these devices degenerate slowly and that, when required, substitution of the prosthesis can be performed electively with low risk is a fallacy, especially in the younger and the older patients. We have seen several asymptomatic or only mildly symptomatic young patients with calcified stenotic bioprostheses die while awaiting elective valve re-replacement.

Mechanical prostheses

In contrast, modern era mechanical valves have generally been proven to be

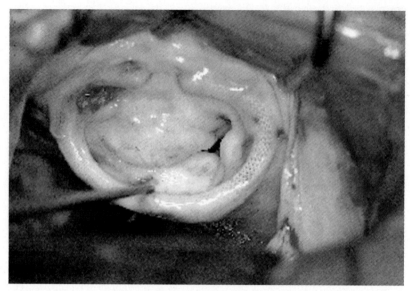

Figure 8.7-2: Intraoperative photograph of a mitral valve, 3 1/2 years after repair in a 13-year old child. The leaflets are scarred and distorted by recurrent acute rheumatic carditis.

remarkably free from structural failure (incidence less than 0.1% per patient year). Nevertheless, there have been some recent examples of valves bedevilled by mechanical failures which have forced definitive or temporary withdrawal from the market, as was the case with the C-C (convexo-concave) Björk-Shiley and Duromedics-Edwards valves. Failures may result from stress fracture of the valve ring, struts and occluders, or from poppet or disc wear, erosion and escape. These are catastrophic events which most often cause the immediate death of the patient or require reoperation on an emergency basis, which also carries a very high mortality.

Elective replacement has been performed for defective Braunwald-Cutter prostheses (21) and for the series 1000 Starr-Edwards valve (22). Even more recently, the problem was again raised by the structural problems of the C-C Björk-Shiley prosthesis. Although elective reoperation has not been considered necessary in all cases (23), it may be justified by the very high rates of structural failure of some batches of these valves which outweigh the morbidity and mortality of elective reoperation (20,24,25) (see also Chapter 9.5).

Valve repair and reconstruction

Reoperation for persistent, recurrent or new regurgitation or stenosis is virtually the only significant complication following mitral valve reconstruction. In rheumatic cases the incidence varies from 2%-4% per patient year (freedom from reoperation, 90% at five years and 80% at 10 years) (26,27), higher in younger than in older patients. Reoperation is required predominantly in the first year after the initial procedure, although a peak is likely to occur again much later in the follow up. It may result from technical error or progression of the rheumatic pathology, especially in younger patients (Fig. 8.7-2) (28).

On the other hand, the rate of valve failure is less than 1% per patient year in patients operated on for degenerative (Barlow's) disease (29). This has been a rather surprising finding since reconstruction fails to eliminate all the valve tissue, leaflets and chordae tendineae, diffusely involved in the pathologic process. Finally, the need for reoperation after repair of ischemic mitral regurgitation is as yet unknown because of the few and usually small reported series.

The indications for and timing of reoperation after valvuloplasty are identical to those accepted for the primary valve operation, but emergent intervention may be required in cases of sudden disruption, such as in rupture of the chordae tendineae and dehiscence of annuloplasty rings.

Prosthetic valve endocarditis

This group includes all cases of infection of the prosthesis and annular tissues, confirmed by preoperative positive blood cultures, echocardiographic evidence of vegetations or prosthetic dysfunction, and/or by intraoperative verification by the surgeon of the signs of active infection. Patients with a past history of endocarditis that has been cured spontaneously or by antibiotic therapy should not be included when they are reoperated for another cause, such as periprosthetic leaks, whether a consequence of the infectious process or not, because the risk and prognosis are different.

Early prosthetic valve endocarditis (within 60 days) is one of the most important causes of morbidity and mortality following valve replacement. It is the result of perioperative contamination of either endogenous or exogenous origin, by aggressive micro-organisms often resistant to antibiotics, of which the most common is staphylococcus epidermidis. The reported incidence averages 1%-4% and the mortality with medical therapy alone reaches 50% (30,31). Early surgery is therefore indicated,

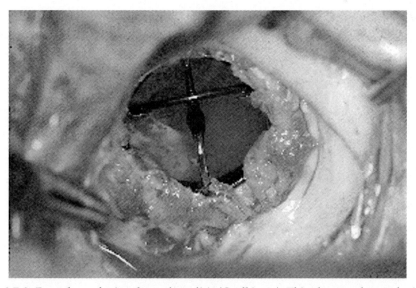

Figure 8.7-3: Fungal prosthetic valve endocarditis (C. albicans). This photograph was obtained 18 days after mitral valve replacement with a Medtronic Hall prosthesis in a patient who had not been infected previously.

especially if there are signs of prosthetic dysfunction. However, patients with positive blood cultures not accompanied by clinical and/or echocardiographic evidence of valve dysfunction may be managed medically, without surgery.

In contrast, late prosthetic valve endocarditis is more frequently caused by Streptococci and gram negative bacilli, usually sensitive to the most commonly used antibiotics. The reported incidence of this complication is 0.5%-1.0% per patient year. The mortality remains high but lower than that which is associated with early prosthetic valve endocarditis. If the diagnosis is made early and there are no signs of prosthetic dysfunction or periprosthetic leakage, a cure may be possible by medical treatment alone. Otherwise, reoperation is indicated and should be performed earlier rather than later as there is no evidence that prior sterilization by antibiotic therapy, even if possible, improves the results. Amongst all etiologies, fungal prosthetic endocarditis (Fig. 8.7-3) carries the poorest prognosis, with a mortality of over 50%, and surgery is always indicated as it usually constitutes the only hope for cure.

Infection often recurs and leads to multiple reoperations. As a matter of fact, the presence of infection at the time of implantation of the prosthesis is the strongest incremental risk factor for prosthetic valve endocarditis (29). The inability to cure the endocarditis is related to the destruction of the annular tissues, which prevents adequate insertion of a new prosthesis. Homograft aortic root replacement probably has one of its best indications here, since these valves are known to be more resistant to infection than other prostheses (32,33). In some cases, however, infection seems to perpetuate and cardiac tissues may be destroyed to such an extent that cardiac transplantation may become the only alternative (34).

Bland periprosthetic leakage

Under this designation are included all non-infected cases, as well as those of infective

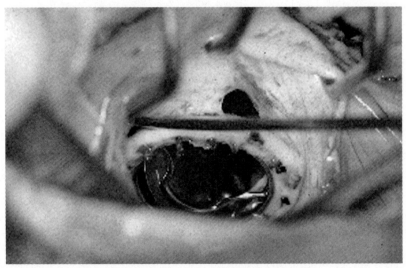

Figure 8.7-4: Periprosthetic leak after mitral valve replacement with a Bjork-Shiley prosthesis using an interrupted suture technique.

origin but which are sterile at the time of surgery. The reported incidence of this complication is 1%-4%, but it is probably underestimated since many minor leaks remain undiagnosed or may close with time. Periprosthetic leakage represents 13%-30% of the causes of reoperation in the larger series (8,35,36). It is also one of the most important causes of multiple reoperations, which accounted for 14% of both our series and that of Husebye et al. (21).

Periprosthetic leaks appear to occur more frequently with mechanical valves than with bioprostheses. They may also be related to the technique of implantation, since they are allegedly more often associated with continuous than with interrupted sutures (37). However, this has not been our experience and we believe that the real factor is accuracy rather than the type or technique (Fig. 8.7-4).

Since the symptomatic status of the patient does not bear a close relationship with the size of the defect (38), the decision to reoperate on perivalvular leaks is a difficult one. Due to the increased risk of prosthetic endocarditis, reoperation is probably indicated in all cases with more than mild regurgitation.

Valve thrombosis and systemic thromboembolism

Together, prosthetic thrombosis (Fig. 8.7-5) and systemic thromboembolism constitute the most important cause of composite mortality and morbidity after mechanical valve replacement. The incidence is variable and may be influenced by many factors, including the type of prosthesis, position, technique of implantation, chamber size and

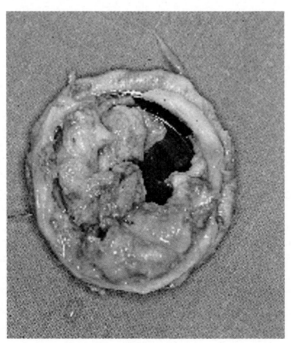

Figure 8.7-5: Thrombosed Medtronic Hall prosthesis. The laminated texture indicates the "chronic" nature of the process.

cardiac rhythm, but the most important is the compliance of the patient with anticoagulation.

The reported incidence of thrombosis, one of the most catastrophic complications of mechanical prostheses, is 0%-1.2% per patient year (average 0.5% per patient year) (39-41). In our experience, it led to the death of the patient in two thirds of cases (12,13). It may evolve slowly, by deposition of successive layers of platelet-rich clot, causing progressive dysfunction of the prosthesis, or rapidly, with formation of fresh red thrombus, often over an older layer of white thrombus (42). In this case the sudden dysfunction causes acute hemodynamic deterioration requiring emergent surgery, while in the other cases a timely diagnosis often permits elective or semi-elective operation.

This complication is thought to be less serious in bileaflet than in tilting disc valves. However, this does not conform to our experience with both compliant and non-compliant populations, where the incidence and respective mortality were identical with the St. Jude Medical and the Medtronic Hall prostheses (43,44).

Although successful thrombolysis has been reported (45-46), we believe that surgery remains the only safe method of treatment of thrombosed aortic and mitral prostheses and is indicated on an emergency basis, as soon as the diagnosis is made, especially when a mitral prosthesis is involved. In principle, the affected prosthesis should be replaced during reoperation. However, in the late 1970s and early 1980s we and others (47) used thrombectomy extensively in patients belonging to an underdeveloped population group. Most of the operations involved tilting disc valves, where it was possible to remove all the clot and leave the prosthetic disc clean and shiny. The method appeared to be very effective, but many patients returned later with thrombosed valves (48). Whether removal of the clot had been incomplete or the patients simply remained non-compliant with anticoagulation therapy is undetermined. Nevertheless, Indian surgeons have recently reported much better results with this technique. Evidently, clot removal may still be an option to consider in some circumstances, as it is a simple procedure which can be performed within very short cross-clamp times. Leaving the prosthesis, which has otherwise been performing well, may help to avoid the risk of periprosthetic leaks and, perhaps, of early prosthetic endocarditis. However, bileaflet prostheses are not suitable for declotting, because it is almost impossible to reach the hinges and eliminate all the clot.

Thrombosis of bioprostheses is much rarer and is usually reported together with degeneration, with which it is often associated (49). The indications for reoperation are also similar to those for degenerated valves (50).

A rare indication for reoperation is repeated systemic thromboembolism originating from cardiac prostheses, a diagnosis which should only be made when other sources of emboli have been excluded, which is often difficult to achieve. In some cases, however, a history of multiple embolic episodes may lead to the diagnosis of prosthetic thrombosis that was obscured by the liberation of fragments of clot, permitting adequate function of the prosthesis. In these cases reoperation is indicated on an urgent basis.

Other causes

Growth of host tissue over the sewing and metal rings is a cause of prosthetic stenosis.

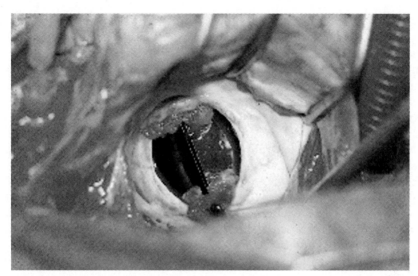

Figure 8.7-6: Thrombosed Standard St. Jude Medical mitral valve. Note the exuberant fibrous tissue overgrowth, which may have been the primary cause of the thrombosis.

We have seen this complication more frequently with standard Björk-Shiley valves, which may simply reflect the time elapsed since implantation, as it appeared to occur with increasing frequency after 10 or 12 years of follow up. The incidence of this complication may be influenced by the type of cloth of which the sewing ring is made (dacron vs. teflon). As the fibrous tissue grows over and encroaches on the valve orifice, it may impair the movement of the occluder and finally cause the valve to thrombose (Fig. 8.7-6) (42). Surgery is indicated when there is evidence of increasing transvalvular gradients and/or of valvular dysfunction.

Patient-valve mismatch, another form of prosthetic stenosis, is an infrequent cause of reoperation. It may be the consequence of either the implantation of a valve too small for the patient's size, especially in the case of some old, relatively inefficient models, or of the growth of the patient subsequent to valve replacement. In either case the indications for programmed replacement of the prosthesis are identical to those for stenosis of the native valves, especially in the aortic position.

Subclinical hemolysis is associated with almost all mechanical prostheses. However, severe hemolysis may occur with apparently normal valves. It may be caused either by the impact of blood jets on sutures and remains of the native valve tissue or by small periprosthetic leaks of otherwise little or no hemodynamic significance (51). Finally, minor irregularities in the valve components may cause significant hemolysis. When other causes of damage to the blood cells are excluded, surgery for replacement of the prosthesis or repair of the leak is indicated.

TIMING OF THE REOPERATION

In most centers, the follow up of patients in whom valve prostheses have been implanted is carried out by their cardiologists, mostly for logistic reasons. Surgeons should, however, be kept informed about the clinical evolution of their patients and be immediately notified of any complications, especially those of a surgical nature. The decision with regards to the indication for and timing of reoperation should essentially be theirs or, at least, be discussed and made jointly with the cardiologist.

The indications for reintervention were discussed for each subset of pathology. In many instances the patients are very symptomatic and require urgent or emergency surgery. However, the operative mortality is much higher after reoperations performed on an emergency basis than after elective procedures, as discussed below.

Based on these considerations we have progressively changed the timing of reoperation in the past decade towards earlier reintervention, before significant deterioration of the symptomatic status of the patient occurs. This applies, for example, to patients with bioprostheses once the signs of degeneration arise, especially if there is regurgitation, which is a sign of eminent disintegration of one or more cusps. It is also applicable in the case of dysfunction of mechanical prostheses, especially that which results from ingrowth of fibrous tissue with increasing transvalvular gradients, even if there is no restriction to the movement of the occluder. When the latter is observed reoperation is urgent as the risk of thrombosis is very high, especially in mitral prostheses.

Elective substitution of certain batches of C-C Björk-Shiley prostheses is indicated because of the higher risk of strut fracture (24). Is is also indicated in the case of some cloth-covered Starr-Edwards prostheses, now relatively rare, with evidence of cloth wear and embolization. Finally, prosthetic replacement may also be required in patients with recurrent systemic embolism when other embolic sources have been excluded.

In contrast, reoperation is perhaps better delayed in the case of periprosthetic leaks or residual valve dysfunction after valvuloplasty in asymptomatic or only mildly symptomatic patients. However, these patients should be careful and closely monitored for early detection of the signs of ventricular dysfunction, in which case surgery should be undertaken without delay.

On the other hand, when patients present in an advanced functional class, reoperation may be indicated on an emergency basis. However, delaying surgery, if possible, may improve the patients' chances of survival. In the past decade we have succeeded in cooling down the pathologic process and improving the functional class of many patients who were subsequently operated on electively or semi-electively with much lower mortality. This was possible in the majority of cases of non-structural prosthetic dysfunction and was achieved by aggressive anti-failure therapy; if a rapid improvement was not observed reoperation was performed immediately. No patient was lost while pursuing this policy which, however, is not applicable to patients with prosthetic thrombosis or mechanical dysfunction, who must be operated on an emergency basis.

Special consideration must be given to the problem of prosthetic valve endocarditis. Patients without signs of prosthetic dysfunction or periprosthetic leakage may be cured medically by antibiotic therapy alone. However, the majority of patients present with partial dehiscence of the prosthesis. In the past it has often been said that there is nothing to gain from waiting in these cases, but we have also modified our approach in recent years. Patients can often be improved symptomatically by aggressive anticongestive therapy. While doing this there is the opportunity to obtain identification of the infective agent and initiate adequate antimicrobial therapy. Most patients currently reach surgery one to two weeks after diagnosis and the results obtained appear to vindicate this policy.

From what was discussed above it appears obvious that virtually no patient is too sick for surgery but that many patients can be markedly improved before the procedure is undertaken. Recently, however, the problem of patients with acquired immuno-deficiency syndrome has caused great controversy. While HIV-positive patients who do not have clinical manifestations of the disease should be offered the benefit of surgical treatment, in our opinion those with full-blown AIDS should probably be managed only medically because the risk to the surgical team is not justified by the short-term benefit to the patient. Finally, drug addicts who present with repeated episodes of prosthetic endocarditis caused by continuous use of intravenous drugs should probably also be refused surgery.

TECHNIQUE OF REOPERATION

Reoperations are certainly more difficult to perform than the initial procedures, mainly because of the pericardial adhesions and the condition of the annulus after removal of the prosthesis (28,52). Nevertheless, the results are not necessarily worse (6). There are a wide variety of concerns, including re-entry into the mediastinum and the pericardial cavity, techniques of cardiopulmonary bypass, access to the faulty prosthesis, treatment or removal of this prosthesis, and hemorrhage and blood saving.

Planning of the operation

Surgeons are often reluctant to reoperate patients who were originally operated on by another surgeon from a different cardiac team, especially if the surgical report is not available (53). Often the patients do not know what surgery was performed. For example, it is important to know whether or not the pericardium was closed. Information about the type and size of the prosthesis and the technique of suture used is also important because it may provide important clues regarding the mode of treatment. A postoperative mediastinal infection is likely to produce more adhesions in the retro-sternal space and, therefore, make reopening more difficult and dangerous unless special precautions are taken. Finally, a chest X-ray may help the surgeon to plan the reoperation (Fig. 8.7-7). It shows the number of wires used previously and whether the right ventricle is distended against the sternum, in which case it may be preferable to institute cardiopulmonary bypass prior to sternal re-entry, as discussed below.

Reopening of the sternum and pericardium

Reopening of the sternum is one of the most difficult and potentially dangerous steps of the procedure (54,55). It can be performed using a technique similar to that used for primary operations. After removal of the wires or sutures closing the sternum, an oscillating saw is used by most surgeons to cut through the external table of the sternum and the intermediate space. The mediastinal or posterior table may also be sawn or cut with scissors under vision, in order to prevent perforation of the right ventricle or the right atrium when they are enlarged (56). Leaving the cut wires in place while sawing through the bone is a useful trick to avoid injury to the underlying structures (57).

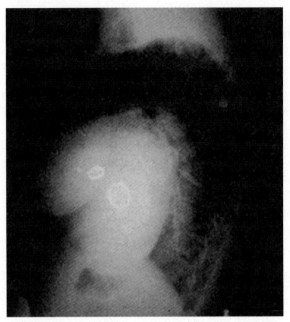

Figure 8.7-7: Lateral view chest X-ray showing the right ventricle adherent to the posterior table of the sternum following a previous aortic and mitral valve replacement with Björk-Shiley prostheses.

However, the stryker saw may be used starting from below. The sub-xiphoid space is dissected with scissors, separating the pericardium and/or the heart from the back of the sternum. While the first assistant pulls the sternum upwards with rake retractors, two to three centimeters of the sternum are sawn at a time, progressing cephalad until it is completely open.

The tissues behind the sternum are dissected further laterally, using scissors or electrocautery. Occasionally, it may be useful to open into the pleural spaces. The pericardial space is then entered. If the pericardium had been closed in the end of the previous operation, there should be a small window in the lower part of the mediastinum where the serosa was not completely closed to give passage to the drain. This window is easily identified because of the bulging of the congested right ventricle. Sometimes the previous suture line can also be seen. However, if the pericardium was not closed during the previous operation, its edges will be found somewhat more laterally.

In order to reduce the incidence of hemorrhagic complications, dissection of the pericardium over the left side of the heart must be kept to a minimum, limited to the area over the aorta and main pulmonary artery, where the aortic cross-clamp is to be applied. We do not consider complete dissection of the heart essential for either adequate exposure of the target valve or deairing of the cardiac cavities at the end of the procedure. On the other hand, complete dissection of the right side, over the lateral wall of the right atrium and venae cavae, to expose the interatrial groove, is essential, especially for mitral valve procedures. It is also necessary for aortic procedures if venting of the left ventricle is done through the right superior pulmonary vein and left atrium, as we routinely do.

If required, cardiopulmonary bypass can also be instituted at this stage. In severely congested patients, the dilated right atrium often complicates dissection and it may be easier to commence bypass with the arterial cannula in the aorta and a single drain in the right atrium to decompress the heart. In emergency situations this may be done as soon as the aorta and the right atrial appendage are exposed. Usually the aorta is easily identifiable and the atrium can also be rapidly reached through the right pleural cavity, entered immediately after the sternal split. In most cases, however, dissection should be completed before heparinization.

Pericardial adhesions are more dense and hemorrhagic from the second to the 6th-9th month postoperatively. Thereafter the adhesions become avascular and looser. Dissection is clearly easier after two or three years. Hence, if reoperation can be delayed, for example for bland periprosthetic leaks, it is best performed after one year.

Cardiopulmonary bypass and access to the cardiac cavities

Cardiopulmonary bypass may be established in several ways. Many surgeons concerned about opening the sternum in the presence of adhesions advocate the routine use of femoral vein to femoral artery bypass before sternal re-entry (55). After moderate cooling, the heart is emptied and as it collapses and pulls away from the sternum, the bone can be opened with the saw without danger to the heart. In our experience, however, this was unnecessary in most cases, and cardiopulmonary bypass was instituted in the classic way, only after sternotomy. Generally, we prefer right atrium-to-aorta cardiopulmonary bypass. A single or double-stage cannula may be used for venous drainage, but two vena cavae cannulae are routinely used for mitral procedures.

If bleeding occurs during reopening, the aorta or the femoral artery are cannulated *in extremis*, while an assistant packs the mediastinum with a large abdominal swab. A drain can then be inserted through the wound of the right ventricle or right atrium. In high risk situations, the femoral or iliac artery only may be preventively cannulated.

The usual oblique or longitudinal incision of the aortic root should be used for access to an aortic prosthesis. The tendency to make this incision too high renders exposure of the prosthesis very difficult. To avoid this, the fat pad of the right ventricular wall must be dissected away from the aortic root, which must also be separated from the right atrial appendage and superior vena cava before the aortic clamp is applied.

In contrast, several approaches have been advocated for the mitral valve, including the classical incision between the interatrial groove and the right pulmonary veins. In reoperations, the exposure of the mitral valve offered by this incision is clearly more limited than that which it gives in primary valve procedures, especially in small atria and where the adhesions of the left side of the heart have not been released. Nevertheless, this classic approach has been adequate in the majority of our patients. In the most difficult cases, wide opening of the left pleural cavity, allowing a leftward rotation of the heart, may be used to improve exposure.

On the other hand, the superior approach through the root of the left atrium, used by some, provides excellent exposure, probably as good as it does in the first operation. A modification of the Dubost technique, recently described (58), starts with the classical approach. If the visualization of the valve is difficult, a T-incision through the right atrial wall and the interatrial septum is carried out, giving a completely unobstructed view of the mitral valve. We have also frequently used a direct transseptal approach via the right atrium in cases with large atria and when a tricuspid valve procedure was also required. However, all these alternative approaches may create additional difficulties, since the surgeon must first dissect and snare the superior and inferior vena cavae. Also, the final integrity of the interatrial septum may be affected.

Finally, a right anterolateral thoracotomy during femoro-femoral bypass without aortic cross-clamping or cardioplegia has been recommended. This gives excellent exposure of the mitral valve, especially for multiple reoperations (59).

Removal of the prosthesis

In some circumstances it may not be necessary to remove the prosthesis. Prosthetic thrombosis, already discussed, may be treated by removal of the clot. Another such situation is tissue overgrowth. In these cases, removal of a ring of fibrous tissue from each side of either or both mitral and aortic prostheses is usually quite simple (Fig. 8.7-8). As in the case of declotting, single disc valves are more amenable to this procedure, because the ventricular aspect of the ring is more readily accessible, especially when the prosthesis can be rotated. Long term results are unavailable at this stage, but the potential advantages of not having to remove the prosthesis also apply here. Finally, small bland periprosthetic leaks can be closed directly within very short aortic cross-clamp periods. Interrupted teflon-pledgeted sutures must be used since the tissues are often weak in the area of the leak.

In the majority of cases, retrieval of the abnormal prosthesis is required and presents some additional technical difficulties. We believe that it is preferable to remove the valve intact. This may be accomplished by cutting the sutures and dissecting the interface between the sewing ring and the tissues, thus leaving the annulus virtually ready for the new sutures and prosthesis (60,61). Others suggest cutting through the sewing ring, first removing the body of the prosthesis, and retrieving the remains of the ring subsequently. It may be simpler, but the risk of embolization by particles left behind is greater. The technique used must be tailored to the circumstances. It is important, however, that utmost care is exercised to preserve the integrity of the patient's annulus, especially in the case of the mitral valve, where the atrioventricular junction may easily be disrupted, with disastrous consequences.

Excision of bioprostheses is more hazardous than that of mechanical valves because larger sizes were usually forced into the annulus and the struts tend to adhere intimately to the ventricular or aortic walls. The native aortic valve and the circumflex artery are particularly at risk during retrieval of a mitral bioprosthesis.

Treatment of annular abscesses in the case of prosthetic valve endocarditis may represent another very delicate technical problem (62). Autologous or bovine pericardial patches have been used to reconstruct the disrupted annular areas (63). Whenever possible, however, aortic root abscesses should be left open to the bloodstream to facilitate sterilization, and the prosthesis should be sutured either to the inferior or superior edge, whichever appears to be more convenient. Nevertheless, if the abscess threatens to rupture into the pericardium or in the case of very extensive annular destruction, homograft aortic root replacement may be the best option. Artificial composite grafts may also be used, but homografts are more resistant to

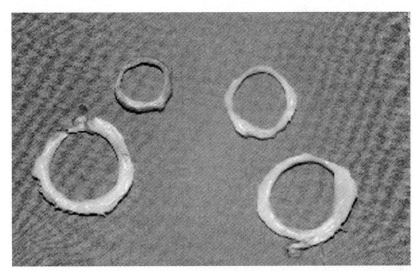

Figure 8.7-8: Fibrous rings removed intraoperatively from both sides of aortic and mitral prostheses without signs of dysfunction other than increasing transvalvular gradients.

reinfection (64,65). We have recently commenced implanting integral aortic valve homografts (valve + aortic sinuses) in the subcoronary position. The proximal suture line is placed in the myocardial walls of the ventricular outflow tract and across the mitro-aortic curtain. It is hoped that maintaining the valve's natural tubular insertion will enhance the durability. Finally, transplantation has also been suggested for situations of uncontrolled infection accompanied by extensive destruction of cardiac tissues (66).

Implantation of a new prosthesis

Choosing a prosthesis for re-replacement is often quite difficult. Is it correct to insert a mechanical valve when reoperating for a degenerated bioprosthesis in a young but non-compliant patient? Or to implant a biological valve in a similar patient reoperated on for a thrombosed mechanical prosthesis? The decision must take into account the individual characteristics of the patient and the surgeon's experience with the population involved. Additionally, the pathology and anatomy of the annulus may influence the decision. Bioprostheses, for example, conform better with annular irregularities and are alledgely more resistant to reinfection (Fig. 8.7-9).

As in the first valve replacement, a continuous suture may be used for mitral valve reimplantation if the annulus is still fairly regular after removal of the previous prosthesis or after a previous valvuloplasty. Often, however, interrupted sutures must be used to ensure that the tissues hold, because the annulus is not as subtle and pliable as in the initial procedure. On the other hand, simple interrupted sutures are usually preferred for aortic valve implantation. The use of teflon pledgets is not always warranted, but when necessary they should be placed on the atrial or aortic side, whatever the case may be, although there may be arguments against this.

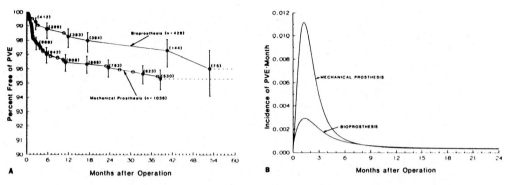

Figure 8.7-9: (A) Actuarial incidence of freedom from prosthetic valve endocarditis after valve replacement with mechanical prostheses and bioprostheses (70% confidence limits). (B) Hazard function in the same groups of patients. (Reproduced from Ivert TSA, et al. Circulation 1984;69:223-232, by permission of the American Heart Association).

Postoperative hemorrhage and blood saving

Contrary to what is commonly believed, in our experience perioperative hemorrhage has not generally been more significant after reoperation than after primary procedures. However, patients reoperated during the first year, while the adhesions remain vascular and edematous, tend to bleed more.

Some aspects of the surgical technique may alter the significance of postoperative hemorrhage. These include limitation of the initial dissection of the pericardium to what is essential for canulation and access to the prosthesis, as discussed above. On the other hand, closure of the pericardial space not only facilitates an eventual re-reoperation but also helps prevent the accumulation of free blood and clots, itself a factor in the perpetuation of the hemorrhage. However, pericardial closure may not be possible, particularly if it was not closed during the first operation. Glutaraldehyde preserved bovine pericardium has been used as a pericardial substitute (67), but the Gore-tex membrane has apparently had better results (68). Recently, artificial absorbable membranes were tested in animals with encouraging results (69). Nevertheless, Loop (54) found no difference in the incidence of catastrophic hemorrhage between patients with open and closed pericardium.

These patients are often on anticoagulation therapy. Additionally, congestive cardiac failure frequently leads to hepatic failure with lower prothrombin activity. Hence, substitution or pharmacologic manipulation of the clotting factors may be important. Recently, high-dose aprotinin (Trasylol) has been shown to reduce perioperative bleeding significantly by preserving or restoring platelet function (70,71). The beneficial effect, initially described for doses of $5-6 \times 10^6$ units (700-850 mg, approximately), was also observed in low-dose protocols (2×10^6 units) (72,73). It may be especially relevant during reoperations. Royston et al. (74) found that blood loss in treated patients was only approximately 20 percent of that in untreated patients who had eight times higher blood transfusion requirements. An identical experience was described by Biagini et al. (75) in a series of 53 patients subjected to valvular reoperations and by Cosgrove et al. (76) in a randomized study of 171 patients who suffered reoperative myocardial revascularization. However, the latter found an increased incidence of myocardial infarction, corresponding to occluded grafts, and of renal dysfunction.

The use of this drug is thus advised in patients with an increased risk of bleeding, such as those who are on anticoagulation or anti-platelet therapy and those with hepatic failure, especially if reoperation is performed early (1-12 months) after the initial procedure. Our experience, albeit limited, also appears to indicate the effectiveness of a low-dose protocol. In these cases a single dose of 2×10^6 units is added to the pump prime. The drug may even be effective if administered in the ICU, when excessive blood loss occurs in patients who were not treated intraoperatively.

Many surgeons now use the cardiotomy reservoir to collect mediastinal and chest tube drainage. The reservoir is simply attached to the drains, using the bypass circuit tubing or a fresh set of tubing, and the collected blood may be retransfused automatically with an electronic pump. We use a very inexpensive and unsophisticated method of reinfusion, made of a regular blood transfusion set and filter interposed between the outlet of the reservoir and one of the three-way tap bridges used during the operation. Blood is reinfused manually with a 50 cc syringe, which should never be detached from the system to avoid infection.

RESULTS

Currently, perioperative and early mortality after reoperation is only slightly higher than that which follows primary valve replacement in most institutions with a significant experience of these procedures. Analysis and comparison of the results is difficult because of the lack of uniformity of the definitions of reoperation in the series published. For example, only 28% of patients included in the series of 1,000 reoperations published from the Cleveland Clinic underwent replacement of a prosthesis (6). As this was a significant risk factor in the series, the global results are bettered by the inclusion of the remaining 72% of patients. In contrast, our own series of 249 mitral and 203 aortic procedures included only cases where isolated replacement of a prosthesis or of a bioprosthesis in one of these positions was performed (4,5).

The analysis is also affected by the very large number of variables involved, making each series unique, and the obvious differences in the statistical methods used. With these limitations, we will attempt to give an overview of the results published over the past decade alone (4-6,17,18,22,23,33-36,60,77,78), since the year of operation was one of the risk factors in most series where this variable was studied, recent procedures showing better results. Nevertheless, other large series published in the late 1970's deserve consideration and will be mentioned occasionally (79,80).

Perioperative mortality

Surgical and early mortality after reoperations varied from 8.7% to 21.3% and is affected by a number of patient factors, including the functional class, by the timing of the procedure and by the pathologic process involved (Table 8.7-I).

Functional class and emergency

The number of patients operated on an emergency basis had a major influence on the results (Table 8.7-II). Hence, the mortality for elective reoperation was 1.3% in the series reported by Husebye et al. (21) from the Mayo Clinic, but this rate was heavily

Table 8.7-I: Significant risk factors for operative mortality

EMERGENCY OPERATIONS
NYHA CLASS IV
PROSTHETIC VALVE ENDOCARDITIS
ASSOCIATED TRICUSPID PROCEDURES
MULTIPLE REOPERATIONS
FEMALE SEX

influenced by the very low mortality of 0.8% (one of 117) in patients operated on for replacement of Braunwald-Cutter valves "which had shown a tendency toward poppet wear and subsequent embolization".

On the other hand, the mortality rate for emergency procedures varied from 24.1% to 45% (28,81). The differences between elective and emergency procedures were also influenced by the classification criteria. Generally speaking, lower mortality rates for elective reoperations go hand in hand with higher rates for emergencies, reflecting the inclusion in the latter group of all patients in a more advanced NYHA functional class. In the report by Husebye et al. (21), only one of 223 patients operated upon electively was in Class IV, whereas 64% of the patients operated on an emergency basis were in this category. Consequently, neither of these two factors had an independent predictive value in the multivariate analysis.

Obviously, the results may be bettered by improving the condition of the patient preoperatively by medical therapy. In our more recent experience this was possible in many critical patients previously operated on as emergencies, with the exception of those with thrombosed valves. Persistent hypoxia and right ventricular failure are the commonest causes of death after cardiopulmonary bypass in patients presenting in pulmonary edema. Aggressive preoperative treatment with inotropes, diuretics and, occasionally, intermittent positive pressure ventilation has enhanced the overall salvage rate. Failing this, reoperation should be performed without further delay.

Age and sex

When analyzed, age was found to be an independent risk factor for patients above 60 years (mortality 16.8%) and more significantly for those above 70 years (32.4%), an important consideration since bioprostheses are being implanted with increasing frequency in elderly patients. Although the durability of these valves is extended in this

Table 8.7-II: Operative mortality (%) according to urgency and functional class.

	Pansini[36] N=183	Antunes[4,5] N=472	Husebye[31] N=617	Bosch[77] N=89	`Lytle[6] N=1000	Wideman[78] N=200
OVERALL	8.7	10.6	8.7	21.3	12.1	5.0
ELECTIVE	2.4	4.5	1.3	19.5	9	-
EMERGENCY	20.0	24.1	45.0	42.9	37	-
NYHA <III		4.4			3	
NYHA IV		29.9		20	23	

age group, a number of reoperations in patients in the eighth to tenth decades of life are inevitable.

Reoperation carried a higher mortality in women than in men, especially in the aortic valve group, although sex was not an independent risk factor in multivariate analyses. This perhaps unexpected finding presumably reflects the higher incidence of associated procedures in the female patient, which were shown to increase the risk to 20% and 24%, respectively, in the experiences of Husebye (21) and Bosch (77) and their coworkers.

Pathology

The perioperative risk was distinctly affected by the different causes of reoperation, again with great variability from series to series (Table 8.7-III).

Dysfunction of mechanical valves was generally not associated with increased risk, the mortality rates varying from 4.5% to 10.3% in elective reoperations. However, the risk depends on the type of malfunction. As mentioned above, Mayo Clinic surgeons (21) were able to electively replace 117 aortic Braunwald-Cutter prostheses with only one death (0.8%), an experience similar to that of the University of Alabama at Birmingham (one death in 65 patients; mortality, 1.5%). On the other hand, emergency reoperations for replacement of convexo-concave Björk-Shiley prostheses with strut fracture and disc embolization carried a much higher mortality (50%) in the experience of Ericsson and the international multi-institutional study group (24).

Degeneration of bioprostheses: Contrary to the opinion commonly expressed, patients with degenerated prostheses may die suddenly or present for surgery in an extremely critical condition (82). Our mortality for re-replacement of bioprostheses was 6%, identical to that reported by Bortolotti et al. (6.1%) (17) and lower than that of Pansini et al. (9.4%) (36). Again, the experience of the surgical team plays an important role in decreasing mortality. Early, programmed substitution of prostheses known to be failing may be accomplished with low risk and is strongly recommended.

Conservative procedures: In our experience, reoperation for failure of conservative procedures carried a much lower risk than reoperation for replacement of a prosthesis (2.4% vs. 10.6%) (6). Lytle and associates (6), of the Cleveland Clinic, registered a mortality rate of 4.0% for reoperation after valvuloplasty which, in their mind, supports

Table 8.7-III: Operative mortality (%) for different types of pathology

	Pansini[36] N=183	Antunes[5,6] N=472	Husebye[21] N=617	Bosch[77] N=89	Lytle[6] N=1000	Wideman[78] N=200
PATHOLOGY						
PVE	16.7	27.9	24.3	62.5	26	19
TO		13.0				
Deg.BIO	9.4	6.0			5	
PV Leaks	5.4	16.3	10.6	23.1	12.9	0
Struct.failure		8.2	9.1	10.3	4.5	
Conservative	2.4		15.4	4.0		

BIO: bioprostheses; PV: perivalvular; PVE: prosthetic valve endocarditis; TO: thrombotic obstruction the continued use of these operations when appropriate. A similar conclusion was arrived at by Niederhauser and colleagues, who reported an 8.8% mortality (83). The absence of the "annular factor", discussed above, is the most likely explanation for the significantly lower mortality.

Prosthetic valve endocarditis: In contrast, prosthetic valve endocarditis always carried the highest mortality, ranging from 24.3% to 62.5%. Lytle et al. (6) reported a higher mortality for aortic prosthetic valve endocarditis (38%), but in our patients the mortality of reoperation for endocarditis of mitral prostheses (35%) was higher than that for aortic valve patients (23%). The early experience usually weighed heavily on the overall results. In the past four years, we were able to reoperate on a series of 18 consecutive patients with prosthetic endocarditis, including 10 early cases, without mortality (84). Cukingnam (85) and Leport (86) and their colleagues were also able to demonstrate improving prognosis in recent years. Here again, the lowest mortality rates were observed in the larger series, thus confirming the importance of the learning curve in the treatment of this type of pathology, where large aortic root abscesses often challenge the surgeons' imagination.

Bland periprosthetic leaks: The risk of reoperation for bland periprosthetic leaks depends on the position and on whether replacement of the prosthesis is required or direct suture closure is feasible. In the case of aortic prostheses, Lytle and colleagues (6) reported a mortality of 14% and 5%, respectively for replacement and repair, but the difference was reversed in the case of mitral periprosthetic leaks (10% and 22%, respectively). In contrast, our patients with periprosthetic leaks of the mitral valve treated by valve replacement had a higher mortality (22%) than did those with leaks of the aortic valve treated similarly (12%).

Thrombotic obstruction: Another lethal complication of mechanical prostheses, thrombotic obstruction, is not reported in most series as it occurs more frequently in non-compliant populations. In our experience (5), mostly with this type of population, the mortality for reoperation (13.0%) did not differ significantly from the global mortality rate of 10.6%, as happened in the experience of Renzulli and colleagues in a different population (42). On the other hand, Martinell and associates (40) reported an operative mortality of 18% in a series of 41 patients with prosthetic valve thrombosis, but this rate was reduced to 4% in their late experience.

Other factors

Generally speaking, aortic reoperations carried a slightly lower risk than mitral reoperations (5.9%-10.9% vs. 8.7%-19.6%), but Bosch and colleagues (77) recorded a much higher mortality for aortic (35.1%) than for mitral (8.7%) procedures (Table 8.7-IV). Also, associated procedures, especially when the tricuspid valve is involved, significantly increase the risk of reoperations. The same is usually true for concomitant coronary artery bypass surgery. However, in the series of Lytle and associates (6) the need for concomitant coronary revascularization increased the risk only slightly in aortic reoperations and not at all in mitral procedures.

Multiple reoperations still represent an increased risk, especially when the tricuspid valve is involved. Our combined mortality for second, third and fourth reoperations was 14.2%, similar to those of Husebye et al. (21) for second reoperations (14.0%) and of Wideman and coworkers (78) for second and third reoperations (15.7%). However, in the experience of Lytle et al. (6) the rates for second and for third to fifth reoperations were 15.0% and 45.0%, respectively.

	Antunes[5,6] N=472	Husebye[21] N=617	Bosch[77] N=89	Lytle[6] N=1000
POSITION				
Aortic	8.9	5.9	35.1	10.9
Mitral	12.0	19.6	8.7	10
ASSOC. PROCEDURES				
Tricuspid valve	23.7			20
Other		23.8	20.0	

Table 8.7-IV: Operative mortality (%) according to the type of procedure.

Finally, it is clear that the risk has decreased with time (35,78). Our mortality rate for the past four years was only 3.1% (two of 64 patients). The introduction of cardioplegia has probably been the most important single technical advance, but this cannot be proved because other variables have also changed. As the experience increased, new technical details were introduced which have also contributed to the much better results of late.

Perioperative morbidity

Other complications, of a non-fatal nature, occur more frequently after reoperations than after primary valve procedures. Sternal re-entry problems, with injury to the heart, occurred in 3.6% of the patients of Lytle and colleagues (6), with a mortality of 36%. Similar incidences were reported by Bortolotti et al. (17) (incidence 2.6%; no mortality) and by Husebye and associates (21) (4%; 8.7%). We had only three cases of laceration of the right ventricle among 472 mitral and aortic reoperations (0.7%; no mortality). Grunwald (56) also had no deaths using a direct-vision technique for sternal re-entry.

However, a survey carried out by Dobell and Jain (87) among American surgeons identified 144 cases of severe hemorrhage with a 37% mortality. They resulted from damage to the right atrium, right ventricle, innominate vein, aorta, coronary arteries, pulmonary artery and vena cavae. Lesions of these structures also occur commonly during dissection of the pericardial adhesions, but these are usually much less serious and can be adequately repaired without significant morbidity.

Another important cause of morbidity is postoperative bleeding during the first few hours in the intensive care unit, which may occasionally cause the death of the patient. Husebye et al. (21) and Pansini et al. (32) found that neither the amounts of blood drained nor the requirement for reintervention because of bleeding and/or cardiac tamponade were different after reoperation and after a primary valve procedure. Our experience confirms their findings. In contrast, Lytle et al. (6) found that reintervention for postoperative hemorrhage was required in 10.4% of their patients, of whom 2.4% died. Their reoperated patients also required greater amounts of blood than did those subjected to primary procedures. However, the use of blood has decreased in their more recent experience. Also, second and subsequent reoperations did not represent an increased risk of bleeding when compared with first reoperations.

During re-exploration for postoperative hemorrhage, specific bleeding sites are often not found. Large amounts of clots originating from diffuse oozing may be present and must be removed. In general, reintervention is curative but intensive replacement of clotting factors may be necessary in a number of patients.

Late results

Bland periprosthetic leaks and prosthetic valve endocarditis, both usually requiring new reoperations, are the factors that most commonly affect late results. Additionally, myocardial dysfunction, whether present preoperatively or a consequence of a long cardiopulmonary bypass or inadequate protection, may be an important factor in late morbidity and/or mortality.

Complications

In these circumstances, prosthetic valve endocarditis may represent either a new infection or reinfection after replacement of an infected prosthesis. The latter, a true complication of the reoperation, occurred in three of 37 cases (8.1%) in the experience of Husebye and coworkers (21). In our own cases, prosthetic valve endocarditis was the most common cause of multiple reoperations but it appeared to have affected only the mortality of the first reoperation, probably because infection was effectively controlled by replacement of the prosthesis and systemic antibiotic therapy. Subsequent procedures were required mostly for correction of periprosthetic leaks with or without minor foci of infection. However, in the experience of Blackstone and Kirklin (2), the actuarial freedom from prosthetic valve endocarditis and periprosthetic leakage was lower after reoperations than after the original procedures.

On the other hand, bland periprosthetic leaks may be more frequent after reoperation than after the initial operation, presumably because of the irregularities of the annulus after removal of the prosthesis. The incidence of this complication varies from 0.8% to 3.0% and may be greater in the mitral than in the aortic position.

Functional status and survival

As for primary valve procedures, functional class (NYHA) improves considerably after reoperations, as most patients return to Classes I and II. In each of the mitral and aortic groups, long term survival is affected by the preoperative functional class. Since there is a much higher percentage of patients undergoing reoperation while in class IV, the global figures of survival are lower than those observed for primary operations. In the experience of Husebye and associates (21), the global seven year survival was 68% and varied between 76% for aortic and 93% for mitral patients in Classes I and II, and 49% for mitral and 60% for aortic patients in Classes III and IV (Fig. 8.7-10). However, patient survival matched by functional class was identical after the primary and secondary operations. Lower actuarial survival rates may be observed after multiple reoperations, probably also influenced by the functional class.

CONCLUSION

Valvular reoperations can be performed electively at no significantly greater risk than

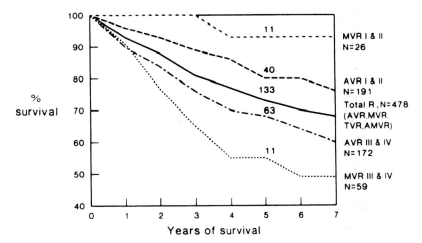

Figure 8.7-10: Relationship between survival after a first reoperation and preoperative class. Patients in Classes I and II had a much better survival rate than those in Classes III or IV. The difference was greatest in patients undergoing mitral valve reoperations (MVR). AMVR: double (aortic and mitral) valve reoperation; AVR: aortic valve reoperation; TVR: tricuspid valve reoperation. (Reproduced from Husebye DG, et al. J Thorac Cardiovasc Surg 1983;86:543-552, by permission of Mosby-Year Book, Inc.)

primary valve procedures. However, a much higher mortality accompanies emergency reoperations performed in patients in NYHA Class IV and with some subsets of pathology, such as prosthetic valve endocarditis. Consequently, repeat surgery for prosthetic complications not treatable medically should be performed early, immediately after the diagnosis is made and, preferably, before significant symptoms arise. On the other hand, many patients presenting in an advanced functional class may be improved by intensive medical care before surgery is undertaken.

Strict adherence to basic surgical principles contributes to the lowering of the operative mortality. Whenever possible, reoperations should be performed by the same surgical team which performed the initial operation and, in each particular team, by the surgeons who have the most experience with this type of procedure.

References

1. Roberts WC. The silver anniversary of cardiac valve replacement. Am J Cardiol 1985;56:503-506
2. Blackstone EH, Kirklin JW. Death and other time-related events after valve replacement. Circulation 1985;72:753-767
3. Magilligan DJ Jr, Lam CR, Lewis JW Jr, Davila JC. Mitral valve - the third time around. Circulation 1987;58(Suppl 1):36-38
4. Antunes MJ, Magalhaes MP. Isolated replacement of a prosthesis or a bioprosthesis in the mitral valve position. Am J Cardiol 1987;59:346-349
5. Antunes MJ. Isolated replacement of a prosthesis or a bioprosthesis in the aortic valve position. Am J Cardiol 1987;59:350-352
6. Lytle BW, Cosgrove DM, Taylor PC, et al. Reoperations for valve surgery: perioperative mortality and determinants of risk for 1,000 patients, 1958-1984. Ann Thorac Surg 1986;42:632-643
7. Edmunds LH, Clark RE, Cohn LH, Miller DC, Weisel RD. Guidelines for reporting morbidity and mortality after cardiac valvular operations. J Thorac Cardiovasc Surg 1988;96:351-353
8. Antunes MJ, Magalhaes MP, Azevedo MG, Baptista AL, Kinsley RH. Reoperations of the mitral and aortic valves. Z Kardiol 1986;75(Suppl 2):163-167
9. Antunes MJ. Bioprosthetic valve replacement in children: long-term follow-up of 135 isolated mitral valve implantations. Eur Heart J 1984;5:913-918

10. Antunes MJ, Santos LP. Performance of glutaraldehyde-preserved porcine bioprosthesis as a mitral valve substitute in a young population group. Ann Thorac Surg 1984;37:387-392

11. Jamieson WR, Allen P, Miyagishima RT, et al. The Carpentier-Edwards standard porcine bioprosthesis: a first-generation tissue valve with excellent long-term clinical performance. J Thorac Cardiovasc Surg 1990;99:543-561

12. Kinsley RH, Antunes MJ, Colsen PR. St. Jude Medical valve replacement. An evaluation of valve performance. J Thorac Cardiovasc Surg 1986;92:349-360

13. Antunes MJ, Wessels A, Sadowski RJ, et al. Medtronic Hall valve replacement in a 3rd world population group. J Thorac Cardiovasc Surg 1988;95:980-993

14. Bloomfield P, Kitchin AH, Wheatley DJ, Walbaum PR, Lutz W, Miller HC. A prospective evaluation of the Bjork-Shiley, Hancock, and Carpentier-Edwards heart valve prostheses. Circulation 1986;73:1213-1222

15. Oakley CM. Investigations before reoperation for acquired heart disease. In: Stark J, Pacifico AD (eds). Reoperations in cardiac surgery. Springer Verlag, Berlin, 1989:17-37

16. Magilligan DJ Jr, Lewis JW, Tilley B, Peterson E. The porcine bioprosthetic valve. Twelve years later. J Thorac Cardiovasc Surg 1985;89:499-507

17. Bortolotti U, Milano A, Mazzucco A, et al. Results of reoperation for primary tissue failure of porcine bioprostheses. J Thorac Cardiovasc Surg 1985; 90:564-569

18. Pelletier LC, Castonguay T, Leclerc T, et al. Reoperation for bioprosthesis: an analysis of 1831 valves over a 12 year period. In: Bodnar E (ed). Surgery for heart valve disease. ICR Publishers, London, 1990:443-451

19. Bortolotti U, Milano A, Guerra F, et al. Failure of Hancock pericardial xenografts: is prophylactic bioprosthetic replacement justified? Ann Thorac Surg 1991;51:430-437

20. Cohn LH. Valve re-replacement in the asymptomatic patient. Ann Thorac Surg 1991;51:357-358

21. Husebye DG, Pluth JR, Piehler JM, et al. Reoperation on prosthetic heart valves. An analysis of risk factors in 552 patients. J Thorac Cardiovasc Surg 1983;86:543-552

22. Grunkemeier GL, Starr A. Late ball variance with the model-1000 Starr-Edwards aortic valve prosthesis: risk analysis and strategy of operative management. J Thorac Cardiovasc Surg 1986;91:918-923

23. Hiratzka LF, Kouchoukos NT, Grunkemeier GL, Miller DC, Scully HE, Wechsler AS. Outlet fracture of the Bjork-Shiley 60° convexo-concave valve; current information and recommendations for patient care. J Am Coll Cardiol 1988;11:1130-1137

24. Ericsson A, Lindblom D, Semb G, et al. Strut fracture with the Bjork-Shiley 70° convexo-concave valve. An international multi-institutional follow-up study. Eur J Cardio-thorac Surg 1992;6:339-346

25. Blackstone EH, Kirklin JW. Recommendations for prophylactic removal of heart valve prostheses. J Heart Valve Dis 1992;1:3-14

26. Antunes MJ, Magalhaes MP, Colsen PR, Kinsley RH. Mitral valvuloplasty. A surgical challenge. J Thorac Cardiovasc Surg 1987;94:44-56

27. Carpentier A. Chirurgie reconstructive de la valve mitrale. In: Acar J (ed). Cardiopathies valvulaires acquises. Flammarion, Paris, 1985:554-561

28. Duran CG. Reoperations on the mitral and tricuspid valves. In: Stark J, Pacifico AD (eds). Reoperations in cardiac surgery. Springer Verlag, Berlin, 1989:325-350

29. Cosgrove DM. Surgery for degenerative mitral valve disease. Semin Thorac Cardiovasc Surg 1989;1:183-193

30. Baumgartner WA, Miller DC, Reitz BA, et al. Surgical treatment of prosthetic valve endocarditis. Ann Thorac Surg 1983;35:87-104

31. Ivert TSA, Dismukes WE, Cobbs CG, Blackstone EH, Kirklin JW, Bergdahl LAL. Prosthetic valve endocarditis. Circulation 1984;69:223-232

32. Donaldson RM, Ross DM. Homograft aortic root replacement for complicated prosthetic valve endocarditis. Circulation 1984;70(Suppl I):178-181

33. Tuna IC, Orszulak TA, Schaff HV, Danielson GK. Results of homograft aortic valve replacement for active endocarditis. Ann Thorac Surg 1990;49:619-624

34. Disesa VJ, Sloss LJ, Cohn LH. Heart transplantation for intractable prosthetic valve endocarditis. J Heart Transplant 1990;9:142-143

35. Cohn LH, Koster JK, Vandevanter S, Collins JJ. The in-hospital risk of rereplacement of dysfunction mitral and aortic valves. Circulation 1982;66(Suppl 1):153-156

36. Pansini S, Ottino G, Forsennati PG, et al. Reoperations on heart valve prostheses: an analysis of operative risks and late results. Ann Thorac Surg 1990;50:590-596

37. Bedderman C, Borst HG. Comparison of two suture techniques and materials: relationship to perivalvular leaks after cardiac valve replacement. Bull Tex Heart Inst 1978;5:534-540

38. Orszulak TA, Schaff HV, Danielson GK, Pluth JR, Puga FJ, Piehler JM. Results of reoperation for periprosthetic leakage. Ann Thorac Surg 1983;35:584-589

39. Cohn LH. Thromboembolism after mitral valve replacement. In: Duran CMG, Angell W, Johnson A, Oury J (eds). Recent progress in mitral valve disease. Butterworths, London, 1984:330-339

40. Martinell J, Fraile J, Artiz V, Cortina J, Fresned P, Rabago G. Reoperation for left-sided low-profile

mechanical prosthetic obstruction. Ann Thorac Surg 1987;43:172-175
41. Grunkemeier GL, Rahimtoola SH. Artificial heart valves. Ann Rev Med 1990;41:251-263
42. Renzulli A, de Luca L, Carusco A, Verde R, Galzerano D, Cotrufo M. Acute thrombosis of prosthetic valves: a multivariate analysis of the risk factors for a life-threatening event. Eur J Cardio-thorac Surg 1992;6:412-421
43. Antunes MJ. Thromboembolic complications and anticoagulants: compliant versus non-compliant patient population. In: Rabago G, Cooley D (eds). Heart valve replacement. Futura Publishers, New York, 1987:307-317
44. Antunes MJ. Clinical performance of St. Jude and Medtronic Hall prostheses: a randomized comparative study. Ann Thorac Surg 1990;50:743-747
45. Boskovic D, Elezovic I, Boskovic D, Simin N, Rolovic Z, Josipovic Z. Late thrombosis of the Bjork-Shiley tilting disc valve in the tricuspid position. Thrombolytic treatment with streptokynase. J Thorac Cardiovasc Surg 1986;91:1-8
46. Roudaut R, Labbe T, Lorient-Roudaut MF, et al. Mechanical valve thrombosis. Is fibrinolysis justified? Circulation 1992;86:II-8-II-15
47. Venugopal P, Kaul V, Iyer KS, et al. Fate of thrombectomized Bjork-Shiley valves. A long-term cinefluoroscopic echocardiographic and hemodynamic evaluation. J Thorac Cardiovasc Surg 1986;91:168-173
48. Antunes MJ. Fate of thrombectomized Bjork-Shiley vales (letter). J Thorac Cardiovasc Surg 1986;92:965
49. Croft CH, Buja LM, Floresca MZ, Nicod P, Estrera A. Late thrombotic obstruction of aortic porcine bioprostheses. Am J Cardiol 1986;57:355-356
50. Mullany CJ, Gersh BJ. Prosthetic heart valves. Annual Cardiac Surg 1990-91:141-149
51. Okita Y, Miki S, Kusuhara K, et al. Intractable hemolysis caused by perivalvular leakage following mitral valve replacement with St. Jude Medical prosthesis. Ann Thorac Surg 1988;46:89-92
52. Pacifico AD. Aortic valve reoperations. In: Stark J, Pacifico AD (eds). Reoperations in cardiac surgery. Springer Verlag, Berlin, 1989:233-247
53. Bahn CH, Annest LS. Reoperation without medical records. Avoidable? J Thorac Cardiovasc Surg 1986;91:139-141
54. Loop FD. Catastrophic hemorrhage during sternal re-entry. Ann Thorac Surg 1984;37:271-272
55. Macmanus A, Okies JE, Philips SJ, Starr A. Surgical considerations in patients undergoing repeat median sternotomy. J Thorac Cardiovasc Surg 1975;69:138-143
56. Grunwald RP. A technique for direct-vision sternal re-entry. Ann Thorac Surg 1985;40:521-522
57. Bortolotti U. The problem of reoperation in bioprosthetic valve recipients. J Heart Valve Dis 1992;1:29-31
58. Campanella C, Cameron E, Feilberg VL. Mitral prosthetic replacement in small left atria. Ann Thorac Surg 1990;50:836-837
59. Praeger PI, Pooley RW, Moggio RA, Somberg ED, Sarabu MR, Reed GE. Simplified method for reoperation on the mitral valve. Ann Thorac Surg 1989;48:835-837
60. Ingram MT, Miller GE Jr. Prosthetic valve replacement using annular preservation technique. Ann Thorac Surg 1985;40:408
61. Bortolotti U, Mazzuco A, Milano A, Galluci V. Technical considerations in reoperation for porcine bioprosthetic valve failure. J Cardiac Surg 1988;3:459-466
62. Cabrol C, Gandjbakkhc I, Pavie A, et al. Surgical treatment of ascending aortic pathology. J Cardiac Surg 1988;3:167-180
63. David TE, Bos J, Christakis GT, et al. Heart valve operations in patients with active infective endocarditis. Ann Thorac Surg 1990;49:694-700
64. Tuna IC, Orszulak TA, Schaff HV, Danielson GK. Results of homograft aortic valve replacement for active endocarditis. Ann Thorac Surg 1990;49:619-624
65. Lau JKH, Robles A, Cherian A, Ross DN. Surgical treatment of prosthetic endocarditis. Aortic root replacement using a homograft. J Thorac Cardiovasc Surg 1984;87:712-716
66. Disesa VJ, Solss LJ, Cohn LH. Heart transplantation for intractable prosthetic valve endocarditis. J Heart Transplant 1990;9:142-143
67. Gallo I, Artinano E, Duran CG. Late clinical results with the use of heterologous pericardium for closure of the pericardial cavity. J Thorac Cardiovasc Surg 1985;89:709-712
68. Revuelta JM, Garcia-Rinaldi R, Val F, Crego R, Duran CMG. Expanded polytetrafluoroethylene surgical membrane for pericardial closure. J Thorac Cardiovasc Surg 1985;89:451-455
69. Fradin D, Causs T, Rabaud M, de Mascarel A, Fontan F. Preliminary experimental results of a new resorbable biomaterial and pericardial substitute. In: Rivera (ed). Actualizacion cardiovascular. Ela. Madrid, 1992:(in press)
70. Bidstrup BP, Royston D, Sapsford RN, Taylor KM. Reduction in blood loss and blood use after cardiopulmonary bypass with high dose aprotinin (Trasylol). J Thorac Cardiovasc Surg 1989;97:364-372
71. Dietrich W, Barankay A, Hahnel C, Richter JA. High-dose aprotinin in cardiac surgery: Three year's experience in 1,784 patients. J Cardiothorac Vasc Anest 1992;6:324-327

72. Mohr R, Goor DA, Lusky A, Lavee J. Aprotinin prevents cardiopulmonary bypass platelet dysfunction. A scanning electron microscope study. Circulation 1992;86(Suppl II):405-409
73. Covino E, Pepino P, Iorio D, Mariano L, Ferrara P, Spampinato N. Low dose aprotinin as blood saver in open heart surgery. Eur J Cardio-thorac Surg 1991;5:414-418
74. Royston D, Bidstrup BP, Taylor KM, Sapsford RN. Effect of aprotinin on need for blood transfusion after repeat open-heart surgery. Lancet 1987;I:1289-1291
75. Biagini A, Comite C, Russo V, et al. High dose aprotinin to reduce blood loss in patients undergoing redo open heart surgery. Acta Anaesthesiol Belg 1992;40:181-186
76. Cosgrove DM, Heric B, Lytle BW, et al. Aprotinin therapy for reoperative myocardial revascularization: a placebo-controlled study. Ann Thorac Surg 1992;54:1031-1038
77. Bosch X, Pomar JL, Pelletier LC. Early and late prognosis after reoperation for prosthetic valve replacement. J Thorac Cardiovasc Surg 1984;88:567-572
78. Wideman FE, Blackstone EH, Kirklin JW, Karp RB, Kouchoukos NT, Pacifico AD. Hospital mortality of re-replacement of the aortic valve. Incremental risk factors. J Thorac Cardiovasc Surg 1981;82:692-698
79. Sandza JG, Clark RE, Ferguson TB, Connors JP, Weldon CS. Replacement of prosthetic valves. A fifteen-year experience. J Thorac Cardiovasc Surg 1977;74:864-874
80. Syracuse DC, Bowman FO, Malm JR. Prosthetic valve reoperations. Factors influencing early and late results. J Thorac Cardiovasc Surg 1979;77:346-354
81. Butchart EG, Breckenridge IM. Prosthetic valve reoperations. In: Starek PJK (ed). Heart valve reoperations and reconstruction. Year Book Medical Publishers, Chicago, 1984:293-304
82. Bortolotti U, Guerra F, Magni A, et al. Emergency reoperation for primary tissue failure of porcine bioprostheses. Am J Cardiol 1987;60:920-925
83. Niderhauser U, Carrel T, Von Segesser LK, Laske A, Turina M. Reoperation after mitral valve reconstruction: early and late results. Eur J Cardio-thorac Surg 1993;7:34-37
84. Antunes MJ, Sanches MF, Fernandes LE. Antibiotic prophylaxis and prosthetic valve endocarditis. J Heart Valve Dis 1993;1:201-205
85. Cukingnam RA, Carey JS, Wittig JH, Cimochowski GE. Early valve replacement in active infective endocarditis. Results and late survival. J Thorac Cardiovasc Surg 1983;85:163-173
86. Leport C, Wilde JL, Bricain F, et al. Fifty cases of late prosthetic valve endocarditis. Improvement in prognosis over a 15 year period. Br Heart J 1987;58:66-72
87. Dobell ARC, Jain AK. Catastrophic hemorrhage during redo sternotomy. Ann Thorac Surg 1984;37:273-278

Chapter 8.8

Heart Transplantation and Valvular Heart Disease

P. Nataf, I. Gandjbakhch, C. Cabrol

Cardiac transplantation for valvular heart disease is rare. The 1992 register of the International Society for Heart and Lung Transplantation (1) listed idiopathic cardiomyopathy in 49% and ischemic heart disease in 41% of all cases; only 4% of heart transplant recipients had valvular disease. In our series of more than 800 cardiac transplantations performed since April 1968 this rate is higher; valvular heart disease represents 8% of the total indications (2,3). The high prevalence of valve disease in France and our special interest in the valvular surgery program may explain this rate.

INDICATION

The primary indication for heart transplantation in valvular heart disease is end-stage cardiac failure with irreversible ventricular dysfunction. Rarely, heart transplantation is indicated after severe myocardial damage due to valvular surgery. Progressive postoperative deterioration despite a fully functional prosthesis or satisfactory repair may also indicate heart transplantation.

Presence of poor prognostic factors for valvular surgery may facilitate the therapeutic choice (4,5). For example, in the case of chronic symptomatic aortic insufficiency with cardiac failure the principal cause of operative mortality is myocardial dysfunction caused by the valvular lesion. This complication is also responsible for most late deaths. In the case of chronic mitral insufficiency, progressive deterioration of the left ventricular systolic function is the cause of a poor prognosis whether surgery is performed or not. Cardiac transplantation is debatable in the case of severe mitral insufficiency with an ejection fraction less than 30%. Repair of the valvular lesion may be considered initially if it is severe and appears to be responsible for the cardiac failure, and transplantation may be envisaged in patients where the valvular lesion does not appear to be fully responsible for the myocardial status. This would be true in the case of a moderate mitral insufficiency of organic origin with severely deteriorated left ventricular function.

In our series of 40 valvular patients operated on between 1988 and 1992, indications for cardiac transplantation were mitral valve disease in 21 patients (12 mitral insufficiency, one mitral stenosis, eight mixed mitral disease), aortic valve disease in nine patients (seven aortic insufficiency, one aortic stenosis, and one with mixed aortic disease), and multiple valve disease in 10 patients. Valvular heart disease was due to rheumatic fever in 25 patients, degenerative lesions in 12 (including three Marfan's disease) and endocarditis in three patients. Thirty-seven patients had had previous valvular operations, nine of them three or more previous operations. Mean preoperative pulmonary artery systolic pressure was 50 ± 20 mmHg and mean pulmonary vascular resistance 3.2 ± 2.2 WU.

Elective transplantation was performed in 39 patients. In one case, a total artificial heart (Jarvik 7) was implanted as an emergency measure due to an acute irreversible cardiac failure until a graft became available.

CONTRAINDICATION

The contraindications to heart transplantation in valvular patients are identical to those of any heart transplantation. Acquired experience allows us to discount certain patients who would not benefit from transplantation. Severe pulmonary hypertension, uncontrolled infection, refractory gastroduodenal ulcer or severe colic diverticulosis, as well as systemic illness, recent malignancies or diffuse amyloidosis, remain absolute contraindications (6). The first and most common is the existence of pulmonary hypertension due to the irreversible elevation of pulmonary vascular resistance. Pulmonary hypertension can be responsible for a severe failure of the right ventricle immediately after transplantation in the operating room or in the intensive care unit.

The degree of acceptable pulmonary arterial hypertension or vascular resistance is difficult to define (7). Our present policy, in the presence of an elevated pulmonary vascular resistance (PVR), is to evaluate its severity as precisely as possible at the first pretransplant examination and to appreciate the importance of a spasmodic factor (a 20% or more fall in PVR after vasodilator tests demonstrates this effect). It is important to carefully and regularly follow its evolution by echo Doppler during the period before transplantation in order to detect any progressive increase which would necessitate urgent transplantation.

If the PVR is equal to or less than six Wood Units (WU) an orthotopic transplantation is performed and is usually successful. A PVR between six and eight WU indicates that an orthotopic procedure using an oversized donor with a vigorous heart (necessitating no drugs) and preferably harvested on site in order to shorten its ischemic time, should be performed. For patients with more than 8-10 WU a heart-lung transplantation is preferable.

Absolute age limits are no longer accepted since newborns and patients up to 70 years have been transplanted, but those older than 60 are usually considered on an individual basis. Although operative mortality is higher (36%), when such patients are carefully selected their long term survival is almost equal to younger patients.

In the spectrum of valvular disease, this concept of age limit makes the indications for transplantation exceptional in the case of a degenerative disease, such as calcified aortic stenosis. Bacterial endocarditis, rheumatic valvular disease and dystrophies remain the most common indications for heart transplantation. Even when the procedure is a repeat operation, as is the case in the majority of valvular candidates for transplantation, this need not be a contraindication despite the major operative risk.

SURGICAL PROCEDURE

The most frequently used surgical procedure remains the original orthotopic transplantation described by Lower and Shumway (8). We perform this procedure with a slight modification that opens the right atrium from the inferior vena cava orifice to the base of the right atrial appendage in order to preserve the integrity and vascularization of the sinus node. In our experience, this modification dramatically lessened the number of atrial arrhythmias and AV blocks observed with Shumway's original technique.

The heterotopic procedure, clinically introduced by Novitsky et al. (9), yielded definitively less satisfactory results. This technique allows a cause of thrombosis to persist in the diseased heart, namely the valvular prosthesis.

The particular technique of cardiac excision in these valvular patients depends on the frequency of previous cardiac interventions. The pericardial fusion in these cases necessitates the dissection of extremely hemorrhagic adhesions. Good surgical hemostasis and optimal control of coagulation are particularly important.

RESULTS AND POSTOPERATIVE COURSE

The postoperative course of these patients is almost identical to that of any heart transplantation. The surgical (30 days) mortality in our series of valvular patients was 35%. This rate may be explained by the frequency of previous operations. The causes of death were infection (n = 8), hemorrhage (n = 2), right heart failure (n = 2), pulmonary edema (n = 1) and gastrointestinal complications (n = 1).

Rejection is rarely observed in the early days post transplantation because 'hyperacute rejection' is avoided either by performing a pretransplant direct cross-match or by detecting the presence and calculating the percentage of reactive antibodies. Recently, however, hyperacute rejection has been observed despite a compatible direct lymphocytotoxic cross-match (10).

Acute rejection is a constant threat from the fifth postoperative day through the first year. In most cases, CsA suppressed the usual clinical, electrical and hemodynamic symptoms of rejection. Presently, the only way to be certain of an ongoing rejection is a histological diagnosis by percutaneous right ventricular endomyocardium biopsies (which unfortunately is an invasive method), which reveal important lymphocyte infiltration and myocyte necrosis.

Serial and two-dimensional echocardiographic findings, considered worthwhile by some groups, seem to correlate with rejection episodes (11). Interestingly, in our experience, early detection of rejection by echo Doppler studies (isovolumic relaxation time and pressure half time) is quite satisfactory and this is now our routine technique for rejection control (12).

Secondary infections, although diminished with CsA, have remained frequent. They mainly take the form of bacterial pneumonia but there are also episodes of fungal infection. Careful donor screening is essential to avoid the frequent transmission of diseases such as toxoplasmosis and cytomegalovirus (CMV) infection.

Another concern in using CsA is nephrotoxicity, which can be acute during the first postoperative days. Renal damage develops rapidly, causing oliguria, anuria and death. This side effect prompted us to follow two principles for immediate immunosuppression therapy as early as 1981; first, delaying the use of CsA until the patient's renal function and hemodynamics improve, and second, the use of low doses of CsA.

Late complications

Careful early use of CsA almost suppressed the early nephrotoxic complications but chronic nephrotoxicity is still observed (50% at two years and 71% at five years). These lesions can be prevented by using low doses of CsA. Nevertheless, if they appear, they are potentially reversible by discontinuing CsA and switching to a more conventional therapy (13).

The systemic hypertension observed at five years in almost all patients (97%) treated with CsA also remains a threat; despite extensive studies by our group and others (14-15), we are unable to find any alteration in the renin-angiotensin system or the aldosterone level, and the only abnormal finding is a persistent hypervolemia. This systemic hypertension is best treated by administration of calcium channel blockers.

Finally, one of the most intriguing and dangerous problems after cardiac transplantation is the secondary occurrence of occlusive coronary lesions. The frequency (35% at five years) and severity of this complication is a major threat to transplantation and deserves future research in which the nutritional status of transplanted patients must be considered. Several other late complications such as rheumatic complications and malignancies were also observed.

Survival

The introduction of CsA in 1981 has been associated with a marked improvement in patient survival. The five year actuarial survival rate was 51%, comparable to that for the entire group (58%) (16). The rate of rejection was 0.09 ± 0.08 event/patient-month. The incidence of infection (early deaths excluded) was 0.42 event/patient-month (16).

CONCLUSION

In conclusion, in the case of patients with acquired heart valve disease, operative risk of cardiac transplantation is increased because of the frequency of previous cardiac surgery and sometimes the age of the patients. However, functional improvement is remarkable in that survivors are leading normal family, social, professional and often physically active lives.

References
1. The Registry of the International Society for Heart and Lung Transplantation: ninth official report. 1992. J Heart Lung Transplant 1992;11:599
2. Cabrol C, Nataf P, Pavie A, et al. Heart transplantation in 1992: the La Pitie[acute] experience. Transplant Proc 1993;25:820-821
3. Nataf P, Gandjbakhch I, Pavie A, et al. Heart transplantation: update. In: Terasaki P (ed). Clinical Transplants 1992. UCLA Tissue Typing Laboratory, Los Angeles, California, 1993;129-135
4. Acar J. Quel traitement pour l'insuffisance aortique chronique. Arch Mal Coeur 1987;80:1297-1305
5. Acar J, Brunet F, Slama M, et al. Le remplacement valvulaire, facteur possible de détérioration myocardique. Arch Mal Coeur 1984;77:1120-1125
6. Conner R, Hosenpud J, Norman D, Pantely G, Cobanoglu MA, Starr A. Heart transplantation for cardiac amyloidosis: successful one-year outcome despite recurrence of the disease. J Heart Transplant 1988;7:165-167
7. Addozissio LJ, Gersony WM, Robbins RC, et al. Elevated pulmonary vascular resistance and cardiac transplantation. Circulation 1987;76(Suppl 5):52-55
8. Lower RR, Shumway NE. Studies on orthotopic homotransplantation of the canine heart. Surgical Forum 1960;11:18-20

9. Novitzky D, Cooper C, Barnard CN. The surgical technique of heterotopic heart transplantation. Ann Thorac Surg 1983;36:476-482
10. Trento A, Hardesty R, Griffith B, Zerbe T, Kormos R, Bahnson H. Role of the antibody to vascular endothelial cells in hyperacute rejection in patients undergoing cardiac transplantation. J Thorac Cardiovasc Surg 1988;95:37-41
11. Hosenpud J, Norman D, Cobanoglu M, Floten H, Conner R, Starr A. Serial echocardiographic findings early after heart transplantation: evidence for reversible right ventricular dysfunction and myocardial edema. J Heart Transplant 1987;6:343-347
12. Desruennes M, Corcos T, Cabrol C, et al. Doppler echocardiography for the diagnosis of acute cardiac allograft rejection. J Am Coll Cardiol 1988;12:63-70
13. Stevens L, Halbrook H, Berron K, Spears C, Hormuth D. Conversion from ciclosporine to azathioprin in heart transplant recipients. J Heart Transplant 1988;7:119-122
14. Rottemburg J, Mattei MF, Cacrol A, et al. Renal function and blood pressure in heart transplant recipients treated with ciclosporine. J Heart Transplant 1985;4:404-407
15. Oyer P, Stinson E, Jamieson S, et al. Cyclosporin A in cardiac allografting: a preliminary experience. Transplant Proc 1983;15:1247-1255
16. Dorent R, Nataf P, Vaissier E, et al. Heart transplantation for valvular heart disease. Transplant Proc 1995;27:1689

Chapter 9.1

Valvular Homografts

Endre Bodnar

It is estimated that about 25,000 homograft valves have been implanted world-wide since the first insertions in 1962 by Donald Ross in London and Brian Barratt-Boyes in Auckland (1,2). The clinical interest, however, has been far from constant. It appears that about 5,000 valves were implanted between 1962 and 1974, not more than about 1,500 between 1974 and 1985 and the rest since 1985.

The reasons for this changing pattern lie in the evolution of heart valve replacement; in the sixties and early seventies, homografts were the biological valve of choice and had great expectations attached to them as compared to the rather thrombogenic first generation of mechanical prostheses. By the early seventies it became apparent that the difficulties in harvesting could not be diminished by the passing of time, and the ultimate failure of the inserted homograft could not be eliminated by any of the preservation methods proposed thus far. The desire for a biological alternative in heart valve replacement, however, remained.

It was against this background that porcine, and later pericardial bioprostheses were introduced to clinical use, and their sweeping early success squeezed homografts out of the front line and back into the hands of only the few faithful. By 1985 the preference had started to shift away from the glutaraldehyde-treated bioprostheses and, at the same time, long term follow up studies with aortic homografts provided reliable data showing excellent patient survival with these valves (3,4). Cryolife, Inc., the first commercial supplier of homografts, was established the same year in the USA and has greatly diminished the harvesting problems for cardiac surgeons in the States. The company has also been instrumental in providing publicity for the good long term results with previous generations of homografts.

The tide was thus stemmed and homografts again became the valve of choice for a selected group of patients. It is easy to anticipate, however, that this 'born again' enthusiasm will decline again in the not too distant future, unless:

- surgical indications for the use of homografts are properly set,
- expectations about the long term performance of these valves are based on realities, and
- the existence of the inherent, complex biological issues are fully recognized.

VIABLE VERSUS NON-VIABLE HOMOGRAFTS

Much confusion has been generated over the years by the fact that widely different series of homografts have been given identical consideration by the general medical public, or even cardiac surgeons at large. Making a distinction between the individual methods of preservation and/or sterilization has been limited to those actively involved in this field. Many important details of harvesting, processing, sterilizing and preserving were not recognized in those days, and as a result these issues were omitted from publications, probably because their respective importance was not completely understood.

A comprehensive terminology defining all pertinent details of homografts, including anatomy, harvesting, transportation, processing, sterilizing and preserving, has recently been published (5), whose terms all relate, to a greater or lesser extent, to the so-called "viability" of these valves. It has been assumed for many years that the long term performance of viable homografts is superior to that of the non-viable valves (6). However, the entire theory of homograft valve viability is currently under review, and it appears that our perception has to be changed fundamentally (7-9).

The choice of the word "viability" introduced ambiguity to our thinking. The true meaning of the word is capability of sustaining life (in a given environment) (10). It has never been proved that homografts, which contain living cells at the time of insertion, are capable of sustaining that cellular life in the recipients' heart. It follows that the expression "living" (at the time of insertion) homograft would be more appropriate.

The problems surrounding viability, however, go far beyond the above semantics. The generally adopted usage of the word implies that the entire inserted valve, as such, is viable, hence normal. This is definitely not the case, and even proponents of the theory of homograft viability define it merely as the presence of living fibroblasts at insertion.

This definition ignores the importance of the endothelium. Indeed, the so called 'viable' valves do not have an intact endothelial cover, and the fibroblasts are not capable of reproducing it. Fibroblasts do not produce elastin, either, and it is inconceivable that the normal structural integrity of the valve could be maintained without continuous reproduction of the elastic fibers. Further, fibroblasts do not produce mucopolysacharides or any other constituents of the extracellular space which, in turn, cannot be assumed to be normal. Finally, fibroblasts do not even produce collagen; they produce procollagen instead, which requires a normal extracellular environment to develop into collagen fibres.

The so called 'viable' valves are, thus, not necessarily normal and most probably not viable either, since it could not be proved so far that those fibroblasts which are alive at insertion would be able to survive, let alone reproduce themselves in the new biological environment.

There is experimental as well as clinical evidence to support the above suggestions (11,12). In a recent study we assessed 639 homografts used for free-hand aortic valve replacement with a maximum follow up of 21 years and a total follow up of 3,416 years. We could not find any difference in the freedom from primary tissue failure whether the valves were sterilized by antibiotics, ethylene oxide or gamma irradiation and were stored in a nutrient solution, were freeze-dried or cryopreserved. The combination of the sterilizing and storage methods yielded two subgroups: those valves which were supposedly viable at insertion (antibiotic sterilization followed by cryopreservation or storage in nutrient solution), and those that were definitely non-viable (chemical sterilization, irradiation, freeze-drying). The difference in long term performance was nil (13).

A question mark about the ultimate validity of the available clinical information on homografts, including our own data, can certainly be raised, because all these studies are only retrospective collations of outcome during widely different time frames. A prospective, randomized trial regarding homograft valves has never been attempted, nor is it underway, to the best of this author's knowledge. This might be at least one of the reasons for the current variety in the methods used world-wide for harvesting, processing and storing homografts.

HARVESTING

Donor selection criteria are the first issue to be decided in the context of harvesting. The heart can be taken from "beating heart donors". They are either recipients of a heart transplant or donors whose hearts were collected for a transplant procedure but not used for some reason. The harvesting takes place under strictly sterile conditions. These valves can be inserted without sterilization immediately or within a few days if kept in Hartman's solution at 4°C, and in either case they are called "homovital valves". If sterilized in a weak antibiotic solution and cryopreserved, they are defined as homografts with a "high cellular viability".

The rest of the valves are collected from mortuaries during forensic or routine hospital autopsies under clean but not sterile conditions. This has been the traditional source of homografts since 1962, and it remains the most practical method for the majority of the non-commercial laboratories. It is interesting to note in this respect that Cryolife, Inc. has recently abandoned their original policy of collecting hearts exclusively from beating heart donors (14).

Donor exclusion criteria are congenital valvular anomalies, pathologic deformation of the valve or surrounding tissues, sepsis or endocarditis. Furthermore, all homograft valves must be screened for Australian antigen (hepatitis) and HIV. The currently accepted age limit is 55 years.

STERILIZATION

All homografts, with the sole exception of homovital valves, are treated in an antibiotic mixture to destroy the contaminating micro-organisms. Colloquially, the method is called 'sterilization', though by definition the antibiotic treatment is not a sterilizing procedure. It follows that every single valve must be sampled for microbiology. The sterility control consists of culturing for aerob and anaerob bacterial, mycobacterial and fungal growths.

Much argument has recently been devoted to the concentration of the antibiotics in the sterilizing solution. All antibiotics are cytotoxic, hence the advocates of high cellular viability tend to use solutions containing only a low concentration of antibiotics. Antibiotic sterilization was introduced by Brian Barratt-Boyes in 1968, and he later modified the originally high concentration to launch the low concentration antibiotic sterilization (15).

The theoretical advantage of lowering the concentration of the cytotoxic antibiotics is obvious. In practice, however, not everyone could confirm the beneficial effects. The University of Washington team attempted to introduce the Auckland antibiotic solution (Brian Barratt-Boyes) but could not duplicate the results (16). At the National Heart Hospital, London, a number of different, high concentration antibiotic mixtures have been used, and the rate of quality control rejection due to contamination has been 3%-4% during the past 18 years. The Barratt-Boyes solution that achieves 98% sterility in Auckland left 62% of the valves non-sterile in London. Furthermore, toxicology studies revealed that, although the low concentration antibiotics are less cytotoxic, both low and high concentration solutions are within the same range of cytotoxicity (17). The practical conclusion appears to be to develop the individual mixture and concentration of the antibiotic/antifungal solution for each homograft center in a pragmatic manner, in order to ensure that the locally prevalent contamination can be safely eliminated. If a high cellular viability is no longer the primary concern (vide supra), there is no trade-off in terms of cytotoxicity.

STORAGE

The storage of homologous heart valves is either 'wet' storage at 4°C (in the past these valves were known as 'fresh') or is accomplished by cryopreservation in liquid nitrogen. Hank's solution or TC 199 tissue culture medium is used for 'wet' storage. DMSO or glycerol is the usual cryoprotectant if the valve is to be kept in liquid nitrogen.

The main difference between 'wet' storage and cryopreservation is the rate of tissue deterioration. It limits the affordable storage period in the former, but remains negligible in the latter case. Due to the limited availability of homografts and the high cost of discarding outdated valves, a feature that is unavoidable with 'wet' storage, cryopreservation has a definite practical advantage for all those who need, or procure and supply valves in relatively large quantities.

Long term clinical experiences at the National Heart Hospital, London did not reveal any difference in the rate of primary tissue failure whether the valves were 'wet' stored or cryopreserved (vide supra). This led us to the inevitable, practical conclusion that cryopreservation should be reintroduced as an alternative to 'wet' storage in 1983 and it has continued to be used since. However, in the opinion of this author, there is no reason why those who are experienced in 'wet' storage and can maintain an adequate level of supply with this method should abandon it.

The addition of fetal calf serum to the tissue culture media or to the cryopreservant solution, as still practised by some, is a controversial issue. It was introduced in 1972 at the National Heart Hospital, London to enhance the cellular viability of valves stored in a nutrient solution (18). Since the laboratory data (corresponding to experiences with tissue culture in general) were able to prove an increase in the number of viable cells when fetal calf serum was added, this method became adopted by almost everybody world-wide.

It was not until 1987 that we realized, and could prove by animal experiments, that the residual calf serum content of the homografts may act as a potent heterologous antigen (19). The experimental results were so persuasive that we decided to abandon the use of calf serum straight away. Although the experimental results and the consequences were questioned by none, some laboratories are still using fetal calf serum as a mandatory adjunct to the cryoprotectant solution. In the practice of the Homograft Department of the National Heart Hospital, however, adequate cryopreservation has been achieved without it.

It is assumed that the reason for this difference lies in the complexity of the extra- and intracellular protection afforded by the various solutions used by the individual laboratories. Glycerol, used in the eighties at the National Heart Hospital, provides both intra- and extracellular protection. DMSO, employed by those who still retain the use of fetal calf serum, does not protect the extracellular structures, or does so only to a negligible degree. Under those circumstances, fetal calf serum or a similar component providing extracellular protection is necessary to achieve adequate cryopreservation. This hypothesis, logical though it may sound, does not have experimental confirmation yet.

ANTIGENICITY

The potential antigenicity of valvular homografts was thoroughly investigated in animal experiments during the early and mid sixties, but the existence of a significant rejection reaction could not be proved (20). Rejection did not appear as a problem in the early clinical experience. Currently available long term experiences with homografts, as compared to those with cardiac transplantation, seem to refute the potential role of immunologic processes as determinants of long term valve performance. Primary tissue failure presents relatively late in the follow up with an increasing rate and/or hazard. Rejection to a transplant has an early peak with a decreasing hazard afterwards. This time-related difference is a strong argument against the potential involvement of the immunologic system in complications following the implantation of valvular homografts.

Nonetheless, clinical evidence has recently emerged that early valve failure can be caused by an acute rejection of the homograft (21). Because (a) this problem has not been encountered before and (b) all rejected valves reported so far have been taken from beating heart donors, it can be postulated that the 'superviable' valves retain a degree of antigenicity that is not present in other homografts. This assumption is supported by studies investigating the behavior of the endothelium; it could be proved that the vast majority of antigen expression is localized to the endothelium, but is almost completely lost during the first 48 hours post mortem (22,23). It appears that the meticulous effort to preserve high cellular viability by collecting hearts from beating heart donors and process them as fast as possible, may be counterproductive in the sense that antigenicity, that could be lost otherwise, is preserved (24). Further clinical experience is expected to provide the final answer.

CLINICAL APPLICATION

Aortic (and pulmonary) homografts are outflow valves, and it would defeat the physiologic way of thinking if one would expect them to behave otherwise and provide the same excellent alternative for atrioventricular replacement as they offer for aortic surgery. Clinical experiences attest to this.

Aortic homografts were first used for aortic valve replacement (1,2), but the early drive to extend the use of biologic valves to every position, in the absence of commercial bioprostheses, led to stentless, 'semi-stented' or stent-mounted (aortic) homograft replacement of the mitral and tricuspid valves (25,26). During the same time frame, they were introduced to replace or bridge the pulmonary outflow tract (27). This remains the most frequent application of aortic homografts today, while they are no longer, or only exceptionally, in clinical use for atrioventricular replacement.

Mitral valve replacement was accomplished either by mounting the aortic homograft on a rigid, metal frame, or inside a Dacron conduit (top hat homograft), with the exception of a few, free hand inserted valves (28). A retrospective analysis, carried out in 1979, found that the long term performance of these valves was unacceptably deficient, and significantly worse than those of free hand-inserted valves in the aortic position (28). The only surgeon who reported better experiences with aortic homografts in the mitral rather than in the aortic position was Magdi Yacoub (29,30). An explanation, however, was not offered for this surprising result, although this is the only clinical experience reported in the medical literature where a biologic or bioprosthetic valve proved itself better in the mitral than in the aortic position.

The aortic root or the main pulmonary artery, containing the respective valves, are probably the best valved conduits available. They also appear to offer versatility. Aortic homografts have been in clinical use for aortic valve replacement since 1962 (1,2), in the pulmonary position since 1965 (27) and for aortic root replacement since 1971 (31). Clinical experiences with pulmonary homografts in the right sided position were first reported in 1985 (32). Currently, there is an increasing tendency to use pulmonary homografts for aortic valve replacement in a number of centers. Long term follow up information, however, to confirm the suitability of pulmonary homografts on the left side of the heart is not yet available.

SURGICAL RESULTS

The immediate and early results are very good in experienced hands, irrespective of whether the homograft is used for aortic valve or aortic root replacement, or inserted in the right sided position. The energy loss across a well seated homograft equals that across the normal, natural valve. This more than outweighs the extra burden put on the patient by the extended time spent on cardiopulmonary bypass, which is longer than would be necessary for implanting a prosthesis that is armed with a convenient sewing ring. Usually, the ease of weaning the patient off bypass and the rapid recovery during the immediate postoperative period are both remarkable. Immediate valve failure is an extreme rarity, and late failure due to surgical technical error affects only about 5% of the free hand inserted valves.

It is more difficult to define the long term results in exact terms. Several authors have reported varying results over several years. In many cases, disappointing experiences were given publicity in the medical literature only when a new sterilization or preservation method had been invented, and the former results could be blamed on the previous method which had been abandoned by the time of the publication.

In a search for comprehensive information, we assessed the long term performance of 619 homografts used for isolated aortic replacement over a 21 year period at the National Heart Hospital (vide supra) (13). To our knowledge, this study analyzed the largest number of valves of this kind followed up for the longest period that has ever been published. The valves were sterilized and stored by one or other of the entire historical variety of relevant methods.

The results are depicted in Figure 9.1-1. The mortality figures are remarkable; more

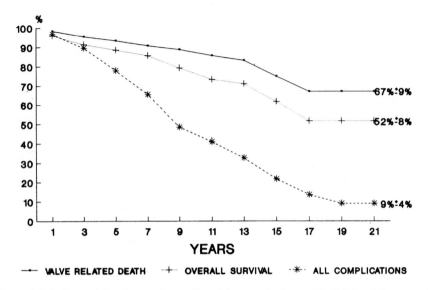

Figure 9.1-1: Actuarial estimate of overall performance indices with 639 aortic homografts. (Reproduced with permission of ICR Publishers from Bodnar E (ed). Surgery for Heart Valve Disease, ICR Publishers, London, 1990.)

than two-thirds of the patient population remained free of valve related death and more than 50% were expected in actuarial terms to be alive 21 years after surgery. However, not more than nine out of 100 originally inserted valves remained functional during the same period, the cause of failure being primary tissue failure in the vast majority of cases.

MITRAL HOMOGRAFTS

The use of a homologous mitral valve for mitral valve replacement was proposed and introduced to clinical practice in the sixties, but the method was soon abandoned because of invariable early failure due to chordal rupture (personal communication, Donald N. Ross, 1996). Recent attempts following an elegant experimental revival of the method (35) appear to be more successful. First the tricuspid valve could be replaced successfully by a mitral homograft (36). This was rapidly followed by successful replacement of the mitral valve with a mitral homograft (37-39). Most recently double mitral and tricuspid valve replacement (40) and partial mitral valve replacement as an ultimate extension of mitral valve repair (41) have been reported. The numbers are, however, small and the available follow up is very short. Further experience is necessary before a final inference could be reached on this issue.

CONCLUSION

In conclusion, it may be pertinent to suggest that homografts are good for the patient but demanding on the surgeon because of the skill that is needed both for insertion and for reoperation. The state of the art in homograft valves encompasses a renewed interest within the surgical and medical community. It is hoped that future results will be even better than the past experience, but overenthusiasm may not be warranted. Proper patient selection, good surgical technique and an ever increasing understanding of the complex biologic issues involved pave the long road which is still ahead.

References

1. Ross DN. Homograft replacement of the aortic valve. Lancet 1962;2:447
2. Barratt-Boyes BG. Homograft aortic valve replacement in aortic incompetence and stenosis. Thorax 1964;19:131-135
3. Bodnar E, Martelli V, Wain W, Ross DN. Lomg-term surgical results with homografts inserted for aortic valve disease. In: Sebening F, Kloevekorn WP, Meisner H, Struck E (eds). Bioprosthetic cardiac valves. Proceedings of the 1979 Bioprosthetic Symposium, Munich. Deutsches Herzzentrum Munich, 1980:135-142
4. Bodnar E, Wain WH, Martelli V, Ross DN. Long term performance of 580 homograft and autograft valves used for aortic valve replacement. Thorac Cardiovasc Surg 1979;27:31-38
5. Bodnar E, Ross DN. Valvular homografts. In: Bodnar E, Frater RWM (eds) Replacement heart valves. Pergamon Press, New York, 1991:287-306
6. Watts LK, Duffy P, Field RB, Stafford EG, O'Brien MF. Establishment of a viable homograft cardiac valve bank: a rapid method of determining homograft viability. Ann Thorac Surg 1976;21:230-234
7. Al-Janabi N, Gibson K, Rose J, Ross DNR. Protein synthesis in fresh aortic and pulmonary allografts as an additional test for viability. Cardiovasc Res 1973;7:247-249
8. McGregor CGA, Bradley JF, McGee GOD, Wheatley DJ. Tissue culture, collagen and protein synthesis in antibiotic sterilised heart valves. Cradiovasc Res 1976;10:389-395
9. Bodnar E, Matsuki O, Parker R, Ross DNR. Viable and non-viable homografts in the subcoronary position: a comparative study. Ann Thorac Surg 1989;47:799-804
10. Sykes JB (ed). The concise Oxford dictionary. Seventh Ed. 1982, Clarendon Press, Oxford
11. Wheatley DJ, McGregor GA. Influence of viability on canine allograft heart valve structure and function. J Cardiovasc Res 1977;11:273-278
12. Bodnar E. Pulmonary autografts, viable and non-viable homografts in the aortic position: a comparative study. In: Yankah AC, Hetzer R, Miller DC et al (eds). Cardiac valve allografts 1962-1987. Steinkopf/Springer, Darmstadt/New York 1987:261-264
13. Bodnar E, Parker R, Davies J, Robles A, Ross DNR. Non viable aortic homografts. In: Bodnar E. (ed). Surgery for heart valve disease. ICR Publishers, London, 1990:497-504
14. Information leaflet, Cryolife, Inc, 1991
15. Barratt-Boyes BG. 25 years' clinical experience in allograft surgery - a time for reflection. In: Yankah AC, Hetzer R, Miller DC et al (eds). Cardiac valve allografts 1962-1987. Steinkopf/Springer, Darmstadt/New York, 1987:347-369
16. Mohri H, Reichenbach DD, Merendino KA. Biology of homologous and heterologous heart valves. In: Ionescu MI, Ross DNR, Wooler GH (eds). Bilogical tissue in heart valve replacement. Butterworths, London, 1972:137-156
17. Bodnar E. Discussion. In: Yankah AC, Hetzer R, Miller DC et al. (eds). Cardiac valve allografts 1962-1987. Steinkopf/Springer, Darmstadt/New York, 1987:379
18. Al-Janabi N, Ross DNR. Enhanced viability of aortic homografts stored in nutrient medium. Cardiovasc Res 1973;7:814-817
19. Bodnar E, Olsen EJG, Florio R, Guerreiro D. Heterologous antigenicity induced in homografts during preservation. Thorac Cardiovasc Surg 1986;34:287-290
20. Lower RR. Laboratory observations on homograft and autograft valve replacement. In: Ionescu MI, Ross DNR, Wooler GH (eds). Biological tissue in heart valve replacement. Butterworths, London, 1972:125-136
21. Campbell DN, Clarke DR, Bishop DA, Shaffer E. Extended aortic root replacement. In: Bodnar E (ed). Surgery for Heart valve disease. ICR Publishers, London, 1990:463-471
22. Yacoub MH, Suitters A, Khagani A, Rose M. Localization of major histocompatibility complex (HLA, ABC and DR) antigens in aortic homografts. In: Bodnar E, Yacoub M (eds). Biologic and bioprosthetic heart valves. Yorke Medical Books, New York, 1986:65-72
23. Yankah AC, Dreyer W, Wottge HU, Mueller-Rucholtz M, Bernhard A. Kinetics of endothelial cells of preserved aortic valve allografts used for heterotopic transplantation in inbred rat strains. In: Bodnar E, Yacoub M (eds). Biologic and bioprosthetic heart valves. Yorke Medical Books, New York, 1986:73-84
24. Barratt-Boyes B. Discussion. In Bodnar E (ed). Surgery for heart valve disease. ICR Publishers, London, 1990:472
25. Ross DN, Somerville J. Mitral valve replacement with stored, inverted pulmonary homograft. Thorax 1972;27:583-586

26. Hamilton DI. Mitral valve replacement. In: Ionescu MI, Ross DNR, Wooler GH (eds). Biological tissue in heart valve replacement. Butterworths, London, 1972:103-124
27. Ross DN, Somerville J. Correction of pulmonary atresia with a homograft aortic valve. Lancet 1966;2:1446-1447
28. Ross DN, Shabbo FP, Wain WH. Long-term results if double valve replacement with aortic homografts. In: Sebening F, Kloevekorn WP, Meisner H, Struck E (eds). Bioprosthetic cardiac valves. Proceedings of the 1979 Bioprosthetic Symposium, Munich. Deutsches Herzzentrum Munich, 1980:143-152
29. Khaghani A, Dhalla N, Penta A, Qureshi S, Theodoropolous S, Esposito G, Yacoub M. Patient status 10 years or more after aortic valve replacement using antibiotic sterilised homografts. In: Bodnar E, Yacoub M (eds). Biologic and bioprosthetic heart valves. Yorke Medical Books, New York, 1986:38-46
30. Mankad P, Khaghani A, Esposito G, Tadjkarimi S, Yacoub M. Late results of mitral valve replacement using unstented, antibiotic-sterilised aortic homografts. In: Bodnar E, Yacoub M (eds). Biologic and bioprosthetic heart valves. Yorke Medical Books, New York, 1986:47-56
31. Lau JKH, Robles A, Cherian A, Ross DN. Surgical treatment of infective endocarditis. Aortic root replacement using a homograft. J Thorac Cardiovasc Surg 1984;87:712-717
32. Kay PH, Livi U, Robles A, Ross DN. Pulmonary homograft. In: Bodnar E, Yacoub M (eds). Biologic and bioprosthetic heart valves. Yorke Medical Books, New York, 1986:58-63
35. Revuelta JM, Cagigas JC, Bernal JM, Val F, Rabasa JM, Lequerica MA. Partial replacement of mitral valve by homograft. An experimental study. J Thorac Cardiovasc Surg 1992;104:1274-1279
36. Pomar JL, Mestres CA. Tricuspid valve replacement using a mitral homograft. Surgical technique and initial results. J Heart Valve Dis 1993;2:125-128
37. Acar C, Farge A, Ramsheyi A, et al. Mitral valve replacement using a cryopreserved mitral homograft. Ann Thorac Surg 1994;57:746-748
38. Acar C, Gaer J, Chauvaud S, Carpentier A. Technique of homograft replacement of the mitral valve. J Heart Valve Dis 1995;4:31-34
39. Kumar AS, Trehan H. Homograft mitral valve replacement - a case report. J Heart Valve Dis 1994;3:473-475
40. Acar C, Iung B, Cormier B, et al. Double mitral homograft for recurrent bacterial endocarditis of the mitral and tricuspid valves. J Heart Valve Dis 1994;3:470-472
41. Dossche K, Vanermen H, Wellens F. Partial mitral valve replacement with a mitral homograft in subacute endocarditis. Thorac Cardiovasc Surg 1994;42:240-242

Chapter 9.2

Pulmonary Autografts

Donald Ross

The first homograft aortic valve replacements seemed to offer an almost perfect valve substitute marred only by the initial difficulties in achieving a competent valve. It was anticipated however that the homologous biological tissue would be incorporated into the structure of the body, probably by being gradually repopulated with host cells, a prospect that has not been fulfilled.

The possibility of an immune reaction was anticipated and was in fact demonstrated both in experimental animals and by the Guy's Hospital immunologists (1,2). The accompanying febrile reaction corresponded with the antibody response and seemed to be transient, so that immunosuppressives were used in the first patients for up to three weeks, but were soon abandoned because of the greater danger of infection. It is interesting to note that febrile reactions, which are still common in the early postoperative period, are only now being restudied as a possible low grade rejection phenomenon (3,4).

We were surprised and disappointed when we examined explanted valves removed for surgical malinsertion within five years of surgery. Without exception these showed acellular cusps and evidence of calcification or primary tissue failure (Fig. 9.2-1). It was abundantly clear therefore that permanent or viable valves could only be achieved by one of two means, namely fresh living valves plus immunosuppression or an immediately transferred autologous pulmonary valve.

The use of low grade or tissue specific immunosuppressives as an alternative still remains a possibility but negates some of the advantages of the trouble-free homograft. A further theoretical prospect could be the deliberate seeding of the homograft stroma with autogenous cells, but the underlying collagen structure would still be vulnerable.

The possibility of using the patient's pulmonary valve was not an entirely irresponsible concept since there had been experimental animal work from Lower and Shumway (5) in 1960 indicating that the excised pulmonary valve would function under a systemic workload. While we had no doubt that the living cusps could adapt, our anxiety was that the cusps would fail under acutely induced systemic pressure. In the event there has never been an acute failure in over 400 patients, but it was not until 1982 that there was biomechanical backing for this factual observation, supplied by workers in Poland (6).

The first patient was operated upon in 1967 (7) and was known to be well in 1995, 28 years later (Fig. 9.2-2). The surgical procedure, although initially protracted, can now be performed routinely in about 100 minutes. Up until 1980 the autograft was inserted in the classical subcoronary position exactly as for homografts. More recently the trend has been to insert them as a free-standing root replacements to avoid distortion, provide an invariably competent mechanism and allow the valve to grow with the patient (Fig. 9.2-3).

Root replacement surgery originated with homografts in 1965. In an attempt to

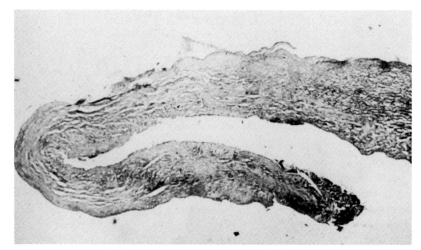

Figure 9.2-1: A typically acellular homograft cusp with reasonable retention of structure.

achieve a competent valve, the valve was inserted as an inclusion cylinder and the coronaries were anastomosed side-to-side (Fig. 9.2-4). The technique is still used and has found favor with a number of autograft surgeons, although it distorts and limits the autograft's ability to grow.

We introduced the free-standing root in 1972, again in homografts, in the treatment of destructive root endocarditis and tunnel obstruction of the left ventricular outflow. We strongly favor this technique and have used also it for autografts since 1986.

The original indication for the autograft operation was to provide a permanent valve replacement for young patients, thus avoiding the need for increasingly dangerous repeat operations with biological valves or the threat of embolism or anticoagulant hemorrhage from mechanical valves throughout the patients' lifetime.

In fact the valve can be used at any age but the increased perfusion time is probably not justified in patients over 50 years. However, there is an increasing application to young children and even infants as a permanent valve replacement with the prospects of growth (8,18).

a.Excise Pulmonary Valve b.Pulmonary Valve To Aorta c.Homograft To Pulmonary Artery

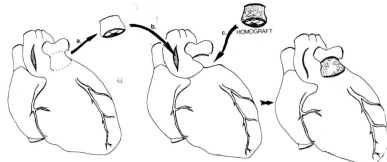

Figure 9.2-2: The principle of the pulmonary autograft operation.

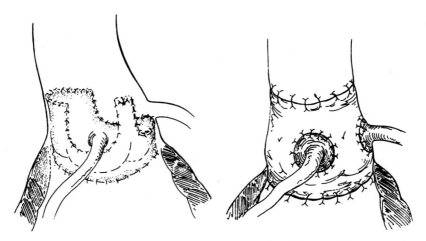

Figure 9.2-3: Conventional subcoronary insertion (a) contrasted with free-standing root replacement (b).

The replacement of the right ventricular outflow tract has been performed using a homograft in the great majority of patients. An aortic homograft was used until 1986, and thereafter we have invariably used a pulmonary homograft (9) which is not only more logical but carries additional benefits like a thinner wall and reduced calcium content. Xenografts, both stented and unstented, have been used in a few cases and in adults can be used with confidence when a homograft is not immediately available. Attempts to have a theoretically ideal completely autogenous replacement with the patient's own living pericardium or fascia lata have been uniformly unsuccessful because of progressive stenosis.

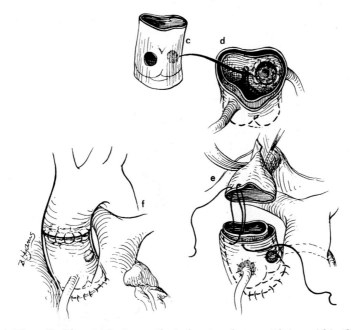

Figure 9.2-4: The cylinder or inclusion method of root replacement lying within the original aorta.

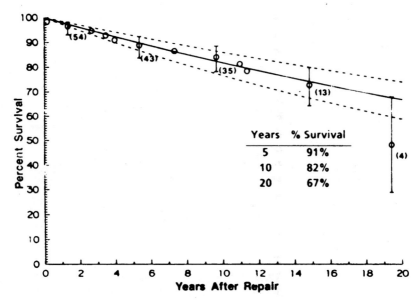

Years	% Survival
5	91%
10	82%
20	67%

Figure 9.2-5: Probability of freedom from valve failure and reoperation after homograft reconstruction of right ventricular outflow.

Studies of the aortic homograft in the right ventricular outflow tract have shown good functional results in 70%-90% of patients at 20 years, and dysfunction of the valve is in no way life-threatening (Fig. 9.2-5) (27). Failure commonly involves regurgitation rather than stenosis.

There have been a number of observed cases of distal suture line stenosis in the right ventricular outflow in our patients and reported by others. It is easy to purse-string this suture line and prophylaxis includes two to three lock stitches and the passage of the

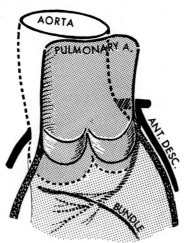

Figure 9.2-6: The first septal artery is closely related to the base of the pulmonary valve and supplies the conducting tissue.

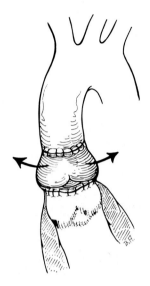 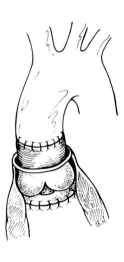

Figure 9.2-7: If the autograft root is attached supra-annually it lacks support and is liable to dilatation. The lower suture line should be at the level of the excised valve.

index finger or appropriate bougie into both pulmonary arteries at surgery. In infants and children under three years of age there is also the possibility of rejection of the homograft (10).

An unexpected complication in our early series was septal infarcts and arrhythmias, some fatal. The problem was eventually traced to the first septal branch of the anterior descending coronary artery (Fig. 9.2-6). The surgical anatomy of this vessel was studied and reported in a key article by Geens (11) This was at a stage before surgeons were familiar with the detailed anatomy of the coronary arteries.

The technical details of the operation have been described both as a subcoronary insertion and a root (12). It is unusual to find a gross discrepancy between the size of the pulmonary and aortic roots, and the elasticity of the pulmonary autograft means it is a very forgiving valve and able to adapt to varying anatomical circumstances. Also, when used as a root, size differences are relatively unimportant, so that a full-sized valve can usually be adapted to a narrow left ventricular outflow. Since we began using root replacement with both homografts and autografts we have never had to use a Konno operation, although Daenen (13) feels the need to combine the two procedures.

The only critical phase of the operation relates to the proximity of the pulmonary root to the first septal branch of the left anterior descending coronary artery. An awareness of the surgical anatomy and careful dissection means that damage to this vessel can be avoided both in removing the valve and in reconstituting the right ventricular outflow with a pulmonary homograft.

The steep early learning curve for the operation was largely the result of damage to the septal artery compounded by our difficulty in achieving a competent subcoronary placement of the valve. Using the free-standing root replacement technique the likelihood of a competent valve is almost certain.

A point of practical importance however is to ensure that the lower suture line is

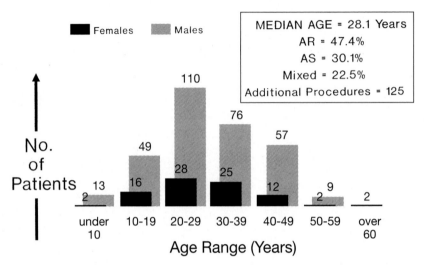

Figure 9.2-8: Age and sex distribution of 403 pulmonary autografts.

attached at the site of the excised aortic valve. This will ensure that the autograft valve will be adequately supported by the left ventricular outflow muscle just as it supports the native aortic valve (Fig. 9.2-7). Attachment to the transsected aorta on a supra-annular attachment means that the valve has little lateral support and may undergo dilatation (14).

CLINICAL APPLICATION

The first clinical assessment of the autograft was a meticulous study of 131 consecutive survivors in the National Heart Hospital. These of course included the traumatic early learning curve of the operation. The cohort was closed at 1984 to ensure that by the time of the reassessment there would have been a minimum 10 years follow up. This was because it was well established from our homograft experience that conventional biological valve deterioration sets in at seven years. The average follow up time for the group was 21 years and the results were reported in 1994 (27).

Ninety-one patients were available for follow up, which was 95% complete. Survival at 10 and 20 years was 86% and 61% respectively, with aortic regurgitation from technical malinsertion at the original operation the main cause of reoperation. Cusp degeneration was not a problem. On the right side they reported a 74% freedom from reoperation or death at 20 years.

Of 72 survivors studied at the time of follow up 59 still had their original autograft and right ventricular homografts in situ. The average NYHA class was 1.2 (range I-III) and judged by transthoracic echocardiography significant stenosis was found in only one autograft, while 30 of the 59 were free of significant regurgitation and where present this was not progressive. In the light of these findings and having passed the learning curve, work proceeded on the autograft with gathering momentum.

There have now been 427 patients operated upon by the same surgeon. The mean

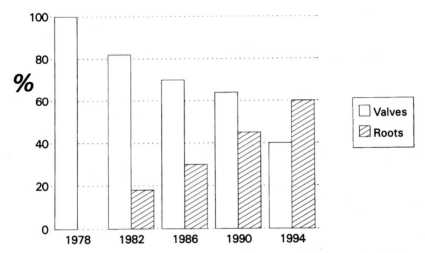

Figure 9.2-9: Histogram showing how root replacement has overtaken conventional subcoronary replacement of the autograft valve since 1982.

age was 28.1 years and the dominant lesion was aortic regurgitation (47.4%). Seventeen percent of the total were children with a median age of 13.2 years, but the tendency has been to operate on younger patients, and there are reports of successful operations in infancy (Fig. 9.2-8) (15,16). Since 1980 an increasing number of autograft roots (free-standing) have been inserted, and this has almost become the standard operation, allowing free growth and avoiding compression from surrounding tissues (Fig. 9.2-9).

Our oldest patient was 64-year-old, but reports have come through including infants and patients as old as 70 years. The procedure can consequently be used at any age but it is sensible to weigh the risks of a more prolonged bypass time against the reduced rate of deterioration in bioprosthetic valves at an advanced age. No anticoagulants or antiaggregants have been used at any stage, and where practicable patients have been reviewed annually.

Event-free analysis was conducted using the method of Kaplan-Meier (17,18). There were 28 operative deaths, giving a 6.5% overall mortality (Fig. 9.2-10). Most of these early deaths occurred in the steep learning phase from hemorrhage, arrhythmias and septal infarcts as a result of involvement of the first septal branch of the anterior

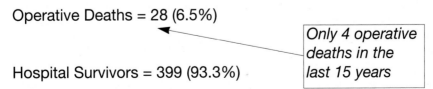

TOTAL NO. OF PATIENTS = 427

Operative Deaths = 28 (6.5%)

Hospital Survivors = 399 (93.3%)

Only 4 operative deaths in the last 15 years

Figure 9.2-10: Most of the operative deaths occurred during the learning curve; most surgeons now record a 2%-3% mortality.

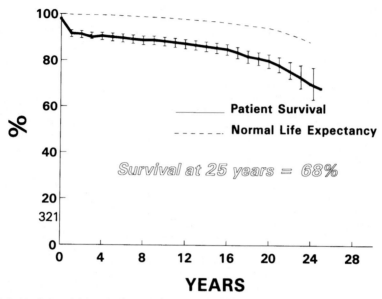

Figure 9.2-11: Actuarial survival runs close to normal life expectancy for the 30 year age group.

descending coronary artery. With four operative deaths during the last 15 years, operative mortality is now low and comparable with any form of aortic valve replacement. There have been 53 late deaths, again chiefly in the first five years of the learning curve and usually the result of technically malpositioned cusps with aortic regurgitation. Actuarial survival including operative deaths is 80% at 20 years, but if equated with the current mortality the curve is close to the normal life expectancy for a similar age group (Fig. 9.2-11).

Forty-six patients were reoperated upon, seven of them early or within a year. Two were for infected right ventricular homografts and five were primarily surgical, including a late bleed from an aneurysm of the right ventricular suture line, two for severe persistent regurgitation from the time of surgery and two from myocardial ischemic damage thought to result from prolapsing cusps obstructing the coronary orifice. Of the remaining 39, persistent regurgitation through the autograft was the cause in 28 and endocarditis in 11. Two of the latter died.

Endocarditis was diagnosed clinically in 13 patients and was proved by blood culture in 11. Six valves classed as 'degenerative' at reoperation showed none of the features of classical degeneration or tissue failure and the consensus was that the localized areas of structural damage probably represented subclinical healed endocarditis. In fact infection of these valves would be the equivalent of native endocarditis on a normal valve. Antibiotic prophylaxis should be rigorously applied in these patients, particularly with dental interventions.

There have been no embolic episodes and, as with the homograft, there does not seem to be a tendency to progressive valve regurgitation.

All explanted cusps showed viable cells, usually with retention of normal structure and even an endothelial lining, which is an important index of retained viability (Fig. 9.2-12).

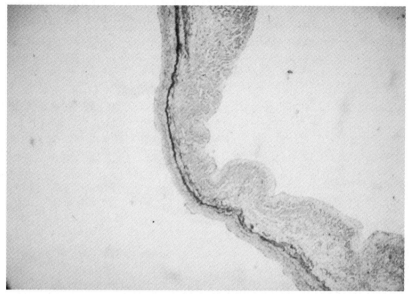

Figure 9.2-12: Histological section of an explanted cusp at three years showing a normal structure and complement of cells plus endothelial layer.

GENERAL REMARKS

The pulmonary autograft incorporates all the advantages of the homograft, including perfect design and the unique structural make-up of the normal cusp tissue. Furthermore it is sterile, non-antigenic and being transferred immediately, needs no preservation or storage techniques.

A remarkable feature is the ability of the pulmonary cusp tissue to withstand the acutely applied systemic diastolic pressure with no evidence of acute failure. It clearly adapts to its new workload and on later inspection seems to thicken slightly and become indistinguishable from normal aortic cusps. Thereafter they do not undergo progressive changes but are presumably susceptible to the normal aging processes.

Sophisticated stress testing first carried out by Polish workers (6) confirms the tensile strength of the pulmonary cusps and almost certainly relates to the fact that the aortic and pulmonary valves arise in common from the truncus arteriosus while subjected to similar pressure loads.

The clinical evidence at present available plus the fact that a number of valves have been fully functional for well over 20 years certainly points to the prospect of a permanent valve replacement. This is supported by the histological finding of fully viable cusp tissue 26 years after insertion. The pathologist reports, "The central fibrosa of all three cusps is retained. They are of normal thickness and normal cellularity."

With retained viability of course goes the possibility of growth, and following the experimental work in puppies from Japan (19) we investigated this in some of our children. Our findings were strongly in favor of growth rather than the simple effect of flow. More recently Elkins (20), in an elegant series of observations, has confirmed this observation.

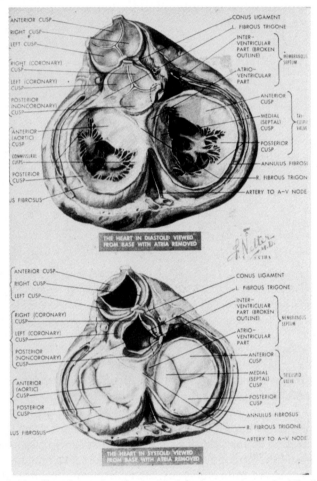

Figure 9.2-13: The fragile pulmonary valve root is largely unsupported while the aortic root is surrounded by left ventricular muscle and valve structures.

The long term prospect plus growth potential mean that the pulmonary autograft becomes the logical valve replacement in children and even infants. Work in this age group is progressing quite rapidly.

The growth prospect underlines the potential advantages of an unimpeded free-standing root replacement as opposed to a subcoronary insertion. There is no good reason why growth should not occur after the subcoronary insertion provided the ventricular outflow and aorta have normal growth potential, which may be deficient in aortic stenosis with a hypoplastic outflow tract.

With the increased use of free-standing root replacement there has been the inevitable anxiety about the possibility of progressive dilatation of the root. There have been sporadic reports pertaining to this (14) and it may equally relate to faulty surgical technique.

Normally the aortic valve lies within the muscular left ventricular outflow tract. As

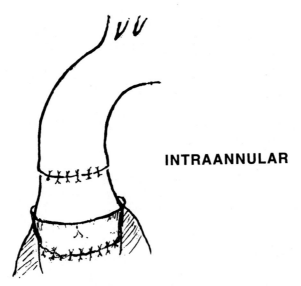

INTRAANNULAR

Figure 9.2-14: The left ventricular muscular support surrounding the transplanted pulmonary valve ring.

such it is well supported and thus able to withstand systemic diastolic pressures (Fig. 9.2-13). The pulmonary valve 'ring' as such had no inherent strength and if transported in isolation to the left side above the level of the excised aortic valve it would be unsupported and liable to leak just as it does on the right side with pulmonary hypertension.

Used as a subcoronary insertion or an inclusion root the transposed pulmonary valve is safe from distension on the left side. Even as a free-standing root, provided the lower suture line coincides with the site of the excised aortic valve and is within the left ventricular muscle support, distension should not occur (Fig. 9.2-14). There is however a tendency for surgeons to transect the aortic wall above the valve ring and interpose the autograft root as an unsupported conduit. It is technically easier but the valve is then vulnerable to lateral distension unless the surrounding tissues supply immediate and close support. Later results will test the validity of this hypothesis.

Other areas of possible contention include the incidence of minor aortic reflux after transfer of the autograft. Diagnostic techniques have become sensitive and sophisticated but it is well known that a number of homografts have shown similar diastolic 'blips' which in general have not been progressive. With a living valve, realignment may become possible and make such findings even less significant (21).

Certainly the planned reflux with most mechanical valves seems to be well tolerated and we have yet to see a comparable study on newly inserted homografts, autografts and bioprostheses. A randomized study on autografts and mechanical valves is at present under way in Copenhagen (Personal communication, Joyce, 1994).

The use of the autograft in the rheumatic age group is probably unwise (22,23), but in some centres, such as Saudi Arabia, with recurring pregnant females it may be justified provided antibiotic prophylaxis is maintained (24).

The autograft technique was avoided in prosthetic endocarditis in our hands because of the possibility of spreading infection to the right ventricular outflow. However, Oswalt (25) in Austin and Joyce (26) logically imply that living tissue is more able to resist infection. This could be one of the important applications of the autograft.

In the presence of Marfan's disease the autograft is almost certainly contraindicated since we are dealing with a generalized disease likely to involve the pulmonary valve. One case (Personal communication, Gunderson, 1992) has been reported in which an autograft root replacement was used in a young adult with medionecrosis and aortic reflux. The patient bled profusely and could only be controlled after replacement of the ascending aorta with Dacron. The excised pulmonary valve had typical Marfan histology and would presumably have failed.

There is little doubt that the pulmonary autograft has an established place in the surgery of aortic valve disease, particularly in children, because of its undoubted long life and growth potential. At the same time it carries a surprisingly low operative mortality, even in adults over sixty years of age. It could in fact become the aortic valve of choice in some centres or take its place with homografts and stentless xenografts as part of a spectrum of biological valve replacements.

Although root replacement is the favored technique of insertion at present, we need to keep an open mind about the possibility of later dilatation. On the other hand we have clear evidence that the autograft can function satisfactorily for at least 25 years in the subcoronary position (27) offering the prospect of a permanent aortic valve replacement.

References
1. Davies H, Lessof MH, Roberts CI, Ross DN. Homograft replacement of the aortic valve. Follow up studies in 12 patients. Lancet 1965;I;926
2. Davies H, Missen KAK, Blandford G, Roberts CJ, Lessof MA, Ross DN. Homograft replacement of the aortic valve: a clinical and patholgoical study. Am J Cardiol 1968;2:195-217
3. Melo JQ, Neves JP, Rands S, Martins AP, Awrade N, Macedo N. The allograft valve in aortic valve replacement and in transplanted patients. Proc AATS meeting, April 27, 1994
4. Yankah AC, Wottge HU, Miller-Rucholtz. Delayed or avert of non-MHC encoded endothelial antigen expression by Cyclosporin A. Third Scientific meeting of the International Association for Cardiac Biological Implants. April 24, 1994
5. Lower RR, Stofer RC, Shumway NH. A study of pulmonary valve autotransplantation. Surgery 1960;48:1090-1100
6. Gorezynski A, Trenker M, Anisurowicz L, Drapella A, Kwatkewska E, D- Suke M. Biomechanics of the pulmonary autograft valve in aortic position. Thorax 1982;37:535-539
7. Ross DN. Replacement of the aortic and mitral valves with a pulmonary autograft. Lancet 1967;II:446-447
8. Gerosa G, McKay R, Ross DN. Replacment of the aortic valve or root with a pulmonary autograft in children. Ann Thorac Surg 1991;51:424-429
9. Livi U, Abdel-Kadir A, Parker R, Olsen E, Ross DN. Viability and morphology of aortic and pulmonary homografts. J Thorac Cardiovasc Surg 1987;93:755-760
10. Clarke DR, Campbell DN, Hayward AR, et al. Degeneration of aortic valve allografts in young recipients. J Thorac Cardiovasc Surg 1993;105:934-941
11. Geens M, Gonzalez-Lavin L, Dawbarn C, Ross DN. The surgical anatomy of the pulmonary artery root in relation to pulmonary valve autografts and surgery of the right ventricular outflow tract. J Thorac Cardiovasc Surg 1971;62:262-267
12. Ross DN. Replacement of the aortic valve with a pulmonary autograft. The "switch" operation. Ann Thorac Surg 1991;52:1346-1350
13. Daenen W, Gewillig M. Extended root replacement with pulmonary autografts. Euro J Cardiothorac Surg 1993;7:42-46
14. Moritz A, Domaig M, Moide P, Simon P, Lauter G, Wolner F. Pulmonary autograft valve replacement in the dilated and asymetric aortic root. Eur J Cardiothorac Surg 1993;7:405-408
15. Matsumi O, Toshikatsuy YM, Yamamoto F, Kawashima Y. Growth potential after root replacement of the right and left ventricular outflow tracts. J Heart Valve Dis 1993;2:308-310
16. Puryear LD, Feliciano SM, Calhoon JH, Ross-Konno. Procedure: a case study of a newborn. Semin Periop

Nurs 1955;4:124-131

17. Kaplan EL, Meier P. Non parametric estimates from incomplete observations. J Am Stat Assoc 1958;53:457

18. Ross DN, Jackson M, Davies J. The pulmonary autograft - a permanent aortic valve. Eur J Cardiothoracic Surg 1992;6:113-117

19. Murata H. A study of autologous pulmonary valve implantation. J Jpn Assoc Thorac Surg 1984;51:424-429

20. Elkins RC, Knott-Craig J, Ward KE, McCue C, Lane M. Pulmonary autograft in children: realized growth potential. Proc Soc Thorac Surg 1994;57:1387-1394

21. Sievers H, Rainer L, Loose R, Gieha M, Petry A, Bernard A. Time course of dimension and function of the autologous pulmonary root in the aortic position. J Thorac Cardiovasc Surg 1993;92:775-780

22. de Vries H, Bogers JC, Schoof PH, et al. Pulmonary autograft failure caused by a relapse of rheumatic fever. Ann Thorac Surg 1994;57:750-751

23. Van Salyen RJ, Schoof PH, Box E, Frohn-Mulder ME, Herzberger C, Thyssen H. Pulmonary autograft failure after aortic root replacement in a patient with juvenile rheumatoid arthritis. Eur J Cardiothorac Surg 1992;6:571-572

24. Kumar N, Prabhkar G, Gometza B, Al-Haless Z, Duran C. The Ross procedure in a young rheumatic population. Early clinical and electrocardiographic profile. J Heart Valve Dis 1993;2:376-379

25. Oswalt JD, Dewar SJ. Aortic infective endocarditis managed by the Ross procedure. J Heart Valve Dis 1993;2:380-384

26. Joyce F, Tingleff J, Pettersson G. Expanding indications for the Ross operation. J Heart Valve Dis 1995;4:352-363

27. Chambers JC, Somerville J, Ross DN. Pulmonary autografts: Results at 26 years. J Am Coll Cardiol. 1994; 23:429A

Chapter 9.3

Bioprosthetic Heart Valves: 25 Years of Development and Clinical Experience

L. Conrad Pelletier, Michel Carrier

Bioprostheses have now been in clinical use for 25 years. Throughout this period, major steps have been accomplished in bioengineering that have improved their design and performance. In this chapter, the development of, as well as the results obtained with the various bioprostheses implanted during the last quarter of a century, will be reviewed.

HISTORICAL BACKGROUND

The introduction of glutaraldehyde by Carpentier and co-workers (1) in 1968 marked the opening of the modern era of biologic devices for heart valve replacement. Although fresh and preserved aortic homografts had been used since 1962 with acceptable long term results, the problem of availability had stimulated the search for alternative tissue valves. Biologic prostheses made of a variety of fresh homologous tissues such as fascia lata, dura mater and pericardium were a disaster and were therefore rapidly abandoned. Others investigated the possibility of using heterografts. The first one was implanted in 1965 by Binet and Carpentier (2), soon to be followed by others. Various methods of sterilization and preservation were applied, with a uniformly low success rate. Out of 23 heterograft implants between 1965 and 1967, Carpentier and his group reported that only 45% to 50% still had good function after one year (1).

This early experience permitted the identification of the various factors which had a major influence on the long term evolution of heterografts, namely the need to protect the graft against cell ingrowth, the necessity of preventing immunologic reactions between host tissue and the heterograft, and finally the prevention of late denaturation of graft collagen (1). Cellular ingrowth was prevented by the use of silicone-impregnated cloth to cover the prosthetic frame. Glutaraldehyde, because of its tanning effect on graft tissue, was found to enhance the formation of collagen covalent cross-linkage bonds, thus increasing tissue strength, and, by rendering the tissue non-viable, it decreased its antigenicity markedly.

The advantages of "heterograft conditioning" were soon confirmed by the observations of a marked increase in graft function preservation after one year, reaching 82% in a group of 30 implants of such heterografts, compared to less than 50% with non-conditioned valves. Whereas non-human tissue valves had been termed "heterografts or xenografts", this new generation of "glutaraldehyde-conditioned valves" was identified by the term "bioprosthesis", to underline the fact that they were made of stabilized inert non-viable biological material, performing as a valvular prosthesis.

Soon after these encouraging results were published, Hancock Laboratories introduced the first glutaraldehyde-treated porcine bioprosthesis, which became available commercially in a full range of sizes in 1970. This heterograft was made from a porcine aortic valve mounted on a rigid stent with partially flexible struts and preserved with glutaraldehyde. In 1976, the valve was modified to improve its effective orifice and became known as the Hancock modified orifice valve. In 1971, Edwards Laboratories developed another porcine bioprosthesis, this one mounted on a fully flexible stent, which became available clinically only in 1975.

In 1971, Ionescu designed a tissue valve constructed of bovine pericardium fashioned into a three-cusp valve, mounted on a cloth-covered rigid titanium frame and treated with glutaraldehyde. Initially this pericardial bioprosthesis was constructed in the laboratories of Leeds General Infirmary, until it was produced commercially by Shiley Laboratories, starting in 1976. In 1980, another pericardial bioprosthesis mounted on a flexible stent was designed and produced by Edwards Laboratories.

It had by then become clear that the single most important factor affecting the durability of bioprostheses was the method of preparation of the tissue, and that, in this regard, glutaraldehyde had played a major role in that it increased collagen strength and stability, and decreased heterologous tissue antigenicity. Since then all biologic valvular heterografts, porcine as well as bovine pericardial, have been prepared and preserved with glutaraldehyde. This significant step forward opened the way to the development and increased popularity of bioprostheses in the treatment of valvular disease, particularly after 1976, their use reaching a peak in the mid-1980's.

BIOENGINEERING

Beside the method of preservation, other determinant factors in the dynamics and durability of tissue valves have been studied in vitro. Various approaches have permitted the improvement of our understanding of mechanical and design characteristics of the different bioprostheses, resulting in better and more durable valves.

Hydrodynamics of transvalvular flow and valve performance

Transvalvular pressure gradients have been studied with pulsatile flows ranging from two to 12 L/min. Significant differences between tissue valves have been found, with the highest pressure drops occurring with porcine valves (Hancock and Carpentier-Edwards), whereas pericardial valves were somewhat less obstructive to flow, the Hancock pericardial valve having the lowest pressure gradient (3,4). In an effort to improve the flow characteristics, the Hancock modified orifice valve was developed, in which the native right coronary cusp was replaced by a muscle-free cusp from another porcine aortic valve (5).

Calculation of the effective orifice area of various bioprosthetic valves has shown a significant improvement between earlier models and more recent prostheses (6). Whereas effective orifice areas of 1.7 to 2.3 cm^2 were obtained with the former, areas of 3 to 4 cm^2 were calculated with more recent valves of the same size, both porcine and pericardial. These data have been used to develop another measurement of valve efficacy, the performance index, which is the ratio of the calculated effective orifice area to the actual valve sewing ring area measured on the prosthesis. The performance index also indicates a clear improvement with newer models from between 0.3 and 0.4 to between 0.5 and 0.7

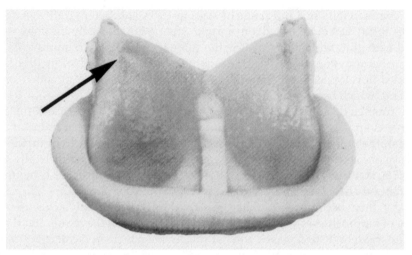

Figure 9.3-1: Ionescu-Shiley bovine pericardial bioprosthesis. The pericardium is wrapped over the valve stent and a commissural holding stitch (arrow) is placed at the summit of the stent to secure the pericardium.

for the same valve size. The search for further improvements in the hemodynamic profile of tissue valves led to the concept of stentless bioprostheses to achieve a better effective orifice area by removing the space-occupying stent of the valve (7).

Dynamic flow testing has shown marked differences in velocity and turbulent shear stress (6). Old designs had higher peak jet velocities and turbulent shear stresses than newer valves. Overall, pericardial bioprostheses had better flow characteristics than porcine valves. The flow velocity profiles of earlier porcine valve models had shown an asynchronous leaflet movement, which has been improved in more recent designs. Despite these improvements, shear stress is still present in newer valves and may be a cause of damage to blood cells and of intravascular hemolysis. On the other hand, the regurgitant flow has also been characterized. It includes two components: the closing regurgitant flow occurring during valve closure, and the leakage flow which continues after the valve has closed (3).

Total regurgitant flow is very similar in all bioprostheses, the closing regurgitant fraction being greater than the leakage regurgitation. This can be expressed in terms of transvalvular energy loss due to heat production and backward blood movement. Overall, total transvalvular energy loss across bioprostheses ranges between 2.5% and 12.3%. It tends to increase at heart rates of 120/min and higher. The energy loss is greatest with the Carpentier-Edwards pericardial valve, whereas the Mitroflow pericardial valve has the lowest. Although not clinically significant, these energy losses can indicate if an acceptable compromise between forward and backward flow performance has been achieved with a specific valve design.

Accelerated fatigue testing and mechanical stress

Durability testing of tissue valves has been performed with accelerated fatigue systems. High speed pulse duplicators are used to determine the number of cycles

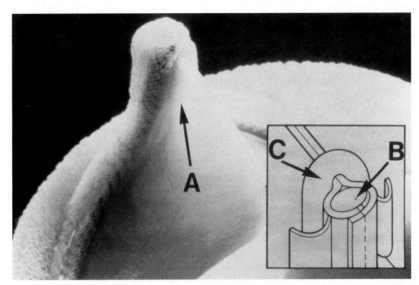

Figure 9.3-2: Carpentier-Edwards bovine pericardial bioprosthesis. The pericardium is mounted inside the stent (arrow A) and is secured in place by a Mylar plug (inset, arrow B) over which the pericardium is fixed. Leaflet coaptation is achieved by the Elgiloy wire (inset, arrow C) of the stent, thus eliminating the need for a holding stitch.

required before fatigue-induced valve lesions occur. Such studies have identified that mechanical and design characteristics are major factors in the development of tissue valve failure (8). Differences in engineering and mounting account for variations in the failure mode of the various valves. While most pericardial valves fail mainly because of stress sustained during closure, porcine valves are damaged during both opening and closing due to their design features (8). The smoothness of the surface of the sewing ring that comes in contact with valve tissue, and the flexibility of the stent to absorb part of the closing energy have been identified as significant factors affecting durability (9).

Fatigue testing of Ionescu-Shiley and Hancock pericardial valves has shown premature leaflet failure due to abrasion of the leaflets by the cloth covering at the edge of the stent during closure of the valve. In addition, these two pericardial valve substitutes, as well as the Mitroflow pericardial valve, all have a similar construction design. The pericardial tissue is wrapped over the stent and a commissural holding stitch is therefore required to secure the pericardium at the summit of the strut (Fig. 9.3-1). This particular point represents a weakness zone, and stress concentration at the support suture causes premature tearing of the leaflet (9).

Characterization of stress areas by finite element analysis on computerized models led to the development of a different mounting concept with the Carpentier-Edwards pericardial valve. The pericardial tissue is mounted inside and underneath the stent, and secured by a Mylar plug introduced within the pericardial fold into the Elgiloy wire frame, thus eliminating the need for an anchor suture at the top of the strut (Fig. 9.3-2). It was believed that such a design would eliminate the commissural stress-induced tissue laceration, a hypothesis which has so far proved to be correct, based on current clinical results with this bioprosthesis.

Stress-induced commissural tears appear to be exacerbated by exposition to the host biological environment (10). Leaflets of pericardial valves that have been implanted become thicker and less extensible than those of unimplanted valves. This observation from explanted valves has been confirmed by subcutaneous implantation in an animal model. These mechanical changes, eventually leading to gross calcification, appear to be linked to collagen fiber disruption associated with leaflet flexure. Initial signs of stress failure have been observed in 60% of Ionescu- Shiley pericardial valves after 17×10^6 cycles, and severe lesions were present after 29×10^6 (11). The tears provoked in vitro were similar to those observed in patients, occurring most often at the tissue attachment to the strut and extending to the top or downward to the base of the cusp. Therefore, these changes are related to valve design, and are exacerbated by a biological environment, suggesting that in vitro accelerated wear testing may actually overestimate the life expectancy of bioprostheses (10).

Among the several modifications proposed in the design of tissue valves to improve their performance and durability and minimize complications due to protrusion of the stent, the low-profile concept has been developed for both the porcine (the Liotta-Bioimplant valve) and the pericardial (the Ionescu-Shiley low-profile valve) bioprostheses (12,13). However, there are indications that a reduction in stent height results in increased stress on the cusps and jeopardizes valve durability (14,15).

A new conceptual design was proposed to improve durability and hydrodynamic performance by constructing a tissue valve with a single leaflet made of glutaraldehyde-preserved bovine pericardium (16). It was thought that the unicusp concept would offer the optimal internal/external diameter ratio and that the wide movement of the leaflet might decrease the propensity to calcify. Extensive in vitro testing and experimental implantations had suggested an increased resistance to fatigue-induced lesions, and a low incidence of calcification, indicating that durability might be better than that of other tissue valves (17). However, an experimental study in sheep disclosed a high calcification rate; after three to five months, 88% of unileaflet mitral and 66% of unileaflet tricuspid valves had calcified, compared to only 25% of porcine valves implanted in the tricuspid position (18). It thus appeared that, despite optimal hemodynamic performance, the unicusp pericardial valve would likely have a limited durability. Explanted valves in the human have shown cusp redundancy, dystrophic calcification, and tears attributed to stretching of the single pericardial leaflet, thus confirming the poor outcome of this design (19).

In porcine valves, mechanical stresses were found to be highest near the commissures of the valve and lowest at the base of the leaflets, which coincide with the sites of maximal and most frequent calcification of the valve, suggesting a possible causative relationship between the magnitude of mechanical stress and leaflet calcification (20). Tissue buckling of glutaraldehyde-treated porcine valves during opening causes compressive stress on the inner surface of the bend because it is less pliable than untreated natural tissue (21). This mechanism has also been suggested as a possible cause of collagen disruption and tissue calcification, which could be alleviated by different designs and preservation techniques.

In addition to valve design, the method of tissue fixation has been found to have an impact on durability. High pressure fixation alters mechanical properties of the tissue by locking the collagen in a stressed state (22). Collagen bundle separation, ultimately leading to fracture at accelerated fatigue-testing, is found in glutaraldehyde treated porcine valves fixed at high pressure (23). Leaflet kinking during opening results from the loss of the crimp in the collagen when fixed at high pressure (24). These sites of kinking are not present in low pressure-fixed valves. More recently, further studies have shown that valves fixed at zero or near zero (1.5 mmHg) pressure, contrary to those fixed at high pressure (80 mmHg), retain a collagen architecture that is virtually identical to that of a fresh porcine valve (25). The zero-pressure fixation used in the preparation of the Medtronic Intact bioprosthesis results in a more natural elastic behavior than low-pressure fixed xenografts and in a better preservation of the stress reducing properties of normal aortic valve tissue (26). Although these studies suggest that the mechanical behavior and pliability are better preserved in valves prepared with zero-pressure fixation than in low-pressure fixed valves, they are not identical to natural aortic valves, and wide variations in leaflet extensibility are observed.

Using bi-axial testing methods to evaluate the mechanical properties of leaflets from second-generation porcine valves, it was found that the new low pressure-fixed valves did not necessarily exhibit more natural leaflet properties than the former high pressure-fixed bioprostheses (27). In the circumferential direction, all tested porcine bioprostheses were highly inextensible, except for the Medtronic Intact valve, which displayed an extensibility similar to that of fresh porcine valves. On the other hand, radial extensibility of all studied valves was significantly lower than that of fresh valves, with the Carpentier- Edwards supra-annular and the Medtronic Intact being more extensible than the others. It was therefore concluded that low-pressure fixation in the second-generation tissue valves did not necessarily improve leaflet mechanical properties, compared to the former high-pressure fixed bioprostheses.

There are indications that the better mechanical properties of the zero-pressure fixed valve may be negated by stent design factors causing an excessive coaptation surface of leaflets during valve closure and compliance mismatch between the rigid stent and the pliable tissue, resulting in no net improvement in durability (28). Despite all these restrictions, low-pressure fixation is now a widely accepted concept in the fabrication of tissue valves. Whether fixation at zero pressure will prove to be superior to low-pressure fixation remains to be established.

Tissue calcification and antimineralization treatment

Calcific degeneration of tissue valves remains a major factor in their eventual failure and limited durability, as repeatedly shown by clinical studies. Several chemical approaches have been proposed to prevent or at least delay the mineralization process of bioprosthetic heart valves. Covalent binding of aminodiphosphonate to residual glutaraldehyde in the pericardial tissue was evaluated experimentally as a method of inhibition of intrinsic tissue calcification (29). A marked decrease in tissue calcification, to 15% of control, without adverse effects on animal growth and bony structure was observed. This inhibition was dependent on the amount of aminodiphosphonate incorporated by the valve tissue.

Another process was based on treating tissue valves with a derivative of oleic acid as an anticalcification method (30). Studies conducted in juvenile sheep, because of their marked propensity for rapid calcification, resulted in a dramatic decrease in the mineralization process of porcine valves compared to untreated controls.

Toluidine blue surface-active agent has been used for the processing of a glutaraldehyde-treated zero pressure-fixed porcine valve, the Medtronic Intact valve. Experimental studies in the sheep have indicated that the toluidine-treated valves had less tendency to calcification than standard untreated porcine valves (31). It was further established that this antimineralization treatment did not alter collagen morphology (25).

Other chemical treatments of tissue valves, such as sodium dodecyl sulphate used in the preparation of the Hancock II valve (32,33), are also presently being investigated. However, clinical studies have so far failed to demonstrate convincingly that current antimineralization treatments have resulted in a significant decrease in tissue calcification of bioprostheses.

PORCINE BIOPROSTHESES

The Hancock porcine valve

The Hancock bioprosthesis is the one for which the available clinical experience is most extensive as regards both total number of patients and length of follow up. It has therefore become the gold standard against which all other tissue valves are compared. Several groups have reported their long term clinical experience with the standard Hancock porcine valve. This initial model is the bioprosthesis with the longest follow up, which now extends up to 15 years. Including all deaths, actuarial survival rates of 65% at 10 and 40% at 15 years following aortic valve replacement, and of 61% and 43% after mitral valve replacement have been reported (34). When only valve-related deaths are accounted for, the respective survival rates are 94% and 86% with aortic, and 90% and 79% with mitral valve replacements. Such excellent survival rates are found in most series (35,36).

Among valve-related complications, endocarditis, hemorrhage due to anticoagulation and perivalvular leaks are rare, with a linearized rate of less than 1%/patient-year each (37). Their hazard function is relatively constant over time, resulting in freedom rates that are almost linear. The incidence of hemorrhage is directly related to the number of patients maintained on anticoagulation therapy. While Bortolotti et al. (36) found the freedom rate from thromboembolic accidents at 15 years to be higher after aortic than following mitral valve replacement, at 92% and 79% respectively, a similar rate of 68% to 70% for both valve positions was reported by Cohn et al. (34).

Structural valve degeneration includes calcification and stenosis of the valve, stenosis by stent creeping, leaflet tear, and valve disruption from the stent. It starts to appear after the sixth year in both aortic and mitral prostheses. With aortic valves, the incidence of degeneration remains low up to 11 to 12 years, after which there is a sudden rise (34). Mitral valves suffer a higher degree of degeneration than aortic valves between seven and 10 years, and the incidence rises still more rapidly after 10 years. Freedom from structural degeneration of aortic valves is 82% at 10 years and 58% after 15 years. For mitral valves, the freedom rates are 75% and 45% respectively (34). Gallucci et al. (37) did not find such a difference in durability with valve position. At 10 years, mitral bioprostheses had a higher freedom rate from degeneration than aortic by more than 20%, but at 15 years both valves had reached similar rates with 41% of mitral and 37% of aortic valves free from degeneration. Bernal and his group (38) also found similar freedom curves for valve deterioration in both positions, with an almost linear

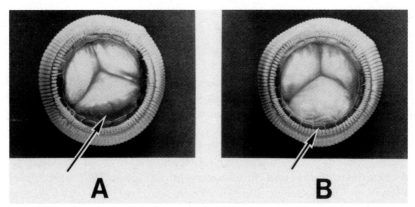

Figure 9.3-3: Hancock porcine bioprostheses. The standard model (frame A) has a leaflet with muscle shelf (arrow). In the modified orifice model (frame B), this leaflet is eliminated and replaced by a non-muscular leaflet from another porcine aortic valve (arrow), thus enlarging the effective orifice area of the valve.

downward slope between six and 14 years, resulting in freedom rates of 44% for aortic and 37% for mitral valves at 14 years.

In the tricuspid position, the Hancock porcine valve has an excellent long term durability record, with a freedom rate from structural valve deterioration of 94% after 10 years (39). Tricuspid bioprostheses retrieved from patients who also underwent implantation of an aortic or mitral bioprosthesis showed less severe degenerative changes than those in the latter positions. Similar observations were made in another study, with freedom from deterioration of 80% at 10 years and 68% at 14 years (40).

The Hancock modified orifice valve

The Hancock modified orifice was designed to improve the flow characteristics of the aortic bioprosthesis, which was deemed necessary particularly for small prosthetic sizes (Fig. 9.3-3). The fabrication of this valve raised questions about its long term durability. A study from DiSesa and colleagues (41) has found excellent results at eight to nine years following aortic valve replacement. Their actuarial survival was 78%, and the respective freedom rates from thromboembolic complications and from intrinsic valve deterioration were 87% and 97%, data which compare favorably with the results of the standard valve design. Therefore, the removal of the muscle shelf leaflet and the suturing of another leaflet do not appear to affect the long term durability of the prosthesis.

The Hancock II valve

Among the major disadvantages of the standard Hancock valve are its high profile, creeping of the stent, which has been responsible for a number of valve failures, and limited durability due to early tissue calcification (42). In an effort to correct some of these deficiencies, the Hancock II valve has been designed. It has a lower profile and an improved and more resistant Delrin stent. The valve is fixed at low pressure and treated with an antimineralization process.

In a study comparing the Hancock modified orifice (or Hancock I) and the Hancock II valves, Oury et al. (32) failed to show any significant differences between the two up to four years, although it was obviously too early to conclude on the effectiveness of the anticalcification treatment on valve durability. In a four-year follow up, Bortolotti et al. (42) reported no instances of structural valve deterioration, and freedom from overall valve failure was 96% for aortic and 91% for mitral and double valve replacements. After eight years, the Hancock II has freedom rates from thromboembolic complications of 93% for aortic and 83% for mitral replacements, and overall freedom rates from structural valve deterioration and from reoperation of 92% and 89% respectively (43). In the latter study, no difference in durability of the bioprosthesis was found as regards valve position.

Comparative data

The results obtained with the Hancock porcine valve have been compared to those of mechanical valve prostheses. No differences in patient survival and in thromboembolic complications between the Hancock valve and the Björk-Shiley mechanical prosthesis was evidenced up to seven years (44). Milano et al. (35) compared the Hancock to the Björk-Shiley and Lillehei-Kaster valves for aortic valve replacement. Up to 15 years, there was no difference in valve-related deaths. During the first six years after implantation, the Hancock bioprosthesis was superior as regards valve-related complications, an advantage that was progressively lost in favor of the two mechanical prostheses as follow up increased, because of the cumulative incidence of intrinsic valve deterioration and reoperation with the tissue valve.

Hemodynamic performance

Hemodynamic evaluation of the mitral standard Hancock valve has shown good performance, with transvalvular gradients of 6 to 9 mmHg and calculated effective orifice areas between 1.4 and 2.2 cm^2 (45,46). In both of these studies however, a significant hemodynamic deterioration was found, with an average increase in the transprosthetic gradient of 3 mmHg and a decrease in effective orifice area of 0.2 to 0.5 cm^2 after six to seven years of implantation. At early postoperative evaluation of the aortic standard Hancock valve, peak systolic aortic gradients averaged between 10 mmHg with 21mm size to 6 mmHg for 27mm size, and effective orifice areas varied from 1.27 cm^2 for 21mm size to 1.97 cm^2 for 27mm size valves (47).

Rossiter and his group compared the aortic standard and modified orifice Hancock valves (48). The average peak systolic gradient of the modified orifice model was almost half that of the standard valve, and mean systolic gradients were lower with the former for all valve sizes, although none of these differences reached statistical significance. No difference in effective orifice area was found between the two models. The changes in the design of the valve therefore appeared to have resulted in a small functional improvement, the clinical significance of which remains uncertain.

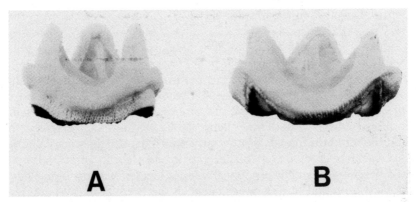

Figure 9.3-4: Aortic Carpentier-Edwards porcine bioprostheses, standard model (A) and supra-annular model (B).

Echocardiographic evaluation of the Hancock II model has shown a mean transvalvular gradient of 7 mmHg for mitral prostheses and 18 mmHg for aortic valves (32). Aortic gradients varied from 11 to 14 mmHg for aortic valve sizes 23 to 29mm, whereas it averaged 23 mmHg for 21mm valves. Peak systolic gradients from 14 to 23 mmHg were reported by David et al. (43) with the Hancock II aortic valve, and mean valve areas ranged from 1.18 cm² for 21mm size to 1.6 cm² for 27mm size. For mitral prostheses, mean valve areas ranged from 2.21 to 3.15 cm², according to valve size. The data obtained for the Hancock II model compare with those of the standard valve, although two different methods of evaluation were used. The hemodynamic performance of both models thus appears adequate.

The Carpentier-Edwards porcine valve

The Carpentier-Edwards porcine valve has also been implanted extensively, although for a shorter period of time. It has a more flexible stent than the Hancock valve, and the muscle shelf is incorporated into the suture line of the sewing ring. The 10- year patient survival is 65% to 69% after aortic valve replacement, and 55% to 62% following mitral replacement (49,50). After 10 years, we have observed freedom rates from thromboembolism of 96% with aortic and 89% with mitral prostheses; those for endocarditis were 95% and 97% respectively (49). Freedom from reoperation for any cause at 10 years varies from 74% to 83% with aortic, and from 53% to 67% with mitral valves (49,50). Up to five years, freedom from intrinsic structural deterioration is virtually 100% for valves in both positions (51). With further postoperative evolution, there is a progressive decrease in freedom from deterioration of mitral prostheses, which tends to accelerate after eight years, resulting in a freedom rate of 54% to 59% at 10 years (49,52). For aortic valves, the fall off of freedom from deterioration is slow until nine years, and seems to accelerate somewhat between nine and 10 years, resulting in a freedom rate of 77% to 82% after 10 years. A similar though less important difference between the two valve positions was also reported by Jamieson and his group (50). In the absence of valve dysfunction, no clinically significant hemolysis occurs with this bioprosthesis (49).

The Carpentier-Edwards supra-annular valve

This is a modification of the design of the standard model to improve the fit of the prosthesis to the native annulus of the patient to minimize the stress-strain on the leaflets, and to obtain better hemodynamic performance, by allowing implantation of the valve in a supra-annular position. The valve has a lower profile, a more flexible stent, and low-pressure fixation is used in the preparation of the tissue (Fig. 9.3-4). Up to five years, no difference was found by Pelletier and associates (52) between the supra-annular and the standard models of the Carpentier-Edwards porcine valve as regards patient survival, reoperation and intrinsic structural deterioration of the valve. No significant differences in patient survival and in the incidence of any of the valve-related complications were found at four years between the two valves by Jamieson and his group (53,54).

Comparative studies

Up to seven to 10 years after implantation, no significant differences between the Hancock standard and the Carpentier-Edwards standard bioprostheses in terms of patient survival, valve-related complications, and structural valve deterioration have been observed (44,55-59). In a tri-institutional study comparing the Hancock, the Carpentier-Edwards, and the Starr-Edwards silastic ball valves, the latter was found superior to tissue valves regarding structural valve deterioration (57). However, using the concept of treatment failure, which includes all permanent valve-related complications, the three valves gave comparative results in the aortic position, while tissue valves displayed a small advantage in the mitral position, after 10 years.

Hemodynamic performance

At postoperative cardiac catheterization, mean pressure gradients ranging from 8 mmHg for sizes 29-31mm aortic prostheses to 13 mmHg for the 21-23mm sizes were measured at rest, the overall gradient averaging 11 mmHg (51). The mean effective aortic orifice areas ranged from 1.14 to 1.93 cm^2. With mitral prostheses, the resting pressure gradient averaged 6 mmHg, ranging from 5 mmHg with larger to 7 mmHg with smaller size valves. Mean effective mitral orifice areas ranged from 2.33 to 2.68 cm^2. Exercise increased pressure gradients, but also the mean effective orifice areas by 12% to 26%, indicating that full opening of the bioprosthesis was flow-dependent.

The improved annulus model was designed to obtain a better hemodynamic performance of the valve, by decreasing the width of the sewing ring, allowing a larger effective orifice area. However, hemodynamic evaluation with cardiac catheterization failed to demonstrate any significant differences in transvalvular pressure gradients and in effective orifice areas between the two valve models (60). Levine et al. (61) reported that the standard Carpentier-Edwards aortic and mitral bioprostheses had a better hemodynamic performance than the Hancock modified orifice valve, with significantly lower transvalvular gradients for all valve sizes, at intraoperative evaluation.

In a study performed intraoperatively comparing the supra-annular and the standard porcine Carpentier-Edwards aortic valves, the supra-annular model had significantly lower systolic pressure gradients than the standard for the 25mm size (62). The effective orifice areas were also improved by 15% to 30% in favor of the former. The 23mm supra-annular valve had a mean orifice area of 1.4 cm^2, close to that of the 25mm size standard valve, which averaged 1.6cm ^{2}. These data therefore suggest that the supra-annular valve is hemodynamically superior to the standard one.

Few studies have specifically addressed the problem of clinical hemodynamic evaluation of small size aortic bioprostheses. Eight patients with an aortic standard Carpentier-Edwards porcine valve were studied by cardiac catheterization within three years of surgery (63). The aortic gradients averaged 33 mmHg for the three valves of 19mm size, and 10 mmHg for the five valves of 21mm size. Valve areas ranged from 0.8 to 1.24 cm^2 (mean: 1.01 cm^2) for the 19mm size, and from 1.06 to 1.70 cm^2 (mean: 1.45 cm^2) for the 21mm size valves, indicating that the 19mm size was slightly obstructive. More recently, the 19mm Carpentier-Edwards supra-annular aortic valve was assessed in 15 patients by echocardiographic studies within four years of surgery (64). The peak aortic pressure gradient at rest averaged 34 mmHg, and the mean effective valve area was 1.1 cm^2, results that are quite similar to those obtained with the standard model in the previous study. Therefore, it appears that the various modifications in valve design have not succeeded in improving the hemodynamic performance significantly, at least in the smallest aortic size.

The Angell-Shiley porcine valve

Although the Angell-Shiley bioprosthesis was introduced soon after the Hancock, very few studies have been published on this valve. It was designed with an asymmetrical valve stent to maintain a more natural configuration and thus optimize leaflet coaptation, decrease tissue stress and valve dehiscence by providing a better adaptation of the stent to the patient annulus (65). Its proponents reported their total experience with more than 700 implanted valves (66). At 10 years, the overall freedom from structural valve deterioration for aortic and mitral valves was similar to that obtained by the same group with the Hancock I porcine valve, with respective rates of 72% and 68%. The fall off of the freedom curve for both valves occurred at a similar rate.

Hemodynamic evaluation

In a hemodynamic study of 45 patients, with cardiac catheterization performed within three years of operation, a mean aortic gradient of 22 mmHg, increasing to 27 mmHg with exercise, was found, with effective orifice areas averaging 1.23 cm^2 at rest and 1.51 cm^2 during exercise (67). The mean diastolic gradient of mitral prostheses averaged 8 mmHg at rest and 12 mmHg during exercise, with respective orifice areas of 1.67 and 2.05 cm^2. Eleven of the 29 aortic valves (38%) had an aortic gradient at rest of 25 mmHg or more, even though all but two of the aortic valves were 25mm size or larger. In the mitral position, eight of the 16 valves (50%) had a gradient of 10 mmHg or more, with all valves but one being 29mm or more in size. This study indicated that this bioprosthesis was significantly stenotic.

This was confirmed in a second study by the same group (68). The hemodynamic evaluation was obtained an average of 14 months postoperatively. The average mitral gradient at rest was 8 mmHg increasing to 27 mmHg at exercise. With aortic valves, the resting gradient was 22 mmHg increasing to 27 mmHg at exercise. A regression analysis model predicted that an aortic stent diameter of less than 25mm would have an effective orifice area smaller than 1.0 cm^2, and that for a mitral valve of less than 30mm the effective area would be under 1.5 cm^2.

It was therefore concluded that this bioprosthesis was suboptimal in its hemodynamic performance, and severely stenotic in the smaller valve sizes. As a consequence, the Angell-Shiley porcine valve was withdrawn from the market in 1982.

The Liotta-Bioimplant porcine valve (St. Jude-Bioimplant)

This bioprosthesis was designed to obtain a better hydrodynamic performance and to take advantage of a low-profile stent in order to decrease the complications due to protrusion of the stent, particularly in the small ventricular cavity of patients with predominant mitral stenosis. Few clinical reports have yet been published on this valve substitute, and only small series are available. In a mid-term report on 184 patients, overall freedom rates at six years were 97% for thromboembolic complications and endocarditis, 92% for valve failure, and 88% for reoperation (69).

However, another group reported a new mode of late failure with this valve in the mitral position (15). Prolapse of the right coronary cusp with eventual commissural rupture and flailed leaflet was found in several of the patients undergoing reoperation because of severe regurgitation. This was attributed to excessive systolic stress on the leaflets due to the low-profile design of the valve. This finding was further substantiated in a long term evaluation of the same series of 71 patients (70). Ten years after implantation of the valve in the mitral position, freedom from thromboembolism was 96%, and that from structural deterioration was 63%. The characteristic low-profile stent configuration was responsible for the particular mode of failure that had been described in the previous study, leading to reoperation in 10 of their patients. Similar findings were reported by another group, who found that structural deterioration of mitral prostheses occurred at a significantly earlier time during follow up with the Liotta-Bioimplant valve compared to the Hancock bioprosthesis (71).

Hemodynamic data

A postoperative hemodynamic evaluation of the valve in 40 patients found excellent results (12). The mean gradient through mitral prostheses averaged 2 mmHg at rest and 5 mmHg with exercise; aortic prosthesis gradients were 14 and 21 mmHg respectively. Mean orifice areas ranged from 1.66 to 4.5 cm^2 for the sizes 28 and 30mm mitral valves, and 1.35 to 2.96 cm^2 for aortic prostheses of 23 to 26mm size. However, no data are available on the small aortic sizes. Despite its excellent hemodynamic characteristics, it appears from these studies that the Liotta-Bioimplant valve does not provide any clear-cut advantages over other standard bioprostheses, and that its low-profile design may even compromise its durability, at least in mitral valve replacement.

The Medtronic Intact porcine valve

The Medtronic Intact valve has a high profile stent, is fixed in glutaraldehyde at zero pressure, and is treated with toluidine blue as an antimineralization process, giving the valve its blue color. This is the main distinctive feature of this bioprosthesis. An initial clinical study on 167 patients reported two cases of ventricular perforation by the struts, believed to be due to the high profile of the valve, and three cases of early calcification of the valve among patients aged less than 20 years, for a three-year calcification rate of 22% (72). However, among patients older than 20 years, there had been no structural deterioration. At three years, the overall freedom from valve deterioration was therefore 78%. Two other early follow up studies reported no primary tissue failure of this valve up to three and four years (73,74). Respective freedom rates were 87% and 85% for thromboembolism, and 90% and 96% for reoperation.

Hemodynamic data

A hemodynamic evaluation obtained in 15 patients with a mitral prosthesis indicated that the 29 and 31mm size valves had acceptable mean diastolic gradients ranging from 4 to 9 mmHg, with valve areas between 1.16 and 3.16 cm^2. However, the 25mm size valves were stenotic, with a mean gradient of 12 mmHg and a valve area always smaller than 1.0 cm^2, averaging 0.88 cm^2 (72). Echocardiographic studies of 32 mitral valves found an average gradient of 4 mmHg and a surface area of 2.2 cm^2 (73). However, all valves were 29mm size or larger. Of the 23 aortic valves studied (sizes 23 to 27mm), the mean pressure gradient averaged 17 mmHg. The 23mm aortic valve was also rather obstructive, with mean and peak aortic gradients averaging 19 and 33 mmHg, respectively.

In a comparative echocardiographic evaluation of 20 to 23mm size allografts, 23mm Medtronic Intact bioprostheses, and 21 or 23mm St. Jude Medical mechanical valves in the aortic position, allograft valves had the best performance (75). Mean aortic gradients at rest averaged 6 to 7 mmHg with allografts, 12 mmHg with the St. Jude valve, and 19 mmHg for the Medtronic Intact. With exercise, respective gradients were 8 to 10, 16, and 28 mmHg. Valve orifice areas ranged from 2.2 cm^2 for allografts to 1.1 cm^2 for the porcine valve. The latter was always more obstructive that the others, even though the valve size used was the largest.

It can therefore be concluded from these reports that the Medtronic Intact valve is somewhat obstructive, and that it should not be used in sizes smaller than 25mm in the aortic position and 29mm for the mitral valve. The antimineralization process is not effective and appears to wash out in a matter of months, according to observations made on explanted prostheses. The high profile of the valve may be deleterious, particularly in patients with a small left ventricle. Finally, cases of leaflet prolapse with major regurgitation, even without tissue laceration, have been observed in our limited experience with this bioprosthesis, leading to early reoperation in three patients.

Other porcine valves

There are other porcine bioprostheses for which the clinical experience is much more limited because they have been restricted, mainly to regional use. Since they have been the object of only few reports, it is difficult to reach a firm opinion regarding the specific valve relative to the more commonly used valves.

The Biocor porcine valve

This tissue prosthesis was developed in Brazil in 1981, and has been in clinical use in that country since then. It is very similar to other porcine valves, and the main characteristics of the Biocor valve are particularly careful harvesting, tanning, and handling of the tissue (76). It is mounted on a low-profile flexible stent. The initial results were satisfactory, although the incidence of valve dysfunction was found to be high in the early experience. This was in part due to implantation in a number of patients less than 15 years of age (76). In a more recent report on 1101 patients with a follow up extending up to eight years, and averaging four years, a high incidence of valve calcification was found, particularly in patients younger than 20 years of age, which represented 20% of the total series (77). However, the eight-year freedom rate from primary valve dysfunction in adult patients was 95% for mitral and 97% for aortic valves, results that are similar to those with other porcine valves. The authors report that the prosthesis is known to be somewhat restrictive, with greater hydrodynamic gradients than those of other tissue valves. They conclude that work continues to be done on this valve to improve its durability, by using a new tanning process without glutaraldehyde, and a new design for better hydrodynamic function.

The Wessex bioprosthesis

Developed in the United Kingdom in 1981, the valve has been implanted in several countries since 1983, but unfortunately the clinical experience has not been published extensively. In 1986, an initial report on early clinical results in 245 patients, pooled from three medical centers in the United Kingdom, indicated satisfactory results after an average follow up duration of one year (78). No primary tissue failure was observed in this short term series. The valve is essentially similar to other porcine bioprostheses, but it is subjected to a more stringent quality control, with individual hydrodynamic testing of each valve, and optimal preservation at the time of harvesting. There are few data on the hemodynamic performance of the valve, none on its long term durability, precluding any valid opinion on its value at this time. Soon after Wessex Medical Ltd. was purchased by Sorin Biomedica, the valve was withdrawn from the market.

The Xenomedica valve

This is yet another porcine bioprosthesis that became available in 1981, and for which only limited and short term information is available. The prosthesis is a composite porcine valve, prepared with low-pressure fixation, and mounted on a low-profile semi-rigid stent. The early experience reported by a British group with 154 patients was also satisfactory, but the follow up averaged only 1.5 years (79). Despite this very limited postoperative follow up, two cases of valve dysfunction occurred, one due to massive thrombosis of an aortic prosthesis 14 months after implantation, the other caused by stiffened leaflets of a mitral valve that required removal. The authors complained about the poor design of the sewing ring, which was difficult to penetrate with the suture needle. A morphologic study of 13 Xenomedica valves explanted between one day and one year after implantation has found changes similar to those reported with the other porcine bioprostheses, with loosening of the spongiosa and loss of proteoglycans;

calcification was present in one of the valves studied (80). No late results are available on this device.

PERICARDIAL BIOPROSTHESES

The Ionescu-Shiley pericardial valve

The standard Ionescu-Shiley pericardial valve became commercially available in 1976, and the low-profile model was introduced in 1981. The initial report by the proponent of the valve was enthusiastic about its clinical performance (81). After five years, the freedom rate from endocarditis was 96%, and that from thromboembolism was 98% for aortic and 92% for mitral prostheses. Freedom from reoperation was 94% with aortic valves and 90% with mitral prostheses, and the respective patient survival rates were 92% and 91%. Similar results were obtained by Gonzalez-Lavin et al. (82) and by Michel and his group (83). In two reviews of his overall experience with the standard model of the valve, Ionescu (84,85) reported a 10-year survival of 73% following aortic and of 72% after mitral replacements. The freedom rates from tissue failure were 88% and 91%, and those from thromboembolism 99% and 96% respectively. These results suggested that this pericardial prosthesis was a safe and reliable valve substitute for up to 10 to 12 years.

It was not until other investigators began to report their own experience that the first signs of alarm regarding the durability of the Ionescu-Shiley valve appeared in the literature. Seven cases of valve degeneration had been found after three to six years following aortic valve replacement with the standard model of the pericardial bioprosthesis in a small series of 65 patients, with a resulting freedom rate from valve deterioration of 79% at seven years (86). This was the first report indicating that the Ionescu-Shiley pericardial valve might be less durable than porcine bioprostheses. This was soon to be confirmed by several other groups. The largest series was no doubt that of Reul et al. (87) with a total of 2,680 patients in whom the standard Ionescu-Shiley valve had been implanted. These authors reported a freedom rate from reoperation at five years of only 82% after aortic replacement and of 87% for mitral valves. The main cause of reoperation was intrinsic degeneration by calcification and leaflet disruption. Their finding did cast serious doubts on the durability of the prosthesis.

There are very few published data on the low-profile model of the Ionescu-Shiley valve. However, from the available results, it appears to be even worse than the standard model. Ravichandran et al. in Leeds (88) observed that leaflet disruption occurred earlier and in a more acute way with the low-profile valve than with the standard model. The mean interval between implantation and explantation was five years with the former compared to 11 years with the standard valve. However, in other studies, both models were found to fail early and by the same mechanism, leaflet tearing from its attachment to the strut of the prosthesis (89-91). A 10-year freedom from tissue degeneration of 77% with aortic valves was reported by Revuelta et al. (92). The first cases of failure occurred between two and three years after implantation, and were due about equally to leaflet disruption and tissue calcification. Even worse results were obtained by Masters et al. (93), with a freedom from structural failure of only 48% with aortic and 44% with mitral valves after 10 years. There was no difference in the risk of degeneration at six years between the standard and low-profile models. The Ionescu-Shiley valve was satisfactory for tricuspid valve replacement, only one instance of degeneration occurring 12 years after implantation among a group of 73 patients (94).

Comparative data

In a comparative study between porcine and pericardial bioprostheses, we had reported similar results in terms of patient survival, thromboembolic complications, and endocarditis, up to six years of follow up (49). The main differences between the two valve types were the rates of reoperation and of structural valve deterioration of mitral bioprostheses, with six-year freedom rates of 92% and 68% for reoperation, and of 92% and 70% for tissue degeneration, in favor of the porcine valves. The higher incidence of structural deterioration among pericardial valves was almost completely due to the Ionescu-Shiley valve, which was responsible for 83% of the failures of pericardial tissue valves in the mitral position. Further analysis indicated that in the aortic position there was no difference in the freedom rate from structural deterioration of Ionescu-Shiley pericardial valves and that of standard Carpentier-Edwards porcine valves up to six years, whereas in the mitral position, it was markedly lower with the Ionescu-Shiley than with the porcine valve, with respective freedom rates of 77% and 93% (52).

On the other hand, Nistal et al. (95) found a higher incidence of primary dysfunction with the Ionescu-Shiley bioprosthesis than with the Hancock valve in the aortic position, with respective freedom rates of 80% and 96% after six years, an experience different from ours. The discrepancy in the results of the two studies may be explained by the difference in the number of patients who were followed for six years or more. In a review of 240 patients undergoing aortic valve replacement using the Ionescu-Shiley bioprosthesis, the 10-year freedom rate from intrinsic tissue failure was 58%. Although the first failures occurred as early as two years, the risk of this complication increased exponentially after the seventh year (96).

Hemodynamic results

The Ionescu-Shiley valve has a very good hemodynamic performance. Mean pressure gradients of 6 mmHg with mitral valves and 10 mmHg for aortic prostheses, with mean effective orifice areas of 1.3 and 1.5cm^2 respectively have been obtained at intraoperative measurements (97). Postoperative evaluation has shown gradients of 10 to 17 mmHg and orifice areas of 1.5 to 1.9 cm^2 for aortic prostheses, and a mean gradient of 5 mmHg and valve areas of 2.7 to 3.1 cm^2 with mitral bioprostheses (98). Even in the small aortic sizes 19 and 21mm, the valve appears very adequate, and is superior to the standard Carpentier-Edwards porcine valve of the same sizes (63). At rest mean aortic pressure gradients average 11 and 6 mmHg for 19 and 21mm size pericardial valves, compared to 33 and 10 mmHg for the porcine ones. With exercise, the gradient of the 19mm pericardial valve increases to 14 mmHg and that of the 21mm size to 16 mmHg. From postoperative catheterization data, effective orifice areas ranging from 1.03 to 2.1 cm^2 for the 19mm size, and 1.5 to 2.65 cm^2 for the 21mm size pericardial valves have been calculated. However, it must be stressed that due to the sizing method used to measure the Ionescu-Shiley prosthesis, the diameter of this prosthesis actually corresponds to that one size larger for most other bioprostheses.

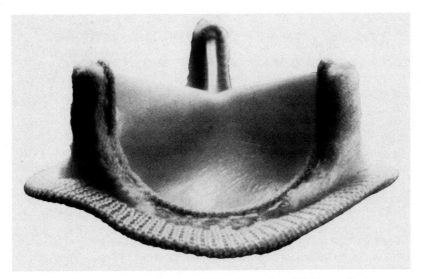

Figure 9.3-5: Carpentier-Edwards bovine pericardial bioprosthesis.

Similar results have been obtained with echocardiographic evaluation of the valve, with a mean gradient of 3 mmHg across mitral and of 11 mmHg across aortic prostheses (99). However, for small aortic sizes, the pressure gradients found at echocardiography were somewhat higher than those reported in the previously cited hemodynamic study, averaging 18 mmHg for 17mm size, 31 and 34 mmHg for 19mm size, and approximately 24 mmHg for 21mm size valves (100,101). Despite excellent hemodynamic characteristics, the poor clinical performance of the valve due to its limited durability prompted discontinuation of its use and its subsequent withdrawal from the market by the manufacturer in 1988.

The Carpentier-Edwards pericardial valve

The Carpentier-Edwards bovine pericardial valve has been in clinical use since 1981 for aortic implantation (Fig. 9.3-5). The mitral model of the valve became available again in 1984, after the initial version had been withdrawn from the market in 1981 following implantation of a few valves only, because of excessive flexibility of the stent. Our initial experience with this valve in 189 patients who underwent aortic valve replacement was favorable (102). The five-year actuarial survival was 82% and the freedom rates from thromboembolic events and reoperation were 91% and 98% respectively. No intrinsic valve deterioration had occurred. No clinically significant hemolysis was shown at hematological evaluation of 77 patients, an average of 18 months after operation.

Further analysis of 284 patients in whom 222 Carpentier-Edwards pericardial valves had been implanted in the aortic position and 77 in the mitral position confirmed earlier results (103). Survival rates after five years were 81% for aortic and 93% for mitral replacements. Three patients developed valve failure in this series; one developed mitral regurgitation due to deformation of the stent because of excessive flexibility of the initial mitral model, one suffered thrombosis of a 19mm size aortic valve, and tissue

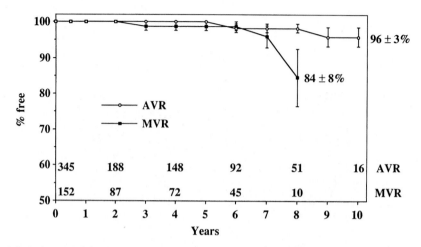

Figure 9.3-6: Actuarial freedom curves from intrinsic structural deterioration in 345 patients with isolated aortic valve replacement (AVR) and in 152 patients with isolated or combined mitral valve replacement (MVR), using Carpentier-Edwards pericardial bioprostheses. Numbers at bottom of the graph indicate number of patients at risk in each group at beginning of period; vertical bars indicate standard error of the mean. Freedom rates shown at 10 years for aortic and at eight years for mitral prostheses.

degeneration with calcification and tear of an aortic prosthesis developed 6.5 years after implantation in the last patient. The overall freedom from valve failure was 96% at six years, and that from reoperation was 92%.

Our total experience now includes more than 500 patients, with a 99% complete follow up extending beyond 10 years. The 10-year patient survival following aortic valve replacement is 69%. Survival eight years after mitral and mitro-aortic valve replacement is 67% and 65% respectively. With aortic prostheses, freedom rates from thromboembolism, endocarditis, and reoperation for any cause are 93%, 95% and 93% respectively after 10 years. At eight years following mitral valve replacement, those freedom rates are 92%, 100% and 77%. Since only 16% of the patients in this series were maintained on long term anticoagulation therapy postoperatively, hemorrhagic events have been rare, with only four minor incidents overall. Intrinsic valve deterioration occurred in three patients with an aortic bioprosthesis, for a freedom rate of 96% after 10 years, and in four with a mitral prosthesis, with a resulting eight-year freedom rate of 84% (Fig. 9.3-6). There has been no primary leaflet tear, and dysfunction has always been due to calcification of the valve.

Others have reported a similar experience with this valve in the aortic position, with a seven-year structural valve deterioration freedom rate of 97%, and an event-free rate for reoperation of 96% (104).

Comparative studies

In a comparative study of different bioprostheses, we had found that up to six years, Carpentier-Edwards porcine and pericardial valves and Ionescu-Shiley pericardial valves in the aortic position had a similar freedom rate from valve degeneration of 98%

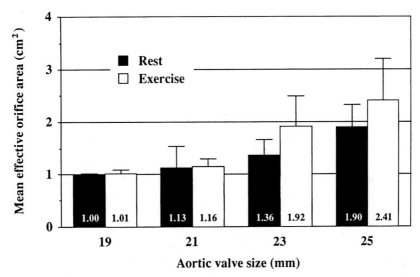

Figure 9.3-7: Mean effective orifice areas at rest and during exercise, in 28 asymptomatic patients with aortic Carpentier-Edwards pericardial valve studied at cardiac catheterization, an average of six months after operation. Data shown as mean ± standard deviation.

(52). In the mitral position, both Carpentier-Edwards bioprostheses had a freedom from deterioration of 97% after five years, contrasting with the rate of 83% for the Ionescu-Shiley valve, a difference which was statistically significant.

Hemodynamic evaluation

Intraoperative hemodynamic measurements following aortic valve replacement have shown excellent hemodynamic results with this valve, even in the small 19mm size (105). Mean transvalvular gradients ranged from 23 mmHg for 19mm size to 13 mmHg for 25mm size, with mean orifice areas from 1.1 to 2.1 cm^2 over the same range. In a comparative study, these authors have also established that the hemodynamic performance of the aortic Carpentier-Edwards pericardial valve was superior to that of the Carpentier-Edwards standard and supra-annular porcine valves (62). For all valve sizes tested, the mean gradient of the pericardial valve was lower with the pericardial than that of either porcine valves, and the effective orifice area was larger, ranging from 1.3 cm^2 for the 21mm valve to 2.2 cm^2 for the 25mm size. The performance index (effective orifice area/sewing ring area) was always better with the former than with either porcine models.

Invasive hemodynamic evaluation of 28 asymptomatic patients, an average of six months after aortic valve replacement, gave very similar results (102). The mean pressure gradients ranged from 24 mmHg for 19mm size to 11 mmHg for 25mm size at rest, increasing to 31 and 13 mmHg respectively with exercise. Calculated mean orifice areas were between 1.0 and 2.4 cm^2 (Fig. 9.3-7). The effective orifice of the 19mm valve did not increase with exercise, whereas that of larger valves increased progressively with size, by as much as 26% with the largest one.

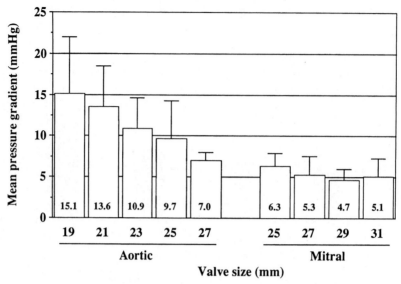

Figure 9.3-8: Mean pressure gradients across Carpentier-Edwards pericardial bioprostheses at postoperative echocardiographic study performed after an average of 15 months in 80 patients with aortic and in 40 patients with mitral prostheses. Data shown as mean ± standard deviation. Overall pressure gradients averaged 12 mmHg for aortic and 5 mmHg for mitral prostheses.

We have also performed echocardiographic studies in 120 patients an average of 15 months after valve implantation. In 80 aortic prostheses, mean transvalvular pressure gradients ranging from 7 to 15 mmHg were measured; in 40 mitral valves, the gradients varied from 5 to 6 mmHg (Fig. 9.3-8). The mean aortic gradients in our series are identical to those reported by Frater et al. (104) from echocardiographic studies performed between one and six years postoperatively. In the latter study, effective orifice areas between 1.0 and 1.8 cm^2 were calculated. Although a significant error factor may be introduced in the valve area calculated from echocardiographic data because of the many assumptions that have to be made, their results compare to ours obtained from postoperative cardiac catheterization (102).

The Mitroflow pericardial valve

The specific characteristic of this bioprosthesis is that each individual unit is submitted to in vitro pulsatile flow testing before it is released for clinical use, to ensure quality control of its hemodynamic performance. Relatively few clinical studies are currently available. In an early report, with a mean follow up of only slightly over 1.5 years in 99 patients, a surprisingly high linearized incidence of 4.1%/patient-year for thromboembolic complications was found (106). This was particularly noticeable with aortic prostheses, whose incidence rose to 7%/patient-year. In addition, structural valve deterioration was also a prominent valve-related complication in this series, with valve failure due to leaflet tear occurring in two patients as early as the third year following mitral valve replacement. The overall freedom from valve deterioration was already decreased to 93% at three years. The three-year freedom rates from valve deterioration and from reoperation for mitral bioprostheses were as low as 83% and 77% respectively. Those results raised questions regarding the durability of the valve in the mitral position and possible thrombogenicity of the aortic prosthesis.

In our comparative study, a similar observation was made regarding the durability of the valve (52). Whereas at four years the deterioration and reoperation-free rates of the Mitroflow were similar to those of other pericardial and porcine valves in the aortic position, they were significantly lower than those of the Carpentier-Edwards porcine and pericardial valves in the mitral position. After four years, 79% of the Mitroflow bioprostheses were free from reoperation and 92% were free from structural deterioration, results that were very close to those obtained with the mitral Ionescu-Shiley valve. As with the latter valve, the cause of failure of the Mitroflow prosthesis was mainly leaflet tear from a commissure downward.

These results were further substantiated in a tri-institutional study gathering a total of 354 patients followed for up to five years (107). Again, early structural deterioration of the prostheses in the mitral position was evidenced by a freedom rate of only 93% and reoperation-free rate of 83% after four years. In this latter study however, the incidence of thromboembolism was similar for both aortic and mitral prostheses. After seven years, an 86% freedom rate from primary tissue failure has been obtained, but four of the five valve failures occurred with mitral prostheses (108).

The hemodynamic performance of the valve has not been studied clinically. From the results currently reported, it appears that the Mitroflow valve will have a clinical evolution similar to that of the Ionescu-Shiley valve. The durability of the mitral prosthesis will most probably be severely compromised at mid-term, and there is a question regarding the thrombogenicity of the aortic model. Therefore, the Mitroflow pericardial valve offers no additional advantages, and its clinical use may be compromised by other tissue valves with a better long term prognosis, particularly for mitral valve replacement.

The Hancock pericardial valve (Vascor)

This valve has not been widely implanted, and the limited clinical experience has been dismal. It became available in 1981. The design of the valve is very similar to that of the Ionescu- Shiley bioprosthesis. The pericardial tissue is wrapped around the struts of the valve and held by a fixation suture at the top of the strut.

As early as two years after implantation, structural deterioration of the valve began to appear, requiring reoperation (109). While the incidence rates of embolic, hemorrhagic, and infective complications were similar to those of other tissue valves, ranging from 0.8 to 1.6%/patient-year, that of structural degeneration of the valve was unduly high, at 5.8%/patient-year. This resulted in a decrease in patient survival to 65% at five years, and to a freedom rate from degeneration of only 74% after five years (110). After a mean follow up of only three years, 16% of all aortic and 33% of the mitral prostheses had already been explanted because of valve failure. In all cases, a longitudinal laceration of the pericardial tissue from the summit of the strut downward, causing leaflet prolapse and regurgitation, was found. Similar results at five years were reported by others (111).

Early degeneration of the valve has also been observed by Bortolotti and his group

(112). The linearized incidence of structural valve deterioration was 10%/patient-year with aortic replacement, 10.6%/patient-year with mitral replacement, and 16.6%/patient-year with double valve replacement. At seven years, the actuarial freedom from degeneration of the valve was 25% after aortic, 29% after mitral, and 0% following double valve replacement. The mechanism of failure was always tearing of the cusps. These authors concluded that the extremely poor clinical results of this valve justified its prophylactic replacement in asymptomatic patients with clinical signs of valve dysfunction. All patients with this valve substitute should be carefully and closely followed for early detection of acute valve failure.

No clinical hemodynamic data are available on this valve substitute. The premature failure of the Hancock pericardial prosthesis was obviously related to its structural design, and its very limited durability justified withdrawal of the device from the market in 1986.

The Meadox-Gabbay unileaflet pericardial valve

The clinical experience with the monocusp pericardial valve is very scanty. Preliminary results seemed encouraging (113). No structural valve deterioration had occurred among 66 patients followed for up to 16 months. Postoperative hemodynamic studies in a small number of patients had shown an excellent early hemodynamic performance in the mitral position, with a mean gradient of 3 mmHg and effective orifice areas ranging from 3.1 to 5.47 cm^2.

However, in a small group of 12 patients with a longer follow up, a very high incidence of valve failure was found (114). After an average follow up of five years, five patients had undergone reoperation because of structural deterioration of the valve between 21 and 81 months postoperatively, and three others had died from congestive heart failure, two of them with signs of major valve dysfunction at echocardiography. Thus, 58% of the patients had developed valve deterioration, and only 33% were still alive and well. Therefore, despite interesting early results, the valve did not live up to expectations, and the extremely poor mid-term durability has made this device totally unsuitable for further clinical use.

Other pericardial valves

A number of new pericardial bioprostheses have been developed in recent years. Their use has remained somewhat limited so far and longer follow up is still needed to determine their late durability.

The Bioflo valve

The Bioflo pericardial valve was designed in 1987, at the Royal Infirmary in Glasgow, Scotland, by Wheatley and his colleagues (115). The frame of the valve is covered with pericardium to prevent leaflet abrasion. The clinical evaluation of this new valve was performed, from 1987 to 1989, in a comparative study with a well established tissue valve, the Carpentier-Edwards supra-annular porcine bioprosthesis, in 145 patients randomly allocated to one of the valves. At this early stage of evaluation, the Bioflo valve was found to perform at least as well as the Carpentier-Edwards porcine valve. No primary tissue failure occurred in this small series with a short follow up. Doppler ultrasound studies performed at two and 51 weeks showed similar hemodynamic characteristics for the two prostheses, both with mitral and aortic valves. Overall mean transvalvular gradients with the Bioflo bioprosthesis were 3 mmHg for mitral and 13 mmHg for aortic valves at two weeks, and were not significantly different at the 51-week evaluation. Due to an epidemic of mad cow disease in the United Kingdom undermining the safety of using bovine material harvested in that country for clinical implant purposes, the manufacturer voluntarily withdraw the valve from the market in 1992.

The Labcor-Santiago valve

This new pericardial valve, developed in Spain in 1989, was designed to minimize mechanical stress and avoid abrasion wear of the tissue by padding of the stent, while preserving the mounting of the pericardium outside of the struts to provide full orifice opening. It is mounted on a low-profile flexible stent. The only clinical study available today reports on implantation of the valve for replacement of the aortic or mitral valve in 40 patients since 1990 (116). No degeneration of the valve has occurred during this short period of evolution. Echo-Doppler assessment of the valve postoperatively has shown an adequate hemodynamic performance, with effective orifice areas of 1.0 to 1.2 cm^2 and mean pressure gradients of 15 to 11 mmHg for size 19 and 21mm aortic valves respectively, and valve areas of 2.0 to 2.3 cm^2 with gradients of 5 and 3 mmHg for size 27 and 29mm mitral prostheses. These results compare to those obtained with other pericardial valves. Only time will tell whether this new valve can achieve its goal of improving the mechanical durability of the pericardial tissue. It is still too early to reach any conclusive evaluation of the Labcor-Santiago valve.

The Sorin-Pericarbon valve

Since its development in Italy in 1989, the Pericarbon valve has been used clinically by several centers, mainly in Europe (117). It is made of two glutaraldehyde-fixed bovine pericardial sheets. The valve leaflets are tailored from a single pericardial sheet shaped by fluid pressure. It is mounted on a second pericardial sheet which is sutured to the sewing ring and serves to cover the Dacron cloth of the stent. It is mounted inside the frame of the sewing ring, in a manner similar to that of the Carpentier-Edwards pericardial valve. The stent is low profile and the fabric coated with a pyrolytic carbon film to prevent invasion of the prosthesis by fibrous tissue pannus. This multi-layer stent was designed to decrease stress concentration and prevent leaflet abrasion by the Dacron fabric (117). Animal experimentation has revealed the absence of cusp tearing or perforation up to 42 months, but tissue calcification was observed in a significant number of prostheses, particularly those implanted in the mitral position (118,119).

The published clinical experience with this new pericardial valve is still very limited. There are several on-going clinical trials in European centers, but the results have yet to be reported. Pathologic examination of 11 bioprostheses explanted more than seven months after implantation found dystrophic calcification with stenosis in five of them (119). No cusp ruptures or commissural tears were observed. This initial clinical experience suggests that the new technical features incorporated in the design of the valve may indeed decrease the incidence of leaflet tearing, but tissue calcification still remains an unsolved problem. Because of the short clinical follow up, no conclusion can be reached as to the eventual durability of the Pericarbon-Sorin valve, and further data with longer observation periods will be needed to compare the clinical and hemodynamic performance of this new device to that of the Carpentier-Edwards pericardial valve, which is becoming the gold standard of evaluation for new-generation pericardial bioprostheses.

AGE OF THE PATIENT AS A FACTOR IN THE DURABILITY OF BIOPROSTHESES

From the previous discussion, it follows that valve preparation and design have a major impact on the durability of tissue prostheses. The site of implantation also appears to play a significant role, since several studies have demonstrated a shorter durability of bioprostheses implanted in the mitral than in the aortic position. Age of the patient at the time of implantation is the only host factor that has so far been shown to have a significant influence on the structural deterioration and late outcome of tissue valves.

In a recent review of our experience with the late follow up of 877 patients who underwent valve replacement with Carpentier-Edwards porcine valves, the effect of patient age at the time of operation on late freedom from structural deterioration of the valve was clearly established (120). The difference between age groups became apparent after the fifth year following implantation, increasing with time. At 10 years, freedom rates from valve degeneration were incremental with each age decade, from 57% for patients younger than 45 years, to 70% between 45 and 54 years, 79% for patients from 55 to 64 years, and 93% for those older than 65 years of age. Similar results were reported by Jamieson et al. (121), with a 10-year freedom rate of less than 30% among patients younger than 30 years of age, to more than 95% beyond 69 years of age.

Furthermore, although we observed a significant difference between age groups for bioprostheses in either the aortic or the mitral position, the difference with the latter was greater than with the former (120). Whereas with aortic prostheses freedom from tissue degeneration after 10 years was 70% for the younger and 93% for the older patients, it was 55% and 95% respectively with mitral valves. Late durability of aortic valves was better over the age of 55 years, whereas the improvement in durability of mitral prostheses seemed to occur after the age of 65 years. A similar finding has been made by others (122).

It has been well known for several years that bioprostheses have a very limited durability in children with dystrophic calcification (123-128). Leaflet calcification occurs early and leads to reoperation in an unduly high proportion of patients within five years of initial operation. In patients under 18 years of age, freedom from re-replacement after five years is only 59% (125). Another study found the survival free from degeneration at six years to be a dismal 20% among 135 patients 20 years old or younger (128). Based on this experience, authors generally agree that the use of bioprostheses should be avoided as much as possible in the young patient.

On the other hand, structural valve degeneration of bioprostheses is a rare event in the elderly patient, and thus they are particularly well suited in this age group (120,129-131). After 10 to 12 years, the freedom rate from tissue degeneration is 87% to 93% among patients 65 years of age or older (120,122). In our series, there has been no tissue

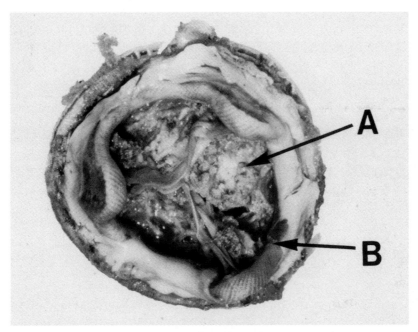

Figure 9.3-9: Dense calcification (arrow A) of a mitral Carpentier-Edwards porcine valve explanted eight years after implantation in a 41-year-old man. Although one leaflet is torn (arrow B), the mode of failure was calcific stenosis with valve obstruction.

degeneration of valves up to 10 years after implantation in patients older than 70 years (120). Recently, Burr et al. (132) reported no valve failure up to 13 years in a group of 79 patients 80 years of age or older at the time of operation. It therefore appears that the age of 60 to 70 years marks the cut-off point after which a bioprosthesis will most probably outlast the patient, both because of the increased durability of the former and of the limited survival of the latter, a conclusion also shared by others (133).

MODES OF VALVE FAILURE

It is now widely recognized that the mode of failure of tissue valves differs according to each valve type (49,52). The clinical presentation of the patient also varies as a consequence of the mechanism of tissue degeneration.

All porcine valves fail because of primary mineralization of the leaflet tissue (134,135). This is particularly prominent in children in whom severe calcification occurs early after valve implantation (124,125,136). The same mechanism prevails in older patients as well (52,137). Although most porcine valves will also display some degree of leaflet laceration, the latter is most often a consequence of the mineralization process and not a primary event (Fig. 9.3-9). In a study of 54 degenerated porcine valves, Stein et al. (138) found that 70% were calcified, and that tears were associated with the mineralization process in 80% of the cases. Gamma-carboxyglutamic acid, a calcium-binding amino acid, has been shown to play a role in the calcification of valve leaflets (124,139). It thus appears to be a chemical as well as a stress-induced lesion (140). It has been postulated

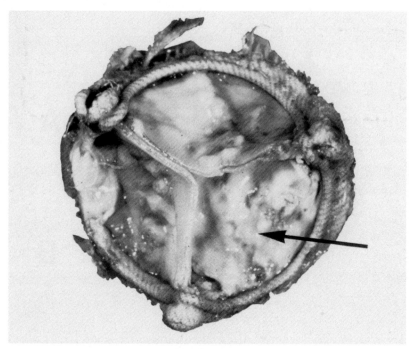

Figure 9.3-10: Carpentier-Edwards pericardial valve showing severe calcific stenosis (arrow) without leaflet tearing at reoperation 11 years after aortic valve replacement in a young man 29 years of age at the time of initial operation. Before explantation, the patient presented with progressive fatigue and dyspnea because of aortic stenosis.

that the higher mineralization rate of tissue valves in children might be related to their more active calcium metabolism with a resulting increase in calcium turnover (123). This hypothesis is supported by experimental work in young calves and sheep (141).

As a result of the failure mechanism involved, the clinical mode of presentation of porcine valve degeneration is pure valve obstruction in nearly 30% of patients and mixed stenosis and regurgitation in 70% (52). The prosthetic dysfunction is relatively well tolerated and is a progressive event that usually need not be taken care of in an urgent manner.

The Carpentier-Edwards pericardial valve's mode of failure is very similar to that of porcine bioprostheses (Fig. 9.3-10). In a recent review of our experience with this valve, we observed seven valves with intrinsic structural degeneration, a linearized incidence rate of 0.39%/patient-year. In six of them, the failure was caused by dense calcification of the leaflets, with or without secondary tearing of the tissue, and the clinical presentation was that of predominant aortic or mitral valve obstruction.

On the contrary, failure of the other pericardial bioprostheses, including Ionescu-Shiley, Mitroflow and Hancock valves, is the result of pure stress-induced tissue laceration, most often originating either from the commissure or from the bottom of the cusp, at the site of flexion of the pericardium where it comes in contact with the cloth of the stent (8-10,142,143). The lesions observed clinically are exactly those that have been provoked with fatigue-testing in vitro, and are clearly related to the specific structural design these three valves have in common (8,11).

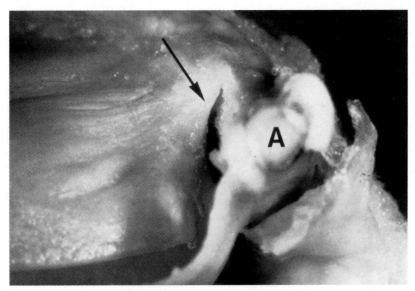

Figure 9.3-11: Commissural leaflet tear (arrow) from the strut (A) of an Ionescu-Shiley pericardial valve explanted 38 months after mitral valve replacement in a woman aged 33 years at initial operation. There is only discrete calcification along the commissure and tear. The patient presented with mitral regurgitation.

Although calcification may also occur in these pericardial valves, it is a secondary stress-induced process, usually limited to the commissures (140,143-145). In addition, tissue degeneration is always present in explanted Mitroflow valves, suggesting that the harvesting or preservation techniques might not be adequate and may participate in the valve failure (144). The predominant failure mechanism remains laceration of the leaflets, particularly with mitral prostheses (Figs. 9.3-11 and 9.3-12). As a result, patients most often develop severe and acute valvular regurgitation, that may be ill-tolerated and require urgent or semi-urgent reoperation. In our own series, more than 80% of the patients with an Ionescu-Shiley or a Mitroflow valve developed acute regurgitation (52). Therefore, patients with any one of these pericardial valves should undergo careful and close follow up for early detection of valve failure because of their higher risk of acute prosthetic dysfunction. However, preventive removal of these valves is not presently indicated (144).

As for the Meadox-Gabbay unicusp pericardial valve, it fails about equally because of either severe calcification and valve stenosis, or progressive valve regurgitation, due to leaflet redundancy caused by stretching of the pericardium, and cusp tearing (114). The multiple modes of clinical failure of this device are similar to those observed in the experimental animal by Shemin et al. (18).

REOPERATION

Indications for replacement of a bioprosthesis include valve thrombosis, endocarditis, paravalvular leaks, and technical failure. It may occasionally be removed prophylactically when performing another cardiac surgical procedure, if the

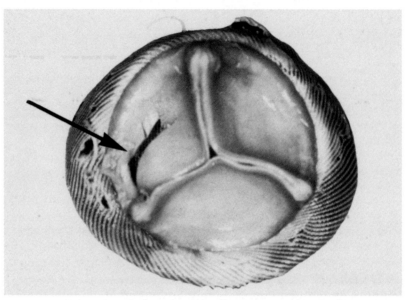

Figure 9.3-12: Commissural tear (arrow) of a Mitroflow pericardial bioprosthesis extending to the bottom of the cusp, without calcification, 34 months after implantation in the mitral position, in a 63-year-old woman who developed acute mitral regurgitation.

bioprosthesis is already aging. However, by far the most frequent indication is structural deterioration of a tissue valve. In our experience and in that of others, it accounts for approximately 75% of all replacements of bioprostheses (49,52,146).

Reoperation for replacement of valvular prostheses carries a significantly higher risk than primary operation. Operative mortality rates of 9% to 21% have been reported (147-149). It is particularly high in patients undergoing multiple valve replacement, urgent operation, and reoperation for prosthetic valve endocarditis (150). In a group of 64 patients who underwent replacement of a bioprosthesis for primary tissue failure, an overall early mortality rate of 12.5% was reported by Bortolotti et al. (146). The 16% mortality rate for replacing an aortic prosthesis was higher than that for a mitral prosthesis, which was 11%.

Several factors may account for the increased risk of reoperation, among which the preoperative clinical status of the patient, the existence of pericardial adhesions, and the difficulty of explanting the prosthesis, particularly with high profile valves and when a large valve had been forced in at first operation. We have experienced repeatedly the problem of explanting large Ionescu-Shiley and Hancock porcine valves with the struts completely embedded in the ventricular or aortic wall, leaving wide gasps after their removal. Uncovering the sewing ring with the use of the electrocautery and peeling off the prosthesis may prevent damage to surrounding structures, but at times this cannot be achieved. It may then become necessary to reconstruct the valve annulus and repair the ventricular or aortic wall with a Dacron patch over which the new prosthesis is sutured.

The timing of surgery may also be of significance in the overall results, the mortality

---

Table 9.3-I: Indications for the use of a bioprosthesis.

- Patient age over 70 years, if anticoagulation is not mandatory
- Medical contraindication to permanent anticoagulation
- Socio-economic contraindications to permanent anticoagulation
- Desire of pregnancy in childbearing age women
- Personal choice of the patient because of life style
- Replacement of the tricuspid valve

---

of elective operation being much lower than that of emergency procedures (150). This is particularly relevant for patients whose bioprosthesis may fail acutely and require urgent operation, as is often the case with Ionescu-Shiley, Mitroflow and Hancock pericardial valves. Because of the extremely high failure rate of the Hancock pericardial valve, it has been suggested that it be removed prophylactically in asymptomatic patients with clinical evidence of valve dysfunction (112). Others prefer a close follow up, delaying surgery until the patient develops symptoms of valve failure (109).

Prophylactic removal of a tissue valve may on occasion be justified in patients who are undergoing another cardiac surgical procedure, and in whom a bioprosthesis has been in place for several years, even though it still appears to be working properly. In such situations, we have opted to remove the bioprosthesis and replace it with a mechanical prosthesis, or with another tissue valve if the patient survival is limited because of their age.

CURRENT INDICATIONS FOR THE USE AND CHOICE OF A BIOPROSTHESIS

The shorter than expected durability of bioprostheses have somewhat restricted their use in recent years (151). Most authors now agree that they should be implanted only in patients with limited survival. We have also modified our approach to valve selection. Whereas up to 1987, tissue valves were the primary choice in most patients, bioprostheses are now implanted in well-selected patients only. As a result, their use has decreased from 71% of our valve implants between 1978 and 1987, to 30% of valve replacements throughout the last six years. The main indication for the selection of a tissue valve is patient age. Although a strict age limit is not determined, bioprostheses are preferred in older patients, unless permanent anticoagulation is necessary because of associated risk factors for thromboembolism, such as chronic atrial fibrillation. There is general agreement that a bioprosthesis is probably the best choice for patients 70 years of age or older. It would probably also be reasonable to consider a bioprosthesis after the age of 65 years, particularly for aortic valve replacement, since the durability of tissue valves in this position appears to be better than in the mitral position (49,52).

Beside the age criteria, bioprostheses may also be selected in other situations (Table 9.3-I). Major contraindications to permanent anticoagulation, either because of associated disease (gastro-intestinal bleeding, cerebral aneurysm, etc.), mental deficiency or psychiatric disorder, or a particular socio-economic situation (living in remote areas, work hazards, etc.), may make a bioprosthesis the best choice given the conditions. The desire for pregnancy in women of childbearing age, and the personal choice of the patient are other specific situations in which a bioprosthesis may have to be considered. Similar selection criteria have been put forward by Louagie and his group (152).

Among the various porcine and pericardial bioprostheses that have been reviewed, several have already been withdrawn from the market as sub-optimal as far as their durability and hemodynamic performance are concerned, and should probably not be considered as adequate valve substitutes. The problems encountered with all these valves are related to their structural design rather than to the biological tissue used as valve leaflets. A few other tissue valves are currently on clinical trial, but the limited experience and scarce available data preclude proper assessment of their eventual clinical value at the present time.

There are currently three bioprostheses available for clinical use, for which the wide experience and extended follow up provide the data necessary to establish a solid understanding of their long term value and performance. All available data indicate that the two porcine valves, the Hancock and the Carpentier-Edwards in their most recent models, give similar adequate long term clinical and hemodynamic results. The Carpentier-Edwards pericardial valve appears to have an advantage as regards hemodynamic performance, particularly for small size aortic valves, and may have a longer durability, at least in the aortic position. Based on present knowledge, the Carpentier-Edwards pericardial valve is currently our bioprosthesis of choice, when the use of a tissue valve is indicated. It should be stressed however that, being the most recent series, more rigorous patient selection criteria (vide supra) have been in force with this bioprosthesis. Longer term experiences are therefore warranted.

NEW IDEAS AND FUTURE DEVELOPMENTS

Future progress in the development of bioprostheses will concern valve design to optimize hemodynamic performance, and tissue preparation to prevent or at least delay the process of tissue mineralization.

The most recent approach to improve the hemodynamics of tissue valves has been the development of the stentless valve design (7). Elimination of the valve stent has no doubt resulted in larger effective orifice areas and better hemodynamic efficacy, as demonstrated at early postoperative echocardiographic studies (153-155). A number of stentless composite aortic valves manufactured from porcine aortic valves, individual porcine aortic leaflets and bovine pericardium are under clinical investigation. Since only small clinical series and short term follow up are as yet available, their durability and long term results are still unknown, and therefore no definitive opinion on these valves can be formulated at the present time. This topic is discussed more thoroughly in Chapter 9.4.

As for the prevention of tissue calcification, no antimineralization process has so far been shown to be effective. Various other chemicals are currently being tested and may soon be the object of clinical trials, but their role in improving the durability of bioprostheses remains to be established. Finally, new methods of tissue preservation, with cross-linking agents different from the currently used glutaraldehyde and with less tendency for calcification, may be another avenue along which future developments in this field will progress. Clinical results with the CarboMedics Photofix pericardial bioprosthesis are eagerly awaited.

References
1.   Carpentier A, Lemaigre G, Robert L, Carpentier S, Dubost C. Biological factors affecting long-term results of valvular heterografts. J Thorac Cardiovasc Surg 1969;58:467-483

2. Binet JP, Carpentier A, Langlois J, Leiva A. Utilisation des homo et heterogreffes dans le replacement de l'appareil aortique chez l'homme. Arch Mal Coeur 1966;10:1570-1572
3. Walker DK, Scotten LN, Brownlee RT. New generation tissue valves. J Thorac Cardiovasc Surg 1984;88:573-582
4. Gabbay S, Kresh JY. Bioengineering of mechanical and biologic heart valve substitutes. In: Morse D, Steiner RM, Fernandez J (eds). Guide to prosthetic cardiac valves. Springer-Verlag Inc., New York, 1985;239-256
5. DiSesa VJ, Collins JJ Jr, Cohn LH. Valve replacement in the small annulus aorta: Performance of the Hancock modified orifice bioprostheses. In: Cohn LH, Gallucci V (eds). Cardiac bioprosthesis. Yorke Medical Books, New York, 1982:552-558
6. Yoganathan AP, Woo YR, Sung HW, Williams FP, Franch RH, Jones M. In vitro hemodynamic characteristics of tissue bioprostheses in the aortic position. J Thorac Cardiovasc Surg 1986;92:198-209
7. David TE, Rotchan GC, Butany JW. Aortic valve replacement with stentless porcine bioprosthesis. J Card Surg 1988;3:501-505
8. Gabbay S, Kadam P, Factor S, Cheung TK. Do heart valve bioprostheses degenerate for metabolic or mechanical reasons? J Thorac Cardiovasc Surg 1988;95:208-215
9. Wheatley DJ, Fisher J, Reece IJ, Spryt T, Breeze P. Primary tissue failure in pericardial heart valves. J Thorac Cardiovasc Surg 1987;94:367-374
10. Trowbridge EA, Lawford PV, Crofts CE, Roberts KM. Pericardial heterografts: Why do these valves fail? J Thorac Cardiovasc Surg 1988;95:577-585
11. Gabbay S, Bortolotti U, Wasserman F, Factor S, Strom J, Frater RWM. Fatigue-induced failure of the Ionescu-Shiley pericardial xenograft in the mitral position. J Thorac Cardiovasc Surg 1984;87:836-844
12. Navia JA, Tamashiro A, Gimenez C, Zambrana Vidal D, Liotta D. Hemodynamic evaluation in valvular patients carrying low profile bioprostheses. In: Cohn LH, Gallucci V (eds). Cardiac bioprostheses. Yorke Medical Books, New York, 1982;104-112
13. Copeland JG, Emery RW, Levinson MM, Copeland J. The Ionescu-Shiley low-profile valve: Early clinical evaluation. In: Bodnar E, Yacoub M (eds). Biologic bioprosthetic valves. York Medical Books, New York, 1986;731-738
14. Hamid MS, Sabbah HN, Stein PD. Influence of stent height upon stresses on the cusp of closed bioprosthetic valves. J Biomech 1986;19:759-769
15. Bortolotti U, Milano A, Thiene G, et al. Mode of late failure of the low-profile (Liotta) porcine bioprosthesis in the mitral position. Am J Cardiol 1988;62:1132-1134
16. Gabbay S, Frater RWM. The unileaflet heart valve bioprosthesis: New concept. In: Cohn LH, Gallucci V (eds). Cardiac Bioprostheses. Yorke Medical Books, New York, 1982;411-424
17. Gabbay S, Bortolotti U, Cipolletti G, Wasserman F, Frater RWM, Factor SM. The Meadox unicusp pericardial bioprosthetic heart valve: New concept. Ann Thorac Surg 1984;37:448-456
18. Sheimin RJ, Schoen FJ, Hein R, Austin J, Cohn LH. Hemodynamic and pathologic evaluation of a unileaflet pericardial bioprosthetic valve. J Thorac Cardiovasc Surg 1988;95:912-919
19. Valente M, Minarini M, Ius P, et al. Durability of glutaraldehyde-fied pericardial valve prostheses: Clinical and animal experimental studies. J Heart Valve Dis 1992;1:216-224
20. Sabbah HN, Hamid MS, Stein PD. Mechanical stresses on closed cusps of porcine bioprosthetic valves: Correlation with sites of calcification. Ann Thorac Surg 1986;42:93-96
21. Vesely I, Boughner D, Song T. Tissue buckling as a mechanism of bioprosthetic valve failure. Ann Thorac Surg 1988;46:302-308
22. Broom ND, Thomson FJ. Influence of fixation conditions on the performance of glutaraldehyde-treated porcine aortic valves: Towards a more scientific basis. Thorax 1979;34:166-176
23. Barratt-Boyes BG. Cardiothoracic surgery in the antipodes. J Thorac Cardiovasc Surg 1979;78:804-822
24. Broom B, Christie GW. The structure/function relationship of fresh and glutaraldehyde-fixed aortic valve leaflets. In: Cohn LH, Gallucci V (eds). Cardiac Bioprostheses. Yorke Medical Books, New York, 1982:476-491
25. Flomenbaum MA, Schoen FJ. Effects of fixation back pressure and antimineralization treatment on the morphology of porcine aortic bioprosthetic valves. J Thorac Cardiovasc Surg 1993;105:154-164
26. Vesely I. Analysis of the Medtronic Intact bioprosthetic valve. J Thorac Cardiovasc Surg 1991;101:90-99
27. Mayne ASD, Christie GW, Smaill BH, Hunter PJ, Barratt-Boyes BG. An assessment of the mechanical properties of leaflets from four second-generation porcine bioprostheses with biaxial testing techniques. J Thorac Cardiovasc Surg 1989;98:170-180
28. Nashef A, Nguyen H, Nguyen T, et al. Low pressure fixation of bioprosthetic tissue: Science and fiction. In: Bodnar E (ed). Surgery for heart valve disease. ICR Publishers, UK, 1990;745-754
29. Webb CL, Benedict JJ, Schoen FJ, Linden JA, Levy RJ. Inhibition of bioprosthetic heart valve calcification with aminodiphosphonate covalently bound to residual aldehyde groups. Ann Thorac Surg 1988;46:309-316

30. Gott JP, Chih P, Dorsey LMA, et al. Calcification of porcine valves: A successful new method of antimineralization. Ann Thorac Surg 1992;53:207-216
31. Valente M, Laborde F, Thiene G, Talenti E, Calabrese F, Gallix P. Medtronic Intact porcine valve: Evidence of mitigation of dystrophic calcification in the growing sheep experimental model. In: Bodnar E (ed). Surgery for heart valve disease. ICR Publishers, UK, 1990:668-678
32. Oury JH, Angell WW, Koziol JA. Comparison of Hancock I and Hancock II bioprostheses. J Card Surg 1988;3(suppl):375-381
33. Lentz DJ, Pollock EM, Olsen DB, Andrews EJ, Murashita J, Hastings WL. Inhibition of mineralization of glutaralehyde-fixed Hancock bioprosthetic heart valves. In: Cohn LH, Gallucci V (eds). Cardiac Bioprostheses. Yorke Medical Books, New York, 1982:306-319
34. Cohn LH, Collins JJ Jr, DiSesa VJ, et al. Fifteen-year experience with 1678 Hancock porcine bioprosthetic heart valve replacements. Ann Surg 1989;210:435-443
35. Milano AD, Bortolotti U, Mazzucco A, Guerra F, Magni A, Gallucci V. Aortic valve replacement with the Hancock standard, Björk-Shiley and Lillehei-Kaster prostheses. J Thorac Cardiovasc Surg 1989;98:37-47
36. Bortolotti U, Milano A, Mazzucco A, et al. The standard Hancock porcine bioprosthesis in the second decade. In: Bodnar E (ed). Surgery for heart valve disease. ICR Publishers, UK, 1990:298-308
37. Gallucci V, Mazzucco A, Bortolotti U, Milano A, Guerra F, Thiene G. The standard Hancock porcine bioprosthesis: Overall experience at the University of Padova. J Card Surg 1988;3(suppl):337- 345
38. Bernal JM, Rabasa JN, Cagigas JC, Echevarria JR, Carrion MF, Revuelta JM. Valve-related complications with the Hancock I porcine bioprosthesis. J Thorac Cardiovasc Surg 1991;101:871-880
39. Kawachi Y, Tominaga R, Hisahara M, Nakashima A, Yasui H, Tokunaga K. Excellent durability of the Hancock porcine bioprosthesis in the tricuspid position. J Thorac Cardiovasc Surg 1992;104:1561-1566
40. Guerra F, Bortolotti U, Thiene G, et al. Long-term performance of the Hancock porcine bioprosthesis in the tricuspid position. J Thorac Surg 1990;99:838-845
41. DiSesa VJ, Allred EN, Kowalker W, Shemin RJ, Collins JJ Jr, Cohn LH. Performance of a fabricated trileaflet porcine bioprosthesis. J Thorac Cardiovasc Surg 1987;94:220-224
42. Bortolotti U, Milano A, Mazzucco A, et al. The Hancock II porcine bioprosthesis. J Thorac Cardiovasc Surg 1989;97:415-420
43. David TE, Armstrong S, Sun Z. Clinical and hemodynamic assessment of the Hancock II bioprosthesis. Ann Thorac Surg 1992;54:661- 668
44. Bloomfield P, Kitchin AH, Wheatley DJ, Walbaum PR, Lutz W, Miller HC. A prospective evaluation of the Björk-Shiley, Hancock and Carpentier-Edwards heart valve prostheses. Circulation 1986;73:1213- 1222
45. Lipson LC, Kent KM, Rosing DR, et al. Long-term hemodynamic assessment of the porcine heterograft in the mitral position. Circulation 1981;64:397-402
46. Ubago JL, Figueroa A, Colman T, Revuelta JM, Ochoteco A, Duran CMG. Hemodynamic evaluation of the Hancock bioprosthesis in the mitral position: A 1-7 years follow up. In: Cohn LH, Gallucci V (eds). Cardiac Bioprostheses. Yorke Medical Books, New York, 1982:79-90
47. Borkon AM, McIntosh CL, Jones M, Lipson LC, Kent KM, Morrow AG. Hemodynamic function of the Hancock standard orifice aortic valve bioprosthesis. J Thorac Cardiovasc Surg 1981;82:601-607
48. Rossiter SJ, Miller DC, Stinson EB, et al. Hemodynamic and clinical comparison of the Hancock modified orifice and standard orifice bioprostheses in the aortic position. J Thorac Cardiovasc Surg 1980;80:54-60
49. Pelletier LC, Carrier M, Leclerc Y, Lepage G, deGuise P, Dyrda I. Porcine versus pericardial bioprostheses: A comparison of late results in 1,593 patients. Ann Thorac Surg 1989;47:352-361
50. Jamieson WRE, Allen P, Miyagishima RT, et al. The Carpentier-Edwards standard porcine bioprosthesis. A first-generation tissue valve with excellent long-term clinical performance. J Thorac Cardiovasc Surg 1990;99:543-561
51. Pelletier C, Chaitman BR, Baillot R, Guiteras Val P, Bonan R, Dyrda I. Clinical and hemodynamic results with the Carpentier- Edwards porcine bioprosthesis. Ann Thorac Surg 1982;34:612-624
52. Pelletier LC, Castonguay Y, Leclerc Y, Lepage G, de Guise P, Dyrda I. Reoperation for bioprostheses: An analysis of 1831 valves over a 12-year period. In Bodnar E (ed). Surgery for heart valve disease. ICR Publishers, UK, 1990:443-453
53. Jamieson WRE, Allen P, Ling H, et al. Carpentier-Edwards porcine bioprostheses: Assessment of clinical performance. Can J Cardiol 1988;4:314-321
54. Jamieson WRE, Munro AI, Miyagishima RT, et al. The Carpentier-Edwards supra-annular porcine bioprosthesis. J Thorac Cardiovasc Surg 1988;96:652-666
55. Nistal F, Artinano E, Gallo I. Primary tissue valve degeneration in glutaraldehyde-preserved porcine bioprostheses: Hancock I versus Carpentier-Edwards at 4- to 7-years' follow up. Ann Thorac Surg 1986;42:568-572
56. Bolooki H, Kaiser GA, Mallon SM, Palatianos GM. Comparison of long-term results of Carpentier-Edwards and Hancock bioprosthetic valves. Ann Thorac Surg 1986;42:494-499
57. Cobanoglu A, Jamieson WRE, Miller DC, et al. A tri- institutional comparison of tissue and mechanical

valves using a patient-oriented definition of "treatment failure". Ann Thorac Surg 1987;43:245-253

58. Spampianato N, Stassano P, Cammarota A, et al. Bioprostheses at twelve years. J Card Surg 1988;(suppl):383-390

59. Perier P, Deloche A, Chauvaud S, et al. A 10-year comparison of mitral valve replacement with Carpentier-Edwards and Hancock porcine bioprostheses. Ann Thorac Surg 1989;48:54-59

60. Pelletier C, Chaitman BR, Bonan R, Dyrda I. Hemodynamic evaluation of the Carpentier-Edwards standard and improved annulus bioprostheses. In: Cohn LH, Galucci V (eds). Cardiac Bioprostheses. Yorke Medical Books, New York, 1982:91-103

61. Levine FH, Carter JE, Buckley MJ, Daggett WM, Akins CW, Austen WG. Hemodynamic evaluation of Hancock and Carpentier-Edwards bioprostheses. Circulation 1981;64(suppl II):192-195

62. Cosgrove DM, Lytle BW, Gill CC, et al. In vivo hemodynamic comparison of porcine and pericardial valves. J Thorac Cardiovasc Surg 1985;89:358-368

63. Bove EL, Marvasti MA, Potts JL, et al. Rest and exercise hemodynamics following aortic valve replacement. J Thorac Cardiovasc Surg 1985;90:750-755

64. Kallis P, Sneddon JF, Simpson IA, Fung A, Pepper JR, Smith EEJ. Clinical and hemodynamic evaluation of the 19-mm Carpentier- Edwards supra-annular aortic valve. Ann Thorac Surg 1992;54:1182-1185

65. Angell WW, Angell JD, Sywak A. The Angell-Shiley procine xenograft. Ann Thorac Surg 1979;28:537-553

66. Angell WW, Infantes-Alcon C, Rivera R, Duran CG. Biodegradation of human and porcine aortic valve tissue. In: Bodnar E (ed). Surgery for heart valve disease. ICR Publishers, UK, 1990;309- 315

67. Rivera R, Infantes C, Delcan JL, Rico M. Clinical and hemodynamic assessment of the Angell-Shiley porcine xenograft. Ann Thorac Surg 1980;30:455-464

68. Delcan JL, Chaitman BR, Lopez-Becos L, Bonan R, Garcia- Dorado D, Rivera R. Hemodynamic evaluation of the Angell-Shiley porcine xenograft. J Thorac Cardiovasc Surg 1982;84:297-305

69. Pavie A, Bors V, Piazza C, et al. Mid-term results of the Liotta-bioimplant low profile bioprostheses. J Card Surg 1988;3(suppl):353-358

70. Bortolotti U, Milano A, Mazzucco A, et al. Influence of prosthetic design on durability of the Liotta porcine valve in the mitral position. Ann Thorac Surg 1990;50:734-738

71. Kazui T, Morikawa M, Yamada O, Komatsu S. Comparative study of primary tissue failure between the Hancock and the Liotta porcine bioprostheses in the mitral position: 8 to 14 year experience. In: Bodnar E (ed). Surgery for heart valve disease. ICR Publishers, UK, 1990:807-814

72. Williams MA. The Intact bioprosthesis - Early results. J Card Surg 1988;3(suppl):347-351

73. Jaffe WM, Barratt-Boyes BG, Sadri A, Gavin JB, Coverdale HA, Neutze JM. Early follow up of patients with the Medtronic Intact porcine valve. J Thorac Cardiovasc Surg 1989;98:181-192

74. Greaves S, Barratt-Boyes BG, Neutze JM. The Medtronic- Intact valve. A clinical follow up extending to 5´ years, including serial echo-Doppler examinations. In: Bodnar E (ed). Surgery for heart valve disease. ICR Publishers, UK, 1990:316-328

75. Jaffe WM, Coverdale HA, Roche AHG, Whitlock RML, Neutze JM, Barratt-Boyes BG. Rest and exercise hemodynamiacs of 20 to 23 mm allograft, Medtronic Intact (porcine), and St. Jude medical valves in the aortic position. J Thorac Cardiovasc Surg 1990;100:167-174

76. Vrandecic MP, Gontijo B, Rabelo S. Clinical experience with a new generation of porcine bioprostheses. In: Bodnar E, Yacoub M (eds). Bioprosthetic valves. Yorke Medical Books, New York, 1986:659- 665

77. Vrandecic MOP, Gontijo Filho BG, e Silva JAP, et al. Clinical results with the Biocor porcine bioprosthesis. J Cardiovasc Surg 1991;32:807-813

78. Reece IJ, Wheatley DJ, Munro JL, et al. Early results with the Wessex porcine bioprosthesis in 245 patients. In: Bodnar E, Yacoub M (eds). Biologic bioprosthetic valves. Yorke Medical Books, New York, 1986:760-767

79. Paphitis CA, Lennox SC. Early experience with the Xenomedica bioprosthetic valve. In: Bodnar E, Yacoub M (eds). Biologic bioprosthetic valves. Yorke Medical Books, New York, 1986:652-658

80. Goffin YA, Hilbert SL, Bartik MA. Morphologic evaluation of 2 new bioprostheses: The Mitroflow bovine pericardial valve and the Xenomedica porcine aortic valve. In: Bodnar E, Yacoub M (eds). Biologic bioprosthetic valves. Yorke Medical Books, New York 1986:366-382

81. Ionescu MI, Tandon AP, Mary DAS, Abid A. Heart valve replacement with the Ionescu-Shiley pericardial xenograft. J Thorac Cardiovasc Surg 1977;73:31-42

82. Gonzalez-Lavin L, Chi S, Blair TC, et al. Five-year experience with the Ionescu-Shiley bovine pericardial valve in the aortic position. Ann Thorac Surg 1983;36:270-280

83. Michel PL, Kassab R, Vahanian A, Belkaid M, Acar J. Resultats a moyen terme du remplacement valvulaire aortique par la bioprothese pericardique de Ionescu-Shiley. A propos de 109 patients. Arch Mal Coeur 1986;79:1046-1051

84. Ionescu MI, Smith DR, Hasan SS, Chidambaram M, Tandon AP. Clinical durability of the pericardial xenograft valve: Ten years' experience with mitral replacement. Ann Thorac Surg 1982;34:265-277

85. Ionescu MI, Tandon AP, Saunders NR, Chidambaram M, Smith DR. Clinical durability of the pericardial

xenograft valve: 11 years' experience. In: Cohn LH, Gallucci V (eds). Cardiac Bioprostheses. York Medical Books, New York 1982:42-60

86. Gallo I, Nistal F, Revuelta JM, Garcia-Satue E, Artinano E, Duran CG. Incidence of primary tissue valve failure with the Ionescu- Shiley pericardial valve. J Thorac Cardiovasc Surg 1985;90:278-280

87. Reul GJ Jr, Cooley DA, Duncan JM, et al. Valve failure with the Ionescu-Shiley bovine pericardial bioprosthesis: Analysis of 2680 patients. J Vasc Surg 1985;2:191-204

88. Ravichandran PS, Kay PH, Kollar A, Murday AJ. Ionescu- Shiley legacy. In: Bodnar E (ed). Surgery for heart valve disease. ICR Publishers, UK, 1990:715-724

89. Walley VM, Keon WJ. Patterns of failure in Ionescu- Shiley bovine pericardial bioprosthetic valves. J Thorac Cardiovasc Surg 1987;93:925-933

90. Walley VM, Bédard P, Brais M, Keon WJ. Valve failure caused by cusp tears in low-profile Ionescu-Shiley bovine pericardial bioprosthetic valves. J Thorac Cardiovasc Surg 1987;93:583-586

91. Daenen W, Noyez L. Lesaffre E, Goffin Y, Stalpaert G. The Ionescu-Shiley pericardial valve: Results in 473 patients. Ann Thorac Surg 1988;46:536-541

92. Revuelta JM, Alonso C, Cagigas JC, et al. Long-term evaluation of the Ionescu-Shiley pericardial xenograft bioprostheses in the aortic position. J Card Surg 1988;3(suppl):391-396

93. Masters RG, Pipe AL, Bedard JP, et al. Long-term clinical results with the Ionescu-Shiley pericardial xenograft. J Thorac Cardiovasc Surg 1991;101:81-89

94. Eng J, Ravichandran PS, Kay PH, Murday AJ. Long-term results of Ionescu-Shiley valve in the tricuspid position. Ann Thorac Surg 1990;51:200-203

95. Nistal F, Garcia-SatuÇ E, Artinano E, Duran CMG, Gallo I. Comparative study of primary tissue valve failure between Ionescu- Shiley pericardial and Hancock porcine valves in the aortic position. Am J Cardiol 1986;57:161-164

96. Gonzalez-Lavin L, Gonzalez-Lavin J, Chi S, Lewis B, Amini S, Graf D. The pericardial valve in the aortic position ten years later. J Thorac Cardiovasc Surg 1991;101:75-80

97. Becker RM, Strom J, Frishman W, et al. Hemodynamic performance of the Ionescu-Shiley valve prosthesis. J Thorac Cardiovasc Surg 1980;80:613-620

98. Vahanian A, Enriquez-Sarano M, Jais JM, et al. Evaluation hemodynamique des bioprotheses pericardiques de Ionescu- Shiley. Arch Mal Coeur 1985;78:119-125

99. Jacobs LE, Parry WR, Kotler MN. Pulsed, continuous, and color flow Doppler echocardiographic assessment of normal and abnormal Ionescu-Shiley pericardial valves. J Card Surg 1988;3(suppl):429-435

100. Teoh KH, Fulop JC, Weisel RD, et al. Aortic valve replacement with a small prosthesis. Circulation 1987;76(suppl III):123- 131

101. Bojar RM, Diehl JT, Moten M, et al. Clinical and hemodynamic performance of the Ionescu-Shiley valve in the small aortic root. J Thorac Cardiovasc Surg 1989;98:1087-1095

102. Pelletier LC, Leclere Y, Bonan R, CrÇpeau J, Dyrda I. Aortic valve replacement with the Carpentier-Edwards pericardial bioprosthesis: Clinical and hemodynamic results. J Card Surg 1988;3(suppl):405-412

103. Pelletier LC, Leclerc Y, Bonan R, Dyrda I. The Carpentier- Edwards bovine pericardial bioprosthesis: Clinical experience with 301 valve replacements. In: Bodnar E (ed). Surgery for heart valve disease. ICR Publishers, UK, 1990:691-701

104. Frater RWM, Salomon NW, Rainer WG, Cosgrove DM III, Wickham E. The Carpentier-Edwards pericardial aortic valve: Intermediate results. Ann Thorac Surg 1992;53:764-771

105. Cosgrove DM, Lytle BW, Williams GW. Hemodynamic performance of the Carpentier-Edwards pericardial valve in the aortic position in vivo. Circulation 1985;72(suppl II):146-152

106. Jamieson WRE, Gerein AN, Ling H, Miyagishima RT, Janusz MT, Tyers FO. The mitral medical pericardial bioprosthesis: New generation bovine pericardial prosthesis. J Card Surg 1988;3(suppl):413-428

107. Jamieson WRE, Pelletier LC, Gerein AN, Pomas J. The Mitroflow pericardial bioprosthesis. Comparison of early clinical performance in aortic and mitral positions. Can J Surg 1992;35:159- 164

108. Revuelta JM, Gaite L, Lequerica MA, et al. Mitroflow pericardial heart valve. A 7-year clinical experience. In: Bodnar E (ed). Surgery for heart valve disease. ICR Publishers, UK, 1990:725- 732

109. Scully H, Goldman B, Fulop J, et al. Five-year follow-up of Hancock pericardial valves. Management of premature failure. J Card Surg 1988;3(suppl):397-403

110. Goldman B, Scully H, Tong C, et al. Clinical results of pericardial xenogrft valves. The Ionescu-Shiley and Hancock valves. Can J Cardiol 1988;4:328-332

111. Dimitri W, Wheatley DJ, Tolland MM, Breeze P. Experience with two pericardial bioprostheses: 5-year analysis. In: Bodnar E (ed). Surgery for heart valve disease. ICR Publishers, UK, 1990:702-714

112. Bortolotti U, Milano A, Guerra F, et al. Failure of Hancock pericardial xenografts: Is prophylactic bioprosthetic replacement justified? Ann Thorac Surg 1991;51:430-437

113. Soots G, Cabrol C, Gandjbakhch I, et al. Preliminary clinical results with Meadox-Gabbay unicusp pericardial heart valve bioprosthesis. In: Bodnar E, Yacoub M (eds). Biologic bioprosthetic valves. Yorke

Medical Books, New York, 1986:699-708

114. Bortolotti U, Ius P, Thiene G, et al. The Meadox-Gabby pericardial xenografts: Failure of the unicusp principle. Ann Thorac Surg 1992;54:952-958

115. Wheatley DJ, Pringle SD, Davidson KG, Tolland MM, Dimitri WR, Cobbe SM. Randomised prospective evaluation of a new heart valve: the Bioflo pericardial bioprosthesis. In: Bodnar E (ed). Surgery for heart valve disease. ICR Publishers, UK, 1990:733-739

116. Garcia-Bengochea JB, Casagrande I, Gonzalez-Juanatey JR, et al. The new Labcor-Santiago pericardial bioprosthesis. J Card Surg 1991;4(suppl):613-619

117. Valente M, Laborde F, Thiene G, et al. Evaluation of Pericarbon valve prosthesis: In vitro, ultrastructural, and animal studies. J Card Surg 1989;4:79-88

118. Thiene G, Laborde F, Valente M, et al. Morphological survey of a new pericardial valve prosthesis (Pericarbon): Long-term experimental model. Eur J Cardiothorac Surg 1989;3:65-74

119. Valente M, Minarini M, Ius P, et al. Durability of glutaraldehyde-fixed pericardial valve prostheses: Clinical and animal experimental studies. J Heart Valve Dis 1992;1:216-224

120. Pelletier LC, Carrier M, Leclerc Y, Dyrda I, Gosselin G. Influence of age on later results of valve replacement with porcine bioprostheses. J Cardiovasc Surg 1992;33:526-533

121. Jamieson WRE, Rosado LJ, Munro AI, et al. Carpentier- Edwards standard porcine bioprosthesis: Primary tissue failure (structural valve deterioration) by age groups. Ann Thorac Surg 1988;46:155-162

122. Jamieson WRE, Tyers GFO, Janusz MT, et al. Age as a determinant for selection of porcine bioprostheses for cardiac valve replacement: Experience with Carpentier-Edwards standard bioprosthesis. Can J Cardiol 1991;7:181-188

123. Geha AB, Laks H, Stansel HC Jr, et al. Late failure of porcine valve heterografts in children. J Thorac Cardiovasc Surg 1979;78:351-364

124. Sanders SP, Levy RJ, Freed MD, Norwood WI, Castaneda AR. Use of Hancock porcine xenografts in children and adolescents. Am J Cardiol 1980;46:429-438

125. Williams DB, Danielson GK, McGoon DC, Puga FJ, Mair DD, Edwards WD. Porcine heterograft valve replacement in children. J Thorac Cardiovasc Surg 1982;84:446-450

126. Miller DC, Stinson EB, Oyer PE, et al. The durability of porcine xenograft valves and conduits in children. Circulation 1982;66(suppl I):172-185

127. Fiddler GI, Gerlis LM, Walker DR, Scott O, Williams GJ. Calcification of glutaraldehyde-preserved porcine and bovine xenograft valves in young children. Ann Thorac Surg 1983;35:257-261

128. Antunes MJ, Santos LP. Performance of glutaraldehyde- preserved porcine bioprosthesis as a mitral valve substitute in a young population group. Ann Thorac Surg 1984;37:387-392

129. Pupello DF, Bessone LN, Hiro SP, Lopez-Cuenca E, Glatterer MS Jr, Ebra G. The Carpentier-Edwards bioprosthesis: A comparative study analysing failure rates by age. J Card Surg 1988;3(suppl):369-374

130. Borkon AM, Soule LM, Baughman KL, et al. Aortic valve selection in the elderly patient. Ann Thorac Surg 1988;46:270-277

131. Jamieson WRE, Burr LH, Munro AI, Miyagishima RT, Gerein AN. Cardiac valve replacement in the elderly: Clinical performance of biological prostheses. Ann Thorac Surg 1989;48:173-185

132. Burr LH, Jamieson WRE, Munro AI, et al. Structural valve deterioration in elderly patient populations with the Carpentier-Edwards standard and supra-annular porcine bioprostheses: A comparative study. J Heart Valve Dis 1992;1:87-91

133. Jones EL, Weintraub WS, Craver JM, et al. Ten-year experience with the porcine bioprosthetic valve: Interrelationship of valve survival and patient survival in 1,050 valve replacements. Ann Thorac Surg 1990;49:370-384

134. Schoen FJ, Kujovich JL, Webb CL, Levy RJ. Chemically determined mineral content of explanted porcine aortic valve bioprostheses: Correlation with radiographic assessment of calcification and clinical data. Circulation 1987;76:1061-1066

135. Schoen FJ, Maranto AR, Webb CL, Levy RJ. Cuspal components in bioprosthetic valve calcification: Elucidation and modification. In: Bodnar E (ed). Surgery for heart valve disease. ICR Publishers, UK, 1990:679-688

136. Curcio CA, Commerford PJ, Rose AG, Stevens JE, Barnard MS. Calcification of glutaraldehyde-preserved porcine xenografts in young patients. J Thorac Cardiovasc Surg 1981;81:621-625

137. Galluci V, Bortolotti U, Milano A, Valfré C, Mazzucco A, Thiene G. Isolated mitral valve replacement with the Hancock bioprosthesis: A 13-year appraisal. Ann Thorac Surg 1984;38:571-578

138. Stein PD, Kemp SR, Riddle JM, Lee MW, Lewis JW Jr, Magilligan DJ Jr. Relation of calcification to torn leaflets of spontaneously degenerated porcine bioprosthetic valves. Ann Thorac Surg 1985;40:175-180

139. Fishbein MC, Levy RJ, Ferrans VJ, et al. Calcification of cardiac valve bioprostheses. J Thorac Cardiovasc Surg 1982;83:602-609

140. Thubrikar MJ, Deck JD, Aouad J, Nolan SP. Role of mechanical stress in calcification of aortic bioprosthetic valves. J Thorac Cardiovasc Surg 1983;86:115-125

141. Harasaki H, Kiraly R, Nose Y. Three mechanisms of calcification in tissue valves. In: Bodnar E, Yacoub M (eds). Biologic bioprosthetic valves. Yorke Medical Books, New York, 1986;433-441

142. Walley VM, Rubens FD, Campagna M, Pipe AL, Keon WJ. Patterns of failure in Hancock pericardial bioprostheses. J Thorac Cardiovasc Surg 1991;102:187-194

143. Michel PL, Vahanian A, Porte JM, et al. Resultats a moyen terme due remplacement valvulaire a l'aide de deux types d'heterogreffes pericardiques. A propos de 208 patients. Arch Mal Coeur 1991;84:785- 791

144. Leandri J, Bertrand P, Mazzucotelli JPH, Loisance D. Mode of failure of the Mitroflow pericardial valve. J Heart Valve Dis 1992;1:225-231

145. Nistal F, Garcia-Martinez V, Fernandez D, Artinano E, Mazorra F, Gallo I. Degenerative pathologic findings after long-term implantation of bovine pericardial bioprosthetic heart valves. J Thorac Cardiovasc Surg 1988;96:642-651

146. Bortolotti U, Milano A, Mazzucco A, et al. Results of reoperation for primary tissue failure of porcine bioprostheses. J Thorac Cardiovasc Surg 1985;90:564-569

147. Bosch X, Pomar JL, Pelletier LC. Early and late prognosis after reoperation for prosthetic valve replacement. J Thorac Cardiovasc Surg 1984;88:567-572

148. Lytle BW, Cosgrove DM, Taylor PC, et al. Reoperations for valve surgery: Perioperative mortality and determinants of risk for 1,000 patients, 1958-1984. Ann Thorac Surg 1986;42:632-643

149. Nallet O, Roger V, Michel PL, Remadi F, Farah E, Acar J. Pronostic des reinterventions pour dysfonction de bioprothese. Arch Mal Coeur 1992;85:303-308

150. Pansini S, Ottino G, Forsennati PG, et al. Reoperations on heart valve prostheses: An analysis of operative risks and late results. Ann Thorac Surg 1990;50:590-596

151. Milano AD, Bortolotti U, Mazzucco A, et al. Performance of the Hancock porcine bioprosthesis following aortic valve replacement: Considerations based on a 15-year experience. Ann Thorac Surg 1988;46:216-222

152. Louagie Y, Noirhomme P, Aranguis E, et al. Use of the Carpentier-Edwards porcine bioprosthesis: Assessment of a patient selection policy. J Thorac Cardiovasc Surg 1992;104:1013-1024

153. David TE, Bos J, Ropchan GC, Pollick C. A stentless porcine aortic bioprosthesis for aortic valve replacement. In: Bodnar E (ed). Surgery for heart valve disease. ICR Publishers, UK, 1990:828-835

154. David TE, Pollick C, Bos J. Aortic valve replacement with stentless porcine aortic bioprosthesis. J Thorac Cardiovasc Surg 1990;99:113-118

155. Casabona R, De Paulis R, Zattera GF, et al. Stentless porcine and pericardial valve in aortic position. Ann Thorac Surg 1992;54:681-685

Chapter 9.4

Stentless Bioprosthetic Valves

Tirone E. David

Stentless bioprosthetic valves are biological devices used for the replacement of diseased heart valves. Unlike stented bioprosthetic valves, which are mounted in a frame, stentless bioprostheses are mounted directly in the recipient's heart in an attempt to reproduce the anatomy and function of the native valve. Although any heart valve can be replaced with a stentless bioprosthesis, the clinical application of this concept has been largely limited to aortic valve replacement. This chapter will cover only the current knowledge and clinical experience with stentless heterografts used for aortic valve replacement. Aortic valve replacement with homografts is discussed elsewhere in this book.

HISTORICAL BACKGROUND

Aortic valve replacement with a stentless aortic valve homograft was first reported by Ross in 1962 (1) and Barratt-Boyes in 1964 (2). These surgeons used the aortic root of the patient to secure the homograft aortic valve in the subcoronary position. In 1965, Binet and associates reported on five patients who had undergone aortic valve replacement with stentless pig and calf aortic valves (3). O'Brien and associates accumulated a formidable experience with aortic valve replacement using formaldehyde-preserved porcine and bovine aortic valves (4-6). With the development of tissue fixation with glutaraldehyde (7), porcine aortic valves became commercially available already mounted in a frame, and the interest in stentless heterograft aortic valves therefore vanished. Because of difficulties in obtaining enough aortic valve homografts for aortic valve replacement in the early 1980's we began to search for ways of improving the hemodynamic characteristics and durability of glutaraldehyde-fixed porcine aortic valves and started using them without a stent for aortic valve replacement in 1987 (8-9). Since then there has been a renewed interest in stentless porcine aortic bioprosthesis.

EXPERIMENTAL STUDIES

The first report on aortic valve replacement with stentless porcine aortic valves in sheep was read at the IV International Symposium on Cardiac Bioprostheses in April 1988 (8). We learned that partial dehiscence of the heterograft with resulting paravalvular leakage was common in the area corresponding to the muscle bar. The outside wall of the stentless porcine aortic valve was covered with a fine Dacron cloth and the problem of paravalvular dehiscence was abolished. The Dacron cloth also facilitated the implantation and explantation of the stentless valve in sheep (8). Hemodynamic assessment of stentless porcine aortic valves in sheep revealed excellent results with effective valve orifices of 1.22 ± 0.29 cm^2 in animals that had valves of 16 to 19 mm

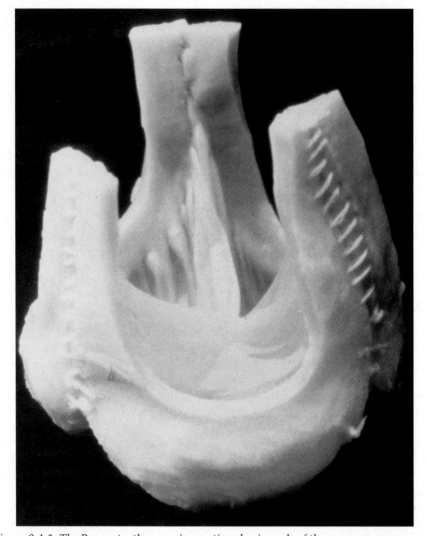

Figure 9.4-1: The Bravo stentless porcine aortic valve is made of three non-coronary cusps.

external diameter (8). Subsequent to this experimental study we began to use this valve in humans (8-9).

Huysmans and Hazekamp (10) compared the performance of stentless porcine aortic valves with stented ones in the aortic position of growing pigs and found that the degree of calcification was less intense in the stentless than in the stented valves.

STENTLESS BIOPROSTHESES FOR AORTIC VALVE REPLACEMENT

The Bravo stentless valve from Bravo Cardiovascular (Irvine, CA), the Freestyle from Medtronic (Minneapolis, MN), the Edwards Prima from Baxter (Irvine, CA), and the Toronto SPV from St. Jude Medical (St. Paul, MN) are some of the stentless valves

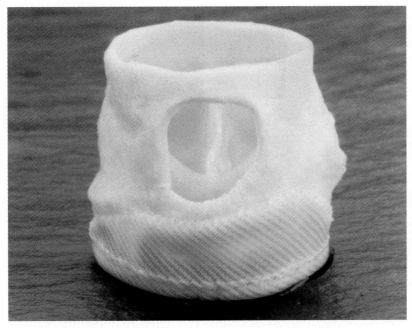

Figure 9.4-2: The Edwards Prima porcine aortic root can be used for aortic root replacement or as a stentless valve after excision of the porcine sinuses.

currently under clinical investigation in North America and Europe.

The Bravo stentless bioprosthesis is a trileaflet valve fashioned from three non-coronary cusps of glutaraldehyde-fixed porcine aortic valves as shown in Figure 9.4-1. This valve was originally designed by Mark O'Brien (6). Since it contains no muscle bar, no Dacron cloth is needed to prevent valve dehiscence. This valve is secured in the recipient's aortic root with a single layer of a continuous suture along the insertion of the leaflets and commissures.

The Prima valve is a glutaraldehyde-fixed porcine aortic root with a strip of Dacron cloth along its inflow. The coronary arteries are excised from the root (Figure 9.4-2). It can be used for replacement of the aortic root, or the aortic sinuses of the pig valve can be trimmed and the valve implanted in the subcoronary position. When this valve is used as a root replacement it probably should not be referred to as a "stentless" valve since the tanned porcine arterial wall functions as a stent. A glutaraldehyde-fixed aortic root is less compliant than most commercially available stented porcine bioprostheses.

The Freestyle valve is a glutaraldehyde-fixed porcine aortic root. The fixation method is rather intriguing; the aortic valve leaflets are fixed at zero-pressure while the aortic sinuses and ascending aorta are subjected to pressures similar to the diastolic pressure of the pig. The result is a tanned aortic root that maintains its normal anatomy, and in which the bending characteristics of the leaflets resemble those of the normal porcine aortic valve (11). The coronary artery stumps are ligated and left in situ. In addition, the valve is treated with alpha-aminooleic acid, an agent that mitigates calcification (12). A photograph of the Freestyle is shown in Figure 9.4-3. The Freestyle valve can be trimmed to be implanted in the subcoronary position as a stentless porcine aortic valve or it can be used as a root replacement. As in the case of the Prima, if the Freestyle is used as a

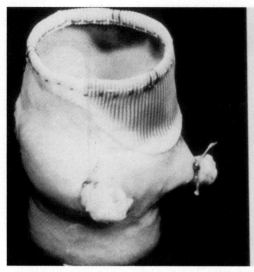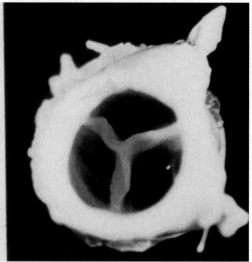

Figure 9.4-3: The Freestyle porcine aortic root can be used for aortic root replacement or as a stentless valve after excising the porcine sinuses.

root replacement it should not be referred to as a "stentless" bioprosthesis.

The Toronto SPV is a glutaraldehyde-fixed porcine aortic valve with its outside wall covered by a fine Dacron cloth, as shown in Figure 9.4-4. Two layers of sutures are needed to secure this valve in the recipient's aortic root, similar to what is done during free-hand implantation of an aortic valve homograft.

Glutaraldehyde fixed bovine pericardium has also been used as leaflet material for stentless aortic valves (13-14). This type of valve is usually tailored in the operating room just before implantation (14). Little is known about the Sorin Pericarbon stentless bovine pericardial valve at the time of this publication.

Hemodynamic assessment of stentless aortic valves

Stentless porcine aortic valves have very good hemodynamic features as assessed by Doppler echocardiography. Table 9.4-I summarizes the hemodynamic data obtained by

Table 9.4-I: Mean systolic gradients, peak systolic gradients, and aortic valve areas in patients with stentless porcine aortic valves (From David TE, et al. (9).

Valve Size (mm)	Mean Gradient (mmHg)	Peak Gradient (mmHg)	Aortic Valve Area (cm^2)
21	1.6 ± 2.8	7.0 ± 5.1	1.63 ± 0.15
23	5.7 ± 0.9	13.7 ± 2.0	1.71 ± 0.15
25	4.7 ± 0.2	12.2 ± 5.0	1.73 ± 0.21
27	3.5 ± 0.3	8.0 ± 3.9	1.87 ± 0.10
29	2.3 ± 2.7	6.0 ± 1.5	2.1 ± 0.38

Values are expressed as mean ± standard deviation.

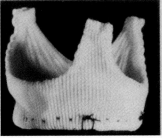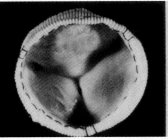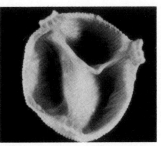

Figure 9.4-4: The Toronto SPV is made of a single porcine aortic valve and its outside wall is covered with a fine Dacron cloth.

Doppler echocardiography in 26 patients who underwent aortic valve replacement with a stentless porcine valve (9).

The hemodynamic data of stentless and stented porcine aortic valves were compared in a cohort study of 22 patients with identical body surface areas and bioprosthetic aortic valve diameters (9). The stentless valves were found to have significantly lower peak systolic gradients and larger effective valve orifices than did the stented valves (9). This should not be surprising because in any given patient it is always possible to implant a larger stentless than stented aortic valve since the size of the latter's effective orifice is restricted by the presence of the stent.

Casabona and co-workers from Italy and Brazil (13) compared the echocardiographic data of 57 patients with stentless aortic valves (30 pericardial and 27 porcine) with two other groups of 30 patients, each with a stented porcine or a single disc mechanical valve. They found an average aortic valve orifice of 1.72 ± 0.2 cm^2 for the stentless pericardial valves, 1.83 ± 0.3 cm^2 for the stentless porcine valves, 1.56 ± 0.1 cm^2 for the stented bioprostheses and 1.38 ± 0.1 cm^2 for the mechanical valves. The stentless valves had orifices significantly larger than did the stented porcine or mechanical valves (13).

One of the problems with stentless aortic valves has been aortic insufficiency. In our initial experience with 28 patients, we encountered trivial or mild aortic insufficiency by Doppler echocardiography in five patients (9). This problem has been largely eliminated by selecting the correct size valve (14). The diameter of the aortic annulus may not be the best way in which to select the size of a stentless valve.

In normal subjects, the diameter of the aortic annulus is 10% to 15% larger than the diameter of the sinotubular junction. Thus in patients with normal aortic roots, the diameter of the aortic annulus is the correct measurement to take for choosing the size of a stentless valve. However, most patients with aortic valve disease have an abnormal aortic root and the relationship between the diameters of the aortic annulus and sinotubular junction may be altered. In these patients, the diameter of the sinotubular junction is more important than is the diameter of the aortic annulus. The upper part of the commissures of a stentless valve is secured at approximately the level of the sinotubular junction and the spatial relationship of the three commissures during diastole determines how well the leaflets coapt.

Every stentless aortic valve probably behaves somewhat differently according to its design. The above considerations are extremely important for aortic valve replacement with the Toronto SPV as well as with free hand sewn pulmonary autografts and aortic

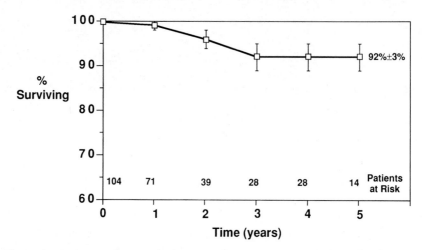

AORTIC VALVE REPLACEMENT WITH TORONTO SPV ACTUARIAL SURVIVAL

Figure 9.4-5: Actuarial survival after aortic valve replacement with the Toronto SPV.

valve homografts. The Toronto SPV is a competent valve when implanted in a normal aortic root or when the disparity between the diameters of the aortic annulus and the sinotubular junction is within 10% to 15%. A greater disparity will result in aortic incompetence either by lack of coaptation (commissures are pulled apart from each other) or by prolapse (commissures are too close to each other). Therefore, for the Toronto SPV, the diameter of the sinotubular junction determines the size of the valve to be implanted. Similar considerations have not yet been determined for other stentless heterografts.

Clinical experience with the Toronto SPV bioprosthesis

We have used the Toronto SPV bioprosthesis for aortic valve replacement in over one hundred patients. The initial experience involved 29 patients and extended from October 1987 to May 1989. The second phase of the this clinical trial started in July 1991 and 75 additional patients have undergone aortic valve replacement with this stentless bioprosthesis. There has been a total of 104 patients whose mean age was 60 years, range 26 to 80 years. Two-thirds of the patients were men. Most patients had aortic stenosis; one-third of the patients also had coronary artery disease. The most common sizes of valves used were 25, 27 and 29 mm (80% of cases).

There was only one operative death. Patients have been followed from one to 84 months. There have been only two late deaths: one patient with a severely impaired left ventricle who also underwent mitral valve repair died of ventricular dysrhythmias 17 months postoperatively; his stentless aortic valve was functioning normally. The other patient was an elderly woman who also underwent a triple coronary artery bypass and died of acute myocardial infarction 32 months postoperatively. Figure 9.4-5 shows the actuarial survival of all patients.

Only one patient developed infective endocarditis three years after surgery and he was successfully treated with antibiotics and repeat surgery because of large vegetations on the valve leaflets. The infection was limited to the leaflets of the valve. The freedom from infective endocarditis at five years was 98% ± 1%. There have been no late strokes, only two transient ischemic attacks. No patient is on oral anticoagulant but approximately one-third of them (mostly those who also underwent coronary artery bypass) are on aspirin.

Patients who underwent aortic valve replacement with the Toronto SPV are being carefully monitored because they have a new type of bioprosthetic heart valve. They are contacted every six months and Doppler echocardiographic studies are performed annually. The peak systolic gradients are very low and the effective valve orifices quite large and have not changed over the years. One of the most remarkable features of this type of biological valve is the low rate of valve-related complications. This feature may explain the exceptionally high actuarial survival shown in Figure 9.4-5.

COMMENTS

Other investigators have described their experiences with stentless aortic valves but all studies have had limited follow up. Batista and associates from Brazil (15) reported a series of 60 patients who underwent aortic valve replacement with a stentless valve constructed with a monopatch of glutaraldehyde-fixed bovine pericardium and sutured directly into the aortic annulus and aortic sinuses. There were six early deaths, none related to the valve. During a maximum follow up of two years, two patients required reoperation because of aortic insufficiency. The other patients did well.

Hofig et al. (15) reported on 12 patients who had undergone aortic valve replacement with a stentless porcine aortic valve containing a sewing ring of Dacron and commissures covered with a fabric. One patient died and one patient had early valve dehiscence because of active infective endocarditis but the other 10 patients did well for up to four years. The transvalvular gradients and the effective valve areas remained stable throughout the follow up period.

Stentless heterograft valves have superior hemodynamic features but the crucial issue is whether they will be more durable than stented porcine and pericardial valves. Although the interactions between the heterograft and the host are important in determining the fate of bioprostheses, mechanical stress is an important determinant of the durability of biological valves (17-18).

The aortic root is probably the best stent for the aortic valve. The anatomy and function of the aortic root may dampen the mechanical stress to which the leaflets are subjected during diastole. This hypothesis is supported by clinical experience with aortic valve homografts. Free-hand sewn aortic valve homografts in the aortic root are significantly more durable than stent-mounted aortic valve homografts used for aortic valve replacement (19-20). The average time for aortic valve homograft failure is approximately 12 years when they are free-hand sewn and eight years when they are mounted in a stent (19). Interestingly, the average time for failure of a stented porcine aortic valve in the aortic position is also eight years (19,21). By extrapolation one could conclude that stentless porcine aortic valves will be more durable than stented porcine valves.

Although our experience with a stentless porcine bioprosthesis extends to just over six years, this valve has excellent hemodynamic features, is associated with a very low risk of valve-related complications and will probably last longer than stented porcine valves.

References

1. Ross DN. Homograft replacement of the aortic valve. Lancet 1962;2:487
2. Barratt-Boyes BG. Homograft aortic valve replacement in aortic valve incompetence and stenosis. Thorax 1964;19:131-150
3. Binet JP, Duran CG, Carpentier A, Langlois J. Heterologous aortic valve transplantation. Lancet 1965;2:1275
4. O'Brien MF, Clareborough JK. Heterograft aortic valve transplantation for human valve disease. Med J Aust 1966;2:228-230
5. O'Brien MF. Heterograft aortic valves for human use. J Thorac Cardiovasc Surg 1967;53:392-397
6. O'Brien MF, Neilson GH, Galea E, et al. Heterograft valves. An analysis of clinical results of valve replacement. Circulation 1970;16 & 17(Suppl II):16-19
7. Carpentier A, Lemaigre G, Robert L, et al. Biological factors affecting long term results of valvular heterografts. J Thorac Cardiovasc Surg 1969;58:467-483
8. David TE, Ropchan GC, Butany JW. Aortic valve replacement with stentless porcine bioprostheses. J Cardiac Surg 1988;3:501-505
9. David TE, Pollick C, Bos J. Aortic valve replacement with stentless porcine aortic bioprosthesis. J Thorac Cardiovasc Surg 1990;99:113-118
10. Huysmans HA, Hazekamp MG. The value of a stentless valve bioprosthesis: Experiments in the growing pig. AustralAs J Cardiac Thorac Surg 1993;2:64-66
11. Vesely I. Analysis of the Medtronic Intact bioprosthetic valve. Effects of "zero-pressure" fixation. J Thorac Cardiovasc Surg 1991;101:90-99
12. Gott JP, Pan-Chih, Dorsey LMA, et al. Calcification of porcine valves: A successful new method of antimineralization. Ann Thorac Surg 1992;53:207-216
13. Casabona R, DePaulis R, Zattera GF, et al. Stentless porcine and pericardial valves in the aortic position. Ann Thorac Surg 1992;54:681-685
14. Batista RJV, Dobrianskij A, Commazzi M Jr., et al. Clinical experience with stentless pericardial aortic monopatch for aortic valve replacement. J Thorac Cardiovasc Surg 1987;93:19-26
15. David TE, Bos J, Rakowski H. Aortic valve replacement with the Toronto SPV bioprosthesis. J Heart Valve Dis 1992;1:244-248
16. Hofig M, Nelessen U, Mahmoodi M, et al. Performance of a stentless xenograft aortic bioprosthesis up to four years after implantation. J Thorac Cardiovasc Surg 1992;103:1068-1073
17. Thubrikar M, Deck JD, Aouad J, Nolan SP. Role of mechanical stress in calcification of aortic bioprosthetic valves. J Thorac Cardiovasc Surg 1983;86:115-125
18. Bromm ND. Fatigue-induced damage in glutaraldehyde-preserved heart valve tissue. J Thorac Cardiovasc Surg 1978;76:202-211
19. Angell WW, Angell JD, Oury JH, Lamberti JJ, Grehl TM. Long term follow up of viable frozen aortic homografts: a viable homograft valve bank. J Thorac Cardiovasc Surg 1987;93:815-822
20. Angell WW, Oury JH, Lamberti JJ, Loziol J. Durability of the viable aortic allograft. J Thorac Cardiovasc Surg 1989;98:48-56
21. Magilligan DJ Jr, Kemp SR, Stein PP, Peterson E. Asynchronous primary valve failure in patients with porcine bioprosthetic aortic and mitral valves. Circulation 1987;76:141-145

Chapter 9.5

Mechanical Valves

Endre Bodnar

The medical and socio-economic impact of mechanical heart valve prostheses is immense; probably more than 100,000 patients receive them each year, while the number who die on the waiting list or from an unrecognized valvular disease in certain geographic areas can only be guessed at. The industry that provides the valves is huge and the price paid by society in terms of the cost of surgical intervention and life-long postoperative care is high. The results, however, seem to justify this.

This chapter highlights the most important features of mechanical prostheses. Not surprisingly, the number of relevant publications can only be measured by the thousands. In January 1996, there were 18,756 publications listed by MEDLINE under the search word "valve", and 12,733 responding to "mechanical valve". Within this vast array of published information, however, results of randomized clinical trials are scarce, and those of prospective randomization when introducing a new device are practically non-existent. The development of consecutive generations of mechanical valves can be defined in summary terms as a continuous series of efforts to eliminate the shortcomings and diminish the complications of previous replacement devices.

HISTORICAL ASPECTS

The first mechanical valve ever inserted was not a 'replacement' valve; it was Hufnagel's ball valve implanted into the descending thoracic aorta to relieve aortic regurgitation (1). Subsequent attempts at orthotopic heart valve replacement tried to mimic the morphology of the natural valve using a variety of synthetic materials. All were unsuccessful, and Lefrak and Starr compared them to man's first attempts to fly; with artificial wings (2).

The true era of heart valve replacement started in 1960, when Dwight Harken reported his first success with orthotopic replacement of the aortic (3) and Albert Starr that of the mitral valve (4), both using caged ball valves. The fortunate partnership of Albert Starr and M. Lowell Edwards took heart valve replacement one step further when M. Lowell Edwards started Edwards Laboratories, Inc. in California and introduced large scale, commercial production of these devices. These two pioneers, Starr and Edwards, laid down the surgical, engineering and manufacturing foundations of current heart valve replacement. The engineering team at Edwards Laboratories became a further source of talent, Don Shiley, and Warren Hancock being the best known among them.

Edwards, Shiley and Hancock Laboratories became the 'Californian arm' of the heart valve industry, while Medical, Inc. with the Lillehei-Kaster, Omniscience and Omnicarbon valves, Medtronic and St. Jude Medical have firmly established Minnesota/St.Paul as a center for replacement valves. Texas entered the scene with

CarboMedics in Austin. The only significant addition to these three states in the USA came from Saluggia, Italy, where Sorin started producing replacement valves about 20 years ago.

The ongoing evolution of mechanical heart valves has been dictated not only by spontaneous human inventiveness, but by the shortcomings of existing devices, design limitations inherent in the available materials, and how great a risk industry was willing to take by adopting and introducing novel concepts.

Regarding design, there have been three major steps in the history of mechanical valves. The first period was characterized by variations on the caged-ball and caged-disc design, the second was the era of the tilting disc valves, and the third, reaching the present, is that of the hinged bileaflet valves.

The first caged-ball valve, the Starr-Edwards valve, was introduced in 1960 (4), and the last such model, the DeBakey-Surgitool valve, in 1970, with more than a dozen variations on the theme in between (5). At present, only the Starr-Edwards model 1260 aortic and 6120 mitral prostheses are still available; all other caged-ball/disc valves had been withdrawn from the market.

The first tilting disc, the Wada-Cutter valve was introduced in 1966, but was short-lived because of the unexpected wear of the Teflon disc (6). The Lillehei-Kaster valve entered the market in 1967 (7), paving the way for the subsequent development of the Omniscience and Omnicarbon valves. This was followed by the successive models of the Björk-Shiley valve (8-12) and in 1977 by the Medtronic Hall valve (13). Since then there has not been a major breakthrough in the field of tilting disc valves. The Medtronic Hall, Omnicarbon/Omniscience, and Monostrut (originally Shiley, currently Sorin) are the best known tilting disc prostheses currently in clinical use.

The first successful hinged bileaflet valve, the St. Jude Medical prosthesis, was released in 1977 (14), and almost all further design developments have been directed towards creating bileaflet alternatives to this valve, which serves today as the "gold standard" for mechanical prostheses.

Regarding materials, it appears that the history can be separated into two main periods, the first before and the second since the introduction of pyrolytic carbon, an achievement of Jack Bokros (15). Metals, however, have been continuously present in one form or another since 1960 (Stellite, Hayes alloy, titanium, Ti6Al4Va alloy).

The interaction between material and design is remarkably demonstrated by the history of mechanical replacement valves. When the caged-ball design was introduced, the necessary synthetic materials and metal alloys were readily available. Pyrolytic carbon was only later applied to this design, but the results were less than satisfactory (16,17). On the other hand, it would be difficult to imagine a bileaflet valve constructed with the synthetic and metal materials of the caged-ball valves; the wear resistance of pyrolytic carbon is a prerequisite for this design. Interestingly, since the discontinuation of the Delrin disc by Shiley, tilting disc valves have remained a combination of metal housing and pyrolytic carbon disc, the only exception being the Omnicarbon valve, which is made entirely from pyrolytic carbon.

The history of mechanical valvular prostheses has been chequered by the failure of some particular devices, with a broad variation in the extent of the consequences. Due to the relatively small numbers implanted, the above mentioned failure of the DeBakey valve (16,17) and disc wear in the first generation Beall valve had few consequences for the overall patient population, but Surgitool, the manufacturer, went out of business as a result. Much larger was the impact of the failure of the Braunwald-Cutter aortic prosthesis due to ball escape, which led to elective reoperation for the removal of the culprit prosthesis world-wide (18). The strut fracture of the Björk-Shiley concavo-convex valve was a similarly major fiasco, details of which will follow in this chapter when describing tilting disc prostheses. Due to the swift and decisive action of Baxter-Edwards in voluntarily withdrawing the valve from the market, the mechanical failure of the Duromedics valve did not have major clinical consequences (vide infra). Despite these structural failures in the past, durability remains the perceived advantage of mechanical as opposed to bioprosthetic replacement valves.

This chapter will review major features of the caged-ball, tilting disc and hinged bileaflet designs and their respective flow characteristics, modes of failure of mechanical valves and the individual valve models currently in clinical use. General aspects of material- and design-related thrombogenicity are detailed in Chapter 10.3.

DESIGN AND FLOW CHARACTERISTICS

The presence of a geometrically perfect, rigid ring is common to all mechanical prostheses. Also universal is a surgical sewing ring attached to the valve housing. The shape of the cross-section and the compound dimension of these two components define the primary orifice available for blood flow. The true effective orifice area is, however, the result of the influence of the closing mechanism on this primary orifice area.

Valve opening and closing is achieved in one of three ways in heart valve prostheses, all of them based on pressure changes during the cardiac cycle. Valve closure can be achieved by a poppet that seals the orifice during closure and drops away downstream to open, as is the case with all caged-ball and caged disc valves and with every variation on this principle (toroidal valve, Cape Town valve, Cooley-Cutter valve, etc.) (5). In the tilting disc valves the disc is retained asymmetrically, thus producing a smaller and a larger surface for the blood pressure to act on and tilt the disc. The result is the creation of a smaller and a larger orifice with less than optimum flow characteristics (vide infra), a setback that cannot be eliminated because a symmetrically retained disc would not act as a valve. Bileaflet valves are intended to overcome this problem. The two leaflets are attached to the housing by hinges, and create three rather than two orifices with improved though still not perfect flow characteristics.

Closing reflux and leakage through the closed valve are also determined by the design. The former is the amount of blood pushed backward through the orifice by the occluder while moving from the open to the closed position. The latter is the amount of blood squeezed through the closed valve between the disc and the ring, also around the hinges in bileaflet devices. The total volume of closing reflux and leakage varies between 2% and 15% of the stroke volume, depending on the design (vide infra). In low cardiac output, however, the retrograde flow may exceed 50% of the stroke volume due to the slow closing movement of the occluder (19). This phenomenon is flow- rather than pressure dependent (19).

Leakage through the closed valve is deliberately created by the designer, and its amount is carefully controlled. This is a low volume-high velocity flow meant to provide "wash-out" and thereby prevent thrombus apposition on the valve surfaces (20).

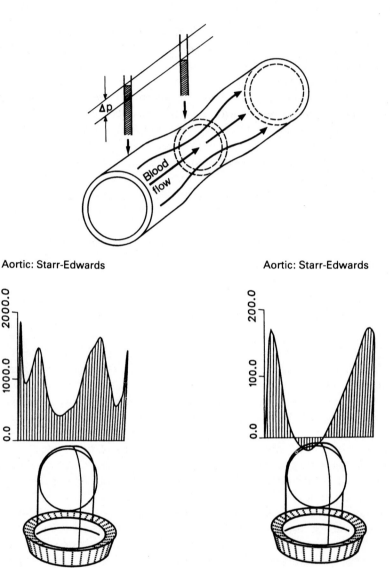

Aortic: Starr-Edwards   Aortic: Starr-Edwards

Turbulent shear stresses in dynes/cm²   Velocities in cm/s

Figure 9.5-1: Flow characteristics of caged-ball valves. Modified with permission from Black MM, Cochrane T, Lawford PV, Reul H, Yoganathan AP. Design and flow characteristics. In Bodnar E, Frater R (eds). Replacement Heart Valves, Pergamon Press, New York, 1991, and from Yoganathan AP, Wick TM, Reul H. The influence of flow characteristics of prosthetic valves on thrombus formation. In Butchart EG, Bodnar E (eds). Thrombosis, Embolism and Bleeding, ICR Publishers, London, 1992

Caged-ball design

The caged-ball design is remarkably reminiscent of that of a bottle stopper which was patented in the USA in 1858 (21). The clear advantage of this prosthesis type is its non-sophisticated nature, lending itself with ease to manufacture, and to surgical insertion, as no particular orientation is necessary in any position. The shortcomings are high profile and obstructive flow characteristics.

High profile is unavoidable with the caged-ball design. The further the bulky ball moves away from the housing ring the less the obstruction to flow will be. However, the distance to which the ball is allowed to drop in these prostheses is limited, because the ability to close must be retained. The actual height of the cage is therefore a compromise between these two design considerations.

The resulting functional orifice is obstructive, creating a high velocity turbulent flow (20). The obstructive nature of the caged-ball design is particularly apparent in the aortic position, where a "secondary" stenosis may develop between the ball and the aortic wall (Fig. 9.5-1A). The central flow that enters the prosthetic annular ring separates symmetrically around the ball, reaching high velocity (Fig. 9.5-1B), and developing high turbulent shear stresses (Fig. 9.5-1C) (20). There is a moderate flow reversal (closing reflux) when the ball moves back to the closed position (Fig. 9.5-1C). The maximum turbulent shear stress created by the Starr-Edwards valve exceeds 3,000 dynes/cm^2, by far the highest among all mechanical prosthesis designs.

Tilting disc design

The development of the tilting disc valves was intended to eliminate, or at least diminish, both major shortcomings of the caged-ball valves by decreasing the profile significantly and improving the flow conditions across the valve. There appear to be two pertinent features which determine the hydrodynamic performance of these valves; the relative size of the large and small orifice areas, and the opening angle of the disc.

The larger the large orifice the more reminiscent of the natural anterior mitral leaflet the opening and closing disc becomes. At the same time the flow across the prosthesis becomes increasingly "central" in nature. However, a parallel decrease in the small orifice size is unavoidable. The consequence is restricted flow through the small orifice and diminishing wash-out, leading to increased thrombogenicity at this point. The position of the tilting axis, which determines the large vs. small orifice ratio, is a compromise between these two design concepts in all tilting disc prostheses. A complete elimination of the small orifice by creating a "toilet seat cover"-like valve was attempted in the sixties, but the design was clinically unsuccessful (5).

The opening angle is that enclosed by the housing ring and the disc in the fully opened position. It is a potential maximum rather than a regular, compulsory degree of disc opening, as it has been established that in atrial fibrillation (22,23), but even without it (24), the disc does not always open to its full potential. The larger the opening angle the larger the effective orifice area, but as the opening angle approaches 90°, disc closure becomes more and more protracted, and the closing reflux as well as the impact of the disc against the housing on closure increase. The former hinders hydrodynamic efficiency, the latter increases cavitation potential (vide infra).

Characteristic of all tilting disc valves is the presence of two high-velocity-jet type flow fields (20) representing the major and minor orifices (Fig. 9.5-2). The velocity is higher above the larger than above the smaller orifice, with flow separation and stagnation

Aortic: Bjørk-Shiley

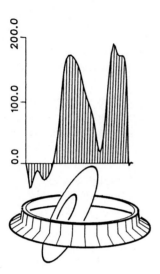

Velocities in cm/s

Figure 9.5-2: Flow characteristics of tilting disc valves. Modified with permission from Yoganathan AP, Wick TM, Reul H. The influence of flow characteristics of prosthetic valves on thrombus formation. In Butchart EG, Bodnar E (eds). Thrombosis, Embolism and Bleeding, ICR Publishers, London, 1992

Aortic: Medtronic-Hall

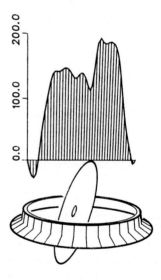

Velocities in cm/s

Aortic: Omnicarbon

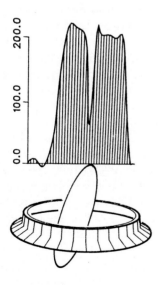

Velocities in cm/s

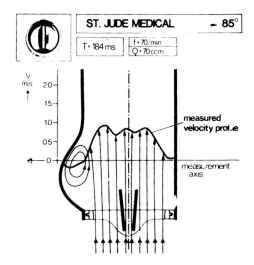

Aortic: St. Jude

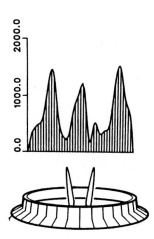

Turbulent shear stresses in dynes/cm²

Figure 9.5-3: Flow characteristics of bileaflet valves. Modified with permission from Black MM, Cochrane T, Lawford PV, Reul H, Yoganathan AP. Design and flow characteristics. In Bodnar E, Frater R (eds). Replacement Heart Valves, Pergamon Press, New York, 1991, and from Yoganathan AP, Wick TM, Reul H. The influence of flow characteristics of prosthetic valves on thrombus formation. In Butchart EG, Bodnar E (eds). Thrombosis, Embolism and Bleeding, ICR Publishers, London, 1992

between the two jets. This flow separation, however, is hardly present in the Medtronic Hall valve (Fig 2C). There is little difference in the magnitude of the developing turbulent shear stress, which varies between 1,000 - 2,000 dynes/cm² (Fig. 9.5-3), reaching the level where platelet damage can occur (25).

With its distinctly asymmetric flow field, i.e. major and minor orifices, the orientation of a tilting disc valve in any position within the heart becomes an important factor. The primary goal, particularly in the mitral position, is to secure free movement of the disc, unimpeded by any surrounding tissue and/or cardiac structure. Within this limitation, the optimum position is the one that provides the best flow pathway between the free edge of the open disc and the left ventricular cavity or the ascending aorta. In the mitral position this appears to be the posterior orientation, i.e. the large orifice placed posteriorly, in which case the disc movement in this orifice resembles that of the anterior cusp of the natural mitral valve. In the aortic position the recommended orientation is to place the large orifice toward the non-coronary segment of the ascending aorta (26).

Hinged bileaflet design

The goal of this concept was to take mechanical valve design one step further by reducing valve profile as compared to tilting disc valves, and by eliminating the inherent disadvantages of the minor orifice. The former objective is particularly well achieved by the St. Jude Medical valve, which has hardly any protrusion into the left ventricular cavity when implanted in the mitral position.

Hinged bileaflet valves have two semicircular leaflets which can be flat (St. Jude Medical, Carbomedics) or curved (Duromedics, Sorin Bicarbon), and which divide the total orifice area into three orifices, two lateral and one central. The result is a flow field which is the closest to that of the natural valves as compared to any other type of mechanical prostheses (Fig. 9.5-3A). The great majority of forward flow passes through the two lateral orifices, developing relatively low turbulent shear stresses (Fig. 9.5-3B) (20).

The weak point of the hydrodynamics of the bileaflet design is valve closure and regurgitation, both of which are inherent in having two rather than one leaflet and four pivot areas which need thorough washout during valve closure. As perfect symmetry, which does not exist in nature, cannot be achieved in any man-made product either, the closure of the two leaflets of any bileaflet mechanical prosthesis is always asynchronous, even in the most meticulously arranged flow chamber (Martin M. Black, Personal communication, 1996). In the beating heart, the actual degree of difference in closure time depends on several factors, such as cardiac rhythm or orientation (27). The regurgitation is a result of (a) the closing movement of the two leaflets, (b) asynchcronous closure, (c) the gap between the closed leaflets and between the leaflets and housing, and (d) washout through the pivot areas, and can be as high as 15% of the forward flow (see Chapter 10.2).

The orientation of a bileaflet valve is defined by the direction of the axis of the leaflets within the heart, or in a flow chamber. Earlier studies could not find any effect of orientation in a pulse duplicator (28,29). Recently, however, with a sophisticated simulation of valve implantation in the mitral position with chordal preservation, the anti-anatomic orientation (valve axis perpendicular to the closing line of the natural valve) was found to be superior with the St. Jude Medical valve (30).

Under clinical conditions, unimpeded leaflet movement must always be reserved, and this sometimes overrules the preferred orientation. There are advocates both of the anatomic (31) and anti-anatomic (32) orientation in the mitral position. The clinical argument for anti-anatomic orientation is to avoid having one leaflet close to the posterior wall of the left ventricle, which may contribute to asynchronous closing. Fontaine et al.'s laboratory findings (30) seem to confirm this concept. In the aortic position interventricular septal hypertrophy may have an effect on valve performance by partially occluding the available prosthetic orifice area, but there is no clear agreement on how to avoid this potential problem (31,32).

MODES OF FAILURE OF MECHANICAL VALVES

Valve failure is an impediment to normal valve function which requires reoperation or leads to prior death (33-35). It can take the form of obstruction, incompetence, or a combination of the two. The possible causes are manifold, and are best categorized as structural and non-structural failure mechanisms. Structural failure is due to wear or fatigue, and is the consequence of flaws in the design or in the materials used in the construction, or in the manufacturing process. Structural failure, however, can be caused by improper handling prior to or during implantation (vide infra). Non-structural failure is the loss of normal function despite an unimpaired morphology (and function) of the explanted valve.

Non-structural failure

Valve thrombosis and pannus ingrowth

Valve thrombosis and pannus ingrowth are by far the most frequent causes of non-structural failure (36). The relevant pathology and anticoagulation management are fully discussed in Chapter 10.3. As far as thrombogenicity of the prosthesis itself is concerned, very little scientifically valid information is available. The only prosthesis which has design-determined protection against pannus ingrowth is the St. Jude Medical valve with its pivot guards. It should be borne in mind that the internationally adopted recommendation to keep the INR between 3.0 and 4.5 is an arbitrarily set target level, which may well serve practical purposes but is not based on any comparative or prospective clinical trial. Again, so far only the St. Jude Medical valve, based on good results arising from a retrospective study (37), has been entered into prospective, randomized clinical trials in France (AREVA study, vide infra) and two years later in Germany (GELIA study) (38) to ascertain the optimum level of anticoagulation with this prosthesis, which appears to be considerably less than the internationally recommended INR of 3.0-4.5.

From a mechanical point of view, both pannus and thrombus may obstruct the valvular orifice, at least partially, and may interfere with occluder function, i.e. ball, disc or leaflet movement, depending on the design. For further details see Chapter 10.3.

Paravalvular leak

Paravalvular leak is not a genuine failure of the device itself, a fact is portrayed in its name; *para*valvular. The cause is a dehiscence, in some cases more than one, between the surgical sewing ring of the prosthesis and the patient's valvular annulus due to torn suture(s) or a weak mitral or aortic annulus which cannot hold the inserting sutures. Paravalvular leak is a frequent consequence of prosthetic endocarditis.

If the paravalvular dehiscence is large, there are major hemodynamic sequelae calling for surgical re-intervention. Smaller leaks may not have hemodynamic consequences yet may become clinically significant by causing a major degree of hemolysis requiring reoperation for this indication. It is a rule in cardiac surgery always to search thoroughly for the existence of hidden, small paravalvular leak(s) when the patient presents with a clinically significant hemolysis.

Impingement

Surrounding cardiac structures or calcific lumps may bulge into the opening and closing pathway of the occluder of any design and prevent full movement in both the mitral and aortic positions. This is called impingement. It may only impair hemodynamic function, or it may cause gross failure either by itself or by provoking secondary valve thrombosis (39,40). Not infrequently, it is caused by inserting an oversized prosthesis (41). Meticulous care during insertion can greatly diminish the potential for impingement. An additional help in this respect is provided by the rotatability of almost all mechanical prostheses.

Entrapment

Long suture ends in any position, and loose chordae in the mitral position can be caught between the occluder and the valve housing. If the consequence is immobilization of the occluder in the closed position, the event is called entrapment. The mechanism is the same as when a door is forcibly shut while a ductile object is held between door and door frame. In the case of a tilting disc valve, the result is instantaneous circulatory collapse and almost invariably sudden death. Survival cannot be expected unless cardiopulmonary bypass is re-established before permanent brain damage occurs (39,42,43).

The smaller the clearance between the closed occluder and valve housing, the greater is the potential for entrapment. Due to inherent design characteristics, tilting disc valves are more prone to entrapment than bileaflet valves (44). All bileaflet valves have in common the advantage that the patient can survive entrapment with one leaflet while the other remains functional until an urgent reoperation can be scheduled.

A particular case of entrapment is when immobilization occurs without an object between the occluder and the valve housing. The cause can be swelling of a polymer disc (44), or distortion of a flexible valve ring (45).

Canting

Every valve design is based on the underlying assumption that the axis of the valve and that of the flow are parallel. If a tilting disc or a bileaflet prosthesis is tilted from this parallel-axis position, regurgitation or complete failure to close may occur. This is sometimes the case when an oversized prosthesis is intentionally implanted in the aortic position by positioning one third of the valve above the non-coronary segment of the annulus (46,47). The larger the opening angle of the disc, the easier it will be for canting to occur.

Structural failure

Structural failure can be caused by degradation of synthetic materials within the blood stream, wear, fatigue, or cavitation damage. Its origin can be limited durability of the materials used for construction, inappropriate combination of materials in a given design, hidden flaws in certain materials, and lack of a truly damage-tolerant design. The ultimate durability of a mechanical prosthetic valve is always the result of the given combination of materials and design.

Material degradation

Material degradation affected only the first generation Starr-Edwards valves causing ball variance through lipid absorption. This mode of failure was quickly eliminated in the sixties by improving the curing process of the silicon rubber ball (44). Biodegradation as a cause of valve failure has not been reported with any other synthetic material. Sporadic reports on problems with the Delrin[R] disc of the Björk-Shiley valve (48,49) were not followed up by confirmation of biodegradation in this material. Delrin, however,

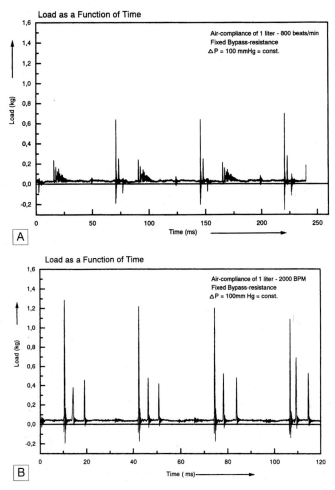

Figure 9.5-4: The effect of frequency changes (and parallel dP/dt changes) on loading conditions in an accelerated wear tester. Reproduced with the permission of ICR Publishers from Reul H, Eichler M, Potthast K, Schmitz C, Rau G. In vitro testing of heart valve wear outside of the manufacturers laboratory - Requirements and controversies. J Heart Valve Dis 1996;5(Suppl. I):S97-S104

does not tolerate autoclave sterilization (50). This limitation was not known during the early clinical series, and a number of valves were submitted to heat sterilization within hospitals leading to swelling or shrinking of the Delrin disc.

Wear

Wear is unavoidable in any mechanical device, including prosthetic heart valves, where two rigid surfaces come into contact repeatedly. If the pulse rate is estimated at a constant 76/min, the number of cardiac cycles per annum is 40 million. If a replacement valve is required to function for 50 years, it must therefore resist 2,000 million cycles. In addition, all this must be done without any "servicing", as this is not possible with

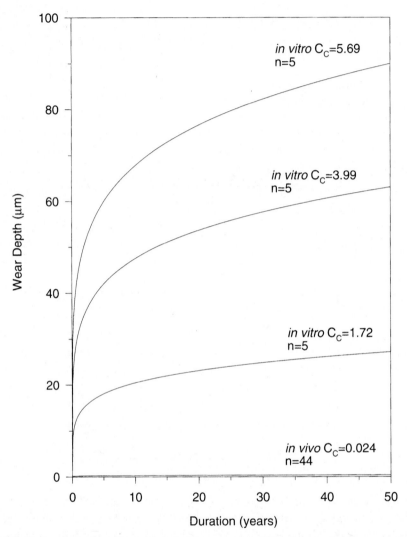

Figure 9.5-5: Comparison of in vitro and and vivo wear rates. Reproduced with the permission of ICR Publishers from Campbell A, Baldwin T, Peterson G, Bryant J, Ryder K. Pitfalls and outcomes from accelerated wear testing of mechanical heart valves. J Heart Valve Dis 1996;5(Suppl. I):S124-S132

implanted prosthetic valves. The expectations are thus very high.

The problem of wear is further increased by the limitations of the laboratory methods that can be used to assess the durability of a replacement valve. Even with known material characteristics the actual design has the ultimate influence on wear rate. It follows that a valid wear test must be completed on the final product, i.e. the valve produced for clinical use. The valve should undergo repeated cycling to achieve full opening and closure of the occluder(s) with pressures kept within the physiologic range (51).

Such a wear test can be carried out in real time, that is the rate kept around 70-80/min

(52). With this method, however, only early effects can be assessed, because of the length of time involved. Therefore, accelerated wear testing became the method of choice, with machines running 10-15 times faster than the physiologic heart rate. The completion of such a test is compulsory for every new valve in order to comply with the FDA, ISO and CE standard regulations (51,53,54).

Recent information makes the interpretation of accelerated wear test data rather difficult. It is now accepted that under accelerated conditions the disc starts vibrating, and instead of one single closing movement hits the ring several times within every cycle. The expected wear is therefore inproportionately higher than it would be in the heart. Furthermore, it was not known until recently that frequency, and the resulting dP/dt changes within the test machine, have a significant effect on wear rate (Fig. 9.5-4) (55). Finally, it has been confirmed that the wear rate in a test machine is incomparably higher than it is during an identical number of cycles in the heart (Fig. 9.5-5) (56).

The conclusion is that accelerated wear tests are only a crude means of estimating valve durability, and the results cannot be extrapolated to predict clinical life expectancy of a replacement valve (57). All these make the careful analysis of clinical explants ever more important.

Synthetic materials: Silicone rubber was the first polymer used successfully in the construction of replacement valves, and it is still in use in the model 1260 and 6120 Starr-Edwards valves. Although the life span of this device stretches over 30 years, there has only been one publication so far reporting on the mechanical degradation of the silicone rubber ball (58). The material proved to be less successful in caged-disc valves (Kay-Shiley, Cross-Jones, Starr-Edwards caged-disc) because of suboptimum wear resistance which led to notching on the disc edge (44). Teflon was tried in some early models (Beall, Wada-Cutter), but its wear resistance proved to be disastrously low, and consequently it was eliminated from the list of polymers with a potential use as a bearing surface in replacement valves. Delrin was found in preclinical testing to have much better wear characteristics (8), and until now wear has not been a major problem with the Delrin-disc Björk-Shiley valves. Despite this it was replaced by a pyrolytic carbon disc in 1971, mainly because of problems with heat sterilization (vide supra).

The Delrin occluder was re-introduced in the St. Vincent tilting disc valve with unknown clinical performance. Otherwise, synthetic materials are no longer used in the construction of prosthetic valves except in the surgical sewing ring.

Metals and metal alloys: Stainless steel, titanium, chromium-cobalt alloy and titanium-aluminium-vanadium alloy have been used in mechanical valves, each one of them with excellent wear resistance. With the only exception of the DeBakey valve, in which significant wear of the titanium housing caused by the pyrolytic carbon ball was reported (44), failure due to wear of the metal/alloy part of a mechanical prosthesis is unknown. The strut fracture of the 60° and 70° Björk-Shiley valves is not caused by wear, it is a fatigue problem, and will be discussed later.

Pyrolytic carbon: Pyrolytic carbon (PyC) has an outstanding wear resistance, and is currently the material of choice for replacement valves. Pure PyC is employed only in the Edwards Tekna (previously Duromedics) and CarboMedics valve housings, otherwise it is used as a 150-250 micron thick coating on a graphite core. Accelerated wear tests predict a clinical durability beyond 100 years. The longest clinical experience is provided by the St. Jude Medical valve, in which PyC wears against PyC. Since its introduction in 1977, there has not been a single valve failure due to wear reported (Personal communication, St. Jude Medical, Inc., 1996, and MEDLINE search, April 1996). The CarboMedics bileaflet valve has a similarly impeccable track record regarding wear (CarboMedics, Inc., 1996, and MEDLINE search, April 1996).

It should be stressed, however, that wear occurs in all PyC valves when implanted in patients (59). It is the low degree of wear which makes these devices apparently so durable. Comparative data show that accelerated wear tests cause a much higher degree of wear than clinical exposure (56) (vide supra).

A unique occurrence of wear has been reported with the Sorin Bicarbon valve, which has a titanium alloy housing coated only by a few microns of turbostratic carbon (Carbofilm^R) deposited at room temperature (60,61). Although the valve was released more than five years ago and over 17,000 units have been implanted so far (60), it was not known until recently that the Carbofilm coating wears off the metal housing after less than two weeks cycling in a real time wear tester (52), as well as under clinical conditions (62). The consequence is continuing wear within a carbon/metal couple which is discussed below.

Carbon/metal couple: The first data in the medical literature on wear in metal/PyC couples was reported by Shim and Schoen in 1974 (63). They compared wear of the PyC component caused by PyC, titanium and chromium-cobalt alloy. Two important conclusions were drawn from this study. Firstly, that the amount of wear for any given combination was linearly related to the sliding distance of the two components. Secondly, that the wear rate in metal/PyC couples was twice as high for metals and more than ten-fold higher for PyC than was found in PyC/PyC couples.

The clinical experience regarding PyC/metal wear does not seem to confirm the above experimental data. With the exception of the Omnicarbon valve, in which both the housing and the disc have a PyC cover on a graphite core, all tilting disc valves have a metal housing and PyC disc. Unlike the DeBakey ball valve (44), valve failure due to wear in either component has not been reported so far with tilting disc valves, and measurements taken on clinical explants predict a 200 - 300 years safety period before critical wear penetration would occur (9,64).

Two important points need to be stressed in this respect. One is that the wear characteristics of the tilting disc valves cannot be extrapolated to hinged bileaflet valves, because in the former case the wear is evenly distributed around the entire circumference by the continuous rotation of the disc, but in the latter case it is localized as both pivots and leaflets have a fixed position. The other is the influence of lubrication, which was not applied in the above experimental work (63), but is provided by the blood flow within the beating heart. Recent data on metal/PyC wear under laboratory conditions provides evidence of the importance of lubrication (60).

It follows that wear in prosthetic heart valves cannot be simplified as a material property, it is the compound result of material characteristics, actual engineering system and lubrication.

Fatigue

Material fatigue in engineering terms describes a situation when small, inconsequential defects increase to a critical size, causing fracture under the effect of repetitive, cyclic loading, the magnitude of which is substantially below the level at which a singular stress would break the given object.

Major clinical consequences of metal fatigue have only been encountered with the 60° and 70° Björk-Shiley valves. The fatigue that develops in the neighbourhood of the welding points causes strut fracture. Unfortunately, there is no diagnostic method available which could predict this fatigue. Recent experience suggests that usually the fractures of the two legs of a strut are consecutive, causing single leg separation followed by total fracture (65). With appropriate radiologic techniques single leg separation can be diagnosed with a high probability, and elective, urgent removal of the (partially) failing prosthesis can be implemented (66). Clinical details of the Björk-Shiley strut fracture are given later in this chapter.

It was commonly held in the past that fatigue would not occur in PyC (44). Most probably due to rather crude methods applied in the investigations, it was thought that mobile dislocation leading to fatigue cannot exist in PyC. Recently, however, Robert O. Ritchie proved beyond doubt the existence of crack propagation under cyclic load in PyC, and recommended a much more rigorous proof test than currently applied in the quality assurance of valve components made of PyC (67). His proposal prompted a thorough scrutiny by industrial and independent scientists (68-73). These studies confirmed the existence of crack propagation in PyC, but at the same time demonstrated the strong relationship between engineering design and material fatigue, which makes the current prosthetic valves safe using the already adopted quality assurance criteria.

From a statistical point of view, there may be a possibility that one Pyc valve component out of a million, perhaps ten million, might fail through fatigue. The increased intensity of compulsory proof tests, as recommended by R.O. Ritchie (67), certainly has the potential of eliminating even this minute probability of fatigue-related failure. However, it would inevitably lead to a manifold increase in the price of mechanical valves. It is the opinion of this author, as well as others (74,75), that incomparably more lives would definitely be lost by a gigantic increase in waiting lists due to financial reasons both in the western world and in developing countries than allowing for one fatigue-failure in a million or more valves.

Cavitation

Cavitation is the formation of micro bubbles in a liquid environment. The life span of these cavitation bubbles is very short, measured only in milliseconds. The energy content however is extremely high, and the sudden release of this energy when the bubbles burst can cause damage to neighbouring structures, in the case of implanted heart valves to the corpuscular elements of the blood and to the valve itself (76).

Cavitation may be generated on closure of the mechanical valves, and the potential for cavitation appears to be inherent in the design (Fig. 9.5-6). In simple terms, the higher the speed of the closing occluder on impact, the higher the potential for creating cavitation bubbles. For practical purposes the critical dP/dt value coinciding with the onset of cavitation is measured (76).

Although the issue of cavitation has received considerable attention recently (77), it appears that its clinical relevance is negligible, because the necessary dP/dt values cannot be generated by the human heart and/or because of the flexible suspension of the

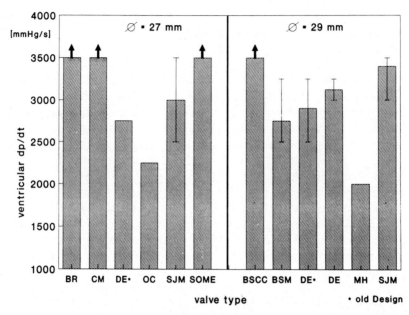

Figure 9.5-6: Comparison of cavitation thresholds of different mechanical prostheses. Reproduced with the permission of ICR Publishers from Graf T, Reul H, Dietz W, Wilmes R, Rau G. Cavitation of mechanical heart valves under physiologic conditions. J Heart Valve Dis 1992;1:131-141

prostheses within the heart (76). The original design Duromedics valve has so far been the only model where valve failure due to cavitation could be assumed in a few cases (78). Nonetheless, a statement on the cavitation threshold must be filed with any FDA application on a new replacement valve in the future, together with a statement on the fatigue resistance of the materials in the given design (51).

MECHANICAL PROSTHESES CURRENTLY IN CLINICAL USE

In the following, the individual valve models that are currently in clinical use are discussed. Due to the large number of patients still alive with the device, the Björk-Shiley range of tilting disc valves is also touched upon.

The major single shortcoming of mechanical heart valves is thrombogenicity, and it is a great loss for clinical science that past experiences cannot be evaluated on a strictly comparative basis because the true level of anticoagulation cannot be established from the vast majority of publications where INR values are not provided, and the important role of patient-related risk factors is not appreciated in past studies (see Chapter 10.3 for details in both respects). The aggregate of valve thrombosis, embolism and anticoagulant-related bleeding (ACH) provides a rough estimate of valve thrombogenicity (and the price of decreasing it), but it must be borne in mind that a prosthesis of low thrombogenicity may be over-anticoagulated by a given team, in which case the above aggregate will unfairly penalize the device. These qualifications apply to each individual model detailed in the following.

Two complications, paravalvular leak and prosthetic endocarditis, do not seem to distinguish between mechanical prosthesis types, therefore they will not be discussed in detail in this chapter. Regarding prosthetic endocarditis, the reader is referred to Chapter 6.3 in this book.

Caged-ball valves

Starr-Edwards valve

The Starr-Edwards valve is the only caged-ball valve currently in clinical use. Since its introduction in 1960, it has undergone several design modifications to eliminate ball variance, which led to structural failure in the early models, and to decrease thrombogenicity. The model 6120 mitral and 1260 aortic prostheses were released in 1966 and are still in clinical use 30 years later. The silastic ball contains barium sulphate to make it radiopaque; the cage is made of Stellite 21, which is a cobalt/chromium/molybdenum/nickel alloy. The valve has an excellent durability record; there has been only one case of a structural failure, a ball fracture, reported so far (58).

Later modifications introducing Stellite ball, cloth cover of the struts and metal tracks within the cloth cover could not provide any real improvement, and were discontinued after seven to nine years in clinical use (79).

Both the model 6120 mitral and 1260 aortic prostheses have a substantially high profile and create a turbulent flow with high shear stresses (vide supra). The result is endomyocardial fibroelastosis in the left ventricle after mitral, and intimal thickening within the aortic root, coronary ostia and proximal coronary arteries after aortic valve replacement with the Starr-Edwards prosthesis (79). In addition, a circular, fibrotic ring may develop around the aortic prosthetic orifice in the left ventricular outflow tract causing a clinically significant stenosis during late follow up.

The hydrodynamic performance of the valve is not spectacular. In in vitro assessments, mean transvalvular gradients of 11.2 mmHg and 16.1 mmHg were found with size 23A and 27A aortic prostheses respectively (80,81), with the simulated cardiac output kept at around 5.0 L/min. With 26M mitral prostheses, mean diastolic gradients of 5.2 mmHg and 16.5 mmHg were recorded with respective simulated cardiac outputs of 5.0 L/min and 9.0 L/min (82).

In vivo hemodynamics show a direct relationship between valve size and obstruction to flow. In the aortic position, peak gradients ranged in a study from 29 mmHg with 21A to 13 mmHg with 27A valves (83). In the mitral position, the diastolic gradient was found to be between 10 mmHg and 6 mmHg for size 26M and 30M valves by the same authors (83). With exercise hemodynamics, the 6.3 mmHg resting diastolic gradient increased to 11.9 mmHg across 30M valves in the mitral position (84). The left atrial pressure in the same patients varied between 15 mmHg at rest and 26 mmHg during exercise.

Clinical performance

Survival: It is reasonable to assume that the overall survival with the Starr-Edwards valves has been influenced by the fact that the majority of these devices were implanted before the 1980s, providing prominence to patient related factors causing mortality. It is important, however, to note that in the Stanford experience, which is one of the largest published long term follow up studies with the Starr-Edwards valve, 13% of the hospital mortality was caused by valve related complications, and in the late mortality spanning over 10 years the proportions of valve related events, sudden death and death due to cerebrovascular accident were 18%, 18% and 10%, respectively, and the actuarial, overall survival at 10 years was only 52% ± 3% (79). Others reported somewhat better overall survival figures, and it is almost certain that the differences are the consequence of differences in the patient populations.

Valve thrombosis: Gross thrombosis of a Starr-Edwards valve is not a frequent event either in the mitral or in the aortic position. Reported incidences are in the range of 0.4% per patient-year (pty) in the aortic and 0.6%/pty in the mitral position (79,85). When thrombosis and/or pannus ingrowth develop, the progress is usually slow, leading to gradually increasing stenosis, and the reoperation can almost invariably be performed on an elective basis. The preferred location of thrombus apposition is the distal end of the cage where the struts meet (86). This was the reason for the Braunwald-Cutter valve eliminating this distal proportion and having an open cage instead. The design, however, did not prove to be safe (vide supra).

Embolism: Considering the relatively low rate of valve thrombosis, the incidence of embolism is disproportionately high with the Starr-Edwards valve in some series. In the aortic position, the linearized rate was 2.7%/pty in the Stanford, and 3.8%-5.0%/pty before and 1.8%-3.4%/pty after 1973 in the Oregon experience (79,85). It is important to note, however, that parallel to the decrease in embolic rate after 1973 in Oregon the incidence of anticoagulant-related bleeding increased from 1.6%/pty to 3.0%/pty. It is obvious that the anticoagulation intensity was increased in 1973 leading to this move of embolism and bleeding rates in opposite directions, particularly that this was the time when the American pharmaceutical industry introduced a new thromboplastin with a much higher ISI value (see Chapter 10.3). It is interesting to note that the sum of embolism and bleeding rates (TEB index) (87) remained virtually identical before and after 1973 in the Oregon series.

In the mitral position, rather disappointing results were reported by the Stanford group. With the model 6120 valve, 35% of 179 patients suffered a first embolic event by the end of the fifth postoperative year, 45% by the end of the 10th and 51% by the end the 14th year after surgery, for a linearized rate of 5.7% ± 0.4% (79). However, if all embolic events, i.e. including repeat embolisms, were entered into the statistics (301 events in 179 patients), the linearized rate was 9.5% ± 0.5%. In the Oregon series, the linearized rate was 6.0%-6.6%/pty before and 0.8%-2.9%/pty after 1973 (85). Similar to the valves in the aortic position, the bleeding incidence increased at the same time from 1.4%/pty to 3.0%/pty. Data published by other groups on embolic incidence fall within these values (79).

Anticoagulant related hemorrhage: The incidence of anticoagulant related hemorrhage (ACH) in patients with the Starr-Edwards valve has seldom been reported, and it varies between 1.4%/pty and 3.7%/pty (vide supra) (79,85). The freedom from this complication has been reported to vary between 67% and 95% at the end of the fifth postoperative year (79,84), providing at least some evidence that a rather high intensity anticoagulation is necessary to keep the incidence of valve thrombosis and embolism within the above range. The current recommendation is an INR of 3.0-4.5, that is full intensity anticoagulation, with Starr-Edwards valves (88).

Hemolysis: Hemolysis was a major problem with the cloth-covered model of the Starr-Edwards valve (vide supra), but with the models currently in clinical use it is only of minor importance. If present, the most likely cause is paravalvular leak or endocarditis. The probability of freedom from clinically significant hemolysis was 92% at 14 years after aortic valve replacement (89).

Composite freedom from valve related mortality and morbidity: This definition, as used by the Stanford group, encompasses all events, including prosthetic endocarditis, paravalvular leak, and reoperation for any reason, some of which complications may not be strictly related to prosthetic performance. It was 25% ± 4% 14 years after mitral valve replacement with the model 6120 device and 51% ± 3% 10 years after aortic valve replacement with the model 1260 device (79).

In summary, the model 1260 aortic and model 6120 mitral Starr-Edwards valves have been in clinical use for 30 years, which makes future results fairly predictable. These valves are durable but rather thrombogenic. The high profile and turbulent flow are additional disadvantages. It cannot be denied, however, that the Starr-Edwards valve provided the firm basis on which heart valve replacement developed to its current stage, and it has by far the longest track record among all replacement valves.

Tilting disc valves

These valves have a ring, or housing, within which a geometrically perfect circular disc is retained in an asymmetrical way. The result is a larger and a smaller orifice in the open position. The retaining strut(s) intrude into the orifice causing additional turbulence, except in the Lillehei-Kaster, Omniscience and Omnicarbon valves where the disc is retained by four small guide lugs located on the ring circumference.

The Björk-Shiley range of valves

The ingenious design engineer Don Shiley approached Viking O. Björk in the late sixties, and as the result of the collaborative work between these two, the first Björk-Shiley valve was released in 1969. The free-floating and continuously rotating disc was retained by two M-shaped struts, one on the inflow and one on the outflow aspect, both welded to the flange, allowing the disc to open 50° to 60°.

In the first model, the disc was made of Delrin. For reasons mentioned above, it was replaced by a PyC disc in 1971. In 1978, the outlet strut was re-designed to allow the disc to fall away from the housing by 2.5 mm in the open position, the inlet strut was machined as an integral part of the flange from one piece of Haynes 25 alloy, and the spherical disc was changed to a convexo-concave disc, the CC model. It was made available in two versions, the 60° and 70° opening angle valves. The former was implanted world-wide, the latter only outside the USA. It is believed that approximately 82,000 60° CC valves were implanted world-wide, and approximately 4,000 70° valves outside the USA. The outlet strut was welded onto the prosthetic ring in both models.

The first reports of fracture of the outlet (minor) strut in both the 60° and 70° models appeared as early as 1982 (90), but the seriousness of the problem was not fully recognized until 1985 (91). The consequence of outlet strut fracture is disc escape with an instantaneous mortality of more 50% in the mitral and almost 100% in the aortic position.

The mode of failure has been identified as fatigue of the outlet strut due to closing forces (91).

All CC valves were withdrawn from the market by 1986. Pfizer sold all remaining Shiley products to Sorin in 1992, but the company did not relinquish its responsibilities towards patients still surviving after valve replacement with a Björk-Shiley CC valve. The major single medical issue was, and remains, the selection of patients for an elective reoperation to remove valves at elevated risk of outlet strut fracture.

A rigorous follow up has been instigated to assess the risk of strut fracture in general, and the individual risk factors affecting a given patient in particular. Two medical advisory committees were formed, one dealing with the 60° and the other with the 70° valves. The Shiley Heart Valve Research Center was established in 1990 to gather and assess data collected world-wide, to analyze in laboratory and animal experiments the exact mechanism(s) leading to fracture, and to develop diagnostic methods for the early detection of valves which may proceed to outlet strut fracture.

This elaborate work identified weld related to manufacturing, valve type (70° > 60°), larger valve size and younger age at surgery as independent risk factors. In addition, certain groups of welders were recently found to be related to an increased risk of fracture. The estimated risk for different patient groups varies between 0.10% and 2.82% per year for 60° valves and between 0.21% and 3.29% for 70° valves. Statistical and epidimiological studies are ongoing, and the estimated risk of strut fracture will be communicated by the company as the rates are revised from time to time. As of 1st June 1996, 589 cases of strut fracture have been reported to Shiley (David W. Wieting, personal communication, Shiley Inc., Irvine, California, June 1996).

The final decision as to whether to indicate an elective reoperation remains, however with the physician and his/her patient.

Another result of the above work has been the recognition of "single leg separation" (SLS), i.e. that the two legs of the outlet strut do not break at the same time, the event is almost invariably sequential (65). Acoustic, but particularly X-ray methods have been developed subsequently to diagnose single leg separation (66). The latter reached clinical significance with a sensitivity of 0.962% and specificity of 0.875%. Full clinical implementation of these new potentials is currently underway. (David W. Wieting, personal communication, Shiley Inc., Irvine, California, June 1996).

Monostrut

This prosthesis was launched in 1981 as the "Björk-Shiley Monostrut" valve, the name was changed to "Monostrut" subsequently, and is currently the "Sorin-Monostrut". The valve itself,, however, has remained identical. The welded outlet strut of previous models is replaced by a heavier single hook and the entire valve machined from one piece of metal in this device, hence the name "monostrut". The disc opens to 70°. The valve is rotatable within its sewing ring.

This valve has been in clinical use for 15 years, and it is estimated that more than 100,000 have been implanted outside the USA. Not one case of structural failure has been reported so far.

Hydrodynamic performance of the Monostrut is better than that of the spherical model with a good annulus-to-orifice ratio. The mean systolic gradient in the simulated aortic position was measured at 6.0 mmHg and the mean diastolic gradient in the simulated mitral position at 4.0 mmHg using #25 mm valves with 6.0 L/min output and 70 bpm rate (92).

In vivo hemodynamics are good; the effective orifice area was measured 1.1 cm^2 for 19 mm and 2.1 cm^2 for 25 mm valves in the aortic, and between 1.8 cm^2 and 2.5 cm^2 for 27 mm and 29 mm valves in the mitral position in a representative invasive study (93). The corresponding pressure gradients at rest varied between 12-16 mmHg in the aortic and 7-4 mmHg in the mitral position. Results published by others are in the same range. Regarding echocardiographic data the reader is referred to Chapter 10.2 in this book.

Clinical performance

Survival: Valve-related events were responsible for not more than seven cases of hospital mortality in 2,726 patients (0.26%) in the Spanish multicenter trial (94). The overall survival after Monostrut implantation is influenced mainly by patient-related factors. Medium term survival figures were reported to be between 92%-96% after aortic and between 82%-87% after mitral valve replacement; long term survival (8-12 years) was reported to be between 89%-91% following aortic and between 78%-82% following mitral valve replacement in the relevant literature (26).

Valve thrombosis: The incidence of valve thrombosis in Monostrut valves is considerably lower than it was in previous generation Björk-Shiley valves, with reported rates ranging around 0.3%/pty (95-97). A statistically valid comparison, however, cannot be made because of the lack of exact information on anticoagulation intensity, as mentioned before. The thrombus build up is usually gradual, leading to a sudden, eventual, gross apposition causing a clinical emergency (86). At reoperation, the thrombotic mass can be removed in some cases (98-100), but valve replacement is usually the preferred method.

Embolism: In the well controlled Glasgow series, the linearized incidence of embolism was 0.5%/pty after aortic and 3.0%/pty after mitral valve replacement (101), accounting for an actuarial freedom of 98% and 92% at five years, respectively. In the above mentioned Spanish multicenter study, the corresponding rates were 1.5%/pty after aortic and 2.1%/pty after mitral valve replacement, with an actuarial freedom of 89.8% and 87.9%, respectively.

Anticoagulation-related hemorrhage and hemolysis: The information regarding these complications with the Monostrut valve is scant. Hemolysis does not seem to be a major problem with this device. The anticoagulation management appears to be optimum or near optimum in the Spanish series, where the above embolic rates were accompanied by a linearized incidence of bleeding of 0.95%/pty after aortic and 1.59%/pty after mitral valve replacement (94).

In summary, early and medium-term results with the Monostrut valve are acceptable. Truly long term follow data is not available. This may be due to the checkered history of the previous range of Björk-Shiley valves, and to the change of ownership of the device. A final conclusion cannot therefore be drawn at this stage.

Medtronic Hall valve

This prosthesis was released for clinical use in 1977. The particular aim of the design was the improvement of the ratio between effective orifice area and external diameter. The movement of the flat PyC disc is guided by a sigmoid strut that passes through a central hole of the disc, which is retained by another strut and two guide lugs projecting from the ring. The maximum opening angle is 75° for aortic and 70° for mitral prostheses. The entire housing is machined from a single piece of titanium. The valve is rotatable within its sewing ring. In 1979, the so called D16 version of the original design was released, in which minor modifications were introduced to the minor strut and the guide lugs to further minimize subclinical hemolysis.

The durability of the Medtronic Hall valve is good. Structural failure has been reported in only seven cases, all of which could be traced back to an uneven PyC cover of the disc in a limited subset (317 valves) of the D16 version (Personal communication, Medtronic, Inc., 1996). This subset was immediately withdrawn from the market, and there have been no known further cases of valve failure due to structural deterioration with the Medtronic Hall valve.

Suture or chordal entrapment has been reported as a potential cause of sudden failure of the Medtronic Hall valves (42,102), as may also happen to other tilting disc valves of full orifice design (44). It has been confirmed, however, that with a meticulous surgical technique that leaves neither loose chordae nor too long suture ends behind, entrapment can safely be avoided (103).

The hydrodynamic performance is good due to the large opening angle and the unusually large smaller orifice. The latter appears to be the reason for the very small or nil flow separation distal to the two orifices (vide supra). Measured mean gradients in the simulated aortic and mitral positions with 25 mm valves vary between 5 mmHg and 3 mmHg, respectively.

Hemodynamic performance assessed by invasive means is also good, and the degree of obstruction appears to be directly related to valve size. In the aortic position, peak pressure gradients were reported to vary between 13 mmHg and 4 mmHg for 21 mm through 25 mm valves, and the end-diastolic gradient in the mitral position was measured in the range of 4 mmHg to 2 mmHg with valve sizes 27 mm through 31 mm (106,107). For small aortic roots, the company made a size 20 mm valve available. Regarding echocardiographic data see Chapter 10.2 in this book.

Clinical performance

Survival: Keenan et al. reported an overall operative mortality of 10.3%. Valve-related mortality, by position, was 5.3% for aortic valves, 6.0% for mitral valves, and 4.0% for multiple valve replacements. Actuarial five-year survival was 68% (106). Valleho et al. reported better results, the hospital mortality was 6.2% and the overall actuarial eight-year survival 77.2% (107). In the experience of Beaudet et al. the early mortality was 7.7%, and the actuarial survival at 7.5 years 74.1% for the total group and 69.0% for those undergoing AVR, 81.0% for those undergoing MVR, and 67.0% for those undergoing double valve replacement (108). In the Oslo experience including 1,104 patients and a maximum of 10 years' follow up, early mortality was 3.8% after AVR, 7.5% after MVR, and 10.0% after DVR. The probability of surviving 10 years after AVR was 72%, after MVR 56%, and after DVR 60% (109).

Valve thrombosis: Valve thrombosis is not a frequent complication with the Medtronic

Hall valve. Current assessment of Butchart's series showed only four cases of thrombosis (0.05%) in Cardiff, all in the presence of a particular trigger factor, after the insertion of more than 2,000 Medtronic Hall prostheses (see Chapter 10.3). Beaudet et al. reported zero incidence of valve thrombosis in their series including more than 300 patients with a total follow up of 1,125 pty (108). In a third-world patient population receiving 1,000 Medtronic Hall valves, Antunes et al. found 1.2%/pty thrombotic obstruction, however, with a 95% actuarial freedom from the event after five years (110). In the Oslo series, the reported incidence of valve thrombosis was 0.1%/pty, 0.1%/pty and 0.2%/pty after aortic, mitral and double valve replacement, respectively (109).

Embolism: Reported rates of embolism vary between 1.3%/pty and 3.3%/pty (106-110), and the actuarial freedom from this event at five years between 85%/pty (110) and 90% (106). In a limited series of patients after aortic valve replacement in Cardiff, embolic events did not occur unless the patient had one or more additional risk factor(s), such as atrial fibrillation, hypertension, smoking, diabetes, etc. (see Chapter 10.3).

Anticoagulant-related hemorrhage and hemolysis: The reported incidence of anti-coagulation-related bleeding varies between 0.39%/pty (107) and 0.7%/pty outside the USA (109,110), and is clearly dependent on the intensity of anticoagulation (111). This is well demonstrated by the excessive rate of 2.3%/pty major and 13%/pty total bleeding in a USA series (106). Little is known about hemolysis with the Medtronic Hall valve. Valleho et al. reported a 0.52%/pty incidence in 1990 (107). It was considered to be high in the initial trials, leading to the introduction of the D16 series (vide supra), but subsequent, long term studies do not seem to demonstrate an unacceptably high rate of hemolysis.

The Lillehei-Kaster, Omniscience and Omnicarbon valves

These three valves, manufactured by Medical, Inc. Minnesota are unique among tilting disc prostheses as they do not have any strut or other retaining structure intruding into the valvular orifice; the PyC disc in each model is retained by two horn-like struts projecting parallel to the blood flow from the outflow aspect of the ring.

The Lillehei-Kaster valve was introduced in 1967 and withdrawn from the market in 1987 when a renewed premarket application was required by the FDA for valves introduced a long time previously, including the Starr-Edwards and Lillehei-Kaster valves. By that time the company had the Omniscience, Omniscience II and Omnicarbon valves on the market, and decided against a cost- and energy consuming FDA application procedure. A considerable number of patients are still alive with this prosthesis which, at some stage, was reported to be highly thrombogenic (112,113). More recent reports, however, have provided low and comparable thromboembolism rates over a truly long term follow up (114,115).

The Omniscience valve was introduced clinically in 1978. The valve has a convexo-concave PyC disc retained asymmetrically by four angled projections of the valvular ring. The housing is machined from a single piece of titanium. The valve can be rotated within its sewing ring.

Controversial results were reported with the first, investigational version (1978-1982) of the Omniscience valve, describing a very high rate of valve thrombosis in the mitral position, 12.8%/pty in one series and 7.6%/pty in another (116,117). The statistical methods used in these two publications were found, however, to be disputable both by this author and by McGoon (118). Nonetheless, the high thromboembolic rates with Omniscience valves in the mitral position were traced to a combination of three factors, i.e. an extremely thin sewing ring allowing very small clearance between the moving disc and ventricular wall, posterior orientation which could exaggerate this small clearance, and the use of large valve sizes which became oversized once the left ventricle recovered from its preoperative dilated status.

The Omniscience II prosthesis, introduced in 1982 and continued up to now, had modifications aimed at the elimination of the above problems. The large mitral valve housings were downsized and the thickness of the sewing ring was increased to create a greater clearance between the disc path and left ventricular structures. This valve received FDA approval in 1985.

The Omnicarbon valve was introduced in 1984. This is the only all-carbon tilting disc valve, because in this model not only the disc but also the housing is made of PyC on a graphite coat. The Omniscience design is further modified in the Omnicarbon valve by the elimination of the previously existing grooves on the inside surface of the housing, intended to decrease thrombogenicity.

The hydrodynamic performance of the Omni design (119) is good due to the 80° opening angle of the disc which inclines 12° on the housing in the closed position, thus travelling only 68° between the fully open and fully closed positions. There is practically no difference between the Omniscience and Omnicarbon valves, and the overall hydrodynamic results place the Omni design in the top rank of tilting disc valves (28,120).

The hemodynamic performance is also good, but not as predictable as data derived from pulse duplicator studies, because the disc does not always reach the fully open position within the heart. In the case of atrial fibrillation it may be no more than 50° (121). Others have found a broad variation of the opening angle between 35° and 80° with a mean of 55° in the aortic and 53° in the mitral position, with a mean systolic gradient of 17.6 mmHg in the aortic and mean diastolic gradient of 6.5 mmHg in the mitral position (122). Regarding echocardiographic assessment the reader is referred to Chapter 10.2.

Clinical performance

Survival: Reported hospital mortality with the Omnicarbon valve varies between 1.6% and 3% (123,124). Valve-related early mortality has not been published in the relevant literature so far. Late survival appears to be, interestingly, better after mitral than after aortic valve replacement with this device. Thevenet and Albat reported 84.3% overall survival nine years after aortic and 88.4% after mitral valve replacement, for a linearized overall mortality incidence of 2.1%/pty and 0.9%/pty, respectively (123). In the experience of Misawa et al. (124), the six-year survival was 85% after aortic and the three-year survival 94% after mitral valve replacement. Prospective randomized comparison of the Omniscience and Omnicarbon devices has not been completed, but in a retrospective study results were marginally better, though not reaching statistical significance, with the Omnicarbon valve (125).

Valve thrombosis: The controversy regarding early reports on the high incidence of valve thrombosis with the first generation Omniscience valve (vide supra) was not confirmed by any one of the subsequent publications reporting on this device. With the Omnicarbon valve, the rate of valve thrombosis was 0.14%/pty (2/1,383pty) in the considerable French experience (123). The freedom from valve thrombosis 10 years after aortic valve replacement varied between 100% and 95% depending on patient characteristics in the experience of Abe et al. (126).

Embolism: It is almost impossible to provide data in a comparable way, because publications on the Omni devices tend to group valve thrombosis and peripheral embolism in the same category of events. This combined 'thromboembolic' incidence including both valve thrombosis and embolism varies between 0.1%/pty and 1.5%/pty after aortic, and between 1.1%/pty and 1.7%/pty after mitral valve replacement in six recent publications on the Omnicarbon valve (123).

Anticoagulant-related bleeding and hemolysis: The incidence of anticoagulant-related bleeding in the above mentioned six publications varies between 0%/pty and 1.2%/pty, demonstrating a very moderate intensity anticoagulation conducted by these groups, resulting in an aggregate of thrombosis, embolism and bleeding of between 2.6%/pty and 0.63%/pty (123). Clinically significant hemolysis has not been reported with the Omnicarbon prosthesis so far.

In conclusion, it appears that the Omniscience valve received a severe early criticism which did not stand up to later scrutiny, and the valve still carries FDA approval. The available clinical information on the Omnicarbon valve is not numerous, but it demonstrates very good overall performance. It is worth mentioning that this valve was originally included in the AREVA trial in France (vide infra) for a prospective randomized assessment of the adequacy of low intensity anticoagulation, and was dropped later only for non-medical, administrative reasons.

Other tilting disc valves

The Sorin tilting disc valve was released for clinical use in 1977. The PyC disc is plano-convex, and it contains a radiopaque tantalum ring. The annular ring and M-shaped struts are machined from a single piece of titanium; structural failure has never been reported with a Sorin tilting disc valve. The maximum opening angle of the disc is 62°. In the current version, *Allcarbon^R*, the valve housing is coated by a very thin, not more than two micron, carbon coating.

Available published information on the Sorin tilting disc and Allcarbon valves is remarkably scant. A Medline search in June 1996 returned not more than four publications on the clinical performance of the Sorin tilting disc prosthesis (with some duplicate publications in the Italian medical literature) (127-130). An additional publication from Italy could also be identified outside the scope of Index Medicus and Medline (131).

According to these data, the operative mortality varies between 2.5% and 11%, and late survival between 70% to 50%, depending on position, at nine years, and 94% at 6.5 years. The number of valve-related deaths is considerable; in Cotrufo's series (129) seven out of nine late deaths were due to valve-related causes. Although the embolic incidence is low, valve thrombosis, particularly in the mitral position is considerable (130).

The Ultracor valve (Aortech Ltd., UK) was released in 1986 for clinical use, and since then it has been sold outside the USA. Published information on this prosthesis does not exist.

Bileaflet valves

It is beyond doubt that, following the sweeping success of the St. Jude Medical valve, bileaflet prostheses have become the most popular heart valve replacement devices during the past 10-15 years. The total number implanted at the time of this chapter going to press is approaching one million. According to data provided by the respective manufacturers, St. Jude Medical has records of 650,000, CarboMedics 170,000, Baxter with the first generation Duromedics valve 20,000, with the second generation Duromedics/Tekna valve 14,000 (August 1995) and Sorin with the Bicarbon valve 17,000 implants. The total is 871,000 bileaflet valves inserted so far with St. Jude Medical taking 74.6% of this total. The bulk of the remaining proportion belongs to CarboMedics with 19.5% of all bileaflet valves implanted up to now. The trend towards using bileaflet valves appears to be continuing, and the market share of these devices is by far the largest as compared to any other type of replacement valve.

St. Jude Medical prosthesis

The St. Jude Medical .bileaflet mechanical prosthesis (SJM) was introduced in 1977, and is currently considered the gold standard which all other mechanical valves are compared to. The valve received FDA approval 1983. The only change to the design of the original, currently called the "standard", SJM valve was made in 1989 when a metal ring was incorporated into the sewing ring for better X-ray visibility. The entire valve is made of PyC deposited on a graphite core. The discs are flat; the maximum opening angle is 85° and the travelling arc between fully open and closed positions is 55-60°. Unique for the SJM valve among all bileaflet valves is the presence of two pivot guards protecting these two delicate areas from interference by adjacent cardiac structures and/or tissue ingrowth. The standard SJM is not rotatable.

In 1991 the sewing ring of the standard model was re-designed, and the HP (Hemodynamic Plus) series released with the new sewing ring. The result has been an about one full size difference in implantability, i.e. the HP model provides a one size larger orifice area than its identically sized standard counterpart (vide infra).

The issue of rotatability was addressed by St. Jude when the company felt confident that the relevant engineering technology had reached the stage that a rotatable design could be introduced without compromising the effective orifice area. The new series, released for clinical use in 1995, is called the "Masters series", its hydrodynamic performance is claimed to be identical to that of the HP series in the aortic and to the standard series in the mitral models. Due to the very low profile, each of the three series (standard, HP, Masters) lends itself with ease to implantation in the mitral position with chordal preservation (vide infra).

The structural integrity of the SJM valve was assessed by us using all existing data from the medical literature and additional information provided by the manufacturer in 1991 (27). On that date there were 10 leaflet escapes due to fracture, of which only four could not be traced back to potential damage during implantation. There were four additional leaflet escapes without fracture, and one case of an intermittently immobilized leaflet was also known. Updated information from the manufacturer's records is not available currently; in the medical literature there has not been any report of structural failure in an SJM valve since 1991 (Medline).

The hydrodynamic characteristics are superior to previous mechanical valve models with an average performance index of 0.66 for standard series valve sizes 21 mm through 27 mm (132). The performance of the HP valves in a flow chamber is practically identical to that of one size larger SJM standard valves with identical cardiac output (133). The weak point of the SJM hydrodynamics is the relatively large closing reflux and leakage across the closed valve (132).

In the hemodynamic evaluation, a clear distinction must be made between invasive results obtained during cardiac catheterization, and non-invasive results derived from echocardiographic measurements, because the latter can lead to overestimation of pressure gradients. This is due to pressure recovery (134), and the reader is referred to Chapter 10.2 for a detailed discussion of the subject. The average resting mean systolic gradient across 23 mm standard SJM prostheses in the aortic position was measured at 9.6 mmHg, and the average mean diastolic gradient across 29 mm standard SJM prostheses in the mitral position at 2.3 mmHg using invasive methods (27). In a recent Doppler echocardiographic study, the hemodynamic performance of the HP 21 mm valve was found to be practically identical to that of the 23 mm standard valve in the small aortic root (135).

Clinical performance

Survival: Reported operative mortality varies around 2% for aortic and between 1.3% and 4.3% for mitral valve replacement (37,136). Valve-related causes do not seem to contribute to early mortality with SJM valves. Late survival seven years after surgery was 90.8% for aortic and 82.1% for mitral implants in Zurich (136), the 10-year survival was 85% after aortic and 78% after mitral valve replacement in Düsseldorf (37). In the former study, the linearized rate of late death was 2.6%/pty after aortic and 2.2%/pty after mitral valve replacement. Within this rate, the incidence of valve-related death (embolism, endocarditis and anticoagulant related bleeding) was 0.7%/pty and 0.3%/pty, respectively (136).

Valve thrombosis: In 1991, based on 26 publications reporting 51,886 patient-years follow up information, we calculated an average rate of valve thrombosis with the SJM valve of 0.28%/pty in the aortic and 0.21%/pty in the mitral position (27). Depending on individual series, the reported range varies from 0%/pty to 0.9%/pty. This is in stark contrast to those pessimistic forecasts that were made by antagonists of the hinged valve design when the SJM prosthesis was first introduced.

Embolism: The reported rate of embolism in large clinical series varies between 0.6%/pty and 2.1%/pty after aortic (137,138) and between 0.4%/pty and 3.9%/pty after mitral valve replacement (137,139). This apparently wide range of incidence is most probably due to the fact that, as in the case of other devices, a statistically valid assessment of embolic incidence stratified according to patient-related risk factors (vide supra) is not available with the SJM valve either, and that the anticoagulation management in the majority of patients has not been based on INR values.

Anticoagulant-related bleeding and anticoagulation management: The incidence of anticoagulant-related bleeding varies between 0%/pty (139) and 6.74%/pty (37), obviously depending on the intensity of oral anticoagulation.

The necessary level of anticoagulation with the SJM valve has long been a debated issue. Early enthusiasm about the low thrombogenicity of the device led some to try not to anticoagulate patients after isolated aortic valve replacement with this valve. Antiplatelet treatment alone, however, did not provide satisfactory results (140).

An alternative solution was proposed by Nair et al. in 1990 when, based on their 10-year experiences, they recommended a moderate level of anticoagulation with the SJM valve, decreasing the INR to between 1.5-2.5 (141). This was, however, only an arbitrary decision. Decisive action was taken one year later by Jean Acar and his co-workers in France by starting a multicenter, prospective, randomized trial, called the AREVA study, comparing low-dose and standard-dose anticoagulation. The outcome of the trial was reported earlier this year. The results are conclusive showing that in patients after isolated aortic valve replacement and without any additional embolic risk factor the SJM valve can safely be managed with low-dose anticoagulation (INR 1.5 - 2.5) leading to a statistically significant decrease in the incidence of bleeding without an increase in the rate of embolism (142,143).

As mentioned before, another prospective, randomized, multicenter trial, the GELIA study was started in Germany in 1993 (38). This trial was prompted by the Düsseldorf experience with the SJM valve. Over the years anticoagulation had been managed according to the Quick time in Germany using a number of different reagents; INR has only recently been adopted. Horstkotte et al. (37) calculated, in a retrospective way, the INR values for their patients from the documented prothrombin times and reagents used. The result was surprising: patients with fairly uniform prothrombin times were separated into three different groups with high, medium and low INR levels due to the different reagents. The best clinical result, i.e. the lowest embolism/bleeding aggregate, was achieved in the low INR group. A large scale, multicenter, prospective randomized trial with three different INR levels after SJM valve implantation was therefore started in Germany.

Hemolysis: Sporadic cases of clinically significant hemolysis have been reported in the absence of valve malfunction or paravalvular leak with the SJM valve in the mitral position; asynchronous leaflet closure has been implied to be a potential causative factor (27). Usually, however, hemolysis is not a clinically important complication of bileaflet prostheses.

In conclusion, the SJM valve opened a new era in heart valve replacement by making full use of PyC in an entirely new design. The impact has been such that all subsequent new valve models since the introduction of the SJM valve follow the bileaflet principle. The valve has excellent hemodynamics and an apparently low thrombogenicity. Recent (AREVA) and still ongoing (GELIA) trials appear to question the justification of full anticoagulation (INR 3.5 - 4.5) with this device. The HP modification improved the hydro- and hemodynamic performance of the standard model. Clinical experience is not yet available to assess the Masters series.

Edwards Tekna (Duromedics) valve

The valve, originally named "Hemex valve", was clinically introduced in 1982, and received FDA approval in 1986. During the first phase of marketing, the assembly was carried out in Scotland by Thackeray Ltd., and the valves were released as Duromedics valves. In 1986 it was bought by Baxter-Edwards, and the name was changed to

Edwards-Duromedics, but the valve itself remained the same under all three names. Due to unexpected leaflet escapes marketing was suspended world-wide in 1986, and a revised version released in 1988 under the same Edwards-Duromedics name. In 1993 the name of the valve was changed to Tekna Edwards to reflect changes in sizers and rotators; the prosthesis remained the same second version of the Duromedics valve.

The housing is made of solid PyC, the leaflets are curved and made of PyC deposited on a graphite core. The opening angle is 73°-77°, the travel arc 71°-75°. The valve is rotatable. In the revised version important design tolerance adjustments were made, both the mitral and the aortic sewing rings were modified to add additional padding, and new quality control inspections were introduced to assess microporosity by dye penetrant inspection, and to confirm seating lip contact and pivot ball position.

There were 12 leaflet escapes reported when Baxter-Edwards decided to suspend marketing of the prosthesis in 1986. By August 1994, the number of known leaflet escapes was 39, by December 1995 it was 46 (manufacturer's data). This latest figure is 0.23% of the estimated 20,000 valves implanted. Using Grunkemeier's method of patient life time simulation (144), the linearized incidence is 0.029%/pty.

In sharp contrast to strut fracture and cusp escape from the Björk-Shiley valves, the mortality of leaflet escape from the Duromedics valve is very low, because the patient can survive with the remaining leaflet still in position and functional. Elective removal of this prosthesis, therefore, has never been proposed. It is interesting, however, to note that similar to the Björk-Shiley valves, male gender and younger age carry a higher probability of valve failure.

The track record of the re-designed model (currently Tekna valve) is much better, of the first 13,700 valves implanted only two leaflet escapes and one leaflet disruption (suspected mechanical injury) had been reported by August 1995 (manufacturer's data).

Despite its 14 years in clinical use, published information is rather scant on the Duromedics valve. (A current Medline search returned only 27 publications under the name "Duromedics", and none for "Tekna". Of the 27 publications, two are letters to the Editor, two are in Italian, one in Japanese, one in German, and eight by the same center in Vienna.)

In terms of hydrodynamics, the curved leaflet design does not seem to have achieved any improvement in performance (145,146). Clinical results with the Duromedics valve are acceptable despite the occasional leaflet escape. In the last update of the experience in Vienna an operative mortality of 6.9% was reported, and 81% late survival after six years. The rate of embolism was 1.1%/pty with a bleeding incidence of 1.9%/pty. The rate of valve-related mortality was 1.5%/pty, and that of all valve related mortality and morbidity 5.3%/pty (147). Other centers in France, Canada and Spain reported similar results (148,149).

A particular feature of the Duromedics valve is its relatively high noise level, apparently the highest among all replacement devices (150).

In conclusion, the Duromedics/Tekna valve was the first rotatable bileaflet prosthesis. It introduced a solid PyC housing, but it failed to improve durability. The history of this device is chequered by occasional leaflet escapes, and fracture of the housing is not unknown. The curved leaflets with a relatively small opening angle and large travelling arc could not surpass the original bileaflet design (SJM) in terms of hydrodynamic performance. The company has not responded so far to the challenge of the SJM and

CarboMedics (vide infra) recently introduced high performance models. It all adds up to a less than superior popularity; not more than 13,700 valves were implanted between June 1990 and August 1995 (manufacturer's data).

The CarboMedics valve

The CarboMedics valve (CMI) was released for clinical use in 1986, and received FDA approval in 1994. The flat leaflets are made of PyC deposited on a graphite core, the housing is solid PyC reinforced by a titanium ring. The valve is rotatable. The leaflets contain 20% tungsten to improve X-ray imaging. The leaflets open to a maximum of 78°, the travel arc is 53°.

The design of the carbon parts has remained unchanged over the years. The sewing ring however, similar to the SJM HP valve, has undergone changes when the R model (reduced outside diameter) and the Top Hat model (for supra-annular insertion) were introduced. The most recent version is called the "Orbis" valve, and has an identical sewing ring design for both aortic and mitral models. The prosthetic valve within these different sewing rings, however, has not been changed.

The structural integrity of the CMI valve is impeccable; no postoperative structural failure has been reported in the medical literature or to the manufacturer so far (manufacturer's data).

The hydrodynamic performance of the standard CMI valve was compared to that of the standard SJM valve by CarboMedics, Inc. using size 29 mm valves (151). Pressure drop, effective orifice area and regurgitation were all marginally better with the SJM valve, but the company concluded that this was a price well worth paying for the increased safety margin inherent in the design changes. Similar results were reported by others, but the 19 mm valve was found to have a relatively high resistance to flow (145,152).

Hemodynamic data on the CMI valve comes mainly from echocardiographic studies, and they appear to confirm the hydrodynamic results. For details the reader is referred to Chapter 10.2. It was shown in a recent study that the Top Hat design increased the implantability in the small aortic root by one size (153).

Clinical performance

Survival: Reported early mortality varies between 4.9% and 12%, depending on patient-related factors (154-158). Late mortality was 2.7%/pty in Napoli (154), overall survival in the international experience (156) 81% after five years, 83.7% in the experience of Fiane et al. (158), and 68.2% after 4.5 years in a young, seriously ill population in Saudi Arabia (157). Freedom from valve-related mortality was 91.5% in the experience of de Luca et al. (154).

Valve thrombosis: Valve thrombosis does not seem to affect CMI prostheses in the aortic position. In the mitral position, it was 0.64%/pty in the international experience (156), and the combined mitral/aortic incidence, which varies around 0.27%-0.3%/pty in the above publications was 0.27% in that series.

Embolism: The reported rate of embolism occurring after the first 30 postoperative days varies between 0%/pty and 1.1%/pty in the aortic and 2.3%/pty in the mitral position (154-158). It should be noted that the two largest clinical experiences with the

CMI valve are multicenter trials in the USA, Canada, and European countries with widely different patient populations and anticoagulation regimes.

Anticoagulation-related bleeding: The five-year actuarial freedom from anticoagulant related bleeding was 92.4% after aortic and 95.2% after mitral valve replacement in the international experience (156), with results published by others falling around this range. Exact data on the intensity of anticoagulation is available from the international experience where the actually achieved (not the target) INR was 3.2 (156).

Hemolysis: Hemolysis is not a clinically important problem with the CMI valve, with a maximum incidence of 0.5%/pty (158) and 99.6% freedom from the event after five years (156).

In conclusion, the main aim of the CMI design was to eliminate structural failure, and this goal has been fully achieved so far. There has not been, however, any improvement in hydro- and hemodynamics accomplished at the same time. The incidence of valve thrombosis in the mitral position appears to be higher than that with the SJM valve, but it has been suggested that the early, high hazard of this event penalizes the relatively short follow up experience (155).

The Sorin Bicarbon valve

This bileaflet prosthesis was introduced in 1990, and 17,000 clinical implants have been completed since (60). Regretfully, although the hydrodynamic performance of the valve is excellent (145), no data has been published on clinical performance whatsoever. If one, hypothetically, would assign a 2.5 year mean follow up duration to the 17,000 implants, it would amount to 42,500 unknown patient-years of information.

The valve has a titanium-aluminium-vanadium alloy housing. The curved leaflets are made of PyC deposited on a graphite core. The metal housing has a two micron turbostratic carbon cover using Sorin's Carbofilm^R technology, which is the deposition of PyC particles at room temperature.

As mentioned above, it has become publicly known only recently that this thin carbon coating wears off, mainly in the hinge area, within weeks in a real time wear test machine or under clinical conditions (60). The result is a metal/carbon wear couple which is unprecedented in clinically used bileaflet valves, and the consequences of which are unknown at present. According to the manufacturer (60), no case of obstructive valve thrombosis or structural failure has occurred so far.

Publication of clinical results with the Sorin Bicarbon valve appears to be imperative after more than 17,000 implants over a 5.5-year period.

Other bileaflet valves

The ATS valve is assembled in Glasgow, and marketed outside the USA. No published information is available on this device.

GENERAL COMMENTS

All mechanical prosthetic valves have three important features in common; (i) their design and material do not resemble those of the natural valves in any way, (ii) they reduce physiologic valve function, particularly in the mitral position, to an entirely passive uni-directional opening and closing sequel without providing a single central orifice, and (iii) they are thrombogenic and therefore require life-long anticoagulation. There appear to be important developments regarding the latter two statements.

Preservation of the chordal apparatus, whether only the posterior or both, has become an increasingly accepted procedure in mitral valve replacement, with profound effects in the case of mitral regurgitation with an enlarged left ventricle. C. Walton Lillehei's original vision (159) has apparently came to fruition after more than three decades. There is no doubt that in another 10 years reports on long term results after mitral valve replacement will depict a different scenario with the chordo-papillary apparatus intact.

The other important current trend is the world-wide acceptance of the INR, and the drive towards low level anticoagulation. If this goal can be achieved, life expectancy after heart valve replacement with a mechanical valve will be further enhanced, and quality of life improved.

The immediate future goals are therefore within sight.

References

1. Hufnagel CA. Aortic plastic valvular prosthesis. Bull Georgetown University Med Cent 1951;4:128
2. Lefrak E, Starr A. Historic aspects of cardiac valve replacement. In: Cardiac valve prostheses. New York, N.Y., Appleton-Century-Crofts, 1979:3-37
3. Harken D, Soroff HS, Taylor WJ. Partial and complete prosthesis in aortic insufficiency. J Thorac Cardiovasc Surg 1960;40:744
4. Starr A, Edwards M. Mitral replacement: clinical experience with a ball valve prosthesis. Ann Surg 1961;154:726-740
5. Roe B. "Extinct" cardiac valve prostheses. In: Bodnar E, Frater RWM (eds). Replacement cardiac valves. New York, N.Y., Pergamon Press, Inc., 1991:307- 332
6. Wada J, Komatsu, S, Ikeda, K. A new hingeless valve. In: Brewer LA III (ed). Prosthetic heart valves. Springfield, Thomas, 1969:304-314
7. Lillehei CW, Kaster RL, Coleman M, Bloch JH. Heart-valve replacement with Lillehei-Kaster pivoting disk prosthesis. New York State J Med 1974;74:1426-1438
8. Björk VO. A new tilting disc valve prosthesis. Scand J Thorac Cardiovasc Surg 1969;3:1-10
9. Björk VO. The pyrolytic carbon occluder for the Björk-Shiley tilting disc valve prosthesis. Scand J Thorac Cardiovasc Surg 1972;6:109-113
10. Björk VO. The improved Björk-Shiley tilting disc valve prosthesis. Scand J Thorac Cardiovasc Surg 1978;12:81-84
11. Björk VO. Optimal orientation of the 60 degrees and the 70 degrees Björk-Shiley tilting disc valves. Scand J Thorac Cardiovasc Surg 1982;16:113-118
12. Björk VO, Lindblom D. The Monostrut Björk-Shiley heart valve. J Am Coll Cardiol 1985;6:1142-1148
13. Hall KV, Kaster RL, Woien A. An improved pivotal disc-type prosthetic heart valve. J Oslo City Hosp 1979;29:3-21
14. Emery RW, Palmquist WE, Mettler E, Nicoloff DM. A new cardiac valve prosthesis: in vitro results. Trans Am Soc Artif Int Org 1978;24:550-556
15. Bokros JC, Gott VL, La Grange LD, Fadall AM, Vos KD, Ramos MD. Correlations between blood compatibility and heparin adsorptivity for an impermeable isotropic pyrolytic carbon. J Biomed Mater Res 1969;3:497-528
16. Paton BC, Pine MB. Aortic valve replacement with the De Bakey valve. J Thorac Cardiovasc Surg 1976;72:652-656
17. Zumbro GL Jr, Cundey PE Jr, Fishback ME, Galloway RF. Strut fracture in De Bakey valve. Successful reoperation and valve replacement. J Thorac Cardiovasc Surg 1977;74:469-470
18. Blackstone EH, Kirklin JW, Pluth JR, Turner ME, Parr GV. The performance of the Braunwald-Cutter aortic prosthetic valve. Ann Thorac Surg 1977;23:302-318
19. Bodnar E, Reul H, Schmitz B. Prosthetic valve function under simulated low cardiac output conditions: preliminary observations. J Heart Valve Dis 1993;2:348- 351
20. Yoganathan AP, Wick TM, Reul H. The influence of flow characteristics of prosthetic valves on thrombus formation. In: Butchart E, Bodnar E (eds). Thrombosis, embolism and bleeding. London, ICR Publishers, 1992:123-148

21. Williams J. United States Patent No 19323. ; February 9, 1858
22. Itzkoff JM, Curtiss EI, Reddy PS, Uretsky BF, Shaver JA. Intermittent mitral regurgitation due to Beall valve dysfunction: analysis of 13 patients with atrial fibrillation. Am J Cardiol 1984;53:1071-1074
23. Bodur G, Friart A. Intermittent regurgitation flow with Björk-Shiley mitral prosthesis in atrial fibrillation. Am Heart J 1993;126:1006-1007
24. Sabbah HN, Stein PD. Relation of maximal opening of disk valves to characteristics of aortic blood flow. J Biomech Eng 1980;102:147-150
25. Brown C III, Lemuth R, Hellums J, Leverett L, Alfrey C. Response of human platelets to shear stress. Trans ASAIO 1977;21:35-39
26. Bain W, Nashef S. Tilting disc valves: historical perspective. In: Bodnar E, Frater RWM (eds). Replacement cardiac valves. New York, N.Y., Pergamon Press, Inc., 1991:187-200
27. Horstkotte D, Bodnar E. Bileaflet valves. In: Bodnar E, Frater RWM (eds). Replacement cardiac valves. New York, N.Y., Pergamon Press, Inc., 1991:201- 228
28. Scotten L, Racca R, Nugent A, et al. New tilting disc cardiac valve prostheses. J Thorac Cardiovasc Surg 1981;82:136
29. Bruss K, Reul H, Van Gilse J, et al. Pressure drops and velocity field at four mechanical heart valve prostheses. Life Support Syst 1983;1:3
30. Fontaine A, He S, Stadter R, Ellis J, Levine R, Yoganathan A. In vitro assessment of prosthetic valve function in mitral valve replacement with chordal preservation techniques. J Heart Valve Dis 1996;5:186-198
31. Nicoloff D, Arom K, Lindsay W, et al. Techniques for implantation of the St. Jude valve in the aortic and mitral positions. In: DeBakey M (ed). Advances in cardiac valves: clinical perspectives. New York, N.Y., Yorke, 1983:191-196
32. Baudet EM, Oca CC, Roques XF, et al. A 5 1/2 year experience with the St. Jude Medical cardiac valve prosthesis. Early and late results of 737 valve replacements in 671 patients. J Thoracic Cardiovasc Surg 1985;90:137-144
33. Clark RE, Edmunds LH Jr, Cohn LH, Miller DC, Weisel RD. Guidelines for reporting morbidity and mortality after cardiac valvular operations. Eur J Cardio-thorac Surg 1988;2:293-295
34. Edmunds LH Jr, Cohn LH, Weisel RD. Guidelines for reporting morbidity and mortality after cardiac valvular operations. J Thorac Cardiovasc Surg 1988;96:351- 353
35. Edmunds L Jr, Clark R, Cohn L, et al. Guidelines for reporting morbidity and mortality after cardiac valvular operations. Ann Thorac Surg 1988;46:293-295
36. Silver MD, Butany J. Mechanical heart valves: methods of examination, complications, and modes of failure. Human Pathol 1987;18:577-585
37. Horstkotte D, Schulte H, Bircks W, Strauer B. Unexpected findings concerning thromboembolic complications and anticoagulation after complete 10 year follow up of patients with St. Jude Medical prostheses. J Heart Valve Dis 1993;2:291- 301
38. Horstkotte D, Bergemann R, Althaus U, et al. German experience with low intensity anticoagulation (GELIA): protocol of a multi-center randomized, prospective study with the St. Jude Medical valve. J Heart Valve Dis 1993;2:411-419
39. Jarvinen A, Virtanen K, Peltola K, Maamies T, Ketonen P, Mannikko A. Postoperative disc entrapment following cardiac valve replacement - a report of ten cases. Thorac Cardiovasc Surg 1984;32:152-156
40. Roberts WC, Hammer WJ. Cardiac pathology after valve replacement with a tilting disc prosthesis (Björk-Shiley type). A study of 46 necropsy patients and 49 Björk-Shiley prostheses. Am J Cardiol 1976;37:1024-1033
41. Jackson GM, Wolf PL, Bloor CM. Malfunction of mitral Björk-Shiley prosthetic valve due to septal interference. Am Heart J 1982;104:158-159
42. Pai GP, Ellison RG, Rubin JW, Moore HV, Kamath MV. Disc immobilization of Björk-Shiley and Medtronic Hall valves during and immediately after valve replacement. Ann Thorac Surg 1987;44:73-76
43. Browdie DA, Agnew RF, Hamilton CS Jr. Poppet jamming during mitral valve replacement (letter). Ann Thorac Surg 1978;26:591
44. Bokros J, Haubold A, Akins R, et al. The durability of mechanical heart valve replacements: past experience and current trends. In: Bodnar E, Frater RWM (eds). Replacement cardiac valves. New York, N.Y., Pergamon Press, Inc., 1991:21-48
45. Ziemer G, Luhmer I, Oelert H, Borst HG. Malfunction of a St. Jude medical heart valve in mitral position. Ann Thorac Surg 1982;33:391-395
46. Antunes MJ, Colsen PR, Kinsley RH. Intermittent aortic regurgitation following aortic valve replacement with the Hall-Kaster prosthesis. J Thorac Cardiovasc Surg 1982;84:751-754
47. Aldrete V. Intermittent aortic regurgitation with tilting disc valves (letter). J Thorac Cardiovasc Surg 1984;88:458-459
48. Björk VO, Henze A, Holmgren A. Five years' experience with the Björk-Shiley tilting-disc valve in isolated

aortic valvular disease. J Thorac Cardiovasc Surg 1974;68:393-404

49. DeWall R. Discussion of Björk VO, Henze A. Ten years' experience with the Björk-Shiley tilting disk valve. J Thorac Cardiovasc Surg 1979;78:341

50. Larmi TK, Karkola P. Shrinkage and degradation of the Delrin occluder in the tilting-disc valve prosthesis. J Thorac Cardiovasc Surg 1974;68:66-69

51. Division of Cardiovascular Respiratory and Neurological Devices, Draft Replacement Heart Valve Guidance. October 14, 1994

52. King MJ, Olin CL, Fisher J. An initial investigation into the wear and damage within the pivots of three types of bileaflet mechanical heart valves. J Heart Valve Dis 1996;5(suppl 1):S112-S115

53. International Organization for Standardization. Cardiovascular implants- cardiac valve prostheses (Revision of second edition (ISO 5840: 1989)). 1995

54. CE marking Directive (93/86/EEC). 1993

55. Reul H, Eichler M, Potthast K, Schimitz C, Rau G. In vitro testing of the heart valve wear outside of the manufacturers laboratory-requirements and controversies. J Heart Valve Dis 1996;5(suppl 1):S97-S104

56. Campbell A, Baldwin T, Peterson G, Bryant J, Ryder K. Pitfalls and outcomes form accelerated wear testing of mechanical heart valves. J Heart Valve Dis 1996;5(suppl 1):S125-S133

57. Bodnar E, Arru P, Butchart EG, et al. Wear in mechanical heart valves: panel discussion. J Heart Valve Dis 1996;5(suppl 1):S150-S156

58. Mazzucco A, Luciani GB, Pessotto R, Piccin C, Faggian G, Chiominto B. Ball fracture with the 6120-model Starr-Edwards mitral valve prosthesis occurring late after implantation. J Heart Valve Dis 1993;2:245-247

59. Haubold AD. On the durability of pyrolytic carbon in vivo. Med Prog Tech 1994;20:201-208

60. Arru P, Rinaldi S, Stacchino C, Vallana F. Wear assessment in bileaflet heart valves. J Heart Valve Dis 1996;5(suppl 1):S134-S144

61. Arru P, Rinaldi S, Stacchino C, et al. Relationship between some design characteristics and wear in the Bicarbon heart valve prosthesis. Int J Artif Org 1994;17:280-293

62. van Swieten HA. Discussion of the previous four articles. J Heart Valve Dis 1996;5(suppl 1):S145-S149

63. Shim HS, Schoen FJ. The wear resistance of pure and silicon-alloyed isotropic carbons. Biomater Med Dev Artif Org 1974;2:103-118

64. Lillehei CW. Heart valve replacement with the pivoting disc prosthesis: appraisal of results and description of a new all-carbon model. Med Instrum 1977;11:85- 94

65. de Mol BA, Kallewaard M, McLellan RB, van Herwerden LA, Defauw JJ, van der Graaf Y. Single-leg strut fractures in explanted Björk-Shiley valves. Lancet 1994;343:9-12

66. O'Neill WW, Chandler JG, Gordon RE, et al. Radiographic detection of single leg separations of the outlet strut of mitral Björk-Shiley Convexo-Concave heart valves. New Engl J Med 1995

67. Ritchie RO. Fatigue and fracture of pyrolytic carbon: a damaged-tolerant approach to structural integrity and life prediction in "ceramic" heart valve prostheses. J Heart Valve Dis 1996;5(suppl 1):S9-S31

68. Cao H. Mechanical performance of pyrolytic carbon in prosthetic heart valve applications. J Heart Valve Dis 1996;5(suppl 1):S32-S49

69. Kepner J, Cao H. Effect of repetitive impact on the mechanical strength of pyrolytic carbon. J Heart Valve Dis 1996;5(suppl 1):S50-S58

70. Ma L, Sines G. Fatigue of isotropic pyrolytic carbon used in mechanical heart valves. J Heart Valve Dis 1996;5(suppl 1):S59-S64

71. Ely JL, Stupka J, Haubold AD. Pyrolytic carbon indentation crack morphology. J Heart Valve Dis 1996;5(suppl 1):S65-S71

72. Gilpin CB, Haubold AD, Ely JL. Finite element analysis of indenation tests on pyrolytic carbon. J Heart Valve Dis 1996;5(suppl 1):S72-S78

73. Richard G, Cao H. Structural failure of pyrolytic carbon heart valves. J Heart Valve Dis 1996;5(suppl 1):S79-S85

74. Taylor KM. A cardiac surgeon's perspective. J Heart Valve Dis 1996;5(suppl 1):S7-S8

75. Yoganathan AP. An enginner's perspective. J Heart Valve Dis 1996;5(suppl 1):S3-S6

76. Graf T, Reul H, Dietz W, Wilmes R, Rau G. Cavitation of mechanical heart valves under physiologic conditions. J Heart Valve Dis 1992;1:131-141

77. Cavitation in mechanical heart valves. Proceedings of the 1st international symposium. Miami, 4-5 December 1994. J Heart Valve Dis 1994;3(suppl):S1-S132

78. Kingsbury C, Kafesjian R, Guo G, et al. Cavitation threshold with respect to dP/dt: evaluation in 29 mm bileaflet, pyrolitic carbon heart valves. Int J Artif Org 1993;16:515-520

79. Fann J, Moreno-Cabral C, Miller D. Caged-ball valves: the Starr-Edwards and Smeloff-Sutter prostheses. In: Bodnar E, Frater RWM (eds). Replacement cardiac valves. Elmsford, NY, Pergamon Press, Inc., 1991:149-186

80. Yoganathan AP, Harrison EC, Corcoran WH. Prosthetic heart valves. Proceedings of a symposium of the 14th Annual Meeting of the Association for the Advancement of Medical Instrumentation. Pasadena, Cal

Tech Press, 1980:181
81. Yoganathan A. Cardiovascular fluid mechanics: I. Fluid dynamics of prosthetic aortic valves. II. Use of the fast Fourier transform on the analysis of cardiovascular sounds. California Institute of Technology, 1978
82. Gabbay S, McQueen DM, Yellin EL, Becker RM, Frater RW. In vitro hydrodynamic comparison of mitral valve prostheses at high flow rates. J Thorac Cardiovasc Surg 1978;76:771-787
83. Pyle RB, Mayer JE Jr, Lindsay WG, Jorgensen CR, Wang Y, Nicoloff DM. Hemodynamic evaluation of Lillehei-Kaiser and Starr-Edwards prosthesis. Ann Thorac Surg 1978;26:336-343
84. Horstkotte D, Haerten K, Seipel L, et al. Central hemodynamics at rest and during exercise after mitral valve replacement with different prostheses. Circulation 1983;68:II-161-II-168
85. Macmanus Q, Grunkemeier GL, Lambert LE, Teply JF, Harlan BJ, Starr A. Year of operation as a risk factor in the late results of valve replacement. J Thorac Cardiovasc Surg 1980;80:834-841
86. Schoen F. Modes of failure and other pathology of mechanical and tissue heart valve prostheses. In: Bodnar E, Frater RWM (eds). Replacement cardiac valves. New York, NY, Pergamon Press, Inc., 1991:99-124
87. Bodnar E. A critical assessment of thrombosis and embolism reporting methods. In: Butchart E, Bodnar E (eds). Thrombosis, embolism and bleeding. London, ICR Publishers, 1992:476-484
88. Gohlke-Barwolf C, Acar J, Burckhardt D, et al. Guidelines for prevention of thromboembolic events in valvular heart disease. Ad Hoc Committee of the Working Group on Valvular Heart Disease, European Society of Cardiology. J Heart Valve Dis 1993;2:398-410
89. Wain WH, Drury PJ, Ross DN. Aortic valve replacement with Starr- Edwards valves over 14 years. Ann Thorac Surg 1982;33:562-569
90. Björk VO. Metallurgic and design development in response to mechanical dysfunction of Björk-Shiley heart valves. Scand J Thorac Cardiovasc Surg 1985;19:1-12
91. van Swieten HA. Metallurgical analysis of the Björk-Shiley convexo- concave valve prosthesis to assess the cause of late outlet strut fracture. In: Bodnar E (ed). Surgery for heart valve disease. 1st Ed. London: ICR Publishers, 1990:616-627
92. UK Department of Health. Medical Devices Evaluation Report; Evaluation of Mechanical Valve Prostheses. MDD/92/46. 1992
93. Nakano S, Kawashima Y, Matsuda H, et al. A five-year appraisal and hemodynamic evaluation of the Björk-Shiley Monostrut valve. J Thorac Cardiovasc Surg 1991;101:881-887
94. Castillon L, Pareja J, Ruiz M, Jimenez M, Infantes C, Duarte EP. Five years experience with the Björk-Shiley monostrut valve in 2726 patients: a Spanish multicentre study. In: Bodnar E (ed). Surgery for heart valve disease. 1st Ed. London, ICR Publishers, 1990:268-285
95. Liem AK, Berreklouw E, Van Straten BH, et al. The Monostrut prosthetic valve. Predictors for valve-related events during an eight years' experience. J Cardiovasc Surg 1993;34:407-414
96. Daenen W, Van Kerrebroeck C, Stalpaert G, Mertens B, Lesaffre E. The Björk-Shiley Monostrut valve. Clinical experience in 647 patients. J Thorac Cardiovasc Surg 1993;106:918-927
97. Aris A, Padro JM, Camara ML, et al. The Monostrut Björk-Shiley valve. Seven years' experience. J Thorac Cardiovasc Surg 1992;103:1074-1082
98. de la Rocha AG, Plume SK, Baird RJ. Thrombosis of Björk-Shiley aortic valve prosthesis: report of three cases. Canadian Med Assoc J 1977;116:1158- 1160
99. Gray LA Jr, Fulton RL, Srivastava TN, Flowers NC. Surgical treatment of thrombosed Björk- Shiley aortic valve prosthesis. J Thorac Cardiovasc Surg 1976;71:429-432
100. Martinell J, Salas J, de Vega NG, Moreno T, Fraile J, Rabago G. Thrombotic obstruction of the Björk-Shiley aortic valve prosthesis. Report of four cases. Scand J Thorac Cardiovasc Surg 1979;13:255-257
101. Bain W, Pollock J, Rodger R. Five years experience of the Björk-Shiley monostrut prosthesis: valve-related events and hemodynmic performance. J Cardiovasc Surg 1988;29:5
102. Trites PN, Kiser JC, Johnson C, Tycast FJ, Gobel FL. Occlusion of Medtronic Hall mitral valve prosthesis by ruptured papillary muscle and chordae tendineae. J Thorac Cardiovasc Surg 1984;88:301-302
103. Akins CW. Review of the global experience with the Medtronic-Hall valve. Eur J Cardio-thorac Surg 1992;6(suppl):S68-S74
104. Nitter-Hauge S, Semb B, Abdelnoor M, Hall KV. A 5 year experience with the Medtronic-Hall disc valve prosthesis. Circulation 1983;68:II-169-II-174
105. Hall KV, Nitter-Hauge S, Abdelnoor M. Seven and one-half years' experience with the Medtronic-Hall valve. J Am Coll Cardiol 1985;6:1417-1421
106. Keenan RJ, Armitage JM, Trento A, et al. Clinical experience with the Medtronic-Hall valve prosthesis. Ann Thorac Surg 1990;50:748-753
107. Vallejo JL, Gonzalez-Santos JM, Albertos J, et al. Eight years' experience with the Medtronic-Hall valve prosthesis. Ann Thorac Surg 1990;50:429-436
108. Beaudet RL, Poirier NL, Doyle D, Nakhle G, Gauvin C. The Medtronic- Hall cardiac valve: 7 1/2 years' clinical experience. Ann Thorac Surg 1986;42:644-650

109. Nitter-Hauge S, Abdelnoor M. Ten-year experience with the Medtronic Hall valvular prosthesis. A study of 1,104 patients. Circulation 1989;80(suppl I):I-43-I-148
110. Antunes MJ, Wessels A, Sadowski RG, et al. Medtronic Hall valve replacement in a third-world population group. A review of the performance of 1000 prostheses. J Thorac Cardiovasc Surg 1988;95:980-993
111. Butchart E, Lewis P, JCoombes, Breckenridge I. Moving towards prothesis- specific anticoagulation. In: Bodnar E (ed). Surgery for heart valve disease. London, ICR Publishers, 1990:174-183
112. Kaster RL, Lillehei CW. A new cageless free-floating pivoting disc prosthetic heart valve: design, development and evaluation. In: Digest of the 7th International Conference of Medical and Biological Engineering 1967:387
113. Lillehei CW, Kaster RL, Starek PJ, Bloch JH, Rees JR. A new central flow pivoting disc aortic prosthesis and mitral prosthesis: initial clinical experience (Abstract). Am J Cardiol 1970;26:688
114. Olesen KH, Rygg IH, Wennevold A, Nyboe J. Aortic valve replacement with the Lillehei-Kaster prosthesis in 262 patients: an assessment after 9 to 17 years. Eur Heart J 1991;12:680-689
115. Stewart S, Cianciotta D, Hicks GL, DeWeese JA. The Lillehei-Kaster aortic valve prosthesis. Long-term results in 273 patients with 1253 patient-years of follow-up. J Thorac Cardiovasc Surg 1988;95:1023-1030
116. Fananapazir L, Clarke DB, Dark JF, Lawson RA, Moussalli H. Results of valve replacement with the Omniscience prosthesis. J Thorac Cardiovasc Surg 1983;86:621-625
117. Cortina JM, Martinell J, Artiz V, Fraile J, Rabago G. Comparative clinical results with Omniscience (STM1), Medtronic-Hall, and Björk-Shiley convexo-concave (70 degrees) prostheses in mitral valve replacement. J Thorac Cardiovasc Surg 1986;91:174-183
118. McGoon DC. Editor's note and addendum in reference to: A scientific critique of an Omniscience clinical paper (letter). J Thorac Cardiovasc Surg 1984;88:309-310
119. DeWall RA, Caffarena Raggio JM, Dittrich H, Guilmet D, Morea M, Thevenet A. The Omni design: evolution of a valve. J Thorac Cardiovasc Surg 1989;98:999-1007
120. Knott E, Reul H, Knoch M, Steinseifer U, Rau G. In vitro comparison of aortic heart valve prostheses. Part 1: Mechanical valves. J Thorac Cardiovasc Surg 1988;96:952-961
121. Hashimoto A, Nagase Y, Koyanagi H. A new tilting valve prosthesis, "Omniscience valve": clinical and hemodynamic evalutions. Artif Org 1982;11:2-8
122. Carrier M, Martineau JP, Bonan R, Pelletier LC. Clinical and hemodynamic assessment of the Omniscience prosthetic heart valve. J Thorac Cardiovasc Surg 1987;93:300-307
123. Thevenet A, Albat B. Long term follow up of 292 patients after valve replacement with the Omnicarbon prosthetic valve. J Heart Valve Dis 1995;4:634-639
124. Misawa Y, Hasegawa T, Kato M. Clinical experience with the Omnicarbon prosthetic heart valve. J Thorac Cardiovasc Surg 1993;105:168-172
125. Kazui T, Yamada O, Yamagishi M, Watanabe N, Komatsu S. Aortic valve replacement with omniscience and omnicarbon valves. Ann Thorac Surg 1991;52:236- 244
126. Abe T, Kamata K, Kuwaki K, Kuwaki S. Ten years' experience of aortic valve replacement with the Omnicarbon valve prosthesis. Ann Thorac Surg 1996;61:1182- 1187
127. Calafiore AM, Santarelli P, Glieca F, et al. Valve replacement with the tilting disc Sorin prosthesis in patients with narrow aortic annulus. J Cardiovasc Surg 1988;29:387-391
128. Milano A, Bortolotti U, Mazzucco A, et al. Heart valve replacement with the Sorin tilting-disc prosthesis. A 10-year experience. J Thorac Cardiovasc Surg 1992;103:267-275
129. Cotrufo M, Festa M, Renzulli A, de Luca L, Sante P, Giannolo B. Clinical results after cardiac valve replacement with the Sorin prosthesis. A 6-year experience. Eur J Cardio-thorac Surg 1988;2:355-359
130. Agozzino L, Bellitti R, Schettini S, Cotrufo M. Acute thrombosis of Sorin tilting disc mitral prostheses. Int J Cardiol 1984;5:351-359
131. Pellegrini A, Peronace B, Marcazzan E, Rossi C, Colombo T. Results of valve replacement surgery with mechanical prostheses. Int J Artif Org 1982;5:27-32
132. Yoganathan AP, Chaux A, Gray RJ, et al. Bileaflet, tilting disc and porcine aortic valve substitutes: in vitro hydrodynamic characteristics. J Am Coll Cardiol 1984;3:313-320
133. Fisher J. Comparative study of the hydrodynamic function of the size 19mm and 21mm St. Jude Medical Hemodynamic Plus Bileaflet Heart valves. J Heart Valve Dis 1994;3:75-80
134. Khan SS. Assessment of prosthetic valve hemodynamics by Doppler: lessons from in vitro studies of the St. Jude valve. J Heart Valve Dis 1993;2:183-193
135. Carrel T, Zingg U, Jenni R, Aeschbacher B, Turina MI. Early in vivo experience with the Hemodynamic Plus St. Jude Medical heart valves in patients with narrowed aortic annulus. Ann Thorac Surg 1996;61:1418-1422
136. Schneider K, Hofer M, Siebenmann R, et al. Aortic, mitral and multiple valve replacement with the St. Jude medical device at the Univeristy Hospital Zurich 1980-1987. In: Bodnar E (ed). Surgery for heart valve disease. 1st Ed. London, ICR Publishers, 1990:286-297

137. Le Clerc J-L, Wellens, Francis, Deuvaert, Frank E, Primo, Georges. Long- term results with the St. Jude Medical valve. In: DeBakey M (ed). Advances in cardiac valves: clinical perspectives. New York, N.Y., Yorke, 1983:33-40

138. Czer LS, Matloff JM, Chaux A, De Robertis M, Stewart ME, Gray RJ. The St. Jude valve: analysis of thromboembolism, warfarin-related hemorrhage, and survival. Am Heart J 1987;114:389-397

139. Duncan JM, Cooley DA, Reul GJ, et al. Durability and low thrombogenicity of the St. Jude Medical valve at 5-year follow-up. Ann Thorac Surg 1986;42:500-505

140. Ribeiro PA, Al Zaibag M, Idris M, et al. Antiplatelet drugs and the incidence of thromboembolic complications of the St. Jude Medical aortic prosthesis in patients with rheumatic heart disease. J Thorac Cardiovasc Surg 1986;91:92-98

141. Nair CK, Mohiuddin SM, Hilleman DE, et al. Ten-year results with the St. Jude Medical prosthesis. Am J Cardiol 1990;65:217-225

142. Iung B, Acar J, Teppe JP, Boissel JP. Comparison of low-dose and standard- dose oral anticoagulant therapy in patients with mechanical prosthesis. J Am Coll Cardiol 1996;27:A37

143. Acar J, Iung B, Samama MM, et al. Multicenter randomized comparison of low-dose anticoagulation in patients with mechanical heart valves. Circulation. 1996;94:(In Press)

144. Grunkemeier GL, Chandler JG, Miller DC, Jamieson WR, Starr A. Utilization of manufacturers' implant card data to estimate heart valve failure. J Heart Valve Dis 1993;2:493-503

145. Reul H, van Son JA, Steinseifer U, et al. In vitro comparison of bileaflet aortic heart valve prostheses. St. Jude Medical, CarboMedics, modified Edwards-Duromedics, and Sorin- Bicarbon valves. J Thorac Cardiovasc Surg 1993;106:412-420

146. Chandran KB, Schoephoerster R, Fatemi R, Dove EL. An in vitro experimental comparison of Edwards-Duromedics and St Jude bileaflet heart valve prostheses. Clin Phys Physiol Measurement 1988;9:233-241

147. Moritz A, Klepetko W, Rodler S, et al. Six-year follow-up after heart valve replacement with the Edwards Duromedics bileaflet prosthesis. Eur J Cardio-thoracic Surg 1993;7:84-90

148. Jamieson WR, Pelletier LC, Pomar JL. Clinical performance of the Duromedics bileaflet pyrolite mechanical prosthesis. Canadian J Surg 1992;35:605-611

149. Baudet E, Roques X, McBride J, Panes F, Grimaud JP. A 8-year follow-up of the Edwards- Duromedics bileaflet prosthesis. J Cardiovasc Surg 1995;36:437-442

150. Moritz A, Kobinia G, Steinseifer U, et al. Noise level and perception of the closing click after valve replacement with Duromedics-Edwards and St. Jude medical bileaflet valve protheses. In: Bodnar E (ed). Surgery for heart valve disease. 1st Ed. London, ICR Publishers, 1990:602-609

151. Richard G, O'Bannon W, More R. An in vitro comparison of 29mm mitral CarboMedics and St. Jude medical artificial heart valves. In: Bodnar E (ed). Surgery for heart valve disease. 1st Ed. London, ICR Publishers, 1990:628-634

152. Butterfield M, Fisher J, Davies GA, Spyt TJ. Comparative study of the hydrodynamic function of the CarboMedics valve. Ann Thorac Surg 1991;52:815-820

153. Roedler S, Moritz A, Wutte M, Hoda R, Wolner E. The CarboMedics "top hat" supra-annular prosthesis in the small aortic root. J Cardiac Surg 1995;10:198-204

154. de Luca L, Vitale N, Giannolo B, Cafarella G, Piazza L, Cotrufo M. Mid-term follow-up after heart valve replacement with CarboMedics bileaflet prostheses. J Thorac Cardiovasc Surg 1993;106:1158-1165

155. Cohn LH. Discussion of: Four-year experience with the CarboMedics valve: the North American experience. North American team of clinical investigators for the CarboMedics prosthetic heart valve. Ann Thorac Surg 1994;58:637-638

156. Copeland JG III. An international experience with the CarboMedics prosthetic heart valve. J Heart Valve Dis 1995;4:56-62

157. Duran CM, Gometza B, Martin-Duran R, Saad E, al-Halees Z. Performance of 96 CarboMedics valve replacements in 75 patients less than twenty-one years of age. Ann Thorac Surg 1994;58:639-645

158. Fiane AE, Saatvedt K, Svennevig JL, Geiran O, Nordstrand K, Froysaker T. The CarboMedics valve: mid-term follow-up with analysis of risk factors. Ann Thorac Surg 1995;60:1053-1058

159. Lillehei CW. New ideas and their acceptance. As it has related to preservation of chordae tendinea and certain other discoveries. J Heart Valve Dis 1995;4(suppl):S106- S114

Chapter 10.1

Follow Up and Rehabilitation

Christa Gohlke-Bärwolf, Helmut Gohlke, Helmut Roskamm

The annual number of valve operations has increased markedly over the past few years in most Western countries. In Germany during 1992, 9284 valve operations were performed, twice as many as in 1982, accounting for 20% of all open heart procedures (1). In 1990, an average of 113 patients per million population underwent valve surgery throughout the European countries (2). As a result, the postoperative management of these patients has gained increasing importance for cardiologists, a skill which requires a thorough knowledge of the possible complications, their diagnosis and treatment, and is best managed by a close co-operation between cardiologists, surgeons, anesthetists and the general practitioners as well as the patients.

Usually, patients are treated for one to two days postoperatively in the surgical intensive care unit. The management during this phase is beyond the scope of this chapter and will therefore not be dealt with.

CLINICAL EVALUATION

Careful history and daily physical examinations of these patients are mandatory during the early postoperative period. Thorough auscultation of the heart allows the identification of the normal sounds and murmurs of the artificial heart valve, together with deviations from the normal auscultatory findings, and is one of the most important and cost-effective examinations during the early and long term follow up of these patients. The initial auscultatory findings are of particular importance and should serve as the patient's own control in the follow up assessment. Pericardial rubs are frequently heard in the early postoperative period and may occasionally make the interpretation of the auscultatory findings difficult.

The opening and closing sound of the artificial heart valves, the clicks, their intensity, character and associated murmurs depend on the type and location of prosthesis, the heart rate and rhythm and the underlying hemodynamic status (3). The central ball occluder prostheses such as the Starr-Edwards valve have easily identifiable opening and closing sounds that coincide with maximal excursion of the ball and subsequent seating.

A loud opening click is produced in the aortic position , usually 0.06 to 0.07 seconds after the first component of the first heart sound, and is louder than the closing click. A great 2/6 early crescendo-decrescendo systolic murmur that radiates into the carotid artery is usually present, caused by turbulent flow or a transvalvular gradient or both. An early diastolic murmur in this type of valve has to be regarded as pathologic and indicative of a paravalvular leak or abnormal seating of the ball.

In the mitral position the prominent opening click usually follows the aortic component of the second heart sound within 0.06 to 0.13 seconds. A systolic murmur should not be heard with a competent valve.

In the monocusp or bicuspid valves such as the Björk-Shiley, St. Jude, Sorin, Carbomedics and Duromedics valves, a closing click is audible. The opening click is usually not audible but may be recorded by phonocardiography (4). A loud, distinct closing click can usually be heard with these valves in the *aortic position*, generally louder than the first heart sound. A soft early to mid-systolic ejection murmur is commonly heard. If a diastolic murmur in the aortic position is heard with a bileaflet valve this is distinctly abnormal and prosthetic paravalvular or valvular leak should be suspected. A mild aortic insufficiency, which is "physiologic" due to prosthesis design and closing volume, may be recorded with color-coded Doppler echocardiography.

In the *mitral position*, both the monocusp and bicuspid valves produce an opening sound which is not usually audible, but can be recorded by phonocardiography at an A_2 mitral valve opening interval of 0.05 to 0.09 sec. A loud mitral valve closing click is audible at the apex. A systolic murmur in the mitral position is a distinctly abnormal finding, suggesting paravalvular leak or valve dysfunction. However, on transesophageal Doppler studies a trivial early systolic closing volume is commonly observed which is not considered pathologic.

Regular auscultation of the heart also allows identification of diastolic extra sounds and pericardial rubs. The auscultation and percussion of the lungs identifies pleural effusions, atelectasis or infiltration. Neck vein distension, hepatomegaly and peripheral edema are important signs of congestion, restriction, heart failure or tamponade which need to be looked for. Daily measurements of weight allow assessment of fluid balance. Regular ECGs are necessary, as are frequent x-rays.

Previously, phonocardiography was used to document the normal opening and closing sounds together with murmurs of the artificial heart valve prosthesis as a basis for follow up and to diagnose valve dysfunction. One of the useful parameters was the A_2 mitral valve opening interval as was the normal amplitude ratio of the opening to closing sound in central ball occluder valves (3). Presently, transthoracic and particularly transesophageal echocardiography and Doppler color flow imaging, both pulsed and continuous wave, have become the most important diagnostic tools in documenting the normal function of the valve at baseline and for follow up (5-13). Echocardiography also helps to identify pericardial effusions and tamponade, early valve dysfunction such as paravalvular leaks, valve obstruction due to thrombosis or pannus, or thrombosis in the left atrium, and assessment of left ventricular function. Differentiation between various causes can be achieved in the case of low cardiac output both by hemodynamic measurements and echocardiography.

Consecutive ECGs and echocardiography allow the assessment of the regression of left ventricular hypertrophy which occurs very rapidly within the first four weeks after surgery in case of aortic stenosis (14). A reduction in left ventricular size and improvement in the left ventricular shortening fraction are of prognostic importance. An early improvement in the ejection fraction conveys an independent subsequent survival benefit in patients after aortic valve replacement (15). Doppler echocardiography is also important for the documentation of valve gradients and areas at baseline and for further follow up. Normal values of Doppler echocardiographic parameters for different valve prostheses have been defined by several authors (8,11,13,16-18).

The role of transesophageal echocardiography as a routine test after valve replacement has not been clarified yet. So far we have used transesophageal echocardiography only for patients with postoperative complications such as thromboembolic events, or clinical suspicion of endocarditis or valve dysfunction. Transesophageal echocardiography is especially helpful in patients after mitral valve replacement and in those with suspected prosthetic valve malfunction (19,20-22).

Transesophageal echocardiography has been suggested as a routine investigation in the early postoperative course of patients undergoing mitral valve replacement (23) to detect latent, clinically asymptomatic valve thrombosis or small abnormal echoes, extending from the prosthesis into the left atrium. These small abnormal echoes seem to be markers of an increased embolic risk and are associated with inadequate anticoagulation.

We also routinely perform a 24-Holter monitoring test before discharge to identify asymptomatic atrial or ventricular rhythm disturbances, which have been found to be of prognostic significance in some studies (24-27). We did not find any correlation with the postoperative incidence of sudden death in patients with aortic stenosis (28), but all our patients with symptomatic or severe arrhythmias were treated with antiarrhythmic medications (see below) and the response was documented with repeat ambulatory ECG.

Right heart catheterization under exercise gives important information on the postoperative improvement of patients with severely impaired left ventricular function and/or pulmonary hypertension preoperatively (29).

In patients with mechanical heart valve failure such as fracture of a Björk-Shiley or Duromedics valve, or valve obstruction by thrombosis or pannus with impaired leaflet opening, fluoroscopy allows a rapid diagnosis.

COMPLICATIONS

Fever

An elevated temperature is almost always present for at least six days after operation and during a normal course of convalescence. In 20% of patients new fever develops after day seven (30). It is the most common clinical sign of a postoperative infection (31). Fever within the first days after operation is attributed to alterations in blood components after cardiopulmonary bypass, inflammation in wound areas, atelectasis, pleuritis or pericarditis.

In addition to infective causes, fever occurring beyond six days is most commonly due to post-cardiotomy syndrome, but drug reactions, phlebitis at the site of i.v. lines, atelectasis or pulmonary emboli can also be responsible.

Blood cultures should be obtained from all postoperative valve patients with newly occurring fever after day six or persisting thereafter to exclude early endocarditis.

Arrhythmias

The most common type of arrhythmia in the postoperative valve patient is atrial fibrillation, occurring in at least 60% of patients (26,32,33). There are two peaks in its incidence; the first between the second and third day postoperatively and the second between 10 - 15 days postoperatively. The electrophysiologic mechanisms underlying perioperative arrhythmias are not well defined, although alterations in autonomic nervous tone, increased circulating catecholamines, transient electrolyte imbalance, mechanical irritation of the heart, atrial ischemia during hypothermic cardioplegia and dispersion of atrial refractory periods have all been discussed (34).

Other predisposing factors for arrhythmias are hypoxia, hypocalemia, hypovolemia, metabolic acidosis or alkalosis, respiratory acidosis, anemia, pericarditis, atelectasis, digitalis intoxication, pulmonary infection, pulmonary emboli, left heart failure, trauma to the atrium and/or the sinus node.

In the later postoperative phase atrial fibrillation occurs or reoccurs frequently in association with the post-cardiotomy syndrome. Patient age, preoperative use of digoxin, history of rheumatic heart disease, chronic obstructive pulmonary disease and longer aortic crossclamp time were found to be risk factors in multivariate analysis associated with an increased incidence of postoperative atrial arrhythmias (26). Postoperative atrial fibrillation is associated with an increased incidence of postoperative stroke (3.3% vs. 1.4%, p<0.0005), increased length of hospitalization in the intensive care unit (5.7 vs. 3.4 days) and postoperative nursing ward (10.9 vs. 7.5 days), increased incidence of postoperative ventricular tachycardia or fibrillation (9.2% vs. 4.0%) and an increased need for a permanent pacemaker (3.7% vs. 1.6%)(26).

Arrhythmias, particularly when they are associated with very rapid or very slow heart rates, can lead to low cardiac output. When the heart rate is more than 130/min, all mechanical heart valves open incompletely.

Treatment is not well standardized in the literature; there are several prospective studies available concerning the prevention of atrial arrhythmias after bypass surgery (35-41), but prevention or treatment of postoperative atrial arrhythmias after valve surgery have not been examined as extensively and therefore no recommendation is available. In France and Belgium, Amiodarone is widely used in the treatment of various perioperative arrhythmias. In atrial fibrillation it slows down the ventricular rate and leads to conversion to sinus rhythm in two thirds of patients (42).

Our management is as follows:

- In case of severe hemodynamic impairment due to rapid ventricular rates in atrial fibrillation, direct current cardioversion is performed. In all other cases the main goal of treatment is the slowing of ventricular rates to levels below 100/min, optimally between 80 and 90/min, initially;
- In patients with normal left ventricular function, cardioselective beta-blockers or Sotalol are given either orally or intravenously (e.g. Metoprolol 5 mg slowly i.v. every five minutes for up to three doses).

There is some as yet unconfirmed evidence from three recent preventive trials that Sotalol might be superior to other beta-blockers in reducing the risk of supraventricular arrhythmias after aorto-coronary bypass surgery in patients with normal left ventricular function (40,41,43). Esmolol, an ultra-short acting cardioselective beta-blocker, has been suggested at a dose of 50-250 µg/kg (36,44) with continuous blood pressure monitoring. Three to four doses of Verapamil 5 mg i.v. every 5-10 minutes can also be given (44). In one study Esmolol was found to be superior to Verapamil as regards conversion to sinus rhythm (38% vs. 12% (36)) in patients with recent onset of atrial fibrillation, independent of surgery;

- In patients with impaired left ventricular function we prefer digitalis and Verapamil for slowing of the ventricular rate in an attempt at medical cardioversion. In patients who maintain very rapid rates in spite of adequate doses of digitalis and Verapamil, Amiodarone is added and Verapamil discontinued;
- We postpone electric conversion in our institution to the third or fourth postoperative week because of the high reoccurrence rate within the earlier time period. Cardioversion is rarely attempted in patients with a low chance of success, for example patients with long standing atrial fibrillation preoperatively (more than two years), or large left atrium (> 60mm). In these patients electric cardioversion may be reconsidered six months after surgery, when resolution of the perioperative changes has occurred and preoperative pathologic conditions such as cardiomegaly, heart failure and enlarged left atrium have improved. In the meantime treatment is directed towards slowing of the ventricular rate to about 70-80/min at rest.

In patients with preoperative atrial fibrillation in whom cardioversion is attempted the reoccurrence rate after successful cardioversion is also relatively high, so that antiarrhythmic drugs should be continued for at least six months postoperatively and then slowly discontinued. In patients without atrial fibrillation preoperatively the chance of recurrence after two months postoperatively is low so that antiarrhythmic medication can be discontinued after two to three months.

For the prevention of thromboembolic events, therapeutic anticoagulation with either heparin or vitamin K antagonists is necessary (45) as long as atrial fibrillation persists and for two months after the occurrence of sinus rhythm. The successful treatment and prevention of atrial and ventricular arrhythmias also requires treatment of the predisposing factors.

The incidence and clinical importance of ventricular rhythm disturbances postoperatively are controversial; in 1971, Acar (33) and in 1992 Michel (46) found a high incidence of ventricular extrasystoles and severe ventricular rhythm disturbances in 50% of patients. In our experience clinically important ventricular ectopic beats and rhythm disturbances are less common after valve surgery. Indications for treatment are the severity of the arrhythmia and hemodynamic disturbances. Only patients with severe ventricular arrhythmias (Lown IVb) or a history of preoperative severe symptomatic ventricular arrhythmias are treated. Beta-blockers are used preferentially in patients with an ejection fraction of more than 30%, otherwise we use Amiodarone. The response to medication should be documented by repeat Holter recordings. Electrophysiologic studies are performed in case of symptomatic recurrent ventricular tachycardia unresponsive to medical therapy.

Bradyarrhythmias and conduction defects

Sinus bradycardia and slow AV-junctional rhythms may be a cause of low cardiac output in the early postoperative period. Patients with heavily calcified native valves, particularly aortic valves, are specifically prone to developing new conduction defects and AV-block, thought to be due to surgical trauma and tissue edema. Usually most conduction disturbances resolve within two weeks. If complete AV-block persists and junctional escape rhythm is not sufficient to maintain adequate cardiac output, permanent pacemaker insertion becomes necessary. The incidence of new conduction disturbances postoperatively was reported to be between 5% and 29%, of which half were transient. They are most frequent in patients after aortic valve replacement (22%-30%), most commonly LBBB.

The occurrence of complete AV-block after aortic valve replacement is rare (33,47-50), requiring permanent pacemaker insertion in less than 1% of patients (50). In a recent study by Brodell of patients after mitral valve replacement in 1991 (51), complete AV-block occurred in 1% of patients.

Pericarditis

In the first days after operation a pericardial rub can usually be heard with or without an additional mediastinal rub. This usually persists for two to three days. A separate clinical syndrome is the post-cardiotomy syndrome, which appears later, usually in the second or third week postoperatively. It is in our experience the most common cause of postoperative fever in the second and third week, commonly presenting with chest pain, pericardial or pleural rubs, leukocytosis, an increase in CRP and sedimentation rate, pericardial and pleural effusions and atrial arrhythmias. Clinical findings of a pericardial rub, which is occasionally only heard in a very circumscribed area, should raise a suspicion of this condition. Neck vein distensions, obliteration of the apical impulse in the left lateral position and dyspnea are indications of the hemodynamic significance of an accompanying pericardial effusion. The diagnosis of pericardial effusion can be confirmed by echocardiography. A rare late complication of pericarditis and post-cardiotomy-syndrome is constrictive pericarditis (52).

Treatment

Pleural and pericardial effusions usually respond well to diuretics (e.g. hydrochlorothiazide 50 mg, together with triamterine or spironolactone). Pericardial pain is treated with diclophenac, which interferes less with anticoagulation than aspirin or indomethacin. Occasionally this medication is not sufficient to relieve pain and steroids are necessary (e.g. Prednisone 40-60 mg daily for one week, followed by a slow decrease). On rare occasions pericardial effusions are so large and accumulate so quickly that tamponade can occur.

Cardiac tamponade

Although postoperative echocardiography has shown that virtually all patients have pericardial effusion after cardiac surgery (53), only three percent develop tamponade (54,55). The important clinical features of tamponade, such as diminished heart sounds and pulsus paradoxus, may be obscured in the postoperative patient. Asymmetrical, localized accumulation of blood clots in the mediastinum and pericardial space may

---

Table 10.1-I: Signs and symptoms suggestive of tamponade.

- appearance of atrial fibrillation
- unexplained dyspnea
- sudden decrease in hematocrit
- increase in heart size within few days without signs of left heart failure
- neck vein distension which are not explained by heart failure
- unexplained increase in creatinine
- unexplained decrease in anticoagulation requirement
- widening of the mediastinum by x-ray
- acute deterioration in the postoperative period with hypotension or shock.

---

cause isolated tamponade of one or two cardiac chambers, producing unusual elevations of diastolic pressures (right atrial tamponade with an elevation of CVP without an increase in right ventricular enddiastolic pressure and pulmonary capillary wedge pressure (54,56,57).

The following symptoms and findings should raise a suspicion of tamponade; sudden onset of atrial fibrillation, unexplained dyspnea, sudden decrease in hematocrit, increase in heart size within a few days without signs of left heart failure and/or neck vein distension which are not explained by heart failure, unexplained increase in creatinine, unexplained decrease in the anticoagulation requirement, widening of the mediastinum on x-ray, acute deterioration in the postoperative period with hypotension or shock (Table 10.1-I). In each case of acute deterioration with hypotension and shock tamponade has to be a prime consideration as the underlying cause in the early postoperative period.

Echocardiography is the most rapid and definite diagnostic method (54,55). Localized tamponade with compression of the left or right heart in the later postoperative period may be difficult to diagnose. Right heart catheterization is helpful in determining a pressure plateau between the right atrium, the diastolic right ventricular and pulmonary pressures and the pulmonary capillary wedge pressure (56-59). In the early postoperative period, tamponade is such an acutely life threatening event in most cases that there is no time or necessity for these hemodynamic evaluations. Urgent therapy with pericardial drainage is necessary.

Left ventricular dysfunction and heart failure

Patients with aortic and mitral valve disease and chronic preoperative left heart failure frequently also have signs of left ventricular dysfunction postoperatively. Whereas left ventricular function in patients with aortic stenosis improves rapidly within the first weeks postoperatively (29,60), this is frequently not the case with aortic and mitral insufficiency and impaired left ventricular function preoperatively. The shortening fraction determined by echocardiography often falls immediately after operation and may improve only slowly, over several months (61-67). Intraoperative myocardial infarction or deficient myocardial protection during surgery can impair left ventricular function (66,67). In these patients, digitalis and diuretics are also usually required after surgery. In addition, vasodilators such as nitrates and ACE-inhibitors may be necessary and can decrease the chances of heart failure (68). The requirement for digitalis, diuretics and vasodilators should be assessed during the first cardiologist out-patient examination.

Nitrates are very useful in patients with marked preoperative pulmonary hypertension during the postoperative period to lower pulmonary pressure and relieve right heart failure (69). Aldactone in addition to furosemide is a very effective diuretic, particularly in patients with right heart failure. Pulmonary hypertension associated with mitral stenosis usually improves after surgery (70-72). In patients with aortic stenosis and pulmonary hypertension, a marked decrease in pulmonary hypertension can occur after surgery, associated with an increase in the ejection fraction (29,73-75).

Infections

Mediastinitis and sternal osteomyelitis are serious postoperative infections and occur in approximately 2% of patients after sternotomy (76). Risk factors for the development of mediastinitis are obesity, diabetes mellitus, malnutrition, advanced age, severe pulmonary disease, prolonged cardiopulmonary bypass time, excessive postoperative bleeding with re-exploration for control of hemorrhage and diminished cardiac output in the postoperative period (44,77). Definite diagnosis requires wound exploration and cultures. CT and MRI scanning have been reported to be helpful in localizing the sites of infection (44). In addition to surgical therapy antibiotics for 10 to 14 days are recommended, in the case of a documented sternal osteomyelitis for four to six weeks (78).

Viral infections

The two most common transfusion-related viral infections after cardiac surgery are non-A, non-B-hepatitis (hepatitis C) and cytomegalovirus (CMV) infections. The incidence of hepatitis was reported to be 5% (79-81) and has decreased to 2% currently (79). This decrease is due to the reduction in the number of transfusions of blood bank products (82), improved screening techniques and preoperative autologous blood donations. Hepatitis C is caused by an RNA virus and is characterized by a protracted course with fluctuating transaminase levels (80). Acquired immuno-deficiency syndrome and malaria are rare complications of cardiovascular surgery (83,84).

CMV infection is a febrile syndrome that typically presents one month postoperatively. It is characterized by high-spiking fevers, abnormalities of liver function tests and arthralgia. A self-limited illness, it is best treated with antipyretics and supportive fluid therapy.

Patients who have received corticosteroids and long courses of antibiotic treatment postoperatively are at increased risk for fungal infection.

Neurologic complications

Up to 20% of patients develop neurologic complications (79,85,86) such as short term memory loss, lack of concentration, disorientation and visual disturbances. The majority of these symptoms improve spontaneously (87-89); about 10% will continue to show deterioration of their neuropsychologic function over the next six months, especially if they occur in patients over 65 years. Strokes occur in 1% to 5% of patients (86). Symptomatic visual defects can result from retinal emboli, occipital lobe infarction or anterior ischemic optic neuropathy (90). Risk factors for cerebral vascular accidents (CVA) or transient ischemic attacks (TIA) include preoperative carotid bruits, previous CVA or TIA, postoperative atrial fibrillation, prolonged cardio-pulmonary bypass (more than two hours) and preoperative left atrial or left ventricular mural thrombus (91-93).

Gastrointestinal complications

Serious gastrointestinal complications occur in about 1% of patients, half of them requiring surgical intervention (94). Most complications occur within seven days of surgery. Patients who are likely to develop gastrointestinal complications are those with circulatory compromise and those who require intra-aortic balloon pump. Postoperative bleeding due to stress ulcer was reported in 0.1% of patients (79).

Stress gastritis and peptic ulcer disease occur most commonly in patients with chronic obstructive pulmonary disease, postoperative hypotension, bleeding and reoperation (95), so providing prophylactic treatment with antacids and H2-receptor antagonists to these high risk groups is recommended. Clinical management consists of early endoscopy if supportive medical care is unsuccessful, with a nasogastric tube, antacids, H2-receptor antagonists and transfusion, as required.

Valve related complications

Thromboembolic events, valve thrombosis and bleeding are among the most serious complications in the early and late postoperative period and account for 75% of complications after valve replacement. These important topics are discussed in Chapter 10.3. The European Society of Cardiology Working Group on Valvular Heart Disease has developed recommendations concerning the prevention of thromboembolic events in patients with native valve disease and after valve replacement (45). Different results and recommendations published in the literature (96-106) are also discussed in detail in Chapter 10.3.

Bacterial endocarditis is of importance, both in the early and long term follow up of patients after valve replacement and is discussed in Chapter 6.3.

Valvular dehiscence

Prosthesis dehiscence can lead to paravalvular leaks resulting in variable degrees of regurgitation and hemolysis. This appears most often in the first months after operation either due to acute infective endocarditis or post-infective changes within the annulus or para-annular area, or due to calcification of the annulus. Patients with connective tissue diseases like Marfan's syndrome are also prone to developing valvular dehiscence (107). The incidence of valvular dehiscence thus depends on the underlying pathologic valve condition, surgical factors and postoperative complications like endocarditis. It was the cause for reoperation in 15% of patients with bioprostheses (108) and 41% of patients with mechanical aortic and 49% of those with mechanical mitral valves (109). In this series the incidence of valve dehiscence was 2% in mitral and 1.7% in aortic prostheses.

The diagnosis of a paravalvular leak can be made on the basis of a newly appearing regurgitant murmur. Of note is that the systolic murmur of a small paravalvular leak in the mitral position may only be heard when the patient is examined in the left lateral position. Auscultation cannot differentiate between paravalvular and valvular regurgitation, though. If the area of dehiscence is large enough and there is an abnormal excursion of the valve ring during fluoroscopy, a paravalvular leak is likely. Doppler echocardiography, sometimes only with transesophageal echo, can document the regurgitant jet.

Laboratory evaluation of LDH, haptoglobin and hemoglobin detect the presence and amount of hemolysis. If hemolysis is severe and requires recurrent transfusion, reoperation is indicated. If hemolysis is well compensated and/or the regurgitation is not hemodynamically significant then patients may be followed conservatively. Mild degrees of hemolysis can also occur in the absence of a paravalvular leak, even in patients with third generation mechanical valves (109).

Structural valve failure

Ball variance, degeneration and fracture of the occluder disc were problems mainly associated with first and second generation mechanical valves (110). Strut fracture of the Björk-Shiley concave-convex 70° and 60° prostheses were reported early and late after operation (111-113). The fracture rate of the Edwards-Duromedics valve was reported to be 0.03% (114). A markedly lower risk of 0.004% was noted with the St. Jude Medical prosthesis (115-118) (see also Chapter 9.5).

The fracture of a single leaflet valve, like all tilting disc valves, is associated with escape of the occluder disc and massive regurgitation. Unless the patient is reoperated immediately he/she will die. The fracture of a bileaflet valve is tolerated better, since usually only one leaflet escapes and the resultant regurgitation is not as massive, being mitigated by the remaining leaflet. However, urgent reoperation is also necessary in these cases. The condition should be suspected in patients who suddenly develop severe symptoms of dyspnoea, pulmonary edema and shock. Valve clicks are absent on auscultation in case of a fractured Björk-Shiley valve and regurgitant murmurs are audible. The diagnosis can be proven by fluoroscopy.

Considerable effort has been directed recently to diagnose single leg fracture in Björk-Shiley valves, the presence of which could help in the indication of an elective removal of the culprit prosthesis (see Chapter 9.5). However, until this method is validated and becomes generally available, the information of the patients, their relatives and caring physicians about the symptoms associated with fracture and the need for an immediate transport to a cardiothoracic surgical centre for operation is mandatory. This is the only way at the present time to reduce the high mortality associated with this type of valve failure (119).

Valve dysfunction due to pannus

Tissue ingrowth into the valve can lead to impaired opening and obstruction soon after surgery. The diagnosis is made on the basis of newly occurring symptoms, murmurs of obstruction and occasionally regurgitation on auscultation, restricted valve opening on fluoroscopy and increased Doppler echocardiographic gradients (120).

Occasionally, a slowly increasing gradient across the prosthetic valve on follow up is the only evidence of increasing obstruction due to pannus. The reason for pannus formation is not known. Another cause of obstruction is thrombus formation. Transesophageal echocardiography is helpful in identifying the mechanical problem, but differentiation between thrombus and pannus cannot usually be made by echocardiography. Frequently, the cause of the obstruction can only be identified intraoperatively (see also Chapter 8.7).

We recently reoperated a patient 13 years after initial double valve replacement. Within half a year of the last examination, at which time a physiologic gradient across the mitral valve was present, a severe obstruction had developed due to proliferating endocardial fibrosis extending into the mitral valve.

Hemolysis

Chronic intravascular hemolysis is one of the complications of valve replacement. It is due to mechanical damage of erythrocytes, caused by turbulent flow, high flow velocities and direct trauma by the valve. The first generation valves caused significant amounts of hemolysis, frequently leading to hemolytic anemia.

The second generation valves built since the 1970's cause markedly less or no hemolysis due to their improved design and materials, so that clinically relevant anemia does not occur unless valvular dysfunction is present. In this case even small paravalvular leaks can lead to excessive degrees of hemolysis and anemia, requiring valve re-replacement (121). This occurred in only one of our patients with a St. Jude mitral valve among more than 4000 valve operations carried out over the last 15 years.

In the absence of a paravalvular leak or other valve dysfunction most second generation valve prostheses do not cause any or only mild degrees of hemolysis (109, pp. 330-334). Defining hemolysis as reticulocytosis and transfusion requirements, DiSesa (122) did not observe any case of hemolysis after aortic valve replacement and a 2% incidence after mitral valve replacement with the St. Jude valve. The latter cases were all associated with paravalvular leaks. Evaluating hemolysis with a very sensitive parameter like haptoglobin, Horstkotte found that patients undergoing mitral valve replacement with Lillehei-Kaster, Starr-Edwards, Omniscience and Duromedics valves usually had subclinical evidence of hemolysis, as did 2/3 of those with Björk-Shiley and Medtronic Hall valves but only half of those with St. Jude or bioprosthetic valves. In patients undergoing aortic valve replacement the percentage was higher, except for those with St. Jude valves (123).

Laboratory diagnosis and quantification of hemolysis

The presence of hemolysis can be diagnosed by determination of haptoglobin and LDH. Haptoglobin is a very sensitive indicator of its presence, but it is not a useful parameter for the quantification of hemolysis. This is possible with determination of LDH; mild degrees of hemolysis are present when LDH is between 220 to 400 U/I, haptoglobin between 10 and 37 mg%, and free hemoglobin is elevated. A marked degree of hemolysis, which is still compensated, is present when LDH is > 800 U/I, haptoglobin is absent, marked elevation of free hemoglobin occurs, fragmentocytes,

Table 10.1-II: Causes of death after valve replacement with the Björk-Shiley prosthesis.

Causes	AVR	MVR	
Non-cardiac	19.6%	9%	
Cardiac		80.4%	91%
CHF, MI, arrhythmias	51.1%	56%	
Sudden death	11%	10%	
Valve-related causes	18.3%	25%	
anticoagulation	8.3%	4%	
paravalvular leak	3%	3%	
embolism	2.7%	3%	
valve thrombosis	2.7%	10%	
structural failure	1.6%	3%	
PVE		2%	

From Lindblom 1988 (119)

AVR: aortic valve replacement; MVR: mitral valve replacement; CHF: congestive heart failure; MI: myocardial infarction; PVE: prosthetic valve endocarditis.

hyperbilirubinemia and reticulocytosis appear and hemosiderin is present in the urine, yet anemia is compensated. Severe uncompensated hemolysis is present when LDH is over 1000 U/I usually > 3000 U/I, haptoglobin is absent and repeat transfusions for severe anemia are required (109). This is usually associated with valve dysfunction and is considered to be an indication for valve replacement. This was the case in only two patients at our institution.

In general, a degree of hemolysis which is more marked than that usually associated with a specific type of valve should raise a suspicion of valve dysfunction (109,123).

Treatment

As long as the degree of hemolysis is mild to moderate and is not associated with hemodynamically significant valve dysfunction no specific therapy is necessary. However, the patient should be followed at regular intervals for early recognition of increase in the amount of hemolysis or valve dysfunction. If the hemolysis leads to transfusion-requiring anemia, reoperation is the therapy of choice.

FOLLOW UP

Valve-related causes account for 18% of deaths after aortic valve replacement and 25% after mitral valve replacement. Although the majority of patients die of cardiac causes (80% of patients with aortic and 90% of patients with mitral valve replacement) the majority die of congestive heart failure, myocardial infarction and arrhythmias (51% and 56% respectively and 11% due to sudden death) (Table 10.1-II). This illustrates the need for careful and expert follow up of these patients after valve surgery for the rest of their lives.

We recommend a routine cardiologic examination six months after surgery and at yearly intervals thereafter, preferably in the center where the patient was diagnosed and operated. In addition, the cardiologist should be consulted when new serious symptoms or changes in the clinical status of the patient or in the Doppler echocardiographic parameters occur. In case of increasing gradients across the artificial valve patients should be followed very closely to determine the need and time for reoperation. Also, patients with bioprostheses should be followed at shorter time intervals once the prosthesis has been in place for more than five years or begins to show structural abnormalities on echocardiography, even in asymptomatic patients. This is based on the accelerated deterioration rate after the fifth year after implantation and once structural abnormalities are documented (124-128).

REHABILITATION

Definition of rehabilitation by the WHO

"Rehabilitation includes all measures that are required to achieve for a cardiac patient the best possible physical, psychological and social conditions that enable him/her to obtain out of his own strength an as normal as possible place in society and to lead an active and productive life." (129). This definition, initially developed for patients with coronary artery disease, applies to most patients with valvular heart disease, particularly after valve replacement, since implantation of a replacement valve is a palliative procedure. Due to the complexity and multiplicity of problems associated with valve surgery and current abbreviated hospital stay these patients are very well suited to comprehensive cardiac rehabilitation. Rehabilitation after heart valve replacement has become an integral part of cardiac rehabilitation in Germany and is practised as institutional rehabilitation instituted by law. The cost of rehabilitating these patients is borne by the retirement funds of those still working and the sickness funds of those who are retired. 80% of patients participate in rehabilitation after surgery.

Purposes and aims of cardiac rehabilitation

The purposes and aims of rehabilitation after valve surgery are optimization and adjustment of medical treatment and early recognition of complications, early ambulation and physical training, assessment and improvement of functional performance, education about valve-specific topics, education and counselling of patient and family about a health conscious life style, psychologic support in adjusting to chronic disease, and vocational counselling (Table 10.1-III).

There are unique features to rehabilitation after valve surgery in that a rapidly increasing number of elderly, multi-morbid patients, particularly female, present for rehabilitative measures. Their medical, physical and psycho-social problems are very complex and divergent, and require intensive individualized management, education and counseling.

There is abundant literature on the effect of rehabilitation after myocardial infarction and bypass surgery and recommendations are available concerning the type and structure of rehabilitation programs (130-135). In contrast, rehabilitation after valve

---

Table 10.1-III: Purposes of cardiac rehabilitation.

optimization and adjustment of medical treatment
early recognition of complications
early ambulation and physical training
assessment and improvement of functional performance
education about valve-specific topics
education about health conscious life style
psychologic support in adjustment to chronic disease
vocational counselling

---

surgery has received little attention and there is no official recommendation available as to the type and structure of the ideal rehabilitation program after valve surgery. Nonetheless, a co-ordinated multidisciplinary cardiac exercise program is essential to overcome the physical and psycho-social problems associated with cardiac surgery.

The known positive effects of training on cardiovasculatory fitness, such as an improvement in general circulatory response to exercise with reduced heart rate and blood pressure, and greater exercise tolerance, make a physical training program for patients after valve replacement specifically advisable since patients commonly present for valve surgery after years of severe restriction of physical activity.

Cardiorespiratory fitness is further impaired by surgical trauma and postoperative bedrest, so patients recovering from successful cardiac surgery can be in a markedly reduced state of cardiorespiratory fitness, especially those with rheumatic heart disease and impairment of cardiac performance.

The effect of exercise training in patients after aortic valve replacement has been examined in only a few studies (136,137). It was shown that exercise training in patients with aortic valve replacement leads to an increase in exercise tolerance. As far as possible risks and complications of exercise training in patients after valve replacement are concerned, there is one study, published by Habel in 1987 (138), which evaluates the effect of exercise training on valve dysfunction and hemolysis in 10 patients after mitral valve replacement. The authors found that slight hemolysis may occur, but no serious valve dysfunction. Cardiovascular fitness also improved in these patients.

Exercise tolerance after valve replacement

We evaluated exercise tolerance in 1270 patients after single valve replacement. Patients after aortic valve replacement have a better exercise tolerance one month after operation than those after mitral valve replacement, both in terms of absolute values (89.7 ± 2.1 vs. 53.9 ± 2; $p<0.01$), and percent of age and weight adjusted normal values (67% vs. 48%; $p<0.01$)(60).

Hemodynamics

Hemodynamics improved significantly at rest and during exercise in 108 patients with aortic stenosis and impaired left ventricular function preoperatively; pulmonary capillary wedge pressure fell from 14 ± 1.3 mmHg at rest to 5 ± 0.5 mmHg and remained within the

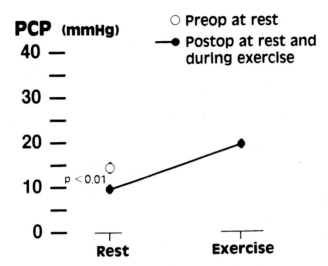

Figure 10.1-1: Pulmonary capillary wedge pressure (PCP) at rest and during exercise after aortic valve replacement in patients with aortic stenosis and impaired left ventricular function; defined as PCP > 12 mmHG, or cardiac index < 2.5 or ejection fraction < 50% (n = 108) (from Gohlke-Bärwolf 1992).

normal range during exercise testing in 60% of patients (Fig. 10.1-1). In contrast, patients after mitral valve replacement not only had a markedly lower exercise tolerance, but also only 40%-60% had normal hemodynamics at rest and only 25% normal hemodynamics during exercise. In patients with mitral stenosis, the pulmonary capillary wedge pressure fell from 24.5 ± 0.2 mmHg at rest preoperatively to 15 ± 0.6 mmHg postoperatively. Patients with mitral stenosis also showed more severe impairment of exercise hemodynamics preoperatively, with a higher pulmonary capillary pressure at lower work load compared to patients with mitral insufficiency. Starting from a lower exercise level, patients with mitral stenosis showed a slightly higher relative improvement in exercise tolerance (+74% vs. +50%) and a slightly greater decrease in pulmonary capillary wedge pressure (-30% vs. -24%) compared to those with mitral insufficiency. Nevertheless, patients with mitral stenosis had a significantly lower exercise capacity at higher wedge pressures than those after valve replacement for mitral insufficiency (Table 10.1-IV).

Between one and six months postoperatively, there is a further increase in exercise tolerance, both in patients with aortic and those with mitral valve replacement, but the

Table 10.1-IV: Exercise hemodynamics before and after mitral valve replacement.

	Preop		Postop	
Mitral regurgitation (N = 50)				
Pulm cap WP (mmHg)	20 ± 2	33 ± 2	12 ±1	25 ± 1
Work load (Watt)	rest	37 ± 5	rest	56 ± 4
Mitral stenosis (N = 85)				
Pulm cap WP (mmHg)	25 ± 1	43 ± 1	15 ± 1	30 ± 1
Work load (Watt)	rest	23 ± 4	rest	40 ± 4

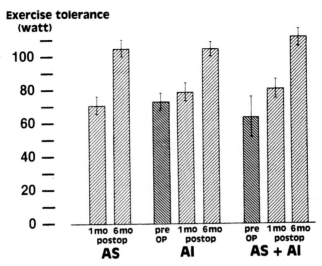

Figure 10.1-2: Exercise tolerance after aortic valve replacement (n = 307) preoperatively, one and six months postoperatively in patients with aortic stenosis (AS), aortic insufficiency (AI) and mixed aortic lesion (AS + AI) (n = 307) (from Gohlke-Bärwolf 1992).

difference in performance is still present (72% vs. 57% of normal) (Fig. 10.1-2).

At six months, patients under 56 years with aortic valve replacement due to aortic stenosis and aortic insufficiency had an exercise tolerance of 105 ± 5 watts and 105 ± 4 watts, respectively. Patients with combined lesions reached 112 ± 5 watts (p = NS). Among patients undergoing mitral valve replacement, those with preoperative mitral insufficiency had the highest exercise tolerance, at 74 ± 4.2 watts, followed by patients with mitral stenosis and combined lesions with a markedly lower exercise tolerance of 62 ± 3.99 watts, and 62 ± 4.64 watts, respectively (Fig. 10.1-3). This level of exercise tolerance was maintained in patients with aortic stenosis during a four year follow up. Therefore, postoperative exercise tolerance depends on the preoperative valve lesion and type of valve replacement, and is maintained at least at a level reached six months postoperatively.

To determine the type of rehabilitative measures, several factors other than hemodynamics need to be taken into account, including the possible risks of training, the postoperative course of regression of left ventricular hypertrophy and any improvement in left ventricular function following correction of the various valve lesions (139).

We addressed the question of possible risks of exercise training in a prospective study in patients after aortic valve replacement for pure aortic stenosis. We took the degree and time course of regression of left ventricular hypertrophy in patients undergoing exercise training using the bicycle ergometer and compared the time course of regression of left ventricular hypertrophy to a previously studied group of patients after aortic valve replacement for aortic stenosis who had not undergone exercise training after surgery (14).

To assess the regression of left ventricular hypertrophy we used the echocardiographic parameter of septal and posterior wall thickness and the cross-sectional area of left ventricular muscle, as well as the Sokolow-Lyon index from the ECG.

Patients who had undergone more vigorous training, including bicycle ergometry, had the same degree of regression of left ventricular hypertrophy as those without

---

Table 10.1-V: Factors influencing exercise recommendations after valve replacement.

---

age of patient
weight
previous level of training
type of cardiac disease and valve replaced
postoperative functional status, determined by

---

exercise testing with and without spiroergometry
measurement of hemodynamics
echocardiographic assessment of left ventricular function
radiographic determination of heart size
Holter-monitoring

---

exercise training. Within four weeks the ECG and echocardiographic parameters of left ventricular hypertrophy, such as Sokolow-Lyon index and cross-sectional area of left ventricular muscle, were comparable in both groups and regression was completed within four weeks postoperatively.

We also performed a prospective randomized study in patients after aortic valve replacement for aortic stenosis, comparing the effect of two different types of reconditioning therapies. The preliminary results of the study show the same trends.

Thus so far there is no evidence that physical exercise has an adverse effect on patients after valve replacement for aortic stenosis, judged by regression of left ventricular hypertrophy.

Recommendations for exercise

Recommendations concerning exercise and recreational activity in patients after valve replacement should also take into account the age of the patient, weight, previous level

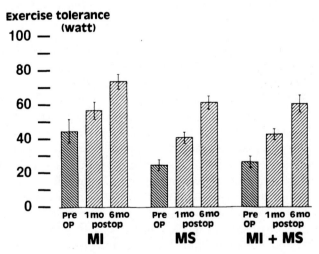

Figure 10.1-3: Exercise tolerance after mitral valve replacement (n = 258) preoperatively, one and six months postoperatively in patients with mitral stenosis (MI) and mixed mitral lesion (n = 258) (from Gohlke-Bärwolf 1992).

of training, type of cardiac disease and valve replaced, postoperative functional status, determined by exercise testing with and without spiroergometry and measurement of hemodynamics, echocardiographic assessment of left ventricular function, radiographic determination of heart size and Holter-monitoring (Table 10.1-V).

As a guide to determination of the ideal training level, the results of the exercise test and, in certain cases, the exercise hemodynamics are very useful. That level of activity or exercise that is still associated with normal hemodynamics can be taken as a guide for leisure time activities. If hemodynamics are not available, a rating of perceived exertion like the Borg scale (140-143) or the so-called "talk test" are valuable measurements of the intensity of exertion. The talk test refers to that level of exertion at which the patient can still lead a conversation.

In general, patients with mitral valve disease have a markedly lower exercise tolerance postoperatively than those with aortic valve disease, and thus are candidates for a different, low level training programme. Patients who can be expected to be candidates for exercise training postoperatively are those with pure aortic stenosis and normal ventricular function, those with aortic insufficiency and preserved left ventricular function pre- and postoperatively and an uncomplicated postoperative course. Patients with isolated mitral valve insufficiency preoperatively on the basis of mitral valve prolapse, especially if they have undergone mitral valve reconstruction, with an uncomplicated postoperative course, can be included in an exercise programme.

Patients with mitral stenosis and combined mitral valve lesion usually have a fairly low exercise tolerance postoperatively. In addition, the residual gradient across the valve and the marked increase in gradient with rising heart rate make an exercise program for these patients particularly challenging. Before conditioning begins, the heart rate needs to be controlled by medication, both at rest and during exercise. A programme specifically designed for these patients, including walking, callisthenics, gymnastics and a low level bicycle ergometry with special consideration of the heart rate achieved, appears to be of particular benefit.

What type of exercise is advisable?

In general the dynamic, aerobic type of exercise like walking, jogging and cycling are preferable to isometric exercise. However, in elderly patients who present with problems of muscle weakness, a high intensity strength training to improve muscle strength and co-ordination has been shown to be of benefit (144). Swimming is associated with an energy requirement equivalent to 100 - 150 watts, as far as the response of heart rate, noradrenalin and lactate levels are concerned (145). Patients should be informed about the amount of energy expenditure associated with different types of exercise and advised about the activities suited to them. A task force of the American College of Cardiology developed recommendations for patients with acquired valvular heart disease concerning sports (146,147).

In conclusion, physical conditioning and individually tailored exercise training are advisable for more patients after valve replacement, taking into account left ventricular function, the type of valve replaced, pulmonary hypertension and heart rate; the general circulatory responses to exercise, like decreased heart rate and blood pressure at a given exercise load, and increased exercise tolerance, are of benefit to most of these patients,

Table 10.1-VI: Univariate analysis of predictors of return to work after valve replacement (n = 375).

	p-value	chi-square
Employment status preop	0.0000	238.67
Sex	0.0000	112.48
Exercise tolerance postop	0.0000	73.36
Type of valve replaced	0.0006	58.09
Heart volume/kg body weight postop	0.0039	8.35
Age (all <56 years)	0.0968	2.76
Bypass duration	0.7997	0.06

and could enable them to participate better in social activities and live a more active and productive life. However, further studies are needed to determine the type, structure, effects and risks of exercise programmes in the various valve lesions.

Educational aspects

One important aspect of rehabilitation in patients with valvular heart disease is the information and education. The patient needs to become an expert on his/her own disease. He/she should know about:

- the type of valve prosthesis and possible complications;
- what to do in case of symptoms and other problems;
- medical therapy;
- oral anticoagulation and the possibility of patient-regulated - anticoagulation and home prothrombin estimation;
- bacterial endocarditis;
- meticulous dental hygiene;
- optimal risk factor control, avoiding smoking, hypertension and obesity, to reduce the risk of thromboembolism;
- the need for reoperation in case of structural valve failure or for newly occurring coronary artery disease, and
- a health-oriented left style.

Table 10.1-VII: Multivariate analysis of predictors of return to work after valve replacement (n = 375).

	p-value	chi-square
Employment status preop	0.000	135.46
Exercise tolerance postop	0.0041	8.23
Sex	0.0148	5.93
Bypass duration	0.1961	1.67
Age (all <56 years)	0.7635	0.09
Heart volume preop	0.8333	0.04
Heart volume postop	0.3997	0.71
Type of valve replaced	0.4428	0.5

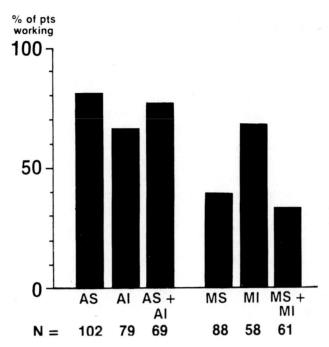

Figure 10.1-4: Employment status after valve replacement in patients under 56 years (n = 448)
(from Gohlke-Bärwolf 1992).

Return to work after valve replacement

Controversial results have been published concerning the influence of valve replacement on the return to work rate; it has been reported to be between 24% and 80% (60,72,148-155). We evaluated the postoperative vocational status of 485 patients undergoing single valve replacement in our institution who were younger than 56 years (139,155). 54% of patients received aortic and 46% mitral valve replacement. The postoperative status was as follows: 62% of patients were working, 2% in education, 16% were housewives, 4% without work, and 16% disabled or retired.

In a univariate and multivariate stepwise logistic regression analysis we evaluated the influence of several factors on return to work. The parameters evaluated were; preoperative occupational status, gender, postoperative exercise tolerance, type and localization of preoperative valve lesion, additional bypass operation, age, and pre- and postoperative heart volume determined by x-ray (Tables VI and VII).

The univariate analysis of these factors showed that the preoperative employment status was most important for the postoperative return to work rate (Table 10.1-VI). Patients who were retired before the operation seldom returned to work postoperatively, in spite of a successful operation. Gender was found to play an important role in return to work; 80% of male patients returned to work, in comparison to 32% of female patients of the same age. The interpretation of these numbers needs to take into account the double task of women in being homemakers and participating in the work force. Also, postoperative exercise tolerance was of great importance for return to work, as was the type and location of the valve replaced.

Patients with aortic valve replacement had a higher return to work rate than those with mitral valve replacement (76% vs. 47%, p<0.02). 82% of patients with aortic stenosis returned to work, as did 67% of those with aortic insufficiency, and 78% of those with combined aortic valve lesions. 40% of patients with mitral stenosis returned to work, and 34% of those with combined mitral valve lesions. However, 69% of patients with isolated mitral insufficiency returned to work (Fig. 10.1-4). The preoperative heart volume determined by x-ray showed a significant correlation with return to work.

An additional bypass operation, or age, recognizing that these patients were all under 56 years, were of no importance.

The results of the multivariate analysis (Table 10.1-VII) showed that beside the preoperative occupational status and gender the postoperative exercise tolerance was the most important determinant of postoperative return to work rate.

Thus return to work after valve replacement is determined by a complex interplay of several medical and non-medical factors; preoperative employment status, gender and functional status after surgery are the most important determinants of postoperative employment. This leads to the conclusion that functional evaluation and improvement should have a high priority in comprehensive cardiac rehabilitation and vocational assessment of patients after valve replacement.

CONCLUSIONS

Successful valve replacement leads to an overall improvement in symptoms, functional performance, quality of life and longevity. The degree of subjective and objective improvement depends on multiple preoperative factors such as NYHA-status, left ventricular function, valve lesion and type of valve replaced, as well as peri- and postoperative factors such as the occurrence of perioperative myocardial infarction, the degree of intraoperative myocardial damage, the type of valve replacement and the speed and degree of postoperative regression of left ventricular hypertrophy and dilatation, together with improvement of left ventricular function.

Exercise tolerance, the ability to return to work and to participate in recreational activities including sports are important parameters which determine quality of life. Early rehabilitation is one important means of improving the degree to which these activities can be performed after surgery. On the other hand, rehabilitation can enable the patient to deal with the palliative aspects of valve surgery and the long term complications associated with this "newly acquired disease".

References
1. Kalmar P, Irrgang E. Cardiac Surgery in the Federal Republic of Germany during 1992. A Report of the German Society for Thoracic and Cardiovascular Surgery. Thorac Cardiovasc Surg 1993;41:202-204
2. Unger F, Hutter J. Open heart surgery in Europe 1990. Eur Heart J 1992;13:1345-1347
3. Kotler MN, Mintz GS, Panidis I, Morganroth J, Segal BL, Ross J. Noninvasive evaluation of normal and abnormal prosthetic valve function. JACC 1983;2:151-173
4. L'Heaff H, Nicolas G, Bouhour G. Etude des phonomecanogrammes chez les malades porteurs d'une prothese de Bjork en position aortique. Arch Mal Coeur 1976;69:143-146
5. Alam M, Rosman HS, Polanco GA, Sheth M, Garcia R, Serwin JB. Transesophageal echocardiographic features of stenotic bioprosthetic valves in the mitral and tricuspid valve positions. Am J Cardiol 1991;68:689-690
6. Alam M, Rosman HS, Sun I. Transesophageal echocardiographic evaluation of St. Jude Medical and bioprosthetic valve endocarditis. Am Heart J 1992;123:236-239

7.   Alton ME, Pasierski TJ, Orsinelli DA, Eaton GM, Pearson AC. Comparison of transthoracic and transesophageal echocardiography in evaluation of 47 Starr-Edwards prosthetic valves. JACC 1992;20:1503-1511
8.   Baumgartner J, Khan S, DeRobertis M, Czer L, Maurer G. Effect of prosthetic aortic valve design on the doppler-catheter gradient correlation: an in-vitro study of normal St Jude, Medtronic-Hall, Starr-Edwards and Hancock valves. JACC 1992;19:324-332
9.   Baumgarnter H, Schima H, Kühn P. Effect of prosthetic valve malfunction on the doppler-catheter gradient relation for bileaflet aortic valve prostheses. Circulation 1993;87:1320-1327
10.   Herrera CJ, Chaudhry FA, Defrino PF, et al. Value and limitations of transesophageal echocardiography in evaluating prosthetic or bioprosthetic valve dysfunction. Am J Cardiol 1992;69:697-699
11.   Nihoyannopoulos P, Kambouroglou D, Athanassopoulos G, Nadazdin A, Smith P, Oakley CM. Doppler hemodynamic profiles of clinically and echocardiographically normal mitral and aortic valve prostheses. Eur Heart J 1992;13:348-355
12.   Pedersen WR, Walker M, Olson JD, et al. Value of transesophageal echocardiography as an adjunct to transthoracic echocardiography in evaluation of native and prosthetic valve endocarditis. Chest 1991;100:351-356
13.   Perin EC, Jin BS, Decastro CM, Ferguson JJ, Hall RJ. Doppler Echocardiography in 180 normally functioning St. Jude Medical aortic valve prostheses; early and late postoperative assessments. Chest 1991;100:988-990
14.   Gohlke-Barwolf C, von Savigny L, Bubenheimer P, et al. Time sequence of regression of left ventricular hypertrophy after aortic valve replacement in patients with pure aortic stenosis. A prospective study. Eur Heart J 1987;9(Suppl 2):441 (Abstr.)
15.   Morris JJ, Schaft HV, Mullany CJ, et al. Determinants of survival and recovery of left ventricular function after aortic valve replacement. Ann Thorac Surg 1993;56:22-30
16.   Deutsch HJ, Bachmann R, Sechtem U, et al. Regurgitant flow in cardiac valve of gradient echo nuclear magnetic resonance imaging in reference to transesophageal 2-dimensional color doppler echocardiography. JACC 1992;19:1500-1507
17.   Gabrielsen FG, Berg-Johansen J, Hoeher M, Eggeling T, Kochs M, Hombach V. Normal hemodynamics of the Medtronics-Hall prosthetic valve in mitral position compared with other mitral valve prostheses as assessed by Doppler echocardiography. Am J Noninvas Cardiol 1992;6:363-366
18.   Reisner SA, Meltzer RS. Normal values of prosthetic valve doppler echocardiographic parameters: a review. J Am Soc Echocardiography 1988;201-210
19.   Malergue MC, Maribas P, Vignon P, Temkine J, Bical O, Gueret P. High incidence of asymptomatic thrombosis of mitral mechanical prostheses in the early postoperative period; demonstration by systematic transesophageal echocardiography (Abstract). Eur Heart J 1992;13(Abstr Suppl):1339,A-237
20.   Van den Brink RBA, Visser CA, Basart DCG, Düren Dr, de Jong AP, Dunning AJ. Comparison of transthoracic and transesophageal color doppler flow imaging in patients with mechanical prostheses in the mitral valve position. Am J Cardiol 1989;63:1471-1474
21.   Daniel WG, Mügge A, Grote J, et al. Comparison of transthoracic and transesophageal echocardiography for detection of abnormalities of prosthetic and bioprosthetic valves in the mitral and aortic positions. Am J Cardiol 1993;71:210-215
22.   Erbel R, Mohr-Kahaly S, Rohmann S, et al. Diagnostische Wertigkeit der transesophagealen Doppler-Echokardiographie. Herz 1987;12:177-186
23.   Iung B, Cormier B, Dadez E, et al. Small abnormal echos after mitral valve replacement with bileaflet mechanical prostheses: predisposing factors and effect on thromboembolism. J Heart Valve Dis 1993;2:259-266
24.   Burckhardt D, Striebel D, Vogt S, et al. Heart valve replacement with St. Jude Medical valve prosthesis: long term experience in 743 patients in Switzerland. Circulation 1988;78(Suppl I):I-18-I-24
25.   Alvarez L, Escudero C, Figuera D, Castillo-Olivares JI. Late sudden cardiac death in the follow-up of patients having a heart valve prosthesis. J Thorac Cardiovasc Surg 1992;104:502-510
26.   Creswell LL, Schuessler RB, Rosenbloom M, Cox JI. Hazards of postoperative atrial arrhythmias. Ann Thorac Surg 1993;56:539-549
27.   Foppl M, Hoffmann A, Amann FW, et al. Sudden cardiac death after aortic valve surgery: incidence and concomitant factors. Clin Cardiol 1989;12:202-207
28.   Gohlke-Barwolf C, Peters K, Petersen J, et al. Influence of aortic valve replacement on sudden death in patients with pure aortic stenosis. Eur Heart J 1988;9:Suppl E):139-141
29.   Gohlke-Barwolf C, Gohlke H, Verlauf. Komplikationen und Prognose der Aortenstenose. In: Roskamm H, Reindell H (eds). Herzkrankheiten. Springer-Verlag, Berlin Heidelberg 1989;3:1264-1266
30.   Livelli FD, Johnson RA, McEnany MT, et al. Unexplained in-hospital fever following cardiac surgery. Natural history, relationship to postpericardiotomy syndrome, and a prospective study of therapy with indomethacin versus placebo. Circulation 1978;57:968-975

31. Verkkala V, Valtonen V, Jarvinen A, Tolppanen EM. Fever, leukocytis and C-reactive protein after open-heart surgery and their value in the diagnosis of postoperative infections. Thorac Cardiovasc Surg 1987;35:78-82
32. Douglas P, Hirshfeld JW, Edmunds H. Clinical correlates of postoperative atrial fibrillation. Circulation 1984;70(Suppl II):165 (Abstr.)
33. Acar J, Hanania G, Lancelin B, Fanjoux J, Auperin A, Kpodunu J. Les modifications electroradiographiques apres chiruregie sous circulation extracorporelle pour remplacement valvulaire. A propos de 95 interventions. Arch Mal Coeur 1971;64:1160-1181
34. Cox JL. A perspective of postoperative atrial fibrillation in cardiac operations. Ann Thorac Surg 1993;56:405-409
35. Johnson LW, Dickstein RA, Fruehan CT, et al. Prophylactic digitalization for coronary artery bypass surgery. Circulation 1976;53:819-822
36. Platia EV, Fitzpatrick P, Wallis D, Antman EM, Michelson EL, Hus TA. Esmolol vs. Verapamil for the treatment of recent-onset atrial fibrillation/flutter; a multicenter study, JACC 1988;11:170A
37. Silverman NA, Wright R, Levitsky S. Efficacy of low-dose propranolol in preventing postoperative supraventricular tachyarrhythmias. Ann Surg 1982;73:196-197
38. Davison R, Hartz R, Kaplan K, et al. Prophylaxis of supraventricular tachyarrhythmias after coronary bypass surgery with oral verapamil: a randomized, double-blind trial. Ann Thorac Surg 1985;39:336-339
39. Suttorp MJ, Kingma JH, Koomen EM, van't Hof A, Tijssen JGP, Lie KI. Recurrence of paroxysmal atrial fibrillation or flutter after successful cardioversion in patients with normal left ventricular function. Am J Cardiol 1993;71:710-713
40. Janssen J, Loomann L, Harink J, et al. Prevention and treatment of supraventricular tachycardia shortly after coronary artery bypass grafting: a randomized open trial. Angiology 1986;37:601-609
41. Forst L, Mälgaard H, Christiansen EJ, Hjortholm K, Paulsen PK, Thomsen PEB. Atrial fibrillation and flutter after coronary artery bypass surgery: epidemiology risk factors and preventive trials. Int J Cardiol 1992;36:253-261
42. Installe E, Schoevaerdts JC, Gadisseux P, Charles S, Tremouroux J. Intravenous amiodarone in the treatment of various arrhythmias following cardiac operations. J Thorac Cardiovasc Surg 1981;81:302-308
43. Peels HOJ, Suttorp MJ, Koomen EM, et al. Supraventricular tachyarrhythmias early after coronary artery bypass graft surgery: analysis of risk factors. JACC 1991;17:211 (Abstr.)
44. Antman EM. Medical management of the patient undergoing cardiac surgery. In: Braunwald E. Heart Disease. W B Saunders Company, Philadelphia, 4th edition 1992;53:1670-1689
45. Gohlke-Barwolf C, Acar J, Burckhardt D, et al. Guidelines for prevention of thromboembolic events in valvular heart disease. J Heart Valve Dis 1993;2:398-410
46. Michael PL, Mandagout O, Vahanian A, et al. Ventricular arrhythmias in aortic valve disease before and after surgery. J Heart Valve Dis 1992;1:72-77
47. Thomas JL, Dickstein RA, Parker FB, et al. Prognostic significance of the development of left bundle conduction defects following aortic valve replacement. J Thorac Cardiovasc Surg 1982;84:382-386
48. Thompson R, Mitchell A, Ahmed T, Towers M, Yacoub M. Conduction defects in aortic valve disease. Am Heart J 1979;98:3-10
49. Fournial JF, Brodaty D, Chomette G, Tereau Y, Cabrol C, Acar J. Troubles conductifs apres remplacement valvulaire aortique. A propos de 200 cas. Arch Mal Coeur 1978;72:4-11
50. Kalusche D, Betz P, Roskamm H, Intraventrikulare Erregungsleitungsstorungen bei Patienten mit kalzifizierten Aortenvitien: Pra- und postoperative Haufigkeit und Einfluss auf die Prognose nach Aortenklappenersatz. Z Kardiol 1986;75:147-150
51. Brodell GK, Cosgrove D, Schiavone W, Underwood DA, Loop FD. Cardiac rhythm and conduction disturbances in patients undergoing mitral valve surgery. Cleveland Clin J Med 1991;58:397-399
52. Kutcher MA, King SB, Alimurung BN, Craver JM, Logue RB. Constrictive pericarditis as a complication of cardiac surgery: recognition of an entity. Am J Cardiol 1982;50:742-748
53. Weitzman LB, Tinker PW, Kronzon I, et al. The incidence and natural history of pericardial effusion after cardiac surgery. Circulation 1984;69:506-511
54. Jones MR, Vine DL, Attas M, et al. Late isolated left ventricular tamponade: clinical hemodynamic and echocardiographic manifestations of a previously unreported postoperative complication. J Thorac Cardiovasc Surg 1979;77:142-145
55. D'Cruz IA, Kensey K, Campbell C, et al. Two-dimensional echocardiography in cardiac tamponade occurring after cardiac surgery. J Am Coll Card 1985;5:1250-1252
56. Bateman T, Gray R, Chaux A, et al. Right atrial tamponade caused by hematoma complicating coronary artery bypass graft surgery: clinical hemodynamic and scintigraphic correlates. J Thorac Cardiovasc Surg 1982;84:413-419
57. Albat B, Picard E, Messner Pellenc P, Thevenet A. Tamponade tardive par compression localisee des cavites gauches apres chirurgie valvulaire. Arch Mal Coeur 1991;84:1961-1964

58. Weeks KR, Chatterjee K, Block S, et al. Bedside hemodynamic monitoring - its value in the diagnosis of tamponade complication cardiac surgery. J Thorac Cardiovasc Surg 1976;71:250-252
59. Shabatai R, Fowler NO, Guntherroth WG. The hemodynamics of cardiac tamponade and constrictive pericarditis. Am J Cardiol 1970;26:480-487
60. Gohlke-Barwolf C, Gohlke H, Samek L, et al. Exercise tolerance and working capacity after valve replacement. J Heart Valve Dis 1992;1:189-195
61. Borer JS, Herrold EM, Hochreiter C, et al. Natural history of left ventricular performance at rest and during exercise after aortic valve replacement for aortic regurgitation. Circulation 1991;84(Suppl):133-139
62. Gaasch WH, Zile MR. Left ventricular function after surgical correction of chronic mitral regurgitation. Eur Heart J 1991;12(Suppl B):48-51
63. Zile MR, Tomita M, Ishihara K, et al. Changes in diastolic function during development and correction of chronic LV volume overload produced by mitral regurgitation. Circulation 1993;87:1378-1388
64. Starling MR, Kirsh MM, Montgomery DG, Gross MD. Impaired left ventricular contractile function in patients with long-term mitral regurgitation and normal ejection fraction. JACC 1993;22:230-250
65. Taniguchi K, Nakano S, Kawashima Y, et al. Left ventricular ejection performance, wall stress, and contractile state in aortic regurgitation before and after aortic valve replacement. Circulation 1990;82:798-807
66. Acar J, Luxereau P, Vahanian A. Criteria for postoperative reversibility of heart failure of valvular origin. Research in Cardiac Hypertrophy and Failure. B Swynghedauw 1990 Inserm/John Libbey Eurotext, pp. 631-646
67. Luxereau P, Herreman F, Carlet F, Lutfalla G, Acar J. Hemodynamic data and left ventricular function of diseased mitral valves replaced by prostheses. The mitral valve D Kalmanson. Action Mass. Publishing Sciences Group Inc 1976
68. Haeusslein EA, Greenberg BH, Massie BM. Does the magnitude of mitral regurgitation determine hemodynamic response to vasodilation in chronic congestive heart failure? Chest 1991;100:1312-1315
69. Ziskind Z, Pohoryles L, Mohr R, et al. The effect of low-dose intravenous nitroglycerin on pulmonary hypertension immediately after replacement of a stenotic mitral valve. Circulation 1985;72(Suppl II):164-169
70. Camara ML, Aris A, Padro JM, et al. Long-term results of mitral valve surgery in patients with severe pulmonary hypertension. Ann Thorac Surg 1988;45:133-136
71. Jegaden O, Rossi R, Delahaye F, et al. Long-term results of mitral valve replacement in patients with severe pulmonary hypertension. Arch Mall Coeur 1991;84:1297-1301
72. Nitter-Hauge S, Froysaker T, Hall KV. Clinical and hemodynamic findings following prosthetic valve replacement for mitral valve disease. Acta Med Scand 1976;200:215
73. Acar J, Luxereau PH, Ducimetiere P, et al. Prognosis of surgically treated aortic valve disease. J Thorac Cardiovasc Surg 1981;82:114-126
74. Tracy GP, Prodor MS, Hizny CS. Reversibility of pulmonary artery hypertension in aortic stenosis after aortic valve replacement. Ann Thorac Surg 1990;50:89-93
75. Jegaden O, Rossi R, Delahaye F, et al. Long-term prognosis of surgically treated aortic valve disease with pulmonary hypertension. A series of thirty-four cases (in French). Arch Mal Coeur 1992;85:33-37
76. Loop FD, Lytle BW, Cosgrove DM, et al. Sternal wound complications after isolated coronary artery bypass grafting: Early and late mortality, morbidity and cost of care. Ann Thorac Surg 1990;49:179-187
77. Demmy TL, Park SB, Liebler GA, et al. Recent experience with major sternal wound complications. Ann Thorac Surg 1990;49:458-462
78. Culliford AT, Cunningham JW, Zeaff RN, et al. Sternal and costochondral infections following open heart surgery. J Thorac Cardiovasc Surg 1976;72:714-726
79. Schlosser V, Graedrich G, Dentz J, Ilgen J, Nguyen LDT. Extrakardiale Organschaden als Komplikation nach Eingriffen am offenen Herzen. Z Herz-, thorax-, Gefasschir 1993;7:1-7
80. Alter HJ, Purcell RH, Shih JW, et al. Detection of antibody to hepatitis C virus in prospectively followed transfusion recipients with acute and chronic non-A, non-B hepatitis. N Engl J Med 1989;321:1494-1500
81. Kellner S, Preiss DU, Betz P, Samek L, Wilhelm K. Post-transfusion hepatitis in cardiac surgical patients. 18th Congress of the International Society of Blood Transfusion. Abstract P1-08. Karger, Basel 1984
82. Preiss DU, Schmidt-Bleibtreu H, Berguson P, Metz G. Blood transfusion requirements in coronary artery surgery with and without the activated clotting time (ACT) technique. Klin Wochenschrift 1985;63:252-256
83. Schiff M, Katz A, Farber B, Kaplan M. Acquired immuno-deficiency syndrome. A complication of cardiovascular surgery. J Thorac Cardiovasc Surg 1989;97:126-129
84. Cohen A, Munoz A, Reitz BA, et al. Transmission of retroviruses of transfusion or screened blood in patients undergoing cardiac surgery. N Engl J Med 1989;320:1171-1176
85. Adrian J, Brankshaw DP, Tiller JW, et al. Effective, cognitive and subjective changes in patients undergoing cardiac surgery - a preliminary report. Anaesth Intensive Care 1988;16:144-149
86. Towns BD. Bashein G, Hornbein TF, et al. Neurobehavioral outcomes in cardiac operations. J Thorac

Cardiovasc Surg 1989;98:774-782

87. Aberg T, Ronquist G, Tyden H, et al. Adverse effects on the brain in cardiac operations as assessed by biochemical psychosomatic and radiologic methods. J Thorac Cardiovasc Surg 1984;87:99-105

88. Cosgrove DM, Loop FD, Lytle BW, et al. Primary myocardial revascularisation. J Thorac Cardiovasc Surg 1984;88:673-684

89. Fish KJ, Helms KN, Sarnquist FH, et al. A prospective randomized study of the effects of prostacyclin on neuropsychological dysfunction after coronary artery surgery. J Thorac Cardiovasc Surg 1987;93:609

90. Shahian DM, Speert PK. Symptomatic visual deficits after open heart operations. Ann Thorac Surg 1989;48:275-279

91. Reed GL, Singer DE, Pilard EH. Stroke following coronary artery bypass surgery. A case control estimate of the risk of carotid bruits. N Engl J Med 1988;319:1246-1250

92. Breuer AC, Franco I, Marzewski D, et al. Left ventricular thrombi seen by ventriculography are a significant risk factor for stroke in open heart surgery. Ann Neurol 1981;10:103-104

93. Taylor GJ, Malik SA, Colliver JA, et al. Usefulness of atrial fibrillation as a predictor of stroke after isolated coronary artery bypass grafting. Am J Cardiol 1987;60:905-907

94. Aranha GV, Pickleman J, Pifarre R, et al. The reasons for gastrointestinal consultation after cardiac surgery. Am Surg 1984;50:301-304

95. Heikkinen L, Alz Kulji K. Abdominal complications following cardiopulmonary bypass in open-heart surgery. Scand J Thorac Cardiovasc Surg 1987;21:1-7

96. BCSH Hemostasis and Thrombosis Task Force. Guidelines on oral anticoagulation (2nd ed). J Clin Pathol 1990;43:177-183

97. Hirsh J, Dalen JE, Deykin D, Poller L. Oral anticoagulants; mechanisms of action, clinical effectiveness, and optimal therapeutic range. Chest 1992;102(Suppl 4):312S-326S

98. Loeliger EA. Therapeutic target values in oral anticoagulation - justification of Dutch policy and a warning against the so-called moderate-intensity regimens. Ann Hematol 1992;64:60-65

99. Poller L. Oral anticoagulants and heparin; standardization of laboratory monitoring. In: Poller L, Thomson JM, (eds). Thrombosis and its management. Churchill Livingstone, Edinburgh, 1993:200-213

100. Samama M, Acar J. Traitements antithrombotiques. Collection de monographies cardiologiques. Masson, Paris, 1993

101. Saour JN, Sieck JO, Mamo LAR, Gallus AS. Trial of different intensities of anticoagulation in patients with prosthetic heart valves. N Engl J Med 1990;322:428-432

102. Turpie AGG, Gunstensen J, Hirsh J, Nelson H, Gent M. Randomisierter Vergleich zweier DosierungsstNrken zur oralen Antikoagulantienthterapie nach Bioklappenersatz. The Lancet (German edition) 1988;2:587-590

103. Altmann R, Rouvier J, Gurfinkel E, et al. Comparison of two levels of anticoagulation therapy in patients with substitute heart valves. J Thorac Cardiovasc Surg 1991;101:427-431

104. Butchart EG, Lewis PA, Bethel JA, Breckenridge IM. Adjusting anticoagulation to prosthesis thrombogenicity and patient risk factors. Circulation 1991;84(Suppl III):61-69

105. Nuşez L, Aguado GM, Larrea JL, Celemin D, Oliver J. Prevention of thromboembolism using aspirin after mitral valve replacement with porcine bioprosthesis. Ann Thorac Surg 1984;37:84-87

106. Turpie AGG, Gent M, Laupacis A, et al. A comparison of aspirin with placebo in patients treated with warfarin after heart-valve replacement. N Engl J Med 1993;329:524-529

107. Rizzoli G, Russo R, Valente S, et al. Dehiscence of aortic valve prosthesis: analysis of a ten-year experience. Internat J Cardiol 1984;6:207-218

108. Schoen FJ, Hobsen EC. Anatomic analysis of removed prosthetic heart valves; causes of failure of 33 mechanical valves and bioprostheses, 1980 to 1983. Hum Path 1985;16:549-558

109. Horstkotte D, Loogen F, unter Mitarbeit von W. Bircks. Erworbene Herzklappenfehler. Urban & Schwarzenberg, München-Wien-Baltimore, 1987;314-315

110. Barnhorst DA, Oxmann HA, Conolly DC, et al. Long-term follow up of isolated replacement of the aortic or mitral valve with the Starr-Edwards prosthesis. Am J Cardiol 1975;35:228-233

111. Van der Graaf Y, de Waard F, van Herwerden LA, Defauw. Risk of strut fracture of Björk-Shiley valves. Lancet 1992;339:257-261

112. Hiratzka LF, Kouchoukos NT, Grunkemeier GL, Miller C, Scully HE, Wechsler AS. Outlet strut fracture of the Bjork-Shiley 60° convexo-concave valve: current information and recommendations for patient care. JACC 1988;11:1130-1137

113. Ostermeyer J, Horstkotte D, Bennet J, et al. The Bjork-Shiley 70° convexo-concave prosthesis strut fracture problem. J Thorac Cardiovasc Surg 1987;35:71-77

114. Dimitri W, Williams BT. Fracture of the Duromedics mitral valve housing with leaflet escape. J Cardiovasc Surg 1990;31:41-46

115. Orsinelli DA, Becker RC, Cuenoud HF, Moran JM. Mechanical failure of a St. Jude medical prosthesis. Am J Cardiol 1991;67:906-908

116. Gunther H-U, Stegmann T. Klappenbruch und Segelembolisation einer St. Jude-Medical-Aortenklappenprothese. Z Herz-. Thorax-, Gefässchir 1987;1:206-208
117. Kratz JM, Crawford FA, Sade RM, Crumbley AJ, Stroud MR. St. Jude prosthesis for aortic and mitral valve replacement: a ten-year experience. Ann Thorac Surg 1993;56:462-468
118. Arom K. St. Jude Medical prostheses: another 10-year follow-up report. Ann Thorac Surg 1993;56:403-404
119. Lindblom D. Long-term clinical results after aortic valve replacement with Björk-Shiley prosthesis. J Thorac Cardiovasc Surg 1988;95:658-667
120. Deviri E, Sareli P, Wisenbaugh T, Cronje SL. Obstruction of mechanical heart valve prostheses: clinical aspects and surgical management. JACC 1991;17:646-650
121. Horstkotte D, Pippert H, Korfer R. Hamolytische Anamie als Folge einer hamodynamisch unbedeutenden paravalvularen Dehiszenz nach St Jude-Medical-Aortenklappenersatz. Z Kardiol 1986;75:502-504
122. DiSesa VJ, Collins JJ, Cohn LH. Hematological complications with the St Jude valve and reduced-dose coumadin. Ann Thorac Surg 1989;48:280-283
123. Horstkotte D, Aul C, Seipel L. Einfluss von Klappentyp und Klappenfunktion auf die chronische intravasale Hamolyse nach alloprothetischem Mitral- und Aortenklappenersatz. Z Kardiol 1983;119
124. Teoh KH, Ivanov J, Weisel RD, Daniel LB, Darcel IC, Rakowski H. Clinical and Doppler echocardiographic evaluation of bioprosthetic valve failure after 10 years. Circulation 1990;82(Suppl IV):110-116
125. Burdon A, Miller DC, Oyer PE, et al. Durability of porcine valves at fifteen years in a representative North American patient population. J Thorac Cardiovasc Surg 1992;103:238-252
126. Hammermeister KE, Sethi GK, Henderson WG, Oprian C, Kin T, Rahimtoola S. A comparison of outcomes in men 11 years after heart-valve replacement with a mechanical valve or bioprosthesis. N Engl J Med 1993; 328:1269-1296
127. Helft G, Tabone X, Georges JL, et al. Resultats Ö moyen terme des bioprotheses apres 65 ans. Arch Mal Coeur 1993;86:1415-1420
128. Pelletier LC, Carrier M, Leclerc Y, Dyrda I, Gosselin G. Influence of age on late results of valve replacement with porcine bioprosthesis. J Cardiovasc Surg 1992;33:526-533
129. Report of the WHO expert Committee on Disability Prevention and Rehabilitation. Disability, prevention and rehabilitation. WHO Tech Ser no 668, World Health Organisation, Geneva 1981
130. Greenland P, Chu JS. Efficacy of cardiac rehabilitation services. With emphasis on patients after myocardial infarction. Ann Intern Med 1988;109:650-663
131. Bruce RA, Larson EB, Startton J. Physical fitness, functional aerobic capacity, aging and responses to physical training or bypass surgery in coronary patients. J Cardiopulmonary Rehabil 1989;9:24-34
132. Oberman A. Does cardiac rehabilitation increase long term survival after myocardial infarction? Circulation 1989;80:416-418
133. O'Connor GT, Buring JE, Yusuf S, et al. An overview of randomized trials of rehabilitation with exercise after myocardial infarction. Circulation 1989;80:234-244
134. Oldridge NB, Guyatt GH, Fischer ME, Rimm AA. Cardiac rehabilitation after myocardial infarction. J Am Med Ass 1988;260:945-950
135. Wenger NK. Rehabilitation of the patient with atherosclerotic coronary heart disease. In: Braunwald E (ed). Heart disease. WB Saunders Company, Philadelphia, 1992;(4th ed)54:1103-1118
136. Newell JP, Kappagoda CT, Stoker JB, Deverall PB, Watson DA, Linden RJ. Physical training after heart valve replacement. Br Heart J 1980;44:638-649
137. Sire S. Physical training and occupational rehabilitation after aortic valve replacement. Eur Heart J 1987;8:1215-1220
138. Habel-Verge C, Landry F, Desaulnier D, et al. L'entrainement physique apres un remplacement valvulaire mitral. Can Med Ass J 1987;136:142-147
139. Gohlke-Barwolf C, Roskamm H. Ergebnisse des Herzklappenersatzes. Prognose - Arbeits-und Leistungsfahigkeit - Berufliche Wiedereingliederung. Versicherungsmedizin 1992;44:163-168
140. Borg G. The perception of physical performance. In: Shephard RJ (ed). Frontiers of fitness. Charles C Thomas, Springfield III, 1971
141. Borg GA. Perceived exertion: a note on history and methods. Med Sci Sports 1973;5:90-93
142. Borg GA. Psychophysical basis of perceived exertion. Med Sci Sports 1982;14:377-381
143. Rutenberg HD, Molla JH, Strong WB, Fischer G, Adams TD. Recommended guidelines for graded exercise resting and exercise prescription for children with heart disease. J Card Rehab 1984;4:10-16
144. Fiatarone MA, Marks EC, Ryan ND, Meredßith CN, Lipsitz LA, Evans WJ. High-intensity strength training in nonagenarians. Effects on skeletal muscle. JAMA 1990;263:3029-3034
145. Samek L, Lehmann M, Keul J, Roskamm H. Ruckwirkungen leichter Schwinnbelastungen bei KHK-Patienten und gesunden Kontrollpersonen aud Kreislaufgrossen, Katecholamine und Laktatspiegel. In: Rieckert H (ed). Sportmedizin - Kursbestimmung. Springer-Verlag, Heidelberg, 1987:912-915

146. Cheitlin MD, Bonow RO, Parmley WW, Roberts WC, Swan HJC, Williams JF. Task force II: Acquired valvular heart disease. JACC 1985;6:1209-1214
147. Mitchell JH, Blomquist CG, Haskell WL, et al. Classification of sports. JACC 1985;6:1198-1199.
148. Gohlke-Barwolf C, Roskamm H. Langzeitergebnisse nach Herzklappenoperation. Massnahmen und Ergebnisse der Rehabilitation. In: Berghoff A (ed). Kardiologische Rehabilitation 1987. Berlin 1988;141-150
149. Carstens V, Behrenbeck DW, Hilger HH. Exercise capacity before and after cardiac valve surgery. Cardiology 1983;70(Suppl 1):41-49
150. Fuhrer U, Both G, Fischer K, et al. Sozialanamnestische und hamodynamische Untersuchungen 4 bis 6 Jahre nach prothetischem Klappenersatz. Z Kardiol 1977;66:251-256
151. Mattern H, Wisshirchen KJ, Fricke G, Bernard A, Belastbarkeit und berufliche Wiedereingliederung nach prothetischem Klappenersatz in Abhangigkeit von der postoperativen HÑmodynamik. Z Kardiol 1979;68:36-40
152. Schwarz F, Baumann P, Manthey J, et al. The effect of aortic valve replacement on survival. Circulation 1982;66:1105-1110
153. Thormann I, Glaser G, Jelavic T, et al. Langzeitergebnisse nach Herzklappenersatz. Z Kardiol 1980;69:625-631
154. Walter PJ, Ibe B, Gottwik M. Return to work after heart valve replacement. In: Walter PJ (ed). Return to work after coronary artery bypass surgery. Springer-Verlag, Berlin Heidelberg New York Tokyo, 1985:125-133
155. Gohlke-Bärwolf C, Gohlke H, Peters K, et al. Welche Faktoren beeinflussen die berufliche Wiedereingliederung nach Herzklappenersatz? Z Kardiol 1990;79(Suppl 1):20

Chapter 10.2

Echocardiographic Assessment of Prosthetic Heart Valves

Richard A. Jones, Alan G. Fraser

Developments in the use of ultrasound for cardiac imaging have made the non-invasive assessment of prosthetic heart valves quick, convenient and accurate. The combination of cross-sectional imaging, color flow mapping and spectral Doppler allows a comprehensive assessment of valvular structure and function to be made. The advent of transesophageal echocardiography has enhanced our ability to assess prosthetic valves, in particular those in the mitral and tricuspid positions. Previously, phonocardiography, cinefluoroscopy and cardiac catheterization provided the main means of assessing valvular function. In certain circumstances the first two techniques may still prove useful, but mostly they have been superseded by echocardiographic assessment. Cardiac catheterization remains the standard invasive method, but it can now be avoided in most patients (1). This is particularly useful in patients with mechanical prostheses, because of problems related to anticoagulation. Furthermore, catheterization is time-consuming, can be technically difficult and carries risks. It is therefore not well suited to the routine follow up of patients with prosthetic valves.

We describe the echocardiographic features of normal prosthetic valves, and the abnormalities that may be found within each class of valve during dysfunction. We also review the uses and limitations of Doppler-derived data in the assessment of prosthetic valves.

ECHOCARDIOGRAPHIC ASSESSMENT

Cross-sectional echocardiography

In skilled hands, this technique can give much information on valve structure and function. The site and orientation of the prosthesis can be seen, and the motion of the occluder in mechanical valves or of the leaflets in bioprosthetic valves can usually be identified. Absence of sharp opening and closing movements raises the suspicion of obstruction. Mechanical mitral valves open rapidly early in diastole and do not exhibit the mid-diastolic partial closure characteristic of normal and bioprosthetic valves. A mitral prosthesis may protrude into the left ventricular outflow tract, and if such protrusion is excessive it may result in obstruction of the outflow tract (2,3).

Cross-sectional echocardiography is useful in demonstrating masses attached to prosthetic valves. Thrombus and vegetations are echogenic and may be identified in continuity with the valve ring, cage or occluding device. However, the limited resolution of precordial cross-sectional echocardiography, and the numerous artifactual echoes created by a metal prosthesis, make it difficult to characterize echogenic structures associated with heart valves. Often it is not clear whether echoes close to or within a valve

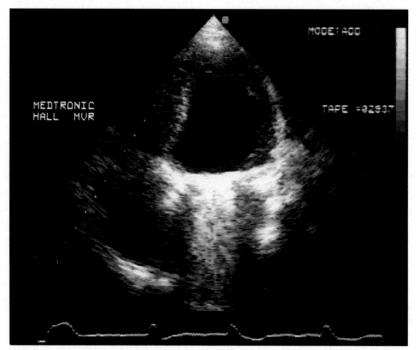

Figure 10.2-1: Apical four-chamber view. A Medtronic Hall prosthesis in the mitral position obscures the left atrium.

are real or artifactual. In addition, from the precordium it is almost impossible to interrogate the atrial aspect of a mitral prosthesis because of acoustic shadowing (Fig. 10.2-1). The proximity of a transesophageal transducer to the heart allows higher frequencies to be used, so the transesophageal approach gives better resolution (typically 0.5 mm axial and 2.0 mm lateral resolution with a 5 MHz transducer). The morphology of solid structures and their attachments may be identified, and movement in relation to the valve during the cardiac cycle studied. Thrombus or vegetations on the atrial aspect of a mitral prosthesis may be seen to prolapse through the valve (Fig. 10.2-2). Individual sutures may be identified as thin relatively immobile structures which are almost uniform in length and regularly spaced (Figs. 10.2-3 & 10.2-4). Recently, some authors have reported that transesophageal echocardiography performed early after mitral valve replacement may demonstrate highly mobile filamentous structures on prosthetic valves (Fig. 10.2-5). The characteristic appearance of these small abnormal echoes, their association with early thromboembolic episodes, and also their frequent disappearance, have been taken to imply that these echoes are caused by strands of fibrin (4).

Many patients with prosthetic mitral valves demonstrate spontaneous echocardiographic contrast in the left atrium or the left atrial appendage, especially when they are imaged from the transesophageal approach. Swirling particulate echoes are seen, with an appearance which has been likened to wisps of smoke. It occurs whenever the velocity of blood flow is very low (less than 20 cm/sec) and shear stress is low, and it may be caused by platelet aggregation as well as by clumping of red blood cells (5). It is also influenced by circulating levels of fibrinogen. Although the

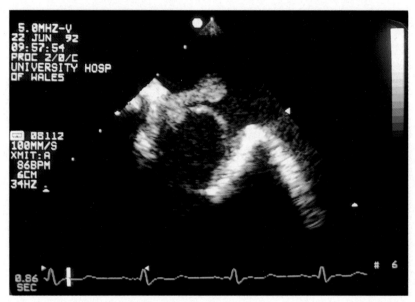

Figure 10.2-2: A large thrombus attached to this bioprosthetic valve is seen prolapsing into the left atrium during systole.

appearances are non-specific in the sense that they are found in patients with normally functioning prostheses as well as in those with dysfunction, the presence of spontaneous echocardiographic contrast is important because it is a marker of increased thromboembolic risk (6). The pattern is sometimes particularly marked in a patient with an obstructed prosthesis. When spontaneous echo contrast is seen, the atrial appendage should be examined carefully for the presence of thrombi.

DOPPLER ECHOCARDIOGRAPHY

Color flow mapping

Color flow maps are useful for guiding alignment of the pulsed wave or continuous wave cursor and for placement of the sample volume for the spectral analysis of transvalvular jets (7). Color flow mapping is also the best technique for identifying the site and estimating the severity of physiologic and pathologic regurgitation (8). From the esophagus, it is particularly useful for identifying the origin of any mitral regurgitant jets and for detecting their extent and timing.

The peak velocity increases as blood crosses any narrowed orifice such as an obstructed prosthesis or a paraprosthetic regurgitant orifice. If the increase in velocity exceeds the limit of the velocity range of the color flow map (the Nyquist limit), then the color display will show 'aliasing' - that is, flow will be displayed as occurring in the opposite direction, with a sharp transition from one color (such as blue) to the opposite one (such as red). Around a prosthetic valve this creates 'convergence zones'. These may be seen with normal prostheses (Fig. 10.2-6), but they are particularly prominent when there is obstruction.

Color flow maps show turbulent flow through and distal to prosthetic valves. Absence

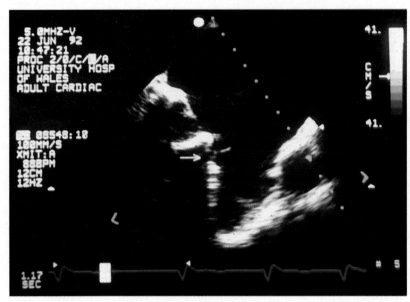

Figure 10.2-3: Transesophageal image of a prosthetic mitral valve, showing a dehisced suture in the left atrium (arrow). There is an accompanying paraprosthetic regurgitant orifice.

of turbulent flow in an area where it is normally expected raises the suspicion of obstruction. For example, the width of each of the two forward jets through the major and minor orifices of the Björk-Shiley valve is about a quarter of the width of the valve ring (9). Absence or a decrease in size of one or both of these jets suggests valvular obstruction.

Convergence zones may also identify blood accelerating towards a regurgitant orifice (10). Their presence around the sewing ring of a mitral prosthesis when it is studied by precordial echocardiography may be taken to imply the presence of a paraprosthetic regurgitant jet, even when this cannot be demonstrated directly because flow within the left atrium is masked by the prosthesis. Color M-mode recordings obtained when the cursor is placed through the area of turbulence allow the timing and duration of regurgitation to be assessed (Fig. 10.2-7).

Spectral Doppler

This technique gives the most precise information about prosthetic valve function since it is possible to measure maximal and mean velocity of flow across a valve, and from these to derive estimated pressure gradients. For valves in the mitral and tricuspid positions, the pressure half-time can be measured and the effective orifice area can be calculated using the Hatle equation (11) (Table 10.2-I). The continuity equation (12) can also be used in conjunction with Doppler-derived data for the assessment of prosthetic function. There are theoretical limitations to the use of these formulae with Doppler ultrasonography in the setting of prosthetic valve disease (13) but acceptable correlations have nonetheless been demonstrated between Doppler- and catheter-derived data (14). It is important not to rely on a single method for deriving valve

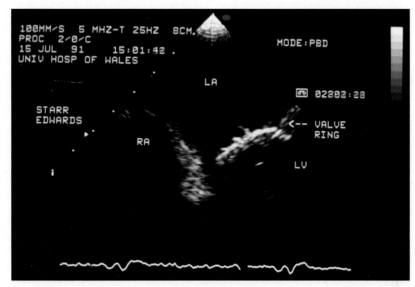

Figure 10.2-4: Transesophageal echocardiogram showing four short regularly spaced sutures attached to the valve sewing ring of this Starr-Edwards prosthesis.

gradient or area, and to study each particular prosthesis using a method that has been validated. For complete assessment, several approaches and different methods of calculation should be used, so that erroneous single measurements can be recognized and discarded.

Doppler assessment of mitral prostheses

Mitral inflow occurs at a relatively low velocity and therefore it can sometimes be interrogated using pulsed-wave Doppler. As for native valves, the sample volume is placed at the tip of the valve leaflets, or in the case of mechanical valves just distal to the valve structure. Bioprosthetic valve flow is central and thus interrogation will be similar to normal. The direction and pattern of flow through mechanical prostheses varies according to their design. Color flow mapping is used to place the sample volume in the area of maximal flow in order to obtain as accurate and reproducible a tracing as possible. With obstruction to forward flow across a mitral prosthesis, the peak diastolic velocity is expected to increase. However, the velocity will also rise when flow is increased by significant mitral regurgitation. In this situation the pressure half-time, which is relatively independent of flow, helps to differentiate between the two. With obstruction, both the velocity and the pressure half-time increase, whereas with increased flow alone, the velocity increases but pressure half-time remains normal (Fig. 10.2-8). Estimated normal values of velocities and pressure half-times for a selection of prostheses are given in Table 10.2-I. These data were obtained from a review of the literature and should be considered as an approximate guide only.

Identification of regurgitation using spectral Doppler from the precordium is difficult because of flow masking of the left atrium by the mechanical valve. Some bioprostheses, although made of animal tissue, are fashioned on a metal stent which can also mask

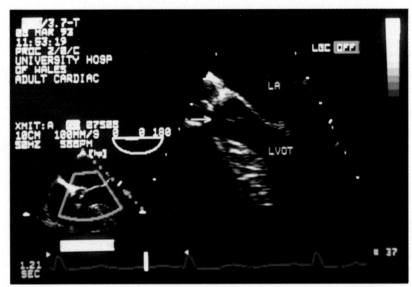

Figure 10.2-5: A fibrin strand attached to an aortic prosthesis is seen in the left ventricular outflow tract (arrow).

regurgitation in the left atrium. The use of color flow mapping has now largely replaced the time-consuming search for regurgitation using pulsed-wave Doppler from the precordium. Transesophageal imaging allows detailed spectral Doppler interrogation of the atria and is therefore used in conjunction with color flow mapping for the detection of regurgitation.

Doppler assessment of aortic prostheses

Continuous-wave Doppler is extremely useful for identifying the velocity across

Table 10.2-I: Doppler characteristics of prosthetic valves in the mitral position

Valve	V max	G max	G mean	t1/2	MVA
Björk-Shiley	1.5	2	6	87	2.5
Carpentier-Edwards	1.8 ± 0.3	13 ± 5	6 ± 1	89 ± 25	2.5
Hancock	1.5	10	3 ± 1	109	2.1
Ionescu-Shiley	1.4 ± 0.5	8	3 ± 1	87 ± 25	2.6
Medtronic Hall	1.9	15	3	76	2.9 ± 0.5
Medtronic Intact	1.5	10	5 ± 2	104	2.0 ± 0.4
Omni/Lillehei-Kaster	1.8 ± 0.3	14	6	119	1.9
Starr-Edwards	1.88	15	5 ± 2	109	2.1
St. Jude	1.5	9.2	4	64	2.9

Velocities are in m/s, gradients in mmHg and areas in cm^2. Where available the standard deviation is given. Vmax: maximal velocity; Gmax: maximal gradient; G mean: mean gradient; t1/2: pressure half-time (ms); MVA: mitral valve area

Table 10.2-II: Doppler characteristics of prosthetic valves in the aortic position

Valve	V max	G max	G mean	EOA
Björk-Shiley	2.4	23	10-18	
Carpentier-Edwards	2.9 ± 0.5	26	17.032	
Hancock	2.5	23	11 ± 2	
Ionescu-Shiley	2.4	22 ± 8	14 ± 4	1.2 ± 0.2
Medtronic Hall	2.28	21 ± 7	10 ± 4	1.5 ± 0.6
Medtronic Intact	2.74	31 ± 11	18 ± 7	1.3 ± 0.2
Omni/Lillehei-Kaster	3.2	40	24	—
Starr-Edwards	3.16	41	25.4	
St. Jude	2.4	24	7-19	1.8 ± 0.7

Velocities are in m/s, gradients in mmHg and areas in cm^2. Where available the standard deviation is given. Vmax: maximal velocity; Gmax: maximal gradient; G mean: mean gradient; EOA: effective orifice area. Data obtained from review of published series.

prosthetic aortic valves (15,16). Acoustic reverberation may disrupt a continuous wave signal from the apex and therefore the suprasternal, right parasternal, supraclavicular and subcostal views should also be used. From the peak velocity, an estimated peak gradient is obtained using the modified Bernoulli equation (Table 10.2-II). It should be noted that the peak Doppler-derived gradient is not the same as the peak catheter-derived gradient. The latter is not instantaneous, but the difference between peak left ventricular and aortic pressures. Doppler-derived mean gradients are more directly comparable to catheter-derived data.

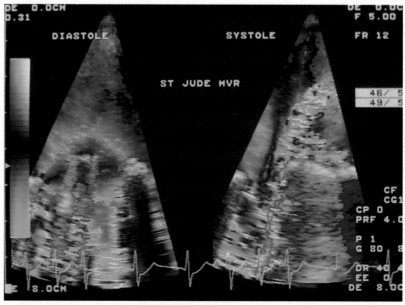

Figure 10.2-6: On the left (diastolic frame) a convergence zone is seen proximal to this St. Jude Medical mitral prosthesis. Transvalvular regurgitation is seen during systole.

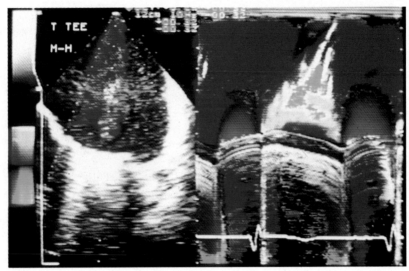

Figure 10.2-7: Color M-mode illustrating the pansystolic timing of regurgitation across a Medtronic Hall mitral prosthesis. The yellow/blue area above the echoes from the valve ring and disc represents the regurgitant flow.

Maximal and mean gradients vary considerably between different valve models with the same quoted valve size. There is also variation between different patients with identical models of the same valve. This reflects the multiple factors affecting valvular gradient including loading conditions, left ventricular function and any associated degree of regurgitation, as well as obstruction. For example, poor left ventricular function decreases flow across an aortic valve so that the effective orifice area may be overestimated. Similarly, in patients with a high cardiac output or stroke volume (for example, secondary to aortic regurgitation) it is possible to overestimate the gradient that would be found in the normal hemodynamic state. Under these conditions it is better to use the continuity equation (12). It is important to relate any given maximal velocity to the valve size (if this is known) before deciding whether the valve is functioning normally or not. What may seem to be a high mean velocity for a 27mm valve may be normal for a 19mm one. A simpler method of assessing aortic obstruction which may be applied to prosthetic valves (17) uses a 'dimensionless Doppler index', which is the ratio of the systolic velocity integral of flow in the left ventricular outflow tract to the systolic velocity integral in the aortic jet. This ratio is particularly useful in the setting of poor left ventricular function as it avoids the confounding factor of low flow. A ratio of 0.3 or less suggests severe obstruction of an aortic prosthesis (18).

Doppler assessment of tricuspid and pulmonary prostheses

Few data are available on echocardiographic assessment of these prostheses. This reflects the much lower rate of disease and implantation of prostheses in these positions. Pye found that pressure half-times were much longer for tricuspid than mitral prostheses (19). The range of pressure half-times for abnormal tricuspid prostheses (237-

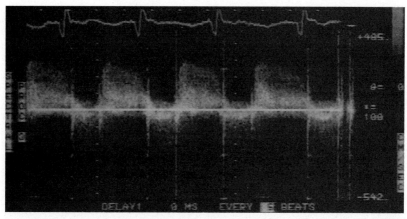

Figure 10.2-8: Doppler recording of an obstructed tilting disc prosthesis in the mitral position. Note the increased maximal (3 m/s) and mean velocities and prolonged pressure half-time.

530 ms) was distinct from apparently normal ones (38-197 ms). Obstruction, as expected, caused an increase in transvalvular velocity. It is suggested that a tricuspid prosthesis with a pressure half-time of greater than 200ms and a peak velocity of greater than 1.6 m/s (in the absence of significant regurgitation) suggests obstruction.

M-MODE ECHOCARDIOGRAPHY

M-mode echocardiography has been superseded by cross-sectional imaging but it can be useful in identifying excursion of the disc or ball. M-mode tracings should show sharp, rapid movements of the occluding poppet (Fig. 10.2-9). The absence of such movements suggests restricted motion which should be confirmed using cross-sectional and Doppler techniques. Similarly, intermittent sticking of the valve may be noted with a normal appearance during one beat and reduced or absent movement during the next. A "curved" upstroke and downstroke of the disc or ball may also indicate a degree of obstruction.

DIAGNOSIS OF COMPLICATIONS OF PROSTHETIC VALVES

Obstruction to forward flow

The commonest factors affecting mechanical valves and leading to obstruction are in-growth of tissue or pannus from the surrounding annulus, and thrombosis. The effect on function varies depending on where the pannus or thrombus forms. For example, thrombus at the apex of a caged-ball prosthesis in the mitral position, may prevent full excursion of the ball during diastole but may allow normal closure during systole (20). In contrast, thrombus formation at the junction of a strut with the valve ring may both obstruct forward flow and prevent normal closure of the valve, either ball or disc, thus allowing regurgitation. In single tilting disc valves the minor aperture is the usual site for thrombosis and this often causes simultaneous obstruction and regurgitation (1). Bioprosthetic valves are less prone to thrombosis, but the cusps tend to thicken and become less pliable (21,22) also leading to a decrease in effective orifice area.

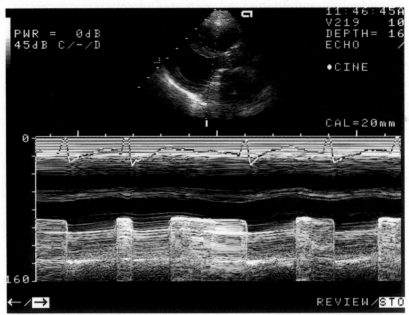

Figure 10.2-9: Parasternal long axis M-mode image of a normally functioning Medtronic Hall prosthesis. Note the sharp vertical disc movement as the valve opens and closes. The patient is in atrial fibrillation.

Echocardiographic techniques can provide evidence of all of these complications, without necessarily revealing the precise nature of the lesion(s) causing any hemodynamic faults.

Regurgitation

It is important to distinguish pathologic transvalvular regurgitation from normal "physiologic" or "built-in" regurgitation (23). Virtually all mechanical valves, including caged-ball prostheses, have some regurgitation (Fig. 10.2-11). This may occur transiently during valve closure or may be pansystolic, depending on the structural design. For example, the central pivotal hole in the Medtronic Hall prosthesis remains patent when the valve is closed, thus allowing pansystolic regurgitation (Fig. 10.2-10). The 'normal' patterns of regurgitation for various types of valve differ. Failure of the occluder to coapt with the valve ring will result in regurgitation within the valve ring (transvalvular regurgitation). Regurgitation occurring outside the valve ring is termed paravalvular. Intermittent sticking of the ball or disc may occur (24). In some earlier models of Starr-Edwards valves, swelling of the silastic ball, probably due to lipid accumulation, led to jamming of the ball within the cage (20,25,26). Uneven wear of balls caused ball variance and regurgitation. Rarely, tilting disc valves have fractured at the junction of the strut with the ring with embolism of the disc and catastrophic consequences. In recent years, this has been a problem only with Björk-Shiley convexo-concave prostheses because they were not fashioned from one solid piece of metal (27).

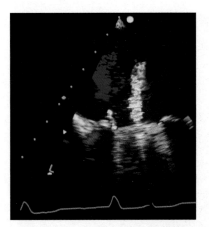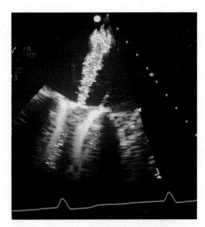

Figure 10.2-10: Transverse (left) and longitudinal views of the central regurgitant jet of the Medtronic Hall prosthesis in the mitral position. The jet is seen to extend deep into the left atrium and to aliase. A smaller peripheral jet (also normal) is seen arising from within the sewing ring.

Color flow mapping is particularly useful in identifying the site and severity of paravalvular regurgitation (Fig. 10.2-12). This may result from the dehiscence of sutures or from the consequences of endocarditis. In our experience, tiny "whiffs" of regurgitation are occasionally seen around the sewing ring at transesophageal echocardiography performed early after surgery. These are narrow in width and short in length. The flow pattern is usually laminar and of low velocity.

Infective endocarditis

Patients with prosthetic heart valves have an increased risk of endocarditis. This can be difficult to diagnose clinically, for example if blood cultures are negative. Echocardiography, particularly from the transesophageal approach, now forms the mainstay of diagnosis as it is able both to image vegetations and detect infective complications. However, the absence of vegetations does not rule out the diagnosis, and complications of endocarditis may be detected without vegetations being imaged.

A vegetation may appear as an echogenic mass of irregular shape attached to the prosthesis or adjacent structures. It may move with the valve or if pedunculated may prolapse with the cardiac cycle. If the sewing ring has been affected then dehiscence may occur. This is detected as a rocking motion of the prosthesis usually with significant paraprosthetic regurgitation. Transvalvular regurgitation may result from infective perforation of a bioprosthetic leaflet or from a vegetation obstructing normal ball or disc motion. Another complication of endocarditis is the formation of abscesses and aneurysms. These are imaged as echo-free spaces adjacent to the prosthesis. Abscesses do not communicate with the cardiac chambers and may contain necrotic material. The aortic valve and perivalvular tissue are most commonly affected, particularly in the area between the aortic root and the mitral annulus, where there is a potential space for infection to localize. The transverse sinus also lies in this area and fluid in it should not be mistaken for an abscess. A pulsatile cavity which, on color flow mapping, is seen to communicate with a cardiac chamber or the aortic root represents

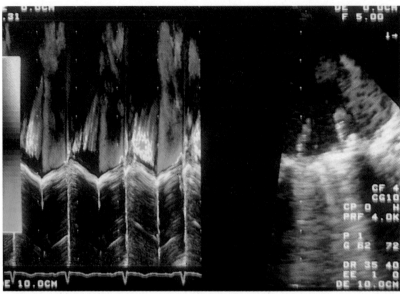

Figure 10.2-11: Two peripheral regurgitant jets are seen originating from a Björk-Shiley mitral prosthesis. The color flow map demonstrates the left hand jet to be pansystolic.

a mycotic aneurysm. Fistulae are recognized as echo-free communications between two chambers (e.g. the aorta and the right atrium) in which color flow mapping demonstrates continuous flow.

Given the far greater sensitivity of the transesophageal approach for the detection of vegetations (28,29) it must be recommended in all prosthetic valve patients in whom the diagnosis is suspected. The investigation should be performed early, as endocarditis is difficult to treat and still carries a high morbidity and mortality.

LIMITATIONS OF DOPPLER ECHOCARDIOGRAPHY

Doppler data seem to give precise values for valvular function but there are pitfalls in their interpretation (13). Understanding the sources of error and the limitations of the formulae used in making Doppler-derived calculations is important. It should encourage the operator to study a given valve by as many means as possible. For example, if a thickened barely-opening aortic valve is visualized using cross-sectional echo but a normal maximal velocity is recorded, then it is likely that the maximal aortic continuous wave signal has not been found.

Factors other than the behavior of the prosthesis may affect Doppler indices. Under conditions of increased flow, such as a high cardiac output or significant valvular regurgitation, the maximal and mean velocities are increased. This translates into increased transvalvular pressures. This should not be taken to imply a degree of obstruction but rather is normal for the hemodynamic state.

Pressure half-time is usually regarded as being relatively independent of flow and thus a good measure of mitral and tricuspid prosthetic function. However, it is affected by flow, atrial and ventricular compliance and also left ventricular preload. In addition,

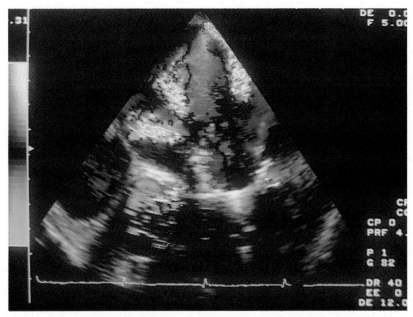

Figure 10.2-12: Four jets of paraprosthetic regurgitation are seen in this transesophageal image of a mechanical mitral prosthesis, obtained from the gastroesophageal junction.

this formula was derived empirically for patients with mitral stenosis (11) and has not been validated in subjects with prostheses. Nevertheless, in practice, the larger the effective valve area the shorter the pressure half-time and vice versa. Pressure half-time is not sensitive at detecting small changes in valve area, but it is abnormal in severe stenosis.

Bioprosthetic valves of a standard size may vary in effective orifice area. They are 'hand made' on an alloy stent and the actual orifice area for any particular ring size may vary from valve to valve. In addition, bioprosthetic leaflets do not open fully at low flow rates and thus a pressure half-time calculation under these conditions will underestimate the real orifice area (13).

Formulae

There are theoretical and practical reasons why some of the formulae used in the calculation of valvular gradients and areas may lead to inaccurate assessment.

The Bernoulli equation is simplified, for ease of application, by discounting the factors referring to flow acceleration and viscous friction. If a prosthetic gradient is estimated using only transvalvular velocity, errors may be introduced. The Bernoulli equation works best for gradients of around 50 mmHg. At low rates of flow, energy losses through viscous friction are relatively increased; estimates of pressure drop across very small orifices such as obstructed valves may be erroneously low if the effect of viscous friction are discounted.

The continuity equation (12) is based on the principle of conservation of mass. It states that if two chambers are in continuity then the volume passing through one orifice in a given time must equal the volume passing through the other in the same time. Significant correlations have been found between the valve area derived using this equation and the actual orifice area but as with all Doppler data the scatter is considerable. For example, in an in vitro study, the 95% confidence limits for difference between planimetered and calculated area was found to be $\pm0.57cm^2$; that is, a large variation exists between the two (30). Errors in using the equation probably stem from estimation of the cross-sectional area in a subvalvular region. Nevertheless in stenotic prostheses the transvalvular velocities tend to be higher and therefore dominate the less accurately measured factors in the equation. Despite these limitations, the equation probably offers the most accurate Doppler method of assessing valve areas.

DIFFERENCES BETWEEN DOPPLER AND CATHETER-DERIVED DATA

These are not directly comparable. Invasive catheterization measures the peak-to-peak gradient (difference between peak left ventricular and peak aortic systolic pressures) while Doppler techniques measure peak instantaneous velocity from which the gradient is calculated. Mean gradients are more directly comparable and therefore more helpful for comparisons. Different hemodynamic states may exist between the catheterization study and the echocardiographic study. Finally, it is important that the Doppler cursor is aligned as closely as possible to the direction of blood flow through the valve. A deviation of more than about 20 degrees results in significant underestimation of velocity.

Despite these shortcomings the regression coefficient for Doppler- versus catheter-derived velocities is good and in clinical practice the Bernoulli equation acts as the mainstay for calculation of aortic valve gradients.

SURVEILLANCE

Since there is considerable variation in echocardiographic parameters between patients, it is strongly recommended that each patient with a newly-implanted prosthetic heart valve should undergo a comprehensive echocardiographic study in the early postoperative period (31). This may best be performed about two to four weeks after operation, once it is possible to again perform a precordial echocardiographic study. In some patients, if imaging is still difficult, then a transesophageal study may even be indicated. These studies provide an individual baseline record of (presumably normal) prosthetic valve function, against which all future results can be compared. In patients with mitral prostheses, an earlier postoperative transesophageal study is recommended by some teams because of the frequency of symptomless non-obstructive thrombus and of small filamentous echoes (4). Not all groups have confirmed this, and there may be a relationship to anticoagulant practice. Perhaps more importantly, an early transesophageal study will detect significant trans- and paraprosthetic regurgitation and give an early assessment of transprosthetic Doppler velocity.

With mitral prostheses, the most useful indices of function are the measured mean velocity and the derived estimated mean transvalvar gradient. The pressure half-time can be measured, if its use has been validated for the valve being studied, but it, and estimates of effective orifice area obtained by applying the Hatle equation have limitations, as already discussed.

For aortic prostheses, estimates of mean velocity and gradient are also most useful. The peak velocity is the simplest Doppler measurement to obtain, and in the individual patient it is reasonable to use this as a guide to valve function, as long as left ventricular function is not significantly impaired. If the peak velocity is low, then clearly valvular function is likely to be normal. When the velocity is high (for example, 3-4 m/sec) then it is important to be able to compare values with previous serial measurements, including those obtained at a baseline postoperative study. When the peak velocity has an intermediate value, then it is important to assess the function of the valve using other methods also. The best measurement is an assessment of effective orifice area using the continuity equation.

MECHANICAL VALVES

Starr-Edwards valve

This was the first prosthetic valve to be used successfully and its simple ball-in-cage design has undergone various modifications. As far as the metal ball version is concerned, in cross-sectional and M-mode echocardiography the movement of the ball may be imaged clearly, but the attenuating properties of the metal in the ball may make it appear non-spherical. When the valve is open there should be no space between the ball and the apex of the cage (20). Such a gap suggests the presence of thrombus. When the valve is open, the ball sits directly in the line of blood flow causing divergent jets and considerable turbulence. Accurate pulsed-wave Doppler interrogation of mitral inflow is difficult because of the absence of a central orifice but the color flow map may be used to guide placement of the sample volume. When the valve closes there is a brief 'whiff' of regurgitation before the ball comes to rest against the orifice ring. In the absence of obstruction there should be no regurgitation thereafter. Regurgitant jets originating outside the sewing ring indicate paraprosthetic leaks secondary to dehiscence or endocarditis. In the aortic position there is a close correlation between the maximal and mean velocities and the size of valve.

Hinged bileaflet valves

Bileaflet valves such as the St. Jude Medical and CarboMedics, have two hemi-discs pivoting inside a pyrolytic steel cage which is attached to a Dacron sewing ring. They have the "best" hemodynamic profile of all the mechanical valves, allowing relatively laminar flow. They also have very low reported rates of thrombosis and the least turbulence on color flow mapping. Each valve has three orifices, two lateral and one central. Values for maximal and mean velocities and gradients for the St. Jude prosthesis in both the mitral and aortic positions are given in Tables I & II.

Bileaflet valves - mitral position

Cross-sectional imaging may show leaflet movement if the ultrasound beams are perpendicular to the long axes of the discs when the valve is open (for example in the parasternal short axis view). From the apex, when the valve is closed there is masking of the left atrium (the bileaflet and Starr-Edwards prostheses are the two most echogenic mechanical valves). During diastole these shadows should change as the valve opens and allows transmission of a portion of the ultrasound beam into the left atrium. Failure to visualize sharp opening and closing of the leaflet or a change in the echogenic shadows produced, raises the suspicion of obstruction. The division of the orifice into three by the twin leaflets may be reflected in the color flow map where three forward flow jets are seen; two lateral, and one smaller central jet. Pulsed or continuous wave Doppler is best aligned to the lateral jets using color flow mapping. The laminar flow is reflected in the color flow map as a rather non-turbulent flow pattern. Deviation from such a pattern under conditions of normal flow suggests valvular obstruction and further confirmation should be sought with spectral Doppler. A transprosthetic velocity of 1.7 m/s or greater raises the suspicion of obstruction.

Bileaflet valves allow a negligible 'closure whiff' of regurgitation and they also demonstrate inherent regurgitation secondary to their design. In any imaging plane, there are usually two small jets located inside the sewing ring, and one larger central jet (23,32). There may also be several small peripheral jets which are variable in their location, for example arising from the pivot points of the disc. All of these jets may be regarded as normal. In common with other such jets they tend to be non-turbulent, of low velocity, and extending for not more than one or two centimeters into the left atrium. They are usually pansystolic and slender or flame-like in shape. Color M-mode is useful in defining the timing and duration of these jets.

Bileaflet valves - aortic position

Mean and peak gradients for these valves have been calculated using the modified Bernoulli equation. Panidis studied 38 patients with normally functioning St. Jude Medical prostheses and found the peak gradient to be 22 ± 12 mmHg and the mean gradient to be 12 ± 7 mmHg. As expected the velocity was highest in the smaller valve sizes (33).

Mild regurgitation may be found on color flow mapping using transesophageal echo, but this should not extend more than about 2 cm from the valve. Larger jets associated with an increased maximal velocity may be due to significant regurgitation. An increased maximal velocity without regurgitation suggests isolated obstruction. The transesophageal approach may allow leaflet motion, morphology and associated lesions to be identified, but it does not contribute additional spectral Doppler information. This is because of the difficulty in achieving good alignment between the continuous wave beam and the outflow jet unless the transgastric long axis view is used. In the presence of a coexisting mitral prosthesis, however, only limited information can be obtained from an esophageal approach about an aortic prosthesis.

Tilting disc valves

These valves include the Björk-Shiley, Omniscience and Medtronic Hall designs. The excursion of the disc can be identified using cross-sectional echocardiography. The single disc divides the valve into major and minor orifices. Color flow mapping shows turbulent flow through both and allows positioning of the Doppler cursor in line with maximal flow. When closed, the pattern of regurgitation depends on the design. The central hole in the disc of the Medtronic Hall prosthesis causes a central, flame-like regurgitant jet extending between 2.0 and 5.5 cm into the left atrium (23). This is of high velocity and so it may be aliased (Fig. 10.2-10). There may also be several much smaller peripheral jets which are of lower velocity and do not alias (23). The Björk-Shiley prosthesis does not have a central orifice but may still have one, or less frequently two regurgitant jets (Fig. 10.2-11). Similarly the Omniscience prosthesis may have several small low-velocity jets.

BIOPROSTHESES

Homografts

When implanted in the aortic position these valves have a similar appearance to native valves. Occasionally, sutures may be seen around the valve annulus. The valve slowly degenerates and this may result in rupture with prolapse of the affected portion (22). This is apparent with cross-sectional imaging and the diagnosis is confirmed using color flow mapping where a turbulent jet is noted in the outflow tract throughout diastole. Rarely, a aortic homografts may rupture spontaneously, leading to severe incompetence. A prolapsing leaflet must be distinguished from a prolapsing suture, which can appear thickened with fibrin deposition. In the latter case there will be little or no regurgitation. Infective endocarditis may lead to valvular or paravalvular regurgitation, and vegetations are not always identified. Aortic homografts may calcify but unlike xenografts the lesions tend to be isolated and discrete (34). Pulmonary autografts in the aortic position have a much lower incidence of degeneration and complications. Their echocardiographic appearance is similar to that of an aortic homograft and transvalvular Doppler velocities are usually in the normal range. Mild regurgitation is common, however, and probably due to mechanical distortion at the time of implantation or dilatation of the pulmonary root secondary to increased systemic pressures (35). Moderate or severe regurgitation is abnormal and suggests dysfunction.

Xenografts

The flexible alloy stents on which these valves are mounted are echogenic and thus they may be imaged in both the mitral and aortic positions. The stent does cast acoustic shadows, making interrogation behind it difficult. The leaflets should be thin and highly mobile (36). Primary degeneration of both pericardial and porcine xenografts results in calcification and thickening which causes valvular stenosis and regurgitation. Degeneration may also cause tearing of a cusp (usually at its site of attachment to the prosthetic annulus) with consequent severe regurgitation (21). Endocarditis may damage either the leaflets or the sewing ring. The latter is suspected when the prosthesis is seen 'rocking' at its point of attachment, often with associated paravalvular regurgitation.

Stented bioprostheses are innately more obstructive than mechanical valves of comparable size, due to encroachment of the stent into the central lumen. This may be reflected in the color flow map, which shows a proximal convergence zone and central turbulent flow through the valve. Planimetry of the valve in the mitral position has been reported to correlate well with the effective orifice area derived by the Gorlin formula (37) and by spectral Doppler.

References

1. Wiseth R, Sande E, Skjaerpe T. Thrombotic disc impediment in a Medtronic Hall aortic valve prosthesis diagnosed by Doppler echocardiography followed by successful operation. J Am Soc Echo 1991;4:645-647
2. Currie PJ, Seward JB, Lam JB, Cerseh BJ, Pluth JR. Left ventricular outflow tract obstruction related to a valve prosthesis: Case caused by a low profile mitral prosthesis. Mayo Clin Proc 1985;60:184-187
3. Rosenzweig MS, Nanda NC. Two-dimensional echocardiographic detection of left ventricular wall impaction by mitral prosthesis. Am Heart J 1983;106:1069-1076
4. Iung B, Cormier B, Dadez B, et al. Small abnormal echos after mitral valve replacement with bileaflet mechanical prostheses: predisposing factors and effect on thromboembolism. J Heart Valve Dis 1993;2:259-266
5. Fraser AG. Ultrasonic detection of increased embolic risk. In: Butchart EG, Bodnar E (eds). Thrombosis, embolism and bleeding (lst ed). ICR Publishers, London, 232-235
6. Daniel WG, Nellessen U, Schroder E, et al. Left atrial spontaneous echo contrast in mitral valve disease: as an indicator of increased thromboembolic risk. J Am Coll Cardiol 1988;11:1204-1211
7. Kapur KW, Fan PH, Nanda NC, Yoganathan AJ, Goyal RG. Doppler color flow mapping in the evaluation of prosthetic mitral and aortic valve function. J Am Coll Cardiol 1989;13:1561-1571
8. Chambers J, Monaghan M, Jackson G. Colour flow Doppler mapping in the assessment of prosthetic valve regurgitation. Br Heart J 1989;62:1-8
9. Dittrich H, Nicod P, Hoit B, Dalton N, Sahn D. Evaluation of Björk-Shiley mitral valves by real-time two-dimensional Doppler echocardiographic flow mapping. Am Heart J 1988;115:133-138
10. Yoshida K, Yoshikawa J, Akasaka T, Nishigami K, Minagoe S. Value of acceleration flow signals proximal to the leaking orifice in assessing the severity of prosthetic valve regurgitation. J Am Coll Cardiol 1992;19:333-338
11. Hatle L, Angelsen B, Tromsdal A. Non-invasive assessment of atrioventricular pressure half-time by Doppler ultrasound. Circulation 1979;60:1096-1094
12. Skjaerpe T, Hegrenaes L, Hatle L. Non-invasive assessment of valve area in patients with aortic stenosis by Doppler ultrasound and two-dimensional echocardiography. Circulation 1985;72:810-818n
13. Chambers J, Deverall P. Limitations and pitfalls in the assessment of prosthetic valves with Doppler ultrasonography. J Thorac Cardiovasc Surg 1992;104:495-591
14. Burstow DJ, Nishimura RA, Bailey KR, et al. Continuous wave Doppler echocardiographic measurement of prosthetic valve gradients. A simultaneous Doppler-catheter correlative study. Circulation 1989;80:504-514
15. Hatle L, Angelsen B. Pulsed and continuous wave Doppler in diagnosis and assessment of various heart lesions. In: Doppler ultrasound in cardiology, (2nd ed). Lea & Febiger, Philadelphia, 1985;188-205
16. Williams GA, Labovitz AJ. Doppler hemodynamic evaluation of prosthetic (Starr Edwards and Björk-Shiley) and bioprosthetic (Hancock and Carpentier-Edwards) cardiac valves. Am J Cardiol 1985;56:325-332
17. Lesbre JP, Tribouilloy C, Boey S, Mirode A. Evaluation des prostheses valvulaires par Doppler. Medecine Sciences, Flammarion, Ch 13:194-220
18. Otto CM, Pearlman AS, Comess KA, et al Determination of the stenotic aortic valve area in adults using Doppler echocardiography. J Am Coll Cardiol 1986;7:509-517
19. Pye M, Weerasana N, Bain WH, Hutton I, Cobbe SM. Doppler echocardiographic characteristics of normal and dysfunctioning prosthetic valves in the tricuspid and mitral position. Br Heart J 1990;63:41-44
20. Nanda NC, Cooper JW, Mahan III AF, Fan P. Echocardiographic assessment of prosthetic valves. Circulation 1991;84(Suppl I):228-239
21. Melacini P, Villanova C, Thiene G, et al. Long term echocardiographic Doppler monitoring of Hancock Bioprostheses in the mitral valve position. Am J Cardiol 1992;70:1157-1163
22. Virdi IS, Monro JL, Ross JK. Eleven year experience of aortic valve replacement with antibiotic sterilised homograft valves in Southampton. Thorac Cardiovasc Surgeon 1986;34:277-282
23. Baumgartner H, Kahn S, DeRobertis M, Czer L, Maurer G. Color Doppler regurgitant characteristics of normal mechanical mitral valve prostheses in vitro. Circulation 1992;85:323-332
24. Sareli P, Chun R. Intermittent intravalvar regurgitation of a mechanical aortic valve prosthesis - diagnosis and clinical implications. A case report. South African Medical J 1991;79:221-222

25. Berndt TB, Goodman DJ, Popp RL. Echocardiographic and phonocardiographic confirmation of suspected caged mitral valve malfunction. Chest 1976;70:221-230
26. Veenendaal M, Nanda NC. Non-invasive diagnosis of mitral prosthesis malfunction. Am J Med 1980;69:458-462
27. Davis PK, Myers JL, Pennock JL, Thiele BL. Strut fracture and disc embolisation in Björk-Shiley mitral valve prostheses: Diagnosis and management. Ann Thorac Surg 1985;40:65- 68
28. Erbel R, Rohmann S, Drexler M, et al. Improved diagnostic value of echocardiography in patients with infective endocarditis by transesophageal approach. A prospective study. Eur Heart J 1988;9:43-53
29. Taams M, Gussenhoven E, Bos E, et al. Enhanced morphological diagnosis in infective endocarditis by transesophageal echocardiography. Br Heart J 1990;63:109-113
30. Chambers JB, Sprigings DC, Cochrane T, Allen J, Black MM, Jackson G. The continuity equation and Gorlin formula compared with directly observed orifice area in native and prosthetic aortic valves. Br Heart J 1992;67:193-199
31. Chambers J, Fraser A, Lawford P, Nihoyannopoulos P, Simpson I. Echocardiographic assessment of artificial heart valves: British society of echocardiography position paper. Br Heart J (Supplement) 1994;71:6-14
32. Hixson CS, Smith MD, Mattson MD, Morris EJ, Lenhoff SJ, Salley RK. Comparison of tranesophageal color flow Doppler imaging of normal mitral regurgitant jets in St Jude Medical and Medtronic Hall cardiac prostheses. J Am Soc Echo 1992;5:57-62
33. Panidis IP, Ross J, Mintz GS. Normal and abnormal prosthetic valve function as assessed by Doppler echocardiography. J Am Coll Cardiol 1986;8:317-326
34. Martinell J, Fraile J, Artiz J, et al. Long term comparative analysis of the Björk-Shiley and Hancock valves implanted in 1975. J Thorac Cardiovasc Surg 1985;90:741-749
35. Kumar N, Prabhakar G, Gometza B, AI-Halees Z, Duran CMG. The Ross procedure in a young rheumatic population: Early clinical and echocardiographic profile. J Heart Valve Dis. 1993;2:376-379
36. Effron MK, Popp RL. Two-dimensional echocardiographic assessment of bioprosthetic valve dysfunction and infective endocarditis. J Am Coll Cardiol 1983;2:597-606
37. Chambers JB, Cochrane T, Black MM, Jackson G. The Gorlin formula validated against directly observed orifice area in porcine mitral bioprostheses. J Am Coll Cardiol 1989;13:348- 353

Chapter 10.3

Thrombogenesis and its Management

Eric G. Butchart

Intracardiac thrombosis and systemic embolism remain the most significant complications for patients with heart valve disease and the most important cause of morbidity and mortality apart from progression of the disease process itself (1,2). A high proportion of symptomatic embolic events involve the brain (1,3) and the associated loss of cerebral function is often devastating, preventing the patient from working and placing great demands on the relatives and the health care system (4).

The reduction of these complications should be the goal of all involved in the care of patients with heart valve disease. It can be brought about only by a better understanding of the mechanisms of intracardiac thrombogenesis and more focused antithrombotic management.

THROMBOGENESIS

It is helpful to examine the problem of thrombogenesis in heart valve disease in terms of the components of Virchow's triad: the surface in contact with the blood, the local flow conditions and the constituents of the blood (5).

Intracardiac Surfaces: Endothelium

Once thought of as a purely passive smooth surface, it is now known that the endothelium is in effect a complex organ with subtle mechanisms that keep the blood in a fluid state under normal circumstances, as well as playing an important role in regulating vascular tone (6). Endothelial cells secrete on their surface a variety of substances which inhibit coagulation (7-10) and platelet adhesion (11,12) and promote fibrinolysis (11,13,14). However, the endothelium also possesses mechanisms to induce thrombosis (14-20).

In health, the balance between the anticoagulant and prothrombotic functions of the endothelium is maintained on the anticoagulant side of the equation, apart from the need to respond to local breaches in its integrity, but a number of local and systemic stimuli may tip the balance towards thrombosis (20-22). High shear stresses in relation to abnormal native valves (23) or prosthetic valves (24) may produce local injury and the stretching effect of abnormally high intracavitary or intravascular pressures (25), for example in the pulmonary vasculature, may induce prothrombotic function (20,26,27). Elevated levels of von Willebrand factor have been reported in patients with pulmonary hypertension, probably as the result of this mechanism (27). Systemic diseases which are associated with procoagulant endothelial function include atherosclerosis (26,28-30), hypercholesterolemia (15), diabetes (31,32) and hypertension (33-35). Continuing

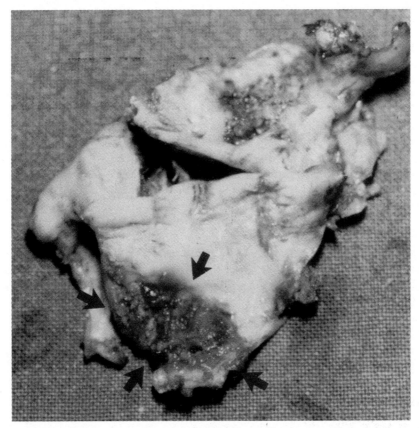

Figure 10.3-1: Excised aortic valve, showing thrombus (arrows) adherent to the outflow surface of the non-coronary cusp.

procoagulant endothelial function is an independent predictor of mortality (36).

Endothelium covering natural heart valves develops procoagulant function in various local (37-40) and systemic (41-47) disease processes and as the result of abnormal flow patterns (23,48). Repeated cycles of thrombus deposition, organization and re-endothelialization can lead to layering and progressive thickening (38,48). Occasionally gross thrombus deposition can be seen on abnormal native valves (Fig. 10.3-1).

Intracardiac surfaces: replacement heart valves

Replacement heart valves present three different types of surface to the flowing blood: sewing ring, biological tissue and mechanical components. Each initiates a different type of reaction and they will therefore be considered separately.

Sewing rings

Incorporation of the sewing ring begins within minutes of implantation with protein adsorption (49,50) followed by platelet deposition (50,51). Using echocardiography, 'filamentous strands' can sometimes be demonstrated extending from the circumference of a mitral prosthesis into the left atrium during the early postoperative period (52-54). The nature of these strands and the conditions which predispose to their formation remain to be clarified. So far they have been reported mainly in association with bileaflet prostheses and appear to be commoner when relative stasis in the left atrium and subtherapeutic anticoagulation co-exist (54). Preliminary studies suggest that their presence is associated with an increased risk of embolism (53-54).

The thrombus which initially covers the surface of the sewing ring becomes organized to avascular fibrous tissue (55). This eventually becomes covered by endothelium, but coverage is usually incomplete and its function is uncertain (56). Whilst the incorporation process is proceeding, and perhaps even after it is 'complete', the sewing ring remains a possible source of embolism. Labeled platelet studies in experimental animals show that microembolism from the sewing ring is a frequent occurrence in the first few weeks (51).

Excessive growth of fibrous tissue on the sewing ring is known as 'tissue ingrowth' or 'pannus formation'. Its etiology is probably multifactoral, with different factors accounting for the varied time of presentation. Although mainly a relatively late phenomenon (57), it has been observed as early as one month after implantation (58). Possible etiologic factors include implantation technique (59), fabric damage (60), locally abnormal flow conditions (61), inadequate early anticoagulation (62,63) and degree of fibrous tissue vascularity (55), foreign body reaction and fibroblast activity (64), the latter possibly accounting, at least in part, for ethnic differences in the incidence of tissue ingrowth (56).

Tissue ingrowth has several adverse effects. In bioprostheses, tissue ingrowth can extend onto the cusps to cause progressive stiffening and stenosis (59,65-67) or cusp retraction (68). Bioprostheses in the tricuspid position are especially prone to this phenomenon (55,65,66,68), probably because low right atrial pressures allow the development of thicker fibrous tissue (55,68). In mechanical valves, tissue ingrowth narrows the effective orifice of the prosthesis, interferes with occluder movement and predisposes to valve thrombosis (69).

Biological tissue

It might be assumed that replacement valves prepared from either human or animal aortic valves would retain their original thromboresistance. Unfortunately, the valve endothelium, on which thromboresistance depends, is largely lost during harvesting, preparation and preservation (70,71), especially in the case of heterografts, and what little remains is lost soon after implantation (70,72-75). Similarly, bioprosthetic valves fashioned from pericardium lose their mesothelial cells (76).

Thus all newly implanted biological valves initially present a foreign, microscopically irregular surface to the blood stream, largely devoid of endothelium and exposing either basement membrane or collagen, both of which soon become covered with a thin layer of fibrin and platelets (70,77,78). This deposition of microthrombus occurs to a greater extent on the outflow (concave) surfaces of the valve cusps (65) probably as the result of lower shear stresses on this side of the valve (70,72) and occasionally progresses to visible thrombus (65,73). Gross thrombus develops in the cusp sinuses of 0.4-1.7% of porcine bioprostheses, leading to thrombotic obstruction (79-83). This complication has not been reported in homografts or pericardial heterografts. Predisposing factors for its development include low cardiac output postoperatively (80), perhaps coupled with asynchronous opening of the cusps (84). Late thrombosis of a porcine valve is sometimes related to structural deterioration and associated cusp stiffness (85) or calcification (79), in keeping with the increased platelet activation and hemolysis seen in association with degenerating porcine valves (86).

In most cases the microthrombus which covers the cusps soon after implantation becomes organized, leading to the formation of a fibrous sheath (77). This varies in thickness and extent, according to the duration of implantation (77), the anatomical site (68,72) and, in the case of homografts, the method of preparation (73,74), but rarely covers the whole cusp (74,85). Subsequent endothelialization occurs only over previously deposited fibrin or fibrous sheath, never over exposed donor collagen (72). Hence biological valve cusps are almost always incompletely endothelialized (72) and sometimes have no endothelial cover whatsoever (72,75). The endothelial cover is greatest on antibiotic treated and fresh homografts (73,74). Porcine heterografts acquire no endothelial cells in the first year after implantation, following which endothelialization increases very slowly so that by five years, up to 70% of valves show some degree of endothelialization, mainly on the outflow (concave) surface of the cusps (72). In the aortic position, where bioprostheses are most commonly implanted, fibrous sheathing and endothelialization are less likely to occur than in the mitral and tricuspid positions (72). Even if endothelium does partly cover the surface of a valve cusp, it is uncertain whether, in this abnormal situation, it possesses any anticoagulant function.

Thus, far from retaining the thromboresistance of the original valve, the newly implanted homograft or heterograft exists in an uneasy equilibrium, with the balance tipped in favor of thrombus deposition, albeit mainly at microscopic level. The fact that this microthrombus is not usually progressive suggests that it undergoes repeated cycles of lysis or microembolism (70,85). This may account for the increased platelet activation and turnover reported in some patients with bioprostheses; both activation and turnover are quantitatively similar to those with some types of mechanical valve (87-89). However, too much reliance should not be placed on cross-sectional data, which cannot distinguish between cause and effect (vide infra). Platelet survival within the normal range has been reported in two studies in homograft recipients (90,91), suggesting that these valves are less thrombogenic than heterografts, although both studies investigated very few patients.

Mechanical components

The materials from which the housing and moving parts of mechanical prostheses are constructed induce a reaction with the constituents of the blood which is initially similar to that induced by the sewing ring, but subsequently differs. Protein deposition begins almost immediately and precedes any platelet deposition (50). Fibrinogen is the dominant protein deposited on a newly implanted surface and the configurational change in the predominantly 'end-on' adherent molecules appears to attract platelets (49). Other proteins are deposited, including fibronectin, von Willebrand factor, thrombospondin and factor XII, all of which also attract platelets.

The layer of proteins adsorbed onto the surface changes with time and according to the nature of the component, some materials being less thrombogenic that others. The thrombogenicity of all materials is at its greatest soon after implantation. Thereafter a process know as passivation of the surface takes place to a greater or lesser extent, as the layer of proteins alters its composition. In general the greater the concentration of albumin, the more passive the surface (49). Materials possessing low thrombogenicity, such as pyrolytic carbon, appear to induce passivation more readily although the exact mechanisms involved remain unclear (49).

The prevention of progressive deposition of thrombus on mechanical components depends not only on the characteristics of the surface but also on blood velocity and coagulability (vide infra). The fact that most modern prostheses do not become covered with thrombus soon after implantation, at a time when anticoagulation is nearly always subtherapeutic, is mainly due to high blood velocity and design characteristics favoring the 'washing' of vulnerable points (24). Throughout its implanted lifespan, a mechanical valve remains in a fragile equilibrium with the blood, always covered with a thin layer of plasma proteins and susceptible to platelet and fibrin deposition if the equilibrium is altered by changes in flow or coagulability of the blood. Unlike the sewing ring, few platelets remain adherent to mechanical components for very long under normal circumstances; rapid flow conditions with high shear rates result in a removal rate which matches the rate of deposition (92). However, dislodged activated platelets may adhere to other surfaces downstream from the prosthesis (56,92). It has been suggested that measurements of platelet kinetics and activation may provide an indirect assessment of prosthesis thrombogenicity (50), but cross-sectional data in this respect are of limited value, since platelet function is influenced by so many other variables (vide infra). Longitudinal data, taking into account preoperative values and non-prosthetic influences may be more useful and prospective studies of this nature should be encouraged.

Intracardiac flood flow

Low flow

Sinus rhythm, normal cardiac output and normal cardiac chamber dimensions and contraction virtually guarantee freedom from intracardiac thrombosis in the presence of normal or mildly diseased heart valves. However the loss of any one of these four cornerstones of normal cardiac function results in locally reduced blood flow or relative stagnation, which disturbs the normally fast flowing suspension of red cells and increases local blood viscosity, due to rouleau formation and red cell aggregation mediated by fibrinogen (93,94). This can be detected clinically by transesophageal echocardiography as 'spontaneous echo contrast' or 'smoke-like echoes' in cardiac chambers exposed to low flow conditions (95).

Stasis brings red cell/fibrinogen aggregates into contact with intracardiac surfaces (96). The potential for subsequent thrombus formation increases with the hematocrit (92,97) but if the surface has a normally functioning intact endothelial layer, the risk of thrombus formation is probably low. However if the coagulation system is up-regulated or if the balance of endothelial function is tipped towards procoagulant function by local or systemic factors or if the surface is devoid of endothelium, as in the case of a prosthetic valve or left atrial fibrosis, the combination of stasis and an abnormal surface will readily lead to thrombus formation (92,97,98).

Disturbed flow

Abnormal flow patterns associated with high velocity flow can also be thrombogenic. The abnormally high shear stresses developed when blood is forced through a narrow orifice lead to endothelial and red cell damage, platelet activation and ADP release (23,99-102), more ADP originating from red cells than platelets (103). ADP activates further platelets which adhere to damaged endothelial cells (11,97). In aortic stenosis, for example, the resulting microthrombus laid down on the surface of the valve and adjacent aortic wall undergoes organization, fibrosis and ultimately calcification, leading to further rigidity of the valve and increasing stenosis (48).

Thrombus deposited under conditions of rapid flow is of a very different nature from that deposited under conditions of stasis. It contains a high proportion of platelets and fibrin with relatively few enmeshed red cells and tends to form slowly (104,105). The thrombus stabilizing protein, factor XIII, binds fibrin molecules rapidly in fast-flowing blood (106). The result is a firm, elastic, insoluble thrombus relatively resistant to fibrinolysis and strongly adherent to the surface (107). This type of thrombus is less susceptible to embolism and probably gives rise to smaller emboli when embolism does

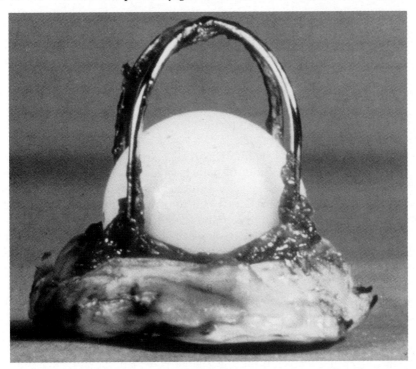

Figure 10.3-2: Thrombosis of Starr-Edwards mitral prosthesis, showing thrombus accumulation around the orifice and on the struts and apex of the cage, from which emboli may be discharged by repetitive ball impact. Reproduced from Ref. #56, with permission.

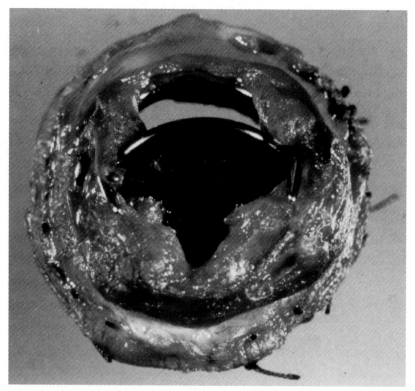

Figure 10.3-3: Thrombosis of Lillehei-Kaster tilting disc mitral prosthesis, occluding the minor orifice and interfering with disc movement. Reproduced from Ref. #56, with permission.

occur. Calcific aortic stenosis, for example, is rarely associated with clinically apparent embolism but in one series more than 25% of patients investigated prior to balloon valvotomy had small silent cerebral infarcts on CT scan (108).

The flow conditions in the vicinity of both mechanical and bioprosthetic valves are highly abnormal (24). Areas of high velocity disturbed flow with vortices coexist with areas of relative stagnation during forward flow (84). In the case of single disc and bileaflet valves, regurgitant jets between the moving parts and the housing also occur when the valve is closed (109-111). The high shear stresses created by both forward and regurgitant abnormal flow patterns damage red cells and activate platelets (23,24,99-102). The shear stresses are greater with mechanical valves than with bioprostheses (24) and further damage to red cells and platelets is caused by the impact of the occluder on the housing with each cardiac cycle. The disturbed flow patterns bring activated platelets into contact with the artificial surface of prosthetic valves and with adjacent endothelium. Nevertheless, thrombosis on most modern mechanical valves is relatively rare if anticoagulation is adequate, a testimony to progressive improvements in heart valve design (56,112).

Despite much progress, all currently available prosthetic valves, including stented bioprostheses, remain imperfect in terms of thrombogenicity. Each design has its Achilles' heel. In caged ball valves, high velocity forward flow occurs peripherally, whilst in the region of the apex of the cage an area of low velocity reverse flow occurs at the point

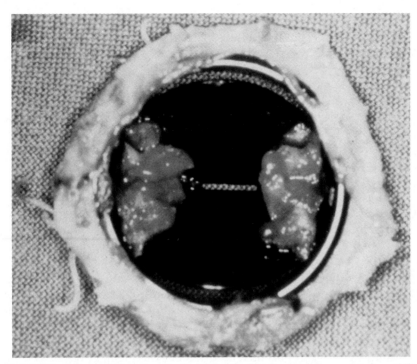

Figure 10.3-4: Thrombosis of St. Jude mitral prosthesis, showing almost complete immobilization of both leaflets by a relatively small volume of thrombus. Reproduced from Ref. #56, with permission.

of full ball travel. This zone of relative stagnation predisposes the apex of the cage to thrombus deposition (113) (Fig. 10.3-2). The major flaws of early tilting disc designs were the low velocity of flow through the minor orifice (61), and lack of clearance between the disc and the housing on full opening (114), defects corrected to some extent in later designs by increasing the relative size of the minor orifice and introducing mechanisms to improve disc clearance (115,116). However in all types of tilting disc valve, the minor orifice remains vulnerable and if thrombosis occurs it usually begins here (Fig. 10.3-3). In bileaflet valves, the hinge mechanism is the site most prone to thrombus formation (69,117) (Fig. 10.3-4) because low velocity reverse flow occurs adjacent to each hinge point even when maximum forward flow is taking place through the two lateral orifices (24).

Stented bioprostheses are associated with abnormal flow characteristics (24,84) imposed by the rigidity of the stent and magnified, in porcine valves, by their relatively stenotic effective orifice areas (110,118). Rapid flow takes place centrally but areas of relative stasis exist in the region of the concavity (outflow surface) of each cusp (84). In the presence of low cardiac output particularly, this relative stasis can contribute to thrombus deposition on that part of the cusp (80).

Blood coagulability

In discussing individual susceptibility to thrombosis, it is convenient to use the word coagulability in its broadest sense to encompass the effect of changes in blood viscosity, platelet function and the fibrinolytic system in addition to the effect of changes in the coagulation system itself. The scope of this chapter does not permit detailed discussion of all these components of coagulability but a brief description is necessary to the understanding of later sections of the chapter.

Blood viscosity depends on hematocrit, plasma viscosity, temperature and shear rate (93). Plasma viscosity in turn is 99% determined by the various plasma proteins, although not in proportion to their concentration. The effect of fibrinogen in particular is disproportionate to its concentration; although normally representing only 4% of the total proteins, it contributes 22% of the viscosity effect because of its large molecular weight and characteristic elongated shape (93).

The increase in viscosity which results from low shear rate is of particular relevance in patients with heart valve disease or replacement valves, where relative stasis of the blood raises local viscosity (93,94). The combination of this local increase in viscosity with a systemically raised viscosity, due to raised hematocrit and fibrinogen levels, as in smokers for example (119-122), increases the risk of thrombus formation further.

Platelets under normal physiological conditions circulate in the blood stream in an inactive state, in which they neither adhere to surfaces nor to each other. Activation involves release of substances from granules within the platelet which promote adhesion to neighboring platelets (aggregation) and to surfaces (16,123-125). It also involves a shape change, exposing specific binding sites (125). Since the principal role of platelets is in plugging breaches in the endothelium, activation is stimulated by substances exposed in the subendothelium, particularly collagen and von Willebrand factor, and by thrombin (11,16,97).

In the context of prosthetic heart valves, platelets are also activated by foreign surfaces (49,50) and by the high shear stresses associated with non-physiological flow patterns (16,24,102). However their subsequent aggregation and adherence may be modified by systemic influences which affect their reactivity.

The thrombogenic potential of platelets is determined by their concentration, their size and reactivity, their degree of activation and their relation to the surface in question (92,126,127). Large platelets are more reactive to ADP and collagen and also release more thromboxane A_2, serotonin and beta-thromboglobulin per unit volume than smaller platelets (127). They are produced following both acute and chronic platelet destruction, as following cardiopulmonary bypass (128), or in immune thrombocytopenic purpura (129) and probably occur in response to the excessive platelet consumption seen with some prosthetic valves also, although this has not yet been fully investigated. Larger platelets also occur in diabetes (130) and chronic hypoxia (131).

A number of systemic influences can cause platelets to become more reactive. Catecholamines are known to potentiate platelet activation (132) and mental stress increases both catecholamine levels and platelet aggregability (133). Raised levels of fibrinogen also increase the responsiveness of platelets to low concentrations of ADP (134). Diets rich in saturated fat (135-138) and increased levels of lipid peroxides, induced by an excess of oxygen free radicals (139), both increase platelet aggregability.

Persistent platelet hyperaggregability of whatever cause probably constitutes a prothrombotic state. In patients with coronary artery disease it is predictive of future coronary events and mortality (140). Its value as a predictor of thrombotic and embolic events in heart valve disease has not been investigated.

Basal procoagulant activity depends on the concentration of certain coagulation factors and their degree of activation, balanced by the effectiveness of natural anticoagulant mechanisms. It determines how readily and to what extent thrombin will be produced by a specific stimulus at a specific site (141,142). The action of thrombin, a serine protease, is to cleave polypeptides from fibrinogen, converting it into fibrin (143). Since fibrinogen is a substrate, unlike the other components of the coagulation cascade (which, when activated, become proteases), its concentration in plasma probably does not directly determine *how much* thrombus will be formed (142). Rather, its overall effect on coagulability is probably mediated through its influence on platelet aggregability (134) and blood viscosity (93), determining *how readily* thrombus will be formed and regulating its growth and viscoelastic properties (143,144). Raised fibrinogen levels are associated with an increased risk of peripheral vascular disease, coronary disease, stroke and TIA (122,145-147) and, in the context of abnormal intracardiac flow conditions due to atrial fibrillation, valve disease or a prosthetic valve, an increased risk of intracardiac thrombosis (98,148).

A prothrombotic state may result from higher circulating levels of inactive precursors of coagulation factors, some degree of pre-activation of precursors, reduced levels of natural anticoagulants or decreased effectiveness of the fibrinolytic system (141). Congenital deficiencies in natural anticoagulants, such as antithrombin III, protein C and protein S result in primary hypercoagulable states which, although important to identify, are comparatively rare (149). Of more relevance to the heart valve patient are the conditions which lead to secondary hypercoagulability, since they are much commoner and in many cases amenable to modification or prevention.

Raised factor VII coagulant activity (VIIc) has a close association with increased plasma lipids, particularly chylomicrons and very low density lipoproteins; even in health, diurnal fluctuations parallel the quantity of fat consumed during a meal, after a lag phase of two to three hours (142). In general, factor VIIc levels increase with age (142) and in conditions, such as diabetes (150), pregnancy (151) and obesity (152), which are associated with hyperlipidemia. Raised levels produce hypercoagulability and are associated with an increased risk of coronary disease (153). Levels are lowered by weight reduction (152) and frequent strenuous exercise (154) and by oral anticoagulation (q.v.).

Von Willebrand factor (vWF) is a huge 'sticky' protein, in effect a biological glue, whose principal role in the hemostatic system is to promote the adherence of platelets to the endothelial surface, to each other and to collagen whenever a breach occurs in the integrity of the endothelium (11,16). However a variety of stimuli, both physical and chemical, release vWF from endothelium and platelets (11,16,17,102). Raised blood levels of vWF are seen in serious infection (155,156), diabetic ketosis (160) and the hypertension of pregnancy (161); they increase the risk of thrombus formation and mortality (26,36,157).

In patients both with and without heart valve disease, there is an association between raised vWF levels and pulmonary hypertension, suggesting that increased pulmonary vascular pressures may stimulate the release of vWF (27). This may have particular relevance in patients with co-existing left atrial stasis (148). vWF is essential for shear-induced platelet aggregation (16,102); raised levels may therefore increase thrombotic risk in the region of valve stenoses and in proximity to prosthetic heart valves.

Secondary hypercoagulability may also result from acquired antithrombin III deficiency (149,162). Of most relevance to patients with heart valve disease or prosthetic valves, is the deficiency of antithrombin III which results from increased consumption (162). Atrial fibrillation, even in the absence of mitral valve disease is reported to decrease antithrombin III levels by about 20%, while the combination of atrial fibrillation with congestive heart failure (with or without mitral stenosis) reduces levels by one third (163). These reduced levels are indicative of the increased flux of the coagulation system as a whole in the presence of abnormal flow conditions (98) although in congestive heart failure, liver dysfunction may contribute to low levels also (163).

Increased consumption of antithrombin III is also seen following major surgery, trauma and sepsis (162,164,165). After major surgery, the fall in antithrombin III concentration parallels the extent of tissue damage and following cardiovascular surgery can fall by two thirds, reaching it lowest point on the third postoperative day (162). In the presence of serious infection, reduced levels persist for much longer (165). Following heart valve replacement, reduced levels of antithrombin III may contribute to the increased thrombotic and embolic risk in the early postoperative period (166).

Another cause of secondary hypercoagulability is a reduction in the efficiency of the fibrinolytic system (149). Fibrin is broken down to its degradation products by plasmin which is generated from its precursor, plasminogen, mainly by the action of tissue plasminogen activator (t-PA) and to a lesser extent by urokinase both of which are synthesized by endothelial cells (14). As with the coagulation system, the fibrinolytic system is enhanced or inhibited by subtle feedback mechanisms. Plasminogen activator inhibitor (PAI-1) is the most important circulating inhibitor of t-PA (14,19). Like t-PA it is produced by endothelial cells but also by liver cells and platelets. It is an acute phase reactant protein (19) and is also the predominant protein in the subendothelial matrix (14). Thrombin stimulates the release of PAI-1 from both endothelial cells and platelets (14,15), an effect which is opposed by nitric oxide (167,168). PAI-1 levels in plasma exhibit diurnal fluctuation (169,170) and are increased in inflammatory conditions (19) by hyperinsulinemia in association with type two (non-insulin dependent) diabetes (31,171), hypertension (33,34,172) and obesity (173,174), and by hypertriglyceridemia (19,31).

Coagulability in heart valve disease

Several studies have examined the effect of abnormal cardiac flow conditions on basal procoagulant activity, platelet activation and activation of the fibrinolytic system. The change from sinus rhythm to atrial fibrillation is accompanied by an increase in hematocrit (175), which is thought to result from fluid loss due to increased secretion of atrial natriuretic peptide (98, 176). Chronic atrial fibrillation, even in the absence of valve disease is associated with raised levels of prothrombin F_{1+2} (177), fibrinogen (148), fibrinopeptide A (178) (a peptide released when fibrinogen is converted into fibrin), vWF (148), factor VIIIc (148), D-dimer (148,179) (a product of fibrinolysis), and beta-thromboglobulin (148) (a platelet release product) and reduced levels of the natural anticoagulant, antithrombin III (178). These changes imply that the coagulation system, natural anticoagulant mechanisms and the fibrinolytic system are all operating at an increased state of flux as a consequence of abnormal flow conditions (98).

The concentration of antithrombin III is also reduced in mitral stenosis complicated by atrial fibrillation and to a lesser extent in mitral stenosis with sinus rhythm (163). Levels of vWF are reported to be higher in the presence of left atrial thrombosis (179) and high plasma levels of D-dimer in patients with mitral stenosis are suspicious of the presence of mobile or freshly evolving left atrial thrombus (180). High levels of tumor necrosis factor (TNF) have been described in patients with severe chronic heart failure (181). TNF stimulates the expression of tissue factor by endothelial cells (182) and monocytes (183) and may contribute to the increased incidence of thrombosis and embolism in congestive cardiac failure (184).

Various coagulation indices have also been studied in patients with prosthetic valves (185,186), but these must be interpreted with caution. Unless preoperative tests have been performed also, it is impossible to separate the effects of the presence of the prosthesis per se from the effects of co-existing abnormalities such as left atrial enlargement, atrial fibrillation, systemic hypertension or residual pulmonary hypertension and congestive heart failure for example.

RISK FACTORS AND TRIGGER FACTORS FOR THROMBOSIS

The risk factors for thrombosis and embolism in heart valve disease are now well-established (1,3). Atrial fibrillation (AF) is probably the most important because of its impact on flow conditions within the left atrium as described above. Its incidence rises progressively with advancing age (187). Even in the absence of valve disease, AF increases the risk of stroke fivefold (188), a risk which is not totally abolished by anticoagulation (189-192). The risk of non-valvular AF can be stratified according to the presence or absence of additional factors which contribute to the risk (176). In the presence of normal left ventricular function and a normal sized left atrium, the incidence of stroke is relatively low, about 1.5% per year (193). Conversely, both significant left atrial enlargement and impaired left ventricular function independently add to the risk of AF, so that the combination of all three in severe degree can raise the risk of stroke to 20% per year (193). The risk appears to be higher soon after the onset of AF (194) or soon after the transition from paroxysmal AF to chronic AF but this increased risk may also be linked to the deterioration which precipitated the AF (176). Long-standing AF alone results in a gradual increase in the size of the left atrium (195) and is associated with histological changes in the atrial myocardium, culminating in fibrosis (196). Left atrial thrombus in patients with rheumatic mitral valve disease in AF has been shown to be localized to sites of maximal fibrosis (197), suggesting either that a procoagulant change occurs in endothelium overlying the fibrosis, or that endothelium is lost altogether.

When left atrial stasis is increased by the combination of rheumatic heart disease with AF, the risk of stroke rises from five-fold to seventeen-fold (198). In the presence of mitral stenosis, an incidence of embolism of 7-14% per year can be expected without anticoagulation (199,200). AF is a more important risk factor in mitral stenosis than the degree of obstruction (200). Hemodynamically important pure mitral regurgitation appears to have some 'protective' role as far as thromboembolic risk is concerned, probably due to its 'stirring' effect, keeping the blood in the left atrium in constant motion (95). However, in rheumatic mitral regurgitation the lesion is often mixed with stenosis and the incidence of embolism in these cases is similar to or even higher than in pure mitral stenosis (200,201).

It is difficult to assess the effect of left atrial enlargement per se on thrombotic and embolic risk since, when moderate or severe, it is usually a secondary phenomenon, occurring as the result of AF, mitral valve disease or impaired left ventricular function or various combinations of these three conditions (193,195,200). Its validity as an *independent* risk factor for left atrial thrombosis and embolism is disputed (2,95,193,200,202-207). There are two probable explanations for the apparently contradictory reports in the literature; 1) the failure to distinguish between primary (q.v.) and secondary dilatation; 2) in secondary dilatation at least, the degree of stasis appears of greater importance than size per se (95). It has been reported that, in mitral stenosis, embolic risk is closely related to the size of the left atrial appendage (208) but this finding has not been confirmed by others (200,201) and it is likely that the contractile function of the appendage is of more importance than its size in estimating risk (208). Amputation or ligation of the appendage does not reduce the risk of embolism postoperatively (201).

Primary left atrial enlargement, usually of minor degree, occurs with advancing age (210). It is hypothesized that it may *cause* AF in the elderly (211) and hence contribute to the risk of embolism in this age group (206,207). However these studies expose the limitations of cross-sectional data and underline the need for longitudinal studies.

Patients with aortic valve disease are at lower risk of thrombosis and embolism than patients with mitral valve disease (200). Most aortic patients are in sinus rhythm and have normal flow conditions in a normally sized left atrium (200), hence avoiding the increased state of flux of the coagulation system associated with sluggish flow conditions (98). Furthermore, following valve replacement the velocity of flow through aortic prostheses is greater than through mitral prostheses, providing more 'washing effect'. Consequently, most series of valve replacement in the literature report lower embolic rates after AVR than MVR (2).

Although thrombotic and embolic episodes in groups of patients with valve disease or valve replacement can often be broadly related to well-established risk factors, the intriguing question remains: what actually triggers a particular event in an individual patient, at a particular moment in time, given that the risk factors have often been present, perhaps relatively unchanged, for many years (202)? Sometimes an event can be linked to the sudden cessation of anticoagulation or a period of poor control (2), but in many cases the patient is either not taking anticoagulants or anticoagulant control has been satisfactory. In these patients it is necessary to search for trigger factors in addition to their risk factors (202).

Changes in coagulability may result from natural diurnal and cyclical variation and as the result of various disease processes, lifestyle influences or drug therapy. These changes may occur acutely or as the result of a gradual increase in prothrombotic conditions until a threshold is reached where anticoagulant and fibrinolytic mechanisms are 'overwhelmed' (Fig. 10.3-5).

Diurnal, cyclical and seasonal variation

Platelet aggregability is at its greatest in the morning, soon after rising (212-214), and has been shown to be associated with the assumption of an upright posture (215). Hematocrit (216,217), plasma viscosity (217), white cell adhesiveness (218) and levels of some clotting factors (219,220) are also at their highest at this time. Fibrinolytic activity

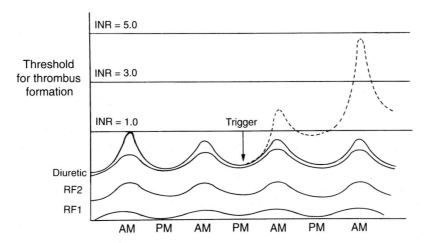

Figure 10.3-5: The relationship between risk factors and trigger factors and intracardiac thrombosis according to anticoagulation level, showing the additive effect of two risk factors and diuretics, diurnal fluctuation and the effect of introducing a trigger factor. Note that anticoagulation may have no effect on some trigger factors (see text).
INR = International Normalized Ratio; RF = Risk Factor

conversely is low in the morning and gradually increases during the day (169,170). Hence the coagulability of the blood is at its greatest between about 8 a.m. and 11 a.m., coinciding with the diurnal peak in the incidence of ischemic stroke (221-223), myocardial infarction (169,220,224) and sudden death (169,225). In examining the effect of circadian rhythm, some investigators have found no significant differences among the different subtypes of cerebral infarction or between patients with and without atrial fibrillation (223), whilst others have found no diurnal variation in the incidence of embolic strokes (221). One would expect the time of heightened coagulability to correspond with the time of *thrombosis* (as in cerebral thrombosis and coronary thrombosis) but not necessarily with the time that a portion of that thrombus breaks loose and *embolises*. Embolism from the left atrium could theoretically take place some hours or even some days after the thrombus was initiated. However, the finding of a morning peak in the incidence of stroke and TIA in mitral valve disease (226) and after mitral valve replacement (202) suggests either that many thrombi embolize soon after they have formed or that many cerebral events labeled as embolic are in fact thrombotic in origin (202).

In pre-menopausal women, fluctuations in coagulability and platelet aggregability occur during the menstrual cycle, both being greatest during the follicular phase of the cycle (days 5-9) (227,228). Greater changes in coagulability take place with the onset of the menopause. Mean levels of factor VIIc, fibrinogen, PAI-1 and cholesterol are higher in post-menopausal women (229-231), although these procoagulant changes are offset to some extent by higher antithrombin III levels (232,233). Women have higher fibrinogen levels than men at all ages but the difference becomes wider after the menopause (235). It has been suggested that procoagulant changes following the menopause may account for the associated increase in ischemic heart disease (229,231) and for the change in pattern of presentation, with a greater proportion of myocardial infarction and sudden death (234), although additional or alternative mechanisms have been proposed (236-238). The relationship between post-menopausal hemostatic variables and thrombosis and embolism in heart valve disease has not been investigated but the risk of valve thrombosis in patients with prosthetic valves appears to be greatest in post-menopausal women (vide infra).

A seasonal variation in fibrinogen and factor VIIc levels occurs among people living in a temperate climate (239-241). Higher levels are seen in the winter months, correlating with the higher mortality from coronary artery disease and stroke at this time of year (222,242,243). Higher fibrinogen levels are associated with the winter rise in infection incidence and are closely related to neutrophil count and C-reactive protein levels (240). Data from the Cardiff Valve Study, on 121 cerebrovascular events following mitral valve replacement (202), have shown a similar seasonal fluctuation with a peak in the winter months, lending support to the hypothesis that infection might be an initiating factor in many episodes of thrombosis and embolism (vide infra). Data from the same study have also shown a winter rise in the incidence of sudden death after valve replacement (244). In looking at seasonal effects, one must also consider the effect of cold per se. Under laboratory conditions mild surface cooling results in small but significant increases in hematocrit, platelet count and blood viscosity (245), and in the community fibrinogen

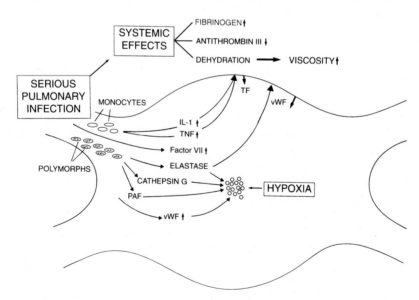

Figure 10.3-6: Diagrammatic representation of the effects of a serious pulmonary infection on conditions in the left atrium. Note that the effects of IL-1, TNF and leukocyte elastase on endothelium, although shown on left atrial endothelium for clarity, probably only occur locally at the site of infection, although concentrations of vWF particularly may be high in left atrial blood as a consequence.
IL-1 = interleukin-1, TNF = tumor necrosis factor, TF = tissue factor, vWf = von Willebrand factor, PAF = platelet activating factor.
The small aggregated circles in the center of the left atrium represent platelets.

levels and platelet aggregability rise progressively as daily air temperatures fall (241), closely paralleling the gradual increase in the incidence of stroke and myocardial infarction (242).

Disease processes

Of the disease processes which increase coagulability, **infection**, both acute and chronic, is probably the most important. Levels of fibrinogen (246) vWF (155,156) and PAI-1 (19) are elevated and levels of antithrombin III depressed (165). Increased levels of other acute phase reactant proteins, such as C-reactive protein and alpha$_2$ macroglobulin, contribute to the raised plasma viscosity (235) predominantly attributable to hyperfibrinogenemia and have direct effects on the procoagulant function of leukocytes (247). Leukocytes and cytokines play a fundamental role in the activation of coagulation (156,182,183,248-252). Many bacterial endotoxins and some viruses can induce platelet aggregation, activate the coagulation system and induce procoagulant function in endothelium (258). Severe infections are also associated with significant fluid loss and reduced fluid intake, which may lead to dehydration, further increasing plasma viscosity (246). Dehydration itself may be an important trigger for thrombus deposition in the presence of abnormal intracardiac flow conditions (98). Pulmonary infections are particularly important since the procoagulant changes are taking place in close proximity to the left atrium (Fig. 10.3-6) and because platelet agregability may be further increased by hypoxia (131,255,256).

The closely interwoven effects of leukocytes, fibrinogen and viscosity are evident in the pathogenesis of arterial disease (257-259). More research work is required on their role in intracardiac thrombosis and cerebrovascular events, but pointers to the importance of infection in patients with valve disease come from two studies. One review of 194 patients suffering embolism in association with rheumatic heart disease over a period of 27 years found that 11% of patients had febrile infections, mainly upper respiratory, within two weeks prior to embolism (197). Since these data were derived retrospectively from hospital records, they may underestimate the true percentage. Among patients in the Cardiff Valve Study suffering cerebrovascular events after mitral valve replacement, 30% reported infections, predominantly pulmonary, immediately prior to their events (202). This is in keeping with the importance of infection as a precursor of cerebral infarction in the general population also (260).

Hypertension increases the susceptibility to thrombosis and embolism as the result of several mechanisms. The endothelial cells of hypertensive blood vessels are larger, bulge into the lumen (35), produce less nitric oxide (261) and are more susceptible to the adherence of leukocytes and platelets (35). Hypertension is also associated with decreased platelet synthesis of nitric oxide (262), increased platelet aggregability (34,263-265), raised fibrinogen levels (33,145) and plasma viscosity (235,266,267) and diminished fibrinolysis due to increased levels of PAI-1 (33,34). Analysis of several studies of the relationship between hypertension and platelet aggregation suggests that increased aggregability may be associated only with mean arterial pressures greater than 120mmHg (264). Correction of hypertension with calcium antagonists or angiotensin converting enzyme (ACE) inhibitors can restore aggregability to normal (34,248) but the use of non-selective beta-adrenergic blockers may actually increase aggregability (34).

PAI-1 levels are raised even in mild hypertension (33), due to the hyperinsulinemia associated with insulin resistance in hypertension (33,172), and can be restored to normal with metformin (174), but not with beta-blockers (34); indeed the use of non-selective beta-blockers may decrease fibrinolytic activity still further (34).

Hypertension is the most important independent stroke risk factor (268), the risk rising progressively with increasing diastolic pressure (269). It also compounds the effect of other risk factors (270-272). Following aortic valve replacement, it is an important predictor of cerebrovascular events, particularly in men (273). Effective treatment of hypertension can be expected to reduce this risk (274).

In **ischemic heart disease** (IHD) hemostatic abnormalities can be demonstrated in many patients, including raised fibrinogen and factor VIIc levels (275), decreased fibrinolytic activity (30) and increased platelet aggregability (140,276,277), in keeping with the increased risk of stroke in IHD (268). Thus many patients with heart valve disease and co-existing coronary disease are at greater risk of cerebrovascular events, an effect which is more readily demonstrable following AVR than MVR. In the Cardiff Valve Study, among AVR patients experiencing minor transient cerebrovascular events, 41% had undergone concomitant coronary surgery in comparison to 20% in patients free of embolism (273). Two studies investigating embolism in patients with St. Jude Medical valves (almost entirely AVR) on antiplatelet therapy alone reported a zero incidence in young patients (mean age 27) with no coronary disease (278) but a 9.2% patient/year incidence in older patients (mean age 57), 45% of whom had coronary and other arterial disease (279).

Diabetes is associated with raised levels of fibrinogen (280,281) and vWF (32,160), reduced endothelial production of prostacyclin (253) and nitric oxide (261) and reduced fibrinolysis (31,171). Platelet function is also abnormal in diabetics with larger platelet volume (130), increased adhesiveness (281) and greater sensitivity to aggregating stimuli (253). **Many chronic inflammatory conditions** are associated with raised fibrinogen levels and these levels may increase during acute exacerbations (246). The anemia of chronic disease is often accompanied by raised fibrinogen, thrombocytosis and increased platelet adhesiveness (282). Patients with **nephrotic syndrome** develop platelet dysfunction, hyperfibrinogenemia and elevated levels of some coagulation factors (149,283). Levels of factor XIII and fibronectin are also raised (284) and levels of antithrombin III reduced (162). **Malignant disease** has a variety of effects on the coagulation system depending on the type of tumor, its pathological stage and the treatment employed. Common abnormalities in many cancers include elevation of fibrinogen and some coagulation factors, thrombocytosis and increased platelet aggregability (41,42). Some tumor cells also activate coagulation directly (42). Anti-endothelial cell antibodies contribute to the endothelial damage of many **autoimmune diseases** (285) and in a number of pathological situations oxygen free radicals can damage endothelium (259,286) and induce platelet activation (139,259).

Lifestyle and environmental influences

Ethnic differences in coagulability have been identified (146,287-291). Whether these differences are genetically determined or due to differences in climate (241,242), diet (291-293), tobacco (q.v.) and alcohol (294) consumption, exercise patterns (q.v.) and the prevalence of chronic disease (287,295,296) has been the subject of much research work. Whatever their pathogenesis, differences in coagulability are almost certainly partly responsible for ethnic differences in stroke incidence (291,295,297,298) and the incidence of intracardiac thrombosis and embolism following heart valve replacement (69,278,299,300).

Dietary fat content influences coagulability. The level of factor VIIc closely parallels total fat intake (142). Diets rich in saturated fat increase platelet aggregability (135-138) and raised lipoprotein(a) levels interfere with normal fibrinolysis on the endothelial cell surface (15). Hypertriglyceridemia is associated with raised fibrinogen and factor X levels and reduced fibrinolytic activity (301). Experimental work in animals suggests that a high fat, high carbohydrate, low protein diet can specifically induce atrial endothelial damage, predisposing to gross atrial thrombus formation (302). Obesity and a sedentary lifestyle are associated with increased blood viscosity (235,290), elevated levels of fibrinogen (235,303,304), factor VII (152,275) and PAI-1 (152,173) and reduced levels of antithrombin III (305). Regular exercise in contrast can reduce levels of factor VII (152,154) PAI-1 (152,306,307) and fibrinogen (154,306,308) and weight reduction in morbid obesity has similar benefits (305,309).

Cigarette smoking has several important effects on coagulability. Procoagulant effects have been demonstrated on all components of the hemostatic system. Raised endothelial cell counts in blood suggest that smoking has a direct toxic effect on endothelium, inducing procoagulant function (310). Fibrinogen levels are elevated in direct proportion to the number of cigarettes smoked per day (120). Indeed chronic cigarette smoking is thought to be the most important cause of raised fibrinogen levels (146) and even ex-smokers have raised levels which only gradually fall towards normal over a ten year period (121). The effect of raised fibrinogen levels on blood viscosity (vide supra) is further enhanced by the raised hematocrit associated with chronic smoking (119). White cell counts are also elevated (121), and platelet adhesiveness increased (311). Reports on platelet aggregability in smokers have been conflicting, some demonstrating increased aggregability (312-315), or reduced sensitivity to prostacyclin (316), others normal (277,317) or reduced aggregability (318,319). This apparent inconsistency is probably explained by differences in methodology and the subjects' age, diet and length of smoking history (312,320) in addition to differences in time elapsed since the last cigarette (312,319). In some subjects, particularly young, healthy people with a short smoking history and those exposed to passive smoking, the effect on platelet aggregability is acute and transient (313-315). High dietary fat intake potentiates this effect (320). The persistently elevated platelet aggregability of long-standing and older smokers (312) may be partly due to raised fibrinogen levels (134), partly due to structural changes in platelets (321), and partly due to excess oxygen free radicals (139). Smoking is also associated with depression of fibrinolytic activity, probably due to increased PAI-1 production secondary to smoking-induced hyperinsulinemia (31,173,322).

The effect of smoking on stroke and coronary risk is dose related. Heavy cigarette smoking approximately doubles the risk of cerebral infarction (272,323), and is synergistic with other risk factors (272,324). It is therefore not surprising to find an influence of smoking on the incidence of cerebrovascular events after valve replacement also. The Cardiff Valve Study has demonstrated a significant relationship between smoking and stroke in patients following both mitral and aortic valve replacement

---

Table 10.3-I: Important drug interactions with oral anticoagulants

---

Enhancement of anticoagulant effect

By inhibition of microsomal enzymes

Allopurinol	Disulfiram	Metronidazole
Amiodarone	Enoxacin	Omeprazole
Azapropazone	Erythromycin	Oxyphenbutazone
Cimetidine	Fluconazole	Phenylbutazone
Ciprofloxacin	Fluvoxamine	Sulphinpyrazone
Co-trimoxazole	Ketoconazole	Sulphonamides

Decreased availability of vitamin K

Aminoglycoside antibiotics	Tetracyclines
Cephalosporins	

Increased catabolism of vitamin-K dependent factors

Thyroid compounds

Mechanisms unknown

Acetyl salicyclic acid	Flurbiprofen	Nalidixic acid
Aminosalicyclic acid	Gemfibrozil	Norfloxacin
Anabolic steroids & androgens	Glucagon	Ofloxacin
Azapropazone	Ifosfamide/Mesna	Phenytoin
Bezafibrate	Indomethacin	Quinidine
Chloramphenicol	Isoniazid	Sulindac
Colfibrate	Itraconazole	Tamoxifen
Danazol	Lovastatin	Topical Salicylates
Diflunisal	Mefenamic acid	Vitamin E
Disopyramide	Miconazole	

Diminution of anticoagulant effect

By induction of microsomal enzymes

Aminoglutethimide	Carbamazepine
Barbiturates/Primidone	Glutethimide
	Rifampicin

By decreasing absorption and/or interruption of enterohepatic circulation

Cholestyramine	Colestipol

Due to decreased catabolism of vitamin K-dependent factors

Carbimazole	Thiouracils

Due to increased synthesis of clotting factors

Oestrogens

Mechanism unknown

Griseofulvin	6-Mercaptopurine
Haloperidol	Phenytoin (may also potentiate)

Reproduced with permission from ref. 333

(202,273). No relationship was found between smoking and TIA following MVR, in keeping with similar findings in medically treated mitral valve disease (226,325). Smoking appears to function mainly as an arterial risk factor (324) and to have little influence in promoting thrombosis under conditions of stasis (326).

Mental stress has several effects on hemostatic variables and has been the subject of much research in connection with ischemic heart disease (327-329). Acute mental stress has been shown to increase platelet aggregability probably through the effects of increased adrenaline secretion (133), while prolonged stress and chronic anxiety states are both associated with raised fibrinogen and blood viscosity (329-331). These changes may have relevance for patients with heart valve disease also, as possible triggering mechanisms in the presence of other risk factors. One series of prosthetic valve thromboses has reported previous depressive illness requiring psychiatric treatment in 21% of cases (332). Experimentally, rats fed on high fat diets are more prone to adrenaline-induced left atrial thrombosis (137).

Drug therapy

Many drugs other than anticoagulants have an influence on coagulability, either directly or indirectly. Perhaps the most common indirect effect is the interaction between oral anticoagulants and other drugs (Table 10.3-I), leading either to enhancement or reduction in effective anticoagulation (333). The unwitting introduction of additional medication which decreases the effectiveness of oral anticoagulation may upset the balance of procoagulant and anticoagulant influences within the left atrium, for example, and result in thrombus deposition. Fortunately most of the drugs which diminish the effect of oral anticoagulants are infrequently required in patients with heart valve disease. The most commonly prescribed additional short-term drugs are antibiotics, but of those which interact with oral anticoagulants, almost all *enhance* the anticoagulant effect (333).

Digitalis preparations at one time were thought to increase coagulability but any effect they might have is probably mediated through the diuresis that they promote in cardiac failure (197). **Diuretic therapy**, by increasing plasma viscosity, enhances coagulability and may play a part in the initiation of intracardiac thrombosis (98). The sodium channel inhibiting diuretic, amiloride, inhibits sodium/hydrogen exchange across the platelet membrane in the early phase of platelet activation and functions as an inhibitor of platelet aggregation, at least in vitro (334). This potential antithrombotic effect may provide further justification for including amiloride in diuretic combinations for patients with heart valve disease.

Beta-adrenergic blockers are commonly prescribed in patients with heart valve disease. Their effects on coagulability are controversial (335). Some studies have demonstrated platelet inhibition (248). Others have shown that non-selective beta blockers increase platelet aggregability (34,336) and leukocyte adhesiveness (337,338) and decrease fibrinolytic activity (24,336). In addition they can cause elevation of plasma triglycerides and reduction in HDL cholesterol (339) which in turn may result in raised levels of fibrinogen and factor X and reduced fibrinolysis (301). Cardioselective beta$_1$ blockers have less of these undesirable effects (34,339,340). **Calcium antagonists** are potentially more suitable for the heart valve patient since they have inhibiting effects on platelet and leukocyte function (248,341) and no adverse effects on lipid metabolism (339).

Corticosteroids have the potential to increase coagulability by stimulating fibrinogen synthesis (342) and inhibiting fibrinolysis (343). Of the non-cardiac drugs which influence coagulability, preparations containing estrogen have aroused the greatest controversy, particularly those used for contraceptive purposes. It is important at the outset to distinguish between the estrogens used in oral contraceptives (which are synthetic, prescribed at relatively high doses and given in conjunction with a synthetic progestogen) and estrogens used as hormonal replacement therapy in post-menopausal women (which are usually natural estrogens given in much smaller doses) (344).

The influence of **oral contraceptive drugs** on coagulability and cardiovascular risk has been extensively reviewed (139,275,326,345). Fibrinogen levels are elevated in many women taking oral contraceptives (346) but the confounding effects of obesity, hypertension and cigarette smoking need to be taken into account (230). Many clotting factors tend to be raised also (139,275) and antithrombin III levels are depressed (162).

Platelet aggregability is also increased, probably due to a direct effect of peroxidized free fatty acids, which result from the change in oxidative status in oral contraceptive users (139). This increased aggregability is potentiated by a high intake of polyunsaturated fatty acids and by smoking. The adverse change in oxidative status in women taking oral contraceptives is due to decreased levels of antioxidants (principally vitamin C and vitamin E), which results in higher levels of oxygen free radicals. In addition to an effect on aggregability, excess oxygen free radicals may also increase platelet clotting activity by modifying the phospholipid composition of the platelet membrane, enhancing its effect in potentiating thrombin formation (139). The hypercoagulable effects of oral contraceptives can be minimized by the avoidance of smoking, by the consumption of a low fat diet and by dietary supplementation with vitamins C and E (139).

The degree of increased stroke risk attributable to oral contraceptive use is closely related to the estrogen content of the preparation, ranging from a factor of almost five in high dose pills down to a factor of two in mini-estrogen pills (30-40µg estrogen) (347). Progestogen only pills appear to carry no excess risk (347). No studies have examined the risk of oral contraceptive use in heart valve patients but either avoidance or prescription of progestogen only pills seems prudent until more data are available.

Hormone replacement therapy (HRT) is widely prescribed for the treatment of menopausal symptoms, osteoporosis and genital atrophy and is taken by some women who wish to remain "feminine forever". Recently interest has centered on possible benefits in reducing cardiovascular risk, but concerns remain about its effects on coagulability (230,344,348,349).

Against the background of altered hemostatic variables and iron metabolism in post-menopausal women (229-238), some of which may be related to changes in lifestyle (more sedentary existence, obesity, dietary changes, etc.), the coagulation data in women taking HRT must be interpreted with care. It has been suggested for example that there may be selection bias, such that any possible protective role attributed to HRT in terms of reduced cardiovascular risk may in fact be due to selection of healthier women to receive HRT (230). Furthermore, assessment of available data is hindered by the fact that among the various published studies, different types and dosages of estrogens have been used both with and without added progestogen. It is perhaps not surprising therefore that some studies have reported adverse effects on coagulation parameters and cardiovascular risk, whilst others have reported either no effect or a beneficial effect. No consistent pattern has so far emerged from these data and large, well-controlled

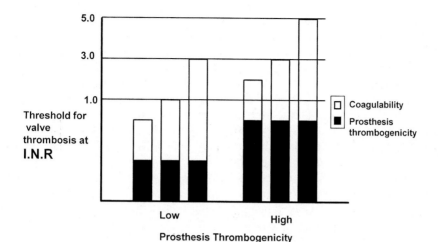

Figure 10.3-7: The additive effect of prosthesis thrombogenicity and coagulability on the risk of prosthetic valve thrombosis in two hypothetical prostheses of different thrombogenicity at different levels of anticoagulation. An increase in coagulability or a fall in anticoagulation intensity creates higher risk in a prosthesis of high thrombogenicity.

prospective randomized studies are clearly required (348). A review of the subject in 1985 concluded that doubt remained about the influence of HRT on coagulability, but that there appeared to be increasing evidence of a protective effect against cardiovascular disease (344). The latter received some confirmation from the 10 year follow up results of the Nurses' Health Study conducted in the USA, which found a significant reduction in the risk of coronary heart disease, but no reduction in the risk of stroke (350). Indeed the relative risk of ischemic stroke, adjusted for age and risk factors, was 1.46 (95% CI 0.85-2.51), which although not considered significant, leans towards the findings of the Framingham study which found an adverse effect of post-menopausal estrogen use on stroke risk (351). Discordance between effects on coronary risk and stroke risk raises the possibility that the excess stroke risk could be due to increased coagulability and greater susceptibility to embolic stroke. Therefore, until further research provides the explanation, it is probably safer to avoid HRT in patients with heart valve disease or prosthetic valves unless there is an overwhelming clinical reason for prescribing it.

Risk factors and trigger factors for prosthetic valve thrombosis

Thrombus forming on a prosthetic valve represents a special situation. Clearly, the most obvious risk factor is the prosthesis itself. Its contribution to the risk is determined by its **inherent thrombogenicity**, a property which is difficult to define in numerical terms since it involves three principal characteristics: its surfaces, its stagnation characteristics and its propensity for activating platelets, through the shear stresses it imposes on flowing blood (vide supra). In addition, 'stenotic' mitral prostheses impose conditions of left atrial stasis (352), a characteristic which must be included in the assessment of prosthetic thrombogenicity. Thus thrombogenicity varies from one type of prosthesis to another, according to construction materials and design features. The assessment of this thrombogenicity in the clinical situation, although a laudable goal, is fraught with difficulties (56) since, in analyzing the incidence of valve thrombosis, it is necessary to allow for the other factors which increase the risk of valve thrombosis and the trigger factors which initiate it. As with intracardiac thrombosis in general, the presence of a risk factor (in this case, the prosthesis) for many years does not result in thrombosis unless a trigger factor alters the balance.

The contribution of each factor to the risk of valve thrombosis may be thought of in diagrammatic terms (Fig. 10.3-7) by envisaging a threshold at which thrombosis occurs. This threshold may be reached by the summation of the various risk factors and trigger factors, the contribution of each varying from prosthesis to prosthesis, from patient to patient and with time. The thrombogenicity of the prosthesis will be highest in the first few months after implantation before endothelialization of the sewing ring occurs (56). This period of increased risk, when combined with the hypercoagulability of the immediate postoperative period (166), and the selective effect of the prosthesis in identifying patients with elevated innate coagulability, probably accounts for the early peak in the hazard function curve for valve thrombosis during the first year after implantation in some series (353). Later, the thrombogenicity of the prosthesis may increase due to structural changes (e.g., mechanical wear (354) or degeneration and calcification in bioprostheses (79)) or tissue ingrowth. Tissue ingrowth is an important predisposing factor for valve thrombosis (61,69,355). The susceptibility of a prosthesis to tissue ingrowth (q.v.), and its vulnerability to secondary valve thrombosis as a result, can be regarded as two further components of its thrombogenicity. Prosthesis thrombogenicity may also vary with size, particularly in tilting disc prostheses, in which the minor orifice has a relatively low flow velocity (24,61), the risk being higher in smaller prostheses (332,356,357).

Returning to Virchow's triad (5), the other factors which influence the risk of valve thrombosis are to be found in intracardiac flow conditions and in the coagulability of the blood. The latter in turn is determined by the patients own coagulability and by overall antithrombotic management and anticoagulation control in particular.

Some degree of relative stasis is a prerequisite for valve thrombosis. Present to a varied amount in different prostheses, including bioprostheses (84), it is enhanced by low **intracardiac flow conditions**, imposed either by low cardiac output (80,358) or by left atrial stasis (355). Atrial fibrillation and left atrial enlargement are reported to increase the risk of mitral valve thrombosis with some prostheses (355) and it has been suggested that advanced NYHA class is a predisposing factor (332).

Hypercoagulability almost certainly contributes to valve thrombosis, both as a risk factor and a trigger factor and may partly account for the higher incidence of valve thrombosis in the early postoperative months (166). Its emergence as a significant factor has probably been obscured in many series of prosthetic valve thrombosis by the dominant etiologic roles of prosthesis thrombogenicity and anticoagulation interruption and by the lack of thorough investigation for possible trigger factors.

In prostheses of low thrombogenicity, valve thrombosis is a rare event and consequently the search for contributing factors is likely to be more rewarding. The Medtronic Hall valve has been shown to be one of the least thrombogenic prostheses (359,360). Analysis of the few valve thromboses which have occurred with this prosthesis in the Cardiff Valve Study reveals the probability that hyperfibrinogenemia

Table 10.3-II: Patient characteristics and anticoagulation status of four patients with obstructive prosthetic valve thrombosis

Patient	#1	#2	#3	#4
Sex	F	F	F	F
Age	72	73	71	72
Obesity	++	+	+	0
Season	W	W	W	W
Infection	+		+	
Valve size (mm)	A20	A20	M23	M27
Anticoagulation interruption	x3		x1 +VIT.K	x1 (4 months duration)

"x" is to say "times" i.e., anticoagulation interuption three times, once, once
F = female, W = winter, A = aortic, M = mitral

Reproduced with permission from ref. 357.
Data derived from the only patients to suffer obstructive valve thrombosis in a series of 1,800 implanted Medtronic Hall valves.

plays a dominant role (357). Raised fibrinogen levels are common to all the possible etiologic factors identified in this study (Table 10.3-II): post-menopausal status (235), obesity (235,303,304), infection (246) and winter origin (239-241). Since these factors occurred in combination in most patients, their effect on fibrinogen is likely to have been additive. In these patients, the combination of small prosthesis size and anticoagulation interruption, when added to hyperfibrinogenemia, was probably sufficient to reach the threshold for valve thrombosis. Careful history taking in future may reveal febrile infections, particularly respiratory, as precursors to many valve thromboses (Fig. 10.3-8). At least one other detailed case report in the literature has recorded such information, although the authors did not comment on its possible significance (361). The hyperfibrinogenemia associated with chronic infection and parasite infestation typical of rural communities in tropical and subtropical Africa (287) may be one explanation for the higher incidence of valve thrombosis in this region (300). Raised fibrinogen levels are known to increase the risk of thrombosis by raising blood viscosity (93) and increasing platelet aggregability (134), effects which are particularly relevant to the abnormal flow conditions associated with prosthetic valves. In the case of infection as a trigger factor, other procoagulant changes (q.v.) probably contribute also.

Anticoagulation interruption or absence of anticoagulation has been identified as a significant factor in may series (278,358,362-365). Of the four cases of obstructive valve thrombosis in the Cardiff Valve Study referred to above, anticoagulation had been interrupted in three patients, in one for several months (357). However, there is no uniformity in the literature on this risk factor, the incidence of anticoagulation interruption in reported series ranging from zero (332) to 100% (358), reflecting the importance of other predisposing factors. Several series of valve thromboses have attributed the complication in many patients to "inadequate" or "poorly controlled"

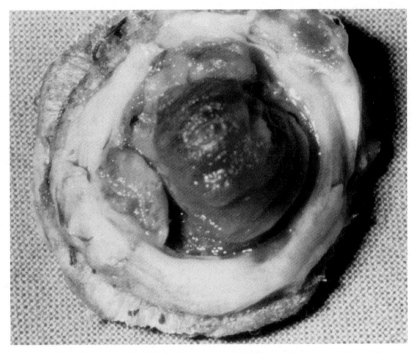

Figure 10.3-8: Thrombosis of Björk-Shiley Standard mitral prosthesis, seen from the ventricular aspect. Progressive symptoms of four weeks duration followed an episode of pneumonia. The rubbery thrombus shows marked lamination, indicating successive layers of thrombus deposition, in keeping with the length of the history.

anticoagulation (69,332,366,367). However, these are meaningless terms unless accompanied by definitions involving numerical data based on anticoagulation levels achieved, and too much reliance should not be placed on *undefined* 'inadequate' anticoagulation as a risk factor. Indeed, the tolerance by a prosthesis of numerically defined low intensity and highly variable anticoagulation with a low risk of valve thrombosis can be regarded as a measure of its low thrombogenicity (359), since detailed analysis shows this type of anticoagulation to be the rule rather than the exception in many centers (368).

Although valve thrombosis rates give a better indication of the thrombogenicity of a prosthesis than embolic rates (q.v.), considerable variation in rates can occur between different series of the same prosthesis, particularly among series of more thrombogenic prostheses (56,360). This variation is almost certainly due to differences in anticoagulation intensity (q.v.), differences in numbers of patients who had their anticoagulation interrupted and differences in patient coagulability and intracardiac flow conditions. In future, reports on valve thrombosis should take these factors into consideration.

EMBOLISM AS AN INDICATOR OF THERAPEUTIC FAILURE

Systemic embolism is a superficially attractive endpoint and its incidence within groups of patients has been used as a means of attempting to distinguish between the effectiveness of different forms of treatment, particularly between different types of prosthesis (1,2,369) and between different regimens of antithrombotic management (369-373). However, it is necessary to sound a note of caution when interpreting embolic incidence, particularly in relation to prosthetic heart valves. In most series, the majority of events reported as "embolism" are cerebrovascular (1,3) and the authors conveniently assume not only that all events are embolic in etiology but that the emboli all originated from the prosthesis. In fact many pathophysiologic mechanisms other than cardioembolism lead to cerebral infarction: in situ arterial thrombosis, artery-to-artery embolism, intrinsic small vessel vasculopathies, various types of arteritis and global hypoperfusion (374). In the general population, only about 15% of ischemic strokes are embolic in origin (375). The proportion of cerebrovascular events due to embolism in patients with prosthetic valves is unknown. It is likely to be higher than 15% but will vary between series according to the age of the patient population and the prevalence of stroke risk factors in addition to the type of prosthesis. Even when the cerebrovascular event is truly cardioembolic, it is often uncertain whether the embolus originated from the prosthesis or from the left atrium.

It is thus meaningless to describe prosthetic valves or indeed therapeutic regimens as having "embolic rates". Only groups of *patients* have embolic rates or, more properly, cerebrovascular event rates, and these are determined not only by their type of prosthesis and their antithrombotic management, but by their age, their stroke and cardiac risk factors, and by trigger factors for thrombosis (vide supra). It is hence not surprising that there is as much variation in embolic rates between reported series of the *same* prosthesis as there is between *different* prostheses (376). Furthermore meta-analysis of reported series (369) merely derives meaningless averages which do nothing to advance understanding of the underlying mechanisms which account for the differences.

When evaluating series of replacement valves in the literature, one should also be suspicious of papers which report a zero incidence of embolism unless the patient population is very young with most patients in sinus rhythm, as in some papers from the Middle East for example (278). There is a 'background incidence' of stroke and TIA in the general population, which gradually rises with age, reaching about 2% per year by the age of 80 in Western populations (297). This incidence may be reduced in some subgroups by anticoagulation (notably in patients with AF) but is never abolished (189-192). Therefore it is impossible that any large valve series which includes elderly patients followed for several years, should not contain some patients who have suffered stroke or TIA. The complete absence of stroke and TIA from any large valve series usually indicates serious defects in the methodology of data collection (377).

THERAPEUTIC CONSIDERATIONS

Numerous factors influence the individual heart valve patient's risk of intracardiac thrombosis and subsequent embolism. Many of these factors relate to intercurrent disease processes, nutritional status and lifestyle and may be just as important to identify as the extent of the heart valve disease and associated cardiac pathology, if progress is to be made in the prevention of thrombosis and embolism. Thus the initial

Table 10.3-III: Coagulation tests required for initial assessment and follow up

Level 1 'Essential' baseline tests

Fibrinogen	-	effects on viscosity and platelets
vWF	-	measure of endothelial procoagulant activity
tPA and PAI-1	-	"balance" of fibrinolytic system
Antithrombin III	-	natural anticoagulant
White cell count	-	evidence of inflammation
Platelet volume	-	association with aggregability

Level 2 Evidence of coagulation and fibrinolytic systems 'in action'

Fibrinopeptide A	-	measure of fibrin production
F_{1+2}	-	measure of thrombin production
D-dimer	-	measure of fibrinolytic activity

NB. The degree of sophistication of coagulation tests is almost unlimited. Basic information sufficient for a useful assessment of the patients coagulability can be obtained from level 1 tests only. F_{1+2} will be influenced by oral anticoagulation.
See text for abbreviations

assessment and regular follow up of the patient with heart valve disease should include a coagulation profile in addition to hemodynamic measurements. The key tests which should allow a useful profile to be constructed are listed in Table 10.3-III.

Because of complications associated with valve replacement, cardiologists have always been reluctant to recommend surgical treatment until the patient's native valve disease has deteriorated to the extent that the symptoms and risk of mortality exceed those associated with valve replacement. This often means that by the time the patient reaches the cardiac surgeon he is already in AF, his left atrium is already significantly dilated or his left ventricular function has deteriorated. The current trend towards greater use of percutaneous balloon valvotomy (Chapter 7.3) and valve repair techniques (Chapters 8.2-8.6) in suitable cases of mitral valve disease, and the current availability of less thrombogenic prostheses, should lead logically to earlier intervention before AF, left atrial enlargement or left ventricular dysfunction supervene. It can be anticipated that a policy of earlier intervention in order to preserve normal cardiac function and prevent pulmonary hypertension would repay a dividend of reduced thromboembolic risk, providing that conservative valve-sparing procedures are used wherever possible and that these are effective in relieving transvalvular gradients or controlling regurgitation. In cases where valve replacement is necessary, the most hemodynamically efficient and least thrombogenic prosthesis should be chosen. If no significant transvalvular gradient remains, cardiac function is normal and the replacement valve is of low thrombogenicity, the risk of embolism will be small and determined mainly by non-cardiac risk factors associated with abnormal hemostatic function and by the antithrombotic management.

Effective antithrombotic management involves much more than simply treating the patient with anticoagulants. It should encompass the performance of the necessary investigations to create a risk factor profile (Table 10.3-III) and where possible the correction of hemostatic abnormalities by eliminating their underlying causes. Thus hypertension, obesity and hyperlipidemia should be treated, cigarette smoking stopped and advice given about diet, exercise and the avoidance of chronic stress and potentially thrombogenic drugs. All infections, but particularly respiratory infections, should be treated promptly.

If hemostatic abnormalities cannot be corrected and intracardiac conditions persist which favor thrombus deposition, antithrombotic treatment will be required. However, wherever possible this should be tailored to the remaining hemostatic abnormalities, the degree of cardiac dysfunction (particularly the degree of left atrial stasis) and the type of prosthetic valve (if present). The smaller the degree of risk, the less intense the regime of antithrombotic treatment that will be required (Fig.10.3-5).

ANTICOAGULATION

Anticoagulation remains the mainstay of antithrombotic prophylaxis and in many patients, no further treatment other than risk factor modification will be required. However, it is important to understand the limitations of anticoagulation and the relationship between intensity of anticoagulation and therapeutic effectiveness. Most space will be devoted to discussion of oral anticoagulation since this form of anticoagulation is of greatest relevance to patients with heart valve disease, but brief mention will also be made of heparin therapy as appropriate.

Oral anticoagulation

Although several oral anticoagulant drugs are in widespread use, all exert their effect by interfering with vitamin K metabolism, thereby decreasing the carboxylation of four coagulation factors and two natural anticoagulants during their synthesis in the liver: factors II (prothrombin), VII, IX and X and proteins C and S (333,378-380). Carboxylation of these proteins is the part of the synthesis which confers their biological activity, enabling them to participate in calcium-dependent reactions on phospholipid surfaces (380). Inhibition of carboxylation results in the production of partially carboxylated proteins (378,380). Already circulating fully carboxylated proteins are unaffected by oral anticoagulants; there is thus a delay in the onset of action of these drugs, proportional to the plasma half-lives of the vitamin-K dependent proteins and their rate of synthesis (333). The activity of protein C is reduced before that of any of the coagulation proteins, resulting in an early increase in coagulability before any drug-induced anticoagulation occurs (9).

The percentage reduction in coagulant activity is related to the reduction in the numbers of carboxylated glutamate residues on prothrombin molecules (378,380). Unfortunately, owing to considerable variation among patients in dietary content of vitamin K, drug absorption and metabolism, intercurrent disease processes and drug interactions, the dose response varies widely from patient to patient (380). It is therefore necessary to have a reliable and reproducible method of measuring the anticoagulation effect, so that a specific intensity of anticoagulation can be prescribed rather than a drug dose.

Measuring the anticoagulation effect

The most widely used method for measuring the effect of oral anticoagulants is the

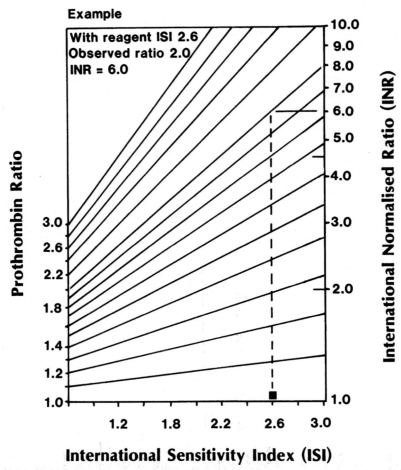

Figure 10.3-9: Nomogram relating International Normalized Ratio (INR) to the measured prothrombin time ratio according to the International Sensitivity Index (ISI) of thromboplastins.

prothrombin time, which provides a means of assessing the extent to which prothrombin and factors VII, IX and X have been inhibited by interference with their carboxylation (380). It does not assess the *effectiveness* of anticoagulation in reducing the generation of thrombin in vivo since this is determined by additional factors which are not affected by oral anticoagulants, for example platelet procoagulant activity (125), the plasma level of antithrombin III (381) and the balance between tissue factor expression and local endothelial production of TFPI which inhibits the activation of factor X by the factor VII/tissue factor complex (7).

The prothrombin time test, originally devised by Quick in 1935 and still in use today, involves the addition of a thromboplastin reagent (usually derived from brain tissue), containing large amounts of tissue factor, to the patient's plasma; calcium is added at zero time and the number of seconds are counted until a clot forms; the prolongation of the clotting time is then compared to a reference plasma pooled from healthy volunteers (382).

This rather crude and deceptively simple test can in fact be dangerously misleading unless the results are expressed in a standardized fashion (383,384). Many different commercial thromboplastins are in use which vary widely in their sensitivity according to the tissue from which they were prepared and the extent to which it was contaminated by blood during preparation (385,386). Some thromboplastins also contain added fibrinogen (386).

Although different thromboplastins yield very similar clotting times when the plasma is *normal*, they can produce widely different clotting times on the same sample of *anticoagulated* plasma because of their different sensitivities. In order to circumvent this dangerous inaccuracy, the concept of the International Sensitivity Index (ISI) was introduced to enable thromboplastin manufacturers to specify the sensitivities of their products and to allow the conversion of the 'raw' prothrombin ratio to a standardized ratio, the International Normalized Ratio (INR) (385). Providing that manufacturers are scrupulous in defining the ISI of their products accurately (387) and providing that allowance is made for potential inaccuracies that can be introduced by different automated coagulation analyzers (385), the use of the INR should allow accurate and reproducible measurement of the extent of the anticoagulant effect *in vitro* permitting much safer anticoagulation management for the individual patient and the opportunity for sensible international communication on the subject of anticoagulation intensity (385). For example, since the rates of prosthetic valve thrombosis and systemic embolism following valve replacement with a particular prosthesis can both be influenced by the

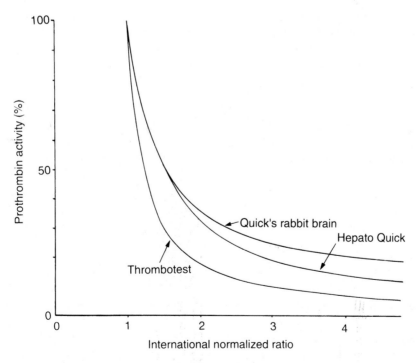

Figure 10.3-10: Graph relating International Normalized Ratio (INR) to percentage prothrombin activity as measured by three commonly used thromboplastins. Reproduced from Ref. #385, with permission.

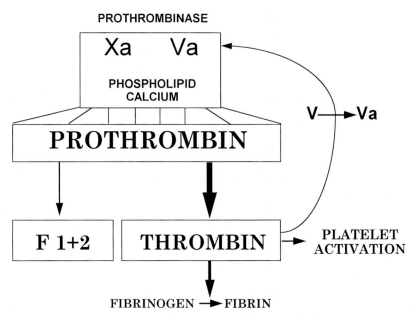

Figure 10.3-11: Diagram showing the fundamental role of thrombin in the coagulation system.

intensity of anticoagulation, reports in the literature which provide rates of these complications without specifying the INR are largely meaningless (166). This is particularly true of reports from the USA which often include the statement that "the prothrombin time was maintained at twice normal". Because of the large number of different thromboplastin reagents in use in the USA, with ISI values ranging from 1.2 to 2.8 (383) a prothrombin time of "twice normal" could be equivalent to an INR anywhere between 2.6 and 7.0 (380). (Fig. 10.3-9).

In Europe, it has been traditional to express the extent of the anticoagulant effect in vitro as the percentage of remaining prothrombin activity. Again different percentages are obtained on the same plasma sample using different thromboplastin reagents, but curves can be drawn for each reagent, relating percentages to INR values (Fig. 10.3-10) (385).

An alternative method for assessing the effect of oral anticoagulants on prothrombin itself is the measurement of the residual quantity of fully carboxylated prothrombin present in the blood. This can be achieved using an antibody, specific for fully carboxylated prothrombin, which does not bind to poorly carboxylated or uncarboxylated prothrombin (388). Using this method, the normal prothrombin level is 90-125µg/ml. It has been suggested that the optimal therapeutic anticoagulant effect probably occurs with levels in the range 12-24 µg/ml, values below this range being associated with a high risk of bleeding and values above being associated with inadequate thromboprophylaxis (388). A prospective randomized trial in the USA, comparing this method with *unstandardized* prothrombin times for monitoring oral anticoagulant therapy revealed significantly fewer bleeding and thrombotic events in the group monitored with blood prothrombin levels; overall an 85% reduction in events was reported (388). However, it should be stressed that unstandardized prothrombin times are acknowledged to be a potentially hazardous method of monitoring anticoagulant therapy, as already discussed, and a comparison between blood prothrombin levels and INR would be more realistic.

The desired effect of anticoagulation, through the inhibition of factor VII, factor X and prothrombin itself, is a reduction in the ability to generate thrombin (Fig. 10.3-11) since thrombin is central to the coagulation process, not only converting fibrinogen into fibrin but also activating platelets and enormously accelerating further thrombin production by activating factor V, a component of the prothrombinase complex (389). When prothrombin is converted to thrombin, part of the molecule is broken off. This fragment (F_{1+2}), unlike thrombin, is relatively stable in plasma and can be measured (390). Levels of F_{1+2} in plasma reflect the amount of thrombin generation and can be used to monitor the anticoagulant effect *in vivo* (381,391,392). This may allow greater precision in anticoagulation control and may lead to safer and more sophisticated tailoring of the anticoagulant effect, once further studies have established the level of F_{1+2} that is consistent with prevention of thrombosis in various situations. It has already been shown that in patients with raised F_{1+2} levels subject to recurrent venous thrombosis, low intensity anticoagulation (INR 1.5) is sufficient to restore F_{1+2} levels to normal (381). In patients with non-valvular AF, the reduction in F_{1+2} levels brought about by low intensity anticoagulation (INR 1.5-2.7) correlates with reduced risk of embolism (393). In patients with prosthetic heart valves, and in other clinical situations, F_{1+2} levels fall in proportion to increasing INR (381,392), unless antithrombin III levels are grossly reduced (381). Preliminary studies in patients with mechanical valves have shown that even low intensity anticoagulation (INR 2.1-2.4) reduces F_{1+2} levels (and hence thrombin levels) to well below the normal range (392). Further research work, correlating F_{1+2} levels to thromboembolic risk in patients with heart valve disease and particular types of prosthetic valve, is required before F_{1+2} levels can be considered as a basis for anticoagulation recommendations. At present, the assay is extremely expensive and it is therefore unlikely that it will supersede the very cheap prothrombin time measurements for routine monitoring purposes.

Limitations of oral anticoagulation.

The most fundamental limitation of oral anticoagulation is that it targets only one of the components of the hemostatic system. It has no direct effect on platelets, endothelial function, the fibrinolytic system or on the prothrombotic effects of activated white cells, although indirect effects may occur on platelets (through reduced thrombin-induced activation) (389) and on the fibrinolytic system (through reduced thrombin-induced release of PAI-1 from endothelium and platelets) (14,19). Trigger factors for thrombosis which exert their effects primarily through these other components of the hemostatic system, for example infection, may thus be largely uninfluenced by a level of anticoagulation considered 'therapeutic' under normal circumstances (Fig. 10.3-5). Furthermore, the role of the various components of the hemostatic system in thrombosis varies according to flow conditions (94), with the coagulation system playing a major role under stagnant 'venous' conditions but a relatively minor role under conditions of high shear stress where the actions of platelets, vWF and other adhesive proteins predominate, to enable the thrombus to resist the high shear stresses (102,394). As a result moderate or low intensity anticoagulation is effective under venous conditions but even high intensity oral anticoagulation cannot totally abolish thrombosis, in the presence of powerful platelet activators such as collagen, under arterial conditions (395).

This difference in effect under different flow conditions has been shown experimentally by drawing anticoagulated human blood at different levels of INR over strips of rabbit aortic subendothelium at rates of flow simulating venous and arterial conditions (395). Much smaller amounts of fibrin were deposited under arterial conditions in comparison to venous conditions either with or without anticoagulation. Under venous conditions even low intensity anticoagulation (INR 2.1) reduced fibrin deposition on this highly thrombogenic surface by about 60%; an INR of 3.5 brought about an 80% reduction and an INR of 5.0 abolished fibrin deposition altogether. However, under arterial conditions the dimensions of *platelet thrombus* were only significantly reduced when the INR reached 5.0 and then only by about 40% (395).

Unfortunately similar studies have never been performed with prosthetic surfaces. However, once a prosthesis is well incorporated, its sewing ring is fully endothelialized and its surface (in the case of mechanical valves) has undergone passivation (49), it may represent a less thrombogenic surface than exposed subendothelium (396), a highly thrombogenic surface, although this is difficult to predict from in vitro studies (396) since much of the 'thrombogenicity' of a prosthesis depends on associated patterns of blood flow in addition to the characteristics of the prosthetic materials (24,56).

The flow conditions associated with mechanical valves (and to a lesser extent with bioprostheses) are a mixture of 'arterial' and 'venous' conditions, the latter occurring in relation to zones of relative stagnation or low velocity reverse flow when the valve is open. In this context, one can define the thrombogenicity of a prosthesis in terms of the two principal flow conditions it creates, since the degree of 'stagnation' will determine the susceptibility to fibrin deposition and the shear stresses caused by non-physiological high velocity flow patterns and associated red cell damage will determine the degree of platelet activation. The latter cannot be controlled by anticoagulation which probably explains why the microembolism of presumed platelet aggregates seen with some mechanical valves in some patients cannot be abolished by increasing the intensity of anticoagulation (397).

Fibrin deposition under 'stagnant' conditions in contrast is readily controlled by anticoagulation (395,398), and from basic principles one would anticipate that the less stagnant the flow conditions, the lower would be the intensity of anticoagulation required to control it. At the other extreme, a prosthesis with high stagnation characteristics would probably need an intensity of anticoagulation capable of virtually abolishing fibrin deposition; extrapolating from the experimental work referred to above, an INR in the region of 5.0 might be required to guarantee freedom from valve thrombosis. This hypothesis is in keeping with clinical reports of valve thrombosis rates in relation to specific anticoagulation levels in the more thrombogenic prostheses (56). Among tilting disc valves of different design, for example, some earlier designs clearly require a higher intensity of anticoagulation to prevent valve thrombosis than more recent designs (56). For this reason, it is important to distinguish between mechanical valves when making recommendations of anticoagulation intensity (166).

The other principal limitation of anticoagulation relates to stability of control. Anticoagulation which is well controlled within a narrow therapeutic band which has been adjusted to the patient's individual needs, should achieve efficient prophylaxis

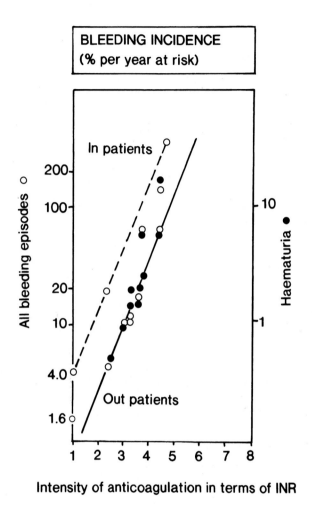

Figure 10.3-12: Graph showing the log-linear relationship between International Normalised Ratio (INR) and the incidence of bleeding. Adapted from Ref. #408, with permission.

against thrombosis, in the absence of overwhelming trigger factors, and expose the patient to a low risk of bleeding. Several studies have established the importance of good control in this respect (399-401). Wide swings in anticoagulation intensity in contrast expose the patient to the risk of thrombosis at one extreme (399) and serious bleeding at the other (400,402). Choice of oral anticoagulation among a range of short-acting, medium-acting and long-acting drugs will influence the quality of control to some extent, most clinicians avoiding short-acting drugs for this reason (333). Proper medical supervision should include dose adjustments to take account of drug interactions (333) (Table 10.3-I) and alterations in metabolism caused by disease processes (403). Computer assistance in these aspects may have a role (404). Patient education is also a vital part of long term anticoagulation, and should include advice about dietary content of vitamin K (378,405).

The target range of anticoagulation intensity also has a bearing on the risk imposed by wide fluctuations in intensity. A low target range will expose the patient to a greater risk

Table 10.3-IV: The management of over anticoagulation

- An INR > 7.0 requires urgent action and admission to hospital is advisable, even if the patient is not bleeding.

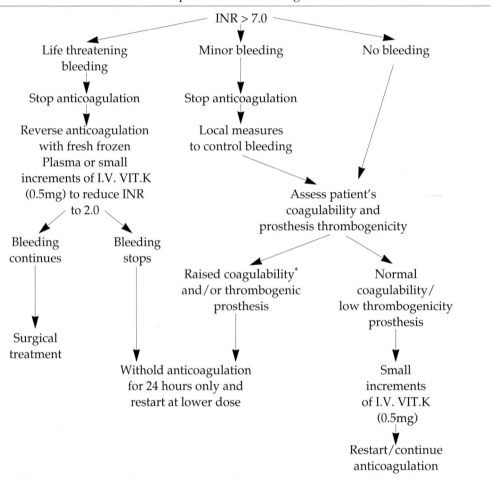

*e.g. hyperfibrinogenemia, presence of pulmonary infection, etc

of episodes of subtherapeutic anticoagulation precipitated by fluctuations in dietary content of vitamin K (378), while a high target range will increase the risk of the intensity reaching dangerously high levels.

Anticoagulant-related bleeding

In assessing the risk of this complication, it should not be forgotten that, as with stroke and TIA, a 'background incidence' of bleeding of all levels of severity exists in the non-anticoagulated population. Data from the placebo arms of several trials reveal that serious bleeding occurs at a rate of 0.7 to 1.6%/patient year (191,406,407). The level of anticoagulation below which the risk of bleeding does not differ significantly from the 'background incidence' remains uncertain because most papers reporting the incidence of bleeding in patients on anticoagulants refer to *target* therapeutic ranges and fail to specify the intensity *achieved* or, more importantly, the INR at the time of bleeding. Furthermore many North American reports are based on unstandardized prothrombin ratios. The risk of serious bleeding increases exponentially as the INR rises (Fig. 10.3-12) (408). Above an INR of 7.0 active measures are required to reduce anticoagulation (Table 10.3-IV) (409,410). At the other end of the scale, an INR around 2.0 or less appears to be associated with a minimal risk of bleeding (408,411,412). Factors which contribute to an increased risk of bleeding include poor anticoagulation control (400,402,413), unstandardized anticoagulation measurement (166,383) and the presence of co-morbid pathological conditions with a tendency to bleed (402,403). Anticoagulation often has an unmasking effect on occult pathology (402), almost certainly explaining the higher incidence of bleeding during the early months of anticoagulation (403,414-416). The risk of major bleeding during the first months of anticoagulation is 10 times higher than the risk after the first year of treatment (403).

The commonest sites of minor bleeding are the nose and mouth, accounting for over one third of episodes (403). The gastro-intestinal tract is the most frequent source of major bleeding, with the majority of events having an underlying pathological source. A previous history of gastro-intestinal bleeding triples the risk of so-called 'anticoagulant-related' bleeding, whereas a previous history of peptic ulcer without bleeding does not appear to increase the risk (403).

Of most concern is the risk of intracranial bleeding and in particular intracerebral hemorrhage (ICH), since it is in this subgroup of patients that most of the fatalities and long term disabilities occur. Fortunately, anticoagulant-related intracranial bleeding is relatively rare, accounting for only 2% of all bleeding episodes (403). In the general population, more than 90% of all ICH occurs in patients who are not on anticoagulants (417). Although the existence of anticoagulant-related ICH as a clinical entity has been recognized for many years, the mechanism remains obscure (417) and its relationship to anticoagulation intensity remains controversial. The risk of ICH in patients on anticoagulants is reported to be between eight and 11 times greater than the non-anticoagulated population (417). Some authors report a relationship between anticoagulation intensity and occurrence (415) and volume of ICH (418), whereas others have found no relationship, suggesting that anticoagulant-related ICH is an all-or-none phenomenon with a low threshold, as yet unidentified (419). However, one review of the subject, whilst acknowledging the difficulty of defining a therapeutic range, concluded that 80% of ICHs were probably related to excessively prolonged prothrombin times (417).

In some series, episodes of ICH have occurred mainly in the first few months after commencing anticoagulation (415,418), suggesting that, in some patients, anticoagulation may have an unmasking effect on pre-existing pathology. Small cerebral vessels may be weakened either by chronic hypertension or by cerebral amyloid angiopathy, a condition of uncertain etiology, the prevalence of which increases with advancing age (420). It is probable that both conditions increase the risk of 'anticoagulant-related' ICH. Some studies have identified hypertension as an independent risk factor for 'anticoagulant-related' ICH whereas others have not (403,417). Similarly there is controversy about the role of previous cerebral infarction as a risk factor for 'anticoagulant-related' ICH (403,417). The different conclusions reached by various reported series may be explicable by differences in anticoagulation intensity and prevalence of risk factors. Until detailed prospective studies on anticoagulant related ICH (with baseline MRI head scans, risk stratification and accurate INR measurements during follow up) clarify the interaction of risk factors, neither hypertension nor previous cerebral infarction should be regarded as contraindications to anticoagulation, although extra vigilance in anticoagulant control and hypertension management would be prudent in hypertensive patients.

Controversy also exists concerning the effect of age on the risk of anticoagulant-related bleeding. The widespread belief that anticoagulation is dangerous for elderly patients has acted as a deterrent to its use in this population group and has consequently influenced the choice between bioprosthetic and mechanical valves. Some series and reviews have reported age to be a risk factor (403,421,422) while others have come to the opposite conclusion (400,406,408,413,423). The discrepancy almost certainly results from the influence of confounding variables and whether they have been allowed for in the analysis. Older patients are more likely to have co-morbid conditions which increase the risk of bleeding and are more likely to be taking a larger number of medications (423). For these reasons they may be more at risk from higher intensities of anticoagulation; it is probably significant that most reports of age as a risk factor come from North America (403,421,422) where dangerously and unpredictably high levels of anticoagulation have been used for many years (383).

Elderly patients should be screened particularly carefully for relevant co-morbid conditions prior to commencing anticoagulation and wherever possible should be managed with low or moderate intensity anticoagulation.

Indications for anticoagulation

The greatest value of anticoagulation is in situations of relative stagnation. In heart valve disease these conditions occur in two situations; in the left atrium and in relation to prosthetic heart valves.

Relatively stagnant conditions occur in the left atrium in the presence of AF, atrial enlargement, mitral valve obstruction or impaired left ventricular function, either singly or in combination (vide supra). It is generally accepted that whenever AF complicates either mitral or aortic valve disease, or whenever there is a history of systemic embolism or evidence of left atrial thrombus, the patient should be anticoagulated without delay (424). Severe pulmonary hypertension is also an indication for anticoagulation in view of the higher incidence of venous thrombosis in the legs (200). However, whilst the patient remains free of thrombosis, retains normal pulmonary vascular resistance and remains in sinus rhythm, the indications for anticoagulation are much less clear cut, since in mitral stenosis for example, the risk of embolism does not correlate with the degree of stenosis (200).

It is therefore necessary to have a scientific basis for the prescription of anticoagulants. Since thromboembolic risk is closely linked to the degree of left atrial stagnation (95), objective assessments of the latter and its effect on coagulability are required. Spontaneous echo contrast (SEC) in the left atrium detected by transesophageal echocardiography provides a semiquantitative assessment of stagnation (95).

Measurement of prothrombin fragment F_{1+2} in plasma gives an indirect assessment of the degree of thrombin generation (390). If SEC is present in the left atrium or F_{1+2} levels are elevated, hypercoagulable conditions almost certainly exist, irrespective of the clinical or hemodynamic findings, and anticoagulation is necessary.

In the case of prosthetic heart valves, all currently available mechanical valves have zones of relative stagnation specific to their particular designs (24). The combination of stagnation and foreign surfaces makes anticoagulation essential for most patients with mechanical valves, although it has to be acknowledged that some prostheses have lower stagnation characteristics than others and that some patients are less coagulable than others. Whether it will be possible for some categories of patients with low thrombogenicity prostheses to be managed without anticoagulation in the future depends on research work currently in progress in this important area. In the meantime it is safer to prescribe anticoagulants for all patients with mechanical valves and for patients with bioprostheses in AF (424). Similarly, following mitral valve repair, anticoagulation will be required if the patient remains in AF (424). Although some cardiac surgeons recommend aspirin therapy in this situation, the inferior results of aspirin in the AF stroke prevention trials (190,191,407), particularly in the subset of cardioembolic strokes (425) and the failure of aspirin to lower F_{1+2} levels in AF (393) suggest that aspirin alone cannot be considered a safe treatment for AF.

Choosing the intensity of anticoagulation

In deciding the intensity of anticoagulation, the most fundamental principle is that the level should only be high enough to combat the degree of activation of the coagulation system imposed either by left atrial stagnation or by the presence of a prosthetic valve (or by both). INR levels within an a safe therapeutic range will not prevent platelet activation or combat the increased coagulability of a serious infection for example (vide supra). Therefore any increase of the INR above that required to reduce thrombin generation to a 'normal' or slightly subnormal level will achieve no additional gain in thromboprophylaxis but will merely increase the risk of bleeding (408).

Although some preliminary work has been done on F_{1+2} levels during oral anticoagulation, insufficient data are currently available on which to base detailed intensity recommendations. Nevertheless, there are already F_{1+2} data which suggest that surprisingly little anticoagulation (INR around 1.5) is required to restore thrombin generation to 'normal' levels under some circumstances (381). This supports the growing clinical trend towards lower anticoagulation levels (424).

In conditions of left atrial stagnation in which AF is the principal factor and the mitral valve is normal, low intensity anticoagulation (mean INR around 2.0) is sufficient to lower F_{1+2} levels to below normal and provide effective embolic prophylaxis (393,426). When the mitral valve is stenotic or a prosthetic mitral valve is in place, the degree of stagnation will be greater in proportion to the degree of obstruction and a higher INR is likely to be necessary. Although SEC can be used as a semiquantitative assessment of the degree of stagnation (95), it cannot be used for monitoring the effects of anticoagulation, since the coagulation system is not involved in its genesis and it does not disappear with increasing anticoagulation. SEC is due to reversible red cell aggregation and serves only as a marker of stagnation (95).

Experimentally, an INR of 5.0 is required to abolish fibrin formation altogether on exposed subendothelium under sluggish flow conditions (395). However, it is unlikely that such extreme flow conditions exist clinically in the left atrium except in the presence of very low cardiac output in terminally ill patients. Indeed, left atrial thrombus has been shown to regress and fibrinopeptide A levels return to normal once a mean INR of 3.0 is achieved in previously non-anticogulated patients with rheumatic valve disease (427). Although there are no studies specifically addressing the question of different levels of anticoagulation in patients with mitral stenosis, the consensus view is that an INR around 3.0 provides adequate prophylaxis for the majority of patients (424). If any doubt remains whether a chosen INR is adequate for a particular patient under particular clinical circumstances, measurement of F_{1+2} may allow an assessment of the efficacy of treatment.

Anticoagulation intensity for the patient with a prosthetic valve. In the past this issue has been shrouded in a fog of confusion due to lack of standardization of anticoagulation measurement (vide supra), a paucity of randomized trials and the assumption that a single intensity of anticoagulation will be required for all prostheses in all patients. The latter assumption is based on two false premises: that all prostheses are equally thrombogenic and that all patients are equally 'coagulable'. Whilst this may be a convenient assumption for those in charge of anticoagulant clinics, the selection of a single high level to cover the worst eventuality inevitably endangers patients of low coagulability with prostheses of low thrombogenicity by subjecting then to unnecessarily high anticoagulation (166).

Two other misapprehensions need to be dispelled; that it is possible to control every patient within a very narrow range of INR and that a particular range of INR, when eventually selected, will protect the patient against thrombosis and embolism under all circumstances. Although it may be possible to set broad recommendations of INR level based on clinical results in large *groups* of patients, *individual* patients often show huge variability in their INR level (368). Furthermore, thrombosis or embolism, if it does occur, often cannot be related to any summary statistic of INR in the *individual* patient (e.g., mean INR, lowest INR, degree of variability of INR, etc.) (368). This suggests that the threshold for thrombus formation varies not only with the INR but also with the degree of thrombophilia imposed by risk factors and trigger factors, many of which exert their effects by *mechanisms unaffected by anticoagulation*. Indeed, many of the cerebrovascular events labeled as embolism are almost certainly non-embolic. It is thus not surprising that several randomized trials of different levels of anticoagulation in patients with prosthetic heart valves have failed to show any difference in 'embolic' incidence (370-372), and that, above a critical level of INR, further increases in anticoagulation intensity, even to dangerously high levels, have no discernible effect on embolic incidence (371).

There are certain fundamentals involved in choosing an anticoagulation intensity for patients with prosthetic valves:

1. Abnormal flow conditions in the left atrium will dictate the lowest safe anticoagulation level. In the presence of AF, left atrial enlargement or a significant residual mitral gradient, an INR in the region of 3.0 should be regarded as the minimum for safety. This recommendation should apply to both MVR and AVR. If flow conditions in the left atrium are normal, the minimum safe INR will be determined by the prosthesis itself.

2. Anticoagulation intensity must also be adjusted to combat the particular stagnation characteristics of the prosthesis. In practice this means selecting the lowest level which will reliably prevent valve thrombosis.

3. The so-called 'embolic' incidence in a group of patients after valve replacement (in effect, the incidence of ischemic cerebrovascular events *of all etiologies)* cannot be used to predict reliably the correct anticoagulation intensity *for the prosthesis* (see section on Embolism as an Indicator of Therapeutic Efficacy). This is particularly the case in patients after AVR, in whom ischemic cerebrovascular events are closely associated with known stroke risk factors, particularly hypertension, cigarette smoking and arterial disease (273), none of which are directly influenced by anticoagulation. In MVR patients, whilst it might be possible to demonstrate differences in embolic incidence with different INRs in the range 1.5-3.0 (428), these differences are inseparable from the effects of anticoagulation on relatively stagnant conditions in the left atrium, i.e., the emboli may have arisen from the left atrium rather than the prosthesis.

For the reasons outlined above, even prospective randomized trials of one type of prosthesis comparing one level of anticoagulation with another must be interpreted with caution if they are based solely on the incidence of ischemic cerebrovascular events (the so-called 'embolic' incidence), unless the patients are also stratified by known stroke risk factors and cardiac risk factors.

Currently available randomized trials are flawed not only by the limitations mentioned above but by mixing prostheses of different thrombogenicity (371), by the addition of antiplatelet agents (372) and by short duration (370,372).

Retrospective studies on patients with Medtronic Hall and St. Jude Medical valves suggest that mean INRs of 2.5 and 3.0 are safe lower limits for AVR and MVR respectively with these prostheses (428,429). Insufficient information is available on other types of prosthesis to make detailed recommendations. Prospective studies with all types of mechanical valve are urgently required to define the safe level of anticoagulation for each. In the meantime, tentative recommendations can be made based on knowledge of left atrial conditions and an approximate assessment of the thrombogenicity of the prosthesis based on published information on valve thrombosis rates (166,359,360) (Table 10.3-IV). It should not be automatically assumed that all 'modern' prostheses are of low thrombogenicity. Until firm published data are available, great caution should be exercised in selecting INR levels for recently introduced valves; in these circumstances, it is probably safer to adhere to the albeit arbitrary, but widely used recommendation of INR 3.0-4.5 (166,424).

Anticoagulation and anti-platelet therapy

All currently available data show that antiplatelet therapy alone gives inadequate protection against left atrial thrombosis, prosthetic valve thrombosis and cardiogenic embolism (278,279,393,430,431), especially in the presence of AF (393,432). Aspirin alone has been recommended as long term prophylaxis for patients with bioprostheses to minimize platelet adhesion (433), but in vitro studies have shown no significant decrease in platelet adherence to bioprosthetic cusps in media containing therapeutic levels of aspirin (78), and it is likely that any therapeutic benefit of aspirin in patients with bioprostheses is mediated through its effect on associated non-prosthetic risk factors (vide infra).

Although the early results of the Stroke Prevention in Atrial Fibrillation (SPAF) study appeared to show a beneficial effect of aspirin in reducing stroke risk in patients with AF (191), subsequent stratification of the patients demonstrated that this beneficial effect was limited mainly to patients at risk of non-cardioembolic stroke (425), suggesting that aspirin was having an impact on 'arterial' risk factors rather than 'venous' risk factors. This is in keeping with the findings of the Copenhagen AFASAK study, in which no benefit was obtained from low dose aspirin in stroke prevention in a group of patients with chronic non-rheumatic AF in whom hypertension was an exclusion criterion (190). The failure of aspirin to prevent thrombus formation within the fibrillating left atrium is due to its lack of any significant effect on the increased flux of the coagulation system typical of left atrial stagnation. This ineffectiveness has been demonstrated recently in patients with chronic AF entered into the Boston Area Anticoagulation Trial for Atrial Fibrillation (BAATAF) study (426); although low intensity anticoagulation (INR 1.5-2.7) lowered F_{1+2} levels significantly, patients taking aspirin had F_{1+2} levels which did not differ from those of control patients taking neither warfarin nor aspirin (393). Despite much evidence to show that antiplatelet drugs have little effect in conditions of relative stasis, an overview of randomized trials of antiplatelet drugs as prophylaxis for venous thromboembolism concluded that some risk reduction was possible with these agents as a group, but individually the least effective drug was aspirin (434).

Although antiplatelet therapy should not be used as a substitute for anticoagulation in patients with valve disease associated with left atrial stagnation or in patients with mechanical valves, there are theoretical advantages to combining certain antiplatelet agents with anticoagulation in some patients with prosthetic valves, to combat platelet adhesion to prosthetic surfaces and inhibit ADP-induced platelet aggregation. A brief description of the sequence of events in ADP-induced platelet aggregation (435) is helpful to the understanding of the pharmacology of platelet antagonists. First ADP becomes attached to a specific receptor on the platelet surface, following which a rapid change of platelet shape occurs from a disc to a sphere with emission of pseudopods. This shape change exposes and activates fibrinogen binding sites (GPIIb/IIIa complex), enabling fibrinogen to bind adjacent platelets together (primary reversible aggregation). At the same time the ability of other agents to stimulate the synthesis of the aggregation inhibitor, cyclic adenosine monophosphate (cAMP) is blocked (vide infra). Primary reversible aggregation does not involve release of substances from the platelet and in vitro occurs only at low concentrations of ADP. With higher concentrations of ADP, the platelet release reaction occurs liberating in particular further ADP (for the recruitment of other platelets) and thromboxane A_2 (TXA_2).

Aspirin, the most commonly prescribed antiplatelet agent, is an irreversible cyclo-oxygenase inhibitor, which blocks the production of TXA_2 from arachidonic acid in the platelet membrane for the lifetime of the platelet (436). TXA_2 is a potent vasoconstrictor and agonist of platelet aggregation, secreted when platelets are activated by any agonist. However because aspirin blocks only this one pathway of aggregation, and because TXA_2 is not indispensable to aggregation, its anti-aggregating activity is easily overcome by increased concentrations of other aggregating stimuli, for example ADP, collagen and thrombin (123,437). Consequently, ADP-dependent shear-induced platelet aggregation is not significantly inhibited by aspirin (438). Furthermore, experimental work in animals shows that aspirin does not prevent platelet adhesion to prosthetic surfaces (439).

Not only are its actions insufficiently focused to enable a strong therapeutic benefit to be envisaged in relation to mechanical valves, aspirin has certain disadvantages also. It reversibly blocks cyclo-oxygenase in endothelial cells, diminishing the synthesis of prostacyclin (123,440), a potent inhibitor of platelet adherence and aggregation (12). It has been suggested that slow-release preparations of aspirin avoid this problem (441,442), but others have shown that even 35mg daily is sufficient to significantly inhibit prostacyclin production (443). Prostacyclin exerts its effect by increasing the levels of cAMP within the platelet by stimulating the activity of adenylate cyclase (436). Cyclic AMP inhibits the final common pathway by which all agonists induce aggregation, i.e., the exposure of the receptor (GPIIb/GPIIIa) which binds to fibrinogen and vWF (435). By in effect reducing platelet cAMP levels, high dose aspirin can virtually abolish the anti-aggregating effect of dipyridamole (444) which works mainly by inhibiting the breakdown of cAMP (vide infra).

Some authors have also reported that, although possessing an anti-aggregating effect, aspirin may actually promote platelet adherence in some circumstances by enhancing (through its inhibition of cyclo-oxygenase) an alternative and quantatively more important pathway of arachidonic acid metabolism which produces 12-HETE (437), a substance which promotes platelet adhesion and enhances the release of tissue factor from stimulated monocytes (445). The production of 12-HETE is further increased in the presence of albumin (437), one of the major proteins which coats prosthetic surfaces (49). Thus there could even be a theoretical case for avoiding aspirin in patients with prosthetic valves. Further research in this important area is required. Finally, perhaps the most important disadvantage of aspirin is the increased risk of bleeding, mediated not only through its anti-aggregant effect and interference with the hemostatic plug but also through the loss of local vasoconstriction normally induced by TXA_2. This risk is increased when aspirin is combined with anticoagulation of moderate or high intensity (446-448). However the combination of low dose aspirin (75mg/day) with an INR of 1.5 is reported to carry a low risk of bleeding (449).

Sulphinpyrazone is also a cyclo-oxygenase inhibitor but unlike aspirin it is a competitive inhibitor of this enzyme and its effects on individual platelets are therefore reversible (436). However, it is probable that it has additional effects on platelet function which are not fully understood since, unlike aspirin, it appears capable of inhibiting the adhesion of platelets to artificial surfaces when used in large doses in experimental animals (439). Studies in patients with older generation caged ball valves have demonstrated normalization of platelet survival with sulphinpyrazone (450) but it has never been evaluated in patients with modern low thrombogenicity prostheses. Its usefulness is limited by its high dosage requirements, by its tendency to exacerbate peptic ulceration and by its uricosuric effect, increasing the risk of uric acid calculi (436). It is no longer widely used.

Antiplatelet agents which increase the concentration of platelet cAMP or cyclic guanosine monophosphate (cGMP) have a theoretical advantage since these substances inhibit the final common pathway of aggregation and thus should have an effect on all agonists (123). Increased levels of platelet cAMP and cGMP may be induced by increased synthesis or by inhibition of natural breakdown mechanisms. Increased synthesis of cAMP is promoted by prostacyclin and its stable analogue, iloprost (436). Both are unsuitable for the long term management of patients with prosthetic valves since they must be given intravenously. Increased synthesis of cGMP is induced physiologically by nitric oxide and pharmacologically by **nitric oxide donors**, such as organic nitrates and **molsidomine** (123). Since free hemoglobin circulating in the plasma zone adjacent to the endothelium, as a consequence of prosthesis-induced hemolysis, inhibits nitric oxide (261,451), nitric oxide donors could be potentially useful in patients with prosthetic valves and clinical trials would appear justified. Of the nitric oxide donors, molsidomine, through its active metabolite SIN-1, is a more effective nitric oxide donor than the organic nitrates since it liberates nitric oxide spontaneously whereas nitric oxide liberation from organic nitrates cannot be performed by platelets (452). The platelet inhibitory effect of organic nitrates are therefore less predictable and are closely linked to the degree of hemodynamic responsiveness, thus limiting their usefulness (453). Molsidomine has been shown to increase t-PA production through inhibition of platelet release of PAI-1, thereby enhancing another important regulatory function of nitric oxide (454). This effect may be of particular value in patients with concomitant ischemic heart disease, many of whom have reduced fibrinolytic activity (30).

Dipyridamole is the most commonly used inhibitor of cAMP breakdown. In addition to inhibiting platelet phosphodiesterase, the enzyme responsible for cAMP breakdown, dipyridamole also increases synthesis of cAMP by stimulating platelet adenylate cyclase both directly and indirectly by increasing plasma adenosine levels (436). Although, as an inhibitor of the final common pathway of aggregation, dipyridamole should theoretically be effective against all agonists, its mechanism of action remains incompletely understood, since its effectiveness varies in response to specific agonists. Animal studies and clinical trials have shown that it does not prevent platelet adhesion or aggregation in response to collagen and that it has little value in arterial injury (455,456). However it does appear active in inhibiting ADP-induced aggregation in vivo (although not in vitro), possibly by augmenting the effect of nitric oxide (457), and in inhibiting platelet adhesion to artificial surfaces in animal experiments (439), both potentially useful mechanisms for patients with prosthetic valves. It has also been suggested that dipyridamole has an effect on the red cell membrane, reducing its propensity for platelet adhesion and subsequent activation following red cell trauma and release of ADP (458). However, if dipyridamole requires the presence of nitric oxide to exert a significant anti-aggregant effect in vivo, as has been suggested, it is possible that significant prosthesis-induced hemolysis may interfere with its activity. This may be an explanation for its ineffectiveness in preventing Doppler-detected microembolism after valve replacement (397). Unlike aspirin and ticlopidine, it does not prolong the bleeding time but drug intolerance occurs in about 10% of patients, mainly because of headache caused by vasodilatation (456).

The inhibition of ADP-induced platelet aggregation is one of the major goals in patients with prosthetic valves. The agents discussed so far achieve this inhibition in an indirect or non-specific way and their inhibition may be overcome by high agonist concentrations. For this reason, specific inhibitors of ADP-induced aggregation may have a particular advantage. **Ticlopidine** is the most widely available and the most extensively evaluated of the agents in this category. It is a potent inhibitor of ADP-induced aggregation even at high concentrations of ADP (459). Its mechanism of action is incompletely understood. It appears not to block ADP-induced shape change but probably prevents the inhibitory effect of ADP on cAMP synthesis and blocks the effect of ADP on the final common pathway of aggregation (GPIIb/IIIa) (435). Since its action appears specific to ADP, its anti-aggregating effects can be overcome by high concentrations of other agonists, notably by thrombin which at higher concentrations is less dependent on ADP for its aggregating effect (435,459).

Ticlopidine requires at least three days of treatment to achieve its maximum effect on platelet function, which is dose related and lasts for the life of the platelet (459). Like aspirin, it prolongs the bleeding time (459,460), but actually prolongs platelet survival when given prior to cardiopulmonary by-pass and, unlike aspirin, has no discernible effect on intraoperative or postoperative blood loss (461), enabling it to be continued safely in the immediate postoperative period. In patients not taking anticoagulants, the long term incidence of bleeding complications is approximately the same with aspirin and ticlopidine, although the development of peptic ulcer is almost four times commoner with aspirin than ticlopidine (460). The theoretical advantages of ticlopidine as a potent inhibitor of ADP-induced platelet aggregation are such that a benefit can be envisaged in patients with prosthetic valves. However, it will be important to assess its safety when used in combination with anticoagulation. Long term studies of ticlopidine in patients with prosthetic heart valves are unavailable at present, but two short-term studies have shown ticlopidine to be more effective than dipyridamole in suppressing ex-vivo platelet aggregability early after valve replacement (166). In terms of platelet adherence to prosthetic materials, ticlopidine has been shown to be at least as effective as a combination of dipyridamole and low dose aspirin in reducing platelet adhesion to vascular grafts (462). A further potential advantage is its modest effect in lowering fibrinogen levels (463,464).

In evaluating **clinical trials of antiplatelet drugs in patients with prosthetic valves**, it is important to appreciate that an apparent benefit may be due to an action on concomitant arterial risk factors rather than a protective role on factors associated with the prosthesis itself. From an assessment of the mechanisms of action of aspirin for example, a marked therapeutic benefit in patients with prosthetic valves would not be anticipated. Yet, in the mid 1970's two randomized studies comparing anticoagulation alone with anticoagulation plus aspirin both showed significantly fewer embolic events among patients treated with aspirin (446,447). These two studies were limited mainly to aortic valve replacement (74% AVR in the first, 100% AVR in the second) and contained predominantly patients with Starr Edwards valves (92% in the first, 100% in the second). No information was given in either study about 'arterial' risk factors in the two groups of patients. This is an important omission because 'arterial' risk factors have been shown to be major determinants of embolic risk following aortic valve replacement particularly (273), and aspirin is known to be effective in reducing the incidence of stroke and TIA in the general population, in the presence of arterial risk factors (425,465). The incidence of gastrointestinal bleeding was four to 5.5 times higher in the aspirin groups (425,465).

In a large study from the Mayo Clinic, reported in 1983, in which almost half the patients had mitral prostheses, no benefit in thromboprophylaxis was demonstrated from the combination of aspirin and warfarin (448). Furthermore, the incidence of serious bleeding with this combination was four times higher than warfarin alone or warfarin plus dipyridamole (448).

A recent randomized, double-blind, placebo-controlled trial, to assess the efficacy of aspirin plus warfarin (with an achieved mean INR of 3.0) after valve replacement appeared to show a benefit from the addition of aspirin, but only when the non-hemorrhagic adverse outcomes were combined as "vascular" events and/or deaths (373). When major systemic embolism alone was compared in the aspirin and placebo groups, the 95% confidence interval on the percentage risk reduction calculation was extremely wide, 1-87%. In this trial, 35% of the patients had ischemic heart disease and almost half the "vascular" deaths were due to myocardial infarction or "acute heart failure". Most of these deaths were in the placebo group. Aspirin is of proven benefit in ischemic heart disease and in stoke prevention in the presence of arterial risk factors (465). It seems likely therefore that the greatest impact of aspirin in this particular trial was on the patients who would have suffered a vascular event or death whether they had a prosthetic valve or not. The trial would have been much more meaningful, in terms of assessing the effect of aspirin on prosthetic valves, if it had included only patients who had normal coronary arteries and no other arterial risk factors (hypertension, diabetes, carotid or peripheral vascular disease and smoking).

The other potentially misleading aspect of this trial (373) concerns the incidence of bleeding in the two groups of patients; although the aspirin group had a higher incidence of bleeding events overall, there was no significant difference in *major* bleeding between the two groups: 8.5% per year in the aspirin group, 6.6% per year in the placebo group. The figure for the aspirin group is not surprising since others have reported bleeding of this magnitude with an aspirin/warfarin combination (448). However, the almost equally high incidence in the placebo group is difficult to understand, given the mean achieved INR in the region of 3.0. With this level of anticoagulation, an incidence of serious bleeding no higher than 1-2% per year would have been expected (360).

The only other antiplatelet agent which has been evaluated in clinical trials in combination with anticoagulation is dipyridamole. Several studies have demonstrated a therapeutic benefit with this drug in patients with prosthetic valves (436). In these studies also, no information was provided about concomitant arterial risk factors, but since dipyridamole is known to be ineffective in the prevention of stroke and myocardial infarction in the general population (455) and because reduction in platelet adherence to artificial surfaces has been demonstrated in animals (439), it is probable that the therapeutic benefit was real. However, all of these studies were performed many years ago on patients with first generation prostheses (mainly caged ball valves), nowadays considered more thrombogenic in comparison to some prostheses of later design. The caged ball valve in particular combines high shear stresses (and associated ADP release) with a zone of stagnation at the apex of the cage (24), favoring the adhesion of activated platelets. From its mode of action, a theoretical benefit could be anticipated from dipyridamole with this particular prosthesis. There are no studies which have examined the effect of dipyridamole in patients with modern tilting disc and bileaflet valves.

In order to formulate firm recommendations, further clinical trials of antiplatelet drugs are required in patients with currently available prosthetic valves, but if they are to have any meaning, the trials must either be limited to patients without concomitant arterial risk factors or the risk factors must be carefully entered into the database and allowance made for them in the analysis. Agents particularly worthy of further trials because of their theoretical advantages are dipyridamole, molsidomine and ticlopidine.

In the meantime, the following *tentative* recommendations can be made, based on currently available evidence (see foregoing discussion and Table 10.3-V):

Table 10.3-V: Tentative mean INR recommendations for patients with prosthetic valves according to left atrial conditions and prosthesis thrombogenicity

	SR LA O MV gr 0 SEC 0	AF LA$^+$ MV gr + Sec +
Prosthesis with low stagnation characteristics	2.5	3.0
Prosthesis with high stagnation characteristics	4.0	4.0
Caged ball prosthesis	3.0 +dp	3.5 +dp

NB. These recommendations apply equally to mitral and aortic prostheses.

Abbreviations:
SR = sinus rhythm, AF = atrial fibrillation, LA O = left atrial size normal, LA$^+$ = left atrium enlarged, Mv gr = mitral valve gradient, SEC = spontaneous echo contrast in left atrium, dp = dipyridamole

1. **Patients with prostheses of proven low thrombogenicity with no arterial risk factors**. No antiplatelet therapy should be necessary for these patients.

2. **Patients with low thrombogenicity prostheses who have arterial risk factors**. In patients with coronary or carotid artery disease, hypertension (even if treated) or diabetes and in those patients who refuse to stop smoking, low-dose aspirin (75mg daily) should reduce the risk of non-prosthetic arterial thrombosis and embolism. However, in order to reduce the risk of bleeding, it should preferably only be combined with low intensity anticoagulation (INR 2.0-2.5). If an INR of 3.0 is required, as in MVR patients, aspirin should be used only in low dose or avoided. It should be avoided altogether in patients with a history of peptic ulcer. A useful alternative, for patients with ischemic heart disease in particular, would be molsidomine.

3. **Patients with caged ball and caged disc valves**. Dipyridamole, 100mg four times a day, should be prescribed (if tolerated), together with moderate intensity anticoagulation (INR 3.0-3.5). If arterial risk factors co-exist, the addition of 75mg aspirin daily should not interfere with the effects of dipyridamole, although an increased risk of bleeding may have to be accepted.

4. **Patients with high thrombogenicity valves**. Valves which are prone to valve thrombosis without higher intensity anticoagulation because of their stagnation characteristics may theoretically benefit from the anti-adherence effect of dipyridamole, but aspirin and ticlopidine should be avoided if INRs of 4.0 or above are being employed, even if arterial risk factors are present.

Anticoagulation during pregnancy.

Confusion and controversy still surround the decisions necessary for the pregnant woman taking oral anticoagulants. As with other aspects of anticoagulation, much of this confusion is due to lack of standardization of anticoagulation measurement and failure to interpret results in relation to anticoagulation intensity. Three important issues need to be addressed: a) the 'hypercoagulability' of pregnancy and the apparent increased risk of prosthetic valve thrombosis, b) the risk of maternal hemorrhage and c) the risk of fetal hemorrhage and embryopathy.

The 'hypercoagulability' of pregnancy. Much has been written about this phenomenon, but recently its existence has been disputed (466,467). A review of the literature has concluded that there is no excess risk of deep vein thrombosis in pregnancy, despite increased venous stasis (466). Throughout pregnancy, levels of many coagulation factors increase progressively (466,467); evidence that the coagulation system is working at an increased flux. This increased flux is thought to result from the constant reparative processes necessary in the growing placenta (466). The fibrinogen level rises gradually during the course of pregnancy, but more rapidly in the last trimester; prior to delivery the level can reach almost twice normal (466), but in many women only modest increases occur (468). This relative hyperfibrinogenemia, together with the increase in platelet aggregability (469) which accompanies it, may be a preparation for the huge demands which are placed on the hemostatic system at the time of delivery. PAI-1 levels are also elevated (19,467,470) but it is thought that inhibition of fibrinolysis is confined to the utero-placental circulation (470), since there is evidence of increased fibrinolysis in the general circulation (467). Overall, the so called procoagulant changes are thus entirely physiological and are balanced by increased cardiac output, lower hematocrit and blood viscosity (468) and increased fibrinolysis (467), making thrombosis a rare occurrence in women with uncomplicated pregnancies and normal cardiac function. However, if the cardiac output cannot increase because of impaired left ventricular function or a stenotic valve or prosthesis, the risk will be higher (471).

It is widely believed that prosthetic valves are at increased risk of thrombotic obstruction during pregnancy (472), but a recent survey of anticoagulant practice during pregnancy among several European centers has shown that the problem of valve thrombosis is largely confined to patients who have been switched to heparin in place of their oral anticoagulants (473). Other authors have reported similar findings (474,475). Heparin is known to be relatively less effective during pregnancy for a number of reasons (476,477): increased protein binding of heparin, increased fibrin binding of thrombin (protecting it from inactivation by heparin/antithrombin III) and increased heparin neutralization by platelet factor four, the levels of which are elevated during pregnancy (478). As a consequence, it has been shown that, to achieve the same degree of thromboprophylaxis, the heparin dosage must be gradually increased during pregnancy, and very carefully monitored for its efficacy, particularly in the last trimester (476). Failure to prescribe adequate doses of heparin probably accounts for most cases of valve thromboses which occur on heparin therapy. Alternatively heparin may simply be unsuitable for long term management of prosthetic valves because of its proaggregatory effect on platelets (479).

Long term heparin anticoagulation is inconvenient and is associated with a 10-12%

Table 10.3-VI: Warfarin embryopathy according to anticoagulation intensity

	Number of pregnancies	INR	% warfarin embryopathy
Ref. 474	39	3.0 - 14.0	29%
Ref. 483	50	2.0 -2.5	4%
Ref. 482	20	2.0	0

risk of maternal hemorrhage (473,480), a 2% risk of osteoporotic vertebral fractures (481) and a 27-33% risk of an abnormal outcome of pregnancy (stillbirth or prematurity) (473,480). The decision to substitute heparin therapy for oral anticoagulation is based on the widespread belief that the latter is even more dangerous for both mother and fetus than heparin. However this view stems from failure to interpret the available data in the literature *according to the intensity of oral anticoagulation employed*. If low intensity anticoagulation is used, the risks are small and there should be no necessity to change to heparin at all.

The risk of maternal hemorrhage. As with hemorrhagic events elsewhere in the body, the risk is closely related to the intensity of anticoagulation. With low intensity oral anticoagulation (INR 2.0-2.5) the risk of antepartum hemorrhage is 0-2% (482,483). Similarly in patients who have continued on oral anticoagulants until the time of delivery, the risk of peripartum hemorrhage appears to be low; in one series with a target INR of 2.0-2.5 there were no cases of excessive bleeding with vaginal delivery (483).

The risk of fetal hemorrhage and embryopathy. It is widely assumed that so-called 'warfarin embryopathy' and stillbirth due to fetal hemorrhage are unavoidable risks if oral anticoagulants are used in the first trimester of pregnancy and many physicians advise switching to heparin therapy during this period. However, this advice is often rather impractical since many women, particularly in 'third world' countries, do not consult a doctor until the end of the first trimester at the earliest. Furthermore, since unmonitored subcutaneous heparin provides inadequate protection against thrombosis and embolism during pregnancy (476), admission to hospital is required so that heparin can be given intravenously and its effects carefully monitored.

These impracticalities demand a closer examination of the risks of simply continuing with oral anticoagulation throughout pregnancy. Careful scrutiny of the literature reveals that these risks have been overstated. Many series reporting complications of oral anticoagulation during pregnancy have given no information about the *intensity* of anticoagulation employed. However, one review of reported cases of warfarin embryopathy contained many cases in which warfarin dosage was high (480), suggesting that high intensity anticoagulation had been employed. Only three series have reported the incidence of warfarin embryopathy and stillbirth according to the intensity of anticoagulation employed (Table 10.3-VI) (474,482,483). These results suggest an association between these complications and INR, with an extremely small risk of embryopathy with low intensity anticoagulation and low dose warfarin (482).

The availability of modern low thrombogenicity prostheses which can be safely maintained on low intensity oral anticoagulation (INR 2.0-2.5) throughout pregnancy should avoid the need for heparin therapy at any stage of pregnancy. With anticoagulation in this range, a very low incidence of both maternal and fetal complications should be expected. With high thrombogenicity prostheses requiring an INR around 4.0, it will be necessary, in discussion with the patient, to balance the risk of warfarin embryopathy against the risk of valve thrombosis if the patient is switched to heparin.

Anticoagulation during non-cardiac surgery

The controversy which surrounds the anticoagulation management of patients undergoing other forms of surgical treatment is in many ways analogous to that associated with anticoagulation management during pregnancy. Much traditional practice in the past has been built on folk-lore, anecdote and prejudice rather than on hard scientific facts. Particularly in the USA, where high intensity anticoagulation has been used for many years, it has been deemed necessary to stop oral anticoagulants in advance of any surgical procedure and to substitute intravenous heparin (484). This practice has resulted from reports of excessive intraoperative bleeding and wound hematomas in some patients in whom high intensity oral anticoagulation was continued (485).

For the patient with a prosthetic heart valve, anticoagulation interruption is potentially hazardous. Most reported series of prosthetic valve thrombosis in the literature reveal that, in the absence of tissue ingrowth as a predisposing factor, anticoagulation interruption (usually for another surgical procedure) is a major trigger factor for valve thrombosis (358,362-365). The risk is higher for patients with mitral prostheses (485). For patients on anticoagulant therapy for untreated valve disease, interruption is associated with an increased risk of embolism, rising in proportion to the severity of the factors necessitating anticoagulant prescription in the first place (486). The risk is particularly high in patients with congestive heart failure (486).

The cessation of oral anticoagulation does not merely restore the status quo in coagulability terms. A period of rebound hypercoagulability occurs during the first four days after withdrawal, with levels of factor VII and factor IX rising more rapidly than those of protein C and protein S, creating an imbalance between coagulation factors and natural anticoagulants, maximal at one week (487). Increased plasma levels of FPA during this period provide evidence of activation of the coagulation system and increased fibrin formation (487). If heparin is substituted, its proaggregatory effect on platelets may compound the problem (479).

In terms of maintaining efficient thromboprophylaxis, much is to be gained by continuing oral anticoagulation during surgical procedures. In Europe, where prescribed anticoagulation intensities have been much lower than in North America, many surgeons have undertaken minor surgical procedures such as dental extraction (488) and ophthalmic operations (489) without discontinuing warfarin and found no significant increase in intraoperative or postoperative bleeding. It has also been shown that low intensity oral anticoagulation (INR 1.5-2.0) does not significantly increase intraoperative or postoperative bleeding in patients undergoing cholecystectomy or gastrectomy (490). If necessary, intravenous warfarin can be given until normal gastrointestinal absorption returns. Most cardiac surgeons are accustomed to performing major operations on patients with an INR in the region of 2.0 and in the majority of patients find that there is no important effect on intraoperative bleeding. Cardiac surgeons should therefore encourage their colleagues in other surgical specialities to overcome their apprehensions

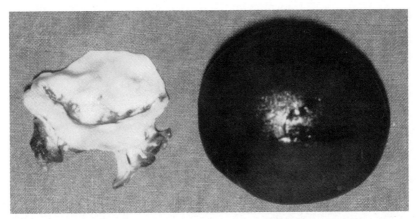

Figure 10.3-13: Left atrial ball thrombus and the stenotic mitral valve with which it was associated.

and reduce the INR no lower than 2.0 in patients with prosthetic valves. Further prospective trials on this important aspect of patient management are urgently required.

THE MANAGEMENT OF INTRACARDIAC THROMBOSIS

The diagnosis of both left atrial thrombosis and prosthetic valve thrombosis is most readily accomplished by transesophageal echocardiography (TEE) supplemented if necessary, in the case of valve thrombosis, by cinefluoroscopy. However, the investigation of the patient with intracardiac thrombosis should also include tests to identify the underlying factors involved in the genesis of the thrombus (see section on risk factors and trigger factors for thrombosis), since modification of these factors must become part of the overall management strategy if recurrent thrombosis is to be prevented.

Left atrial thrombosis

Left atrial thrombus usually comes to light during the investigation of a patient who has suffered a recent embolic event. Occasionally, it is an incidental finding during the routine echocardiographic assessment of mitral valve disease. The commonest site of attachment is the left atrial appendage, although the body of the atrium is almost as common, with the posterior wall the most frequent aspect (197). Very rarely, thrombosis occurs as an unattached ball thrombus when first seen (Fig. 10.3-13) Such thrombi require emergency surgical treatment since they can totally obstruct the mitral valve and cause sudden death (491).

The management of a newly diagnosed left atrial thrombus depends on its maturity and size and on the associated underlying conditions. Recently formed thrombi are often mobile, insecurely attached and at great risk of liberating emboli (180,492). Larger, immobile thrombi with a broad base of attachment pose less risk and organized thrombi pose negligible immediate threat, although the roughened surface of old calcified thrombus predisposes to fresh thrombus deposition (Fig. 10.3-14). Neovascularity on angiography and calcification on plain X-ray or computerized tomography (CT) are evidence of organization (see Chapter 3.5).

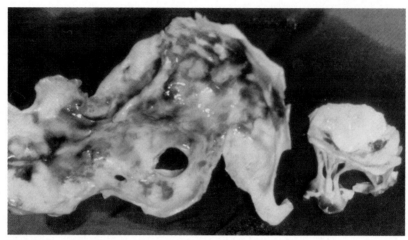

Figure 10.3-14: Complete cast of the left atrium in old, organized and partly calcified thrombus and the stenotic mitral valve with which it was associated. Note the patches of recent, fresh thrombus also.

Fresh, mobile thrombus requires immediate treatment. If the patient is already on oral anticoagulant therapy, the INR should be optimized; if not this treatment should be commenced immediately. It has been shown that with an INR of 3.0, most small mobile thrombi will regress rapidly and FPA levels fall to normal levels (427). In larger, immobile thrombi of greater maturity, the response to anticoagulation is much less predictable and a proportion may not respond (492). If the patient has suffered a recent cerebral infarction, this should not be regarded as a contra-indication to anticoagulation, but several reports and reviews have advised delaying the onset of anticoagulation for 2-3 days to reduce the risk of hemorrhagic transformation of the infarct, on the basis that, in the first few days, this risk is higher in terms of cerebral damage than the risk of recurrent embolism (3,493,494).

If a large thrombus fails to respond to anticoagulation within an acceptable therapeutic range (INR 3.0-4.5), surgical treatment should be contemplated only if there is an associated lesion amenable to surgical correction. In the majority of cases of left atrial thrombosis, the associated lesion will be mitral stenosis. Because the risk of thromboembolism in mitral stenosis does not correlate with the degree of stenosis (200), surgical treatment in the presence of thrombus can only be justified if the valve is suitable for valvotomy or if the degree of stenosis is such that a prosthetic valve, if required, will provide a larger effective orifice area. There is no evidence that ligation of the left atrial appendage decreases the risk of subsequent thrombosis and embolism (201).

Prosthetic valve thrombosis

In discussing the management of this problem, it is important to distinguish between obstructive thrombosis which interferes with the mechanism of the prosthesis and narrows the effective orifice and the type of minor thrombus attachment, usually to the sewing ring, which is discovered as an incidental finding during echocardiography. The former is often a life-threatening emergency whereas the latter can be managed more conservatively. The incidence of minor thrombus attachment is probably underestimated. Early postoperative TEE shows that it is not uncommon at this time of ineffective anticoagulation (54). Optimization of anticoagulation can result in the regression of even quite large thrombi of this type, but careful monitoring with repeated TEE is required. The remainder of this section will be devoted to the more difficult problem of obstructive thrombosis.

Obstructive thrombosis is always symptomatic although the symptoms of decreasing cardiac output are often surprisingly insidious, developing over weeks or even months in some instances as thrombus slowly accumulates (56). Progression of symptoms tends to be more rapid with bileaflet valves than with tilting disc valves because in the former even quite small quantities of thrombus at the hinge points can immobilize both leaflets; with prostheses of this type symptoms tend to develop over days rather than weeks, even when cases of obstruction of one leaflet only are included in the comparison (56). When considering the diagnosis of valve thrombosis, it is important to remember that even bioprosthetic valves are not immune from obstructive thrombosis, the incidence in porcine valves *without* anticoagulation approaching that of the least thrombogenic mechanical valves *with* anticoagulation (56).

The choice of treatment for obstructive thrombosis lies between surgery and thrombolysis. Although there has been a resurgence of interest in thrombolytic therapy recently, it remains controversial. In formulating a logical approach, it is necessary to take into account the underlying cause of the valve thrombosis in each case. If obstruction is due to a combination of tissue ingrowth and thrombosis, thrombolysis will not be successful. Similarly long-standing valve thrombosis demonstrates repeated layers of thrombus deposition, is of firm, rubbery consistency and is resistant to thrombolysis (Fig. 10.3-8).

The place of thrombolytic therapy

Long-standing valve thrombosis (several weeks) or valve thrombosis secondary to tissue ingrowth are not suitable for thrombolysis. Similarly, if valve thrombosis appears primarily related to the high thrombogenicity of the prosthesis and occurs despite well controlled anticoagulation, it is better to take the opportunity to replace the prosthesis with another of lower thrombogenicity in order to prevent recurrence of the problem. It is logical therefore to consider thrombolytic therapy only in patients with recent thrombosis related to non-existent or inadequate anticoagulation or to temporary factors which have increased coagulability (see section on risk factors and trigger factors for prosthetic valve thrombosis). Preservation of occluder mobility has also been proposed as a selection criterion (495). In order for the thrombolysis to have time to work, the patient must also be reasonably stable, and certainly not in extremis (496). An exception to these simple rules would be the patient whose age and generally frail condition would preclude any type of surgical intervention under any circumstances.

Because of their lightweight construction and the vulnerability of the hinge points to thrombosis, bileaflet valves are susceptible to leaflet immobilization by relatively small amounts of thrombus. Hence the time interval between thrombosis and presentation is usually short. As the thrombus is usually recent and its volume small, bileaflet valve thrombosis may be particularly suitable for thrombolytic therapy, as emphasized by a series of valve thromboses recently reported from one American institution (365). The duration of symptoms in most cases was 14 days or less. Out of 17 patients, 10 patients whose INR had been less than 1.5-1.7 received thrombolytic therapy with either streptokinase or urokinase. Although marked improvement of leaflet motion occurred in most patients, it remained incomplete in some, suggesting residual thrombus or tissue ingrowth, and rethrombosis occurred in two patients within a few months, in one patient several times. There were no deaths associated with treatment, but one transient embolic event and four bleeding events occurred.

This report is of particular interest because it demonstrates that even under relatively favorable circumstances, with small quantities of recent thrombus, thrombolysis gives imperfect results (365). Better results have been obtained by restricting thrombolysis to prostheses with occluders that are still mobile (495). Other series of unselected patients have reported much less satisfactory results with significant mortality, high rates of recurrent or residual thrombosis (38%), and an overall incidence of embolism of about 18% (497). Mortality is particularly high following surgery for failed thrombolytic therapy (30%) (497). Individual series are difficult to compare because of differences in selection criteria, thrombolytic therapy, type of prosthesis, size and maturity of thrombus and patients' NYHA class at the time of treatment. No randomized studies have been carried out comparing thrombolysis to surgery but these would be difficult, if not impossible, to organize. Small numbers would necessitate a multicenter trial and, given the emergency nature of valve thrombosis, inclusion and exclusion criteria would be difficult to enforce.

Thrombolytic therapy has been defended by its proponents mainly on claims of lower mortality rates in comparison to reoperation for valve thrombosis (365,495). However, the mortality of reoperation is closely related to the NYHA class at the time of surgery (498). With the widespread diagnostic availability of cinefluoroscopy and TEE, no patient with valve thrombosis should be allowed to deteriorate to the extent that they are in extremis prior to surgery. 'Elective' reoperation on valve thrombosis in its early stages should be a low risk procedure. The slower progression of symptoms of valve thrombosis in tilting disc and caged ball valves in comparison to bileaflet valves may give an additional margin of safety in this respect.

Thrombolytic therapy has also been advocated on the grounds that it can be used as an initial therapy and, if unsuccessful, surgical treatment can follow (365). The flaw in this argument is the greatly increased risk of bleeding if it is necessary to carry out a reoperation shortly after thrombolytic therapy, as may be the case if the patient's condition is deteriorating rapidly. The risk of bleeding is less following the use of fibrin-specific 'second generation' fibrinolytic agents such as tPA, which has a short half life and is less likely to cause generalized fibrinolysis (499). Although the plasmin-inhibitor, aprotinin, is extremely useful in ameliorating the risk of bleeding during surgery in the presence of generalized fibrinolysis (500), the risk remains high.

Because of the increased risk of surgery following thrombolysis, the decision to administer a thrombolytic agent should be made in conjunction with a cardiac surgeon. Furthermore, thrombolytic treatment should only be carried out in hospitals with full cardiac surgical facilities.

Surgical treatment of valve thrombosis

Once the thrombosed valve has been assessed at operation, a choice must be made between thrombectomy and replacement. If the thrombus has resulted from inadequate or non-existent anticoagulation or from other correctable or temporary factors which have increased coagulability on a transient basis, thrombectomy may be appropriate, providing that access to both surfaces of the prosthesis is sufficient to permit complete removal of all traces of thrombus. Undoubtedly some of the failures of thrombectomy are due to incomplete removal of thrombus. Because of problems with visualization, thrombectomy is easiest to perform on tilting disc valves in the aortic position, especially if they can be rotated in situ to allow thorough inspection of the subvalvular area. Results with aortic prosthesis thrombectomy are correspondingly better (496). Mitral prostheses are more problematical; from the atrial aspect large quantities of thrombus may remain hidden on the ventricular surface of the prosthesis (Fig. 10.3-8). This difficulty can be overcome to some extent by opening the aorta and inspecting the ventricular surface through the aortic valve. However if the visualization is poor and the prosthesis cannot be rotated to facilitate inspection, it is safer to proceed to replacement. If thrombectomy alone is being considered as the definitive treatment, it is important to be certain that any hypercoagulability can be corrected and that reliable anticoagulation can be ensured postoperatively. Otherwise a bioprosthesis may be preferable.

If anticoagulation has been well controlled and the underlying cause is tissue ingrowth, it is probably safer to replace the valve. Some surgeons have reported simply excising the excess fibrous tissue (69) but long term follow up data on sufficient numbers of patients to evaluate this technique are not available. The principal concern about tissue ingrowth is its etiology; if it has formed once, it can form again. Some have suggested that it is a prosthesis design-related phenomenon and that particular flow characteristics favor its formation (61). On this basis there would be an argument for replacing the prosthesis with one of a different design. However, almost certainly tissue ingrowth is a multifactoral problem, as discussed earlier in this chapter, and a thorough investigation for possible etiologic factors should be carried out in each case.

If anticoagulation has been well controlled in a range appropriate to the thrombogenicity of the prosthesis and there is no evidence that transient or correctable hypercoagulability or tissue ingrowth has contributed to valve thrombosis, it must be assumed that the prosthesis itself is at fault and it should be replaced either with a less thrombogenic mechanical valve or with a bioprosthesis.

THE MANAGEMENT OF EMBOLISM

All embolic events should be taken seriously and not merely dismissed as the inevitable consequences of either heart valve disease or the presence of a prosthetic valve. It should not be assumed that all cerebral events are ischemic nor that all ischemic events are embolic. Patients who suffer such an event merit CT or MRI brain scan. They should also be thoroughly investigated for underlying risk factors and trigger factors, as outlined earlier in this chapter, so that measures can be taken to minimize the risk of further events. This approach is particularly important in patients who have suffered recurrent embolism. Investigations should include TEE to search for residual thrombus in the left atrium or on the prosthesis. Unfortunately patients with minor transient events are not usually referred to hospital with the result that a golden opportunity is missed to assess coagulability *at the time of the event*. Progress will only be made if more data are collected at this critical time.

The treatment of visceral and limb embolism is well established. However the immediate treatment of cerebral embolism with thrombolysis and the management of recurrent embolism both remain controversial.

Thrombolysis for cerebral embolism

Thrombolytic therapy for acute ischemic stroke was first employed in the late 1950's but attracted little enthusiasm over the succeeding decades (501). However following the advent of CT scanning, enabling more precise diagnosis, and with the availability of more fibrin-specific thrombolytic agents, enthusiasm has been rekindled in recent years, leading to the publication of several randomized trials. A recently published overview of these trials (501), which included cerebral thrombosis as well as cerebral embolism, concluded that the results were sufficiently encouraging to warrant further evaluation of the technique. Four trials in which CT evaluation was employed revealed a significant reduction in the risk of death or deterioration. Analysis of all published studies showed no excess risk of hemorrhagic transformation or severe cerebral edema. The rate of cerebral hematoma formation was 5%, the same as that in the natural history of cerebral infarction. Similar benefit with low risk has been demonstrated in a multicenter trial limited to embolic stroke (502).

Although further research is required to define subsets of patients likely to benefit most, these encouraging results suggest that thrombolysis should be more widely used in the acute treatment of cerebral embolism, under the guidance of an experienced neurologist. It is essential that treatment is commenced within six hours, not only to obtain greatest benefit, but to avoid increasing the risk of hemorrhagic transformation (501). From currently available data, this risk appears to be higher after six hours. Hypertension and a low-density area already visible on CT scan are also thought to be risk factors for symptomatic intracerebral hematoma formation (501) and should probably be regarded as contraindications to thrombolysis until further ongoing trials clarify the situation.

Management of recurrent embolism

In patients with recurrent embolism, the need for full investigation including coagulability assessment cannot be over-emphasised. The traditional practice of merely increasing the anticoagulation intensity and/or adding an antiplatelet agent is insufficient. These measures may be necessary if risk factors and/or trigger factors cannot be eliminated, but their prescription should if possible be scientifically based (see appropriate sections of this chapter). For example, if the patient is discovered to have carotid stenosis or aortic atheromatous plaques, the combination of aspirin with low intensity anticoagulation is likely to be the most beneficial approach. If, on the other hand, excessive stagnation in the left atrium is the problem, raising the intensity of the anticoagulation may decrease the risk and an antiplatelet agent would not be indicated.

Information should also be sought on anticoagulation compliance, if necessary checking serum warfarin levels in addition to frequent INR estimations. Non-compliance with anticoagulation is a major cause of recurrent embolism. Sometimes the problem can be solved by education and by involving the patient more in his own anticoagulation control (401). If the problem is one of forgetfulness or fecklessness, the administration of medication should be entrusted to a relative. Non-compliance alone should never be a justification for replacement of a mechanical valve with a bioprosthesis.

The principal controversy in recurrent embolism after valve replacement centers on the role of the prosthesis. To what extent, if any, is it the source or the cause of the embolism and is it necessary to replace it? These questions can only be answered by full investigation. If the patient is compliant with anticoagulation in an appropriate range and is in sinus rhythm, is normotensive, non-diabetic, of normal nutritional status, is a long-standing non-smoker, has no evidence of arterial disease on Doppler and TEE and has no evidence of thrombophilia, the finger of suspicion must point at the prosthesis. The type of prosthesis must also be taken into account. The caged ball valve is more likely than tilting disc or bileaflet valves to discharge emboli when it becomes thrombosed (Fig. 10.3-2) (56). Therefore recurrent embolism with this prosthesis during a short time period should raise suspicion of valve thrombosis; if proven the prosthesis should be removed. With other types of valves, providing that no thrombus can be detected on the prosthesis on TEE, treatment with appropriate antiplatelet therapy (q.v.) should be instituted as a first step. If repeated embolism continues, the prosthesis should be replaced with one of lower thrombogenicity.

References

1. Abernathy WS, Willis PW. Thromboembolic complications of rheumatic heart disease. Cardiovasc Clin 1973;5:131-175
2. Edmunds LH Jr. Thrombotic and bleeding complications of prosthetic heart valves. Ann Thorac Surg 1987;44:430-445
3. Cerebral Embolism Task Force. Cardiogenic brain embolism. The second report of the Cerebral Embolism Task Force. Arch Neurol 1989;46:727-743
4. WHO Task Force on Stroke and Other Cerebrovascular Disorders: Stroke 1989; recommendations on stroke prevention diagnosis and therapy. Stroke 1989;20:1407-1431
5. Virchow R. Gesammelte abhandlungen zur Wissenschaftlichen medizin. IV Thrombose und embolie. Gefassentzundung und Septische Infektion, Frankfurt, Meidinger 1856
6. Jaffe EA. Physiologic functions of normal endothelial cells. In Loscalzo J, Creager MA, Dzau VJ, (Eds): Vascular Medicine. Boston, Little Brown 1992:3-46
7. Broze GJ. The role of tissue factor pathway inhibitor in a revised coagulation cascade. Semin Hematol 1992;29:159-169
8. Bauer KA, Rosenberg RD. Role of antithrombin III as a regulator of in vivo coagulation. Semin Hematol 1991;28:10-18
9. Esmon CT. The regulation of natural anticoagulant pathways. Science 1987;235:1348-1352
10. Esmon NL. Thrombomodulin. In Coller BS (Ed): Progress in Hemostasis and Thrombosis Vol. 9. Philadelphia, WB Saunders 1989:29-55
11. Ware JA, Heistad DD. Platelet-endothelium interactions. N Engl J Med 1993;328:628-635
12. Lewis MJ, Smith JA. Platelets, thrombosis and the endothelium. In Rubanyi GM (Ed). Cardiovascular Significance of Endothelium-Derived Vasoactive Factors. Mount Kisco, Futura 1991:293-306
13. Hajjar KA. Assembly of the fibrinolytic system on endothelial cells. In Haber E, Braunwald E (Eds): Thrombolysis - Basic Contributions and Clinical Progress. St. Louis, Mosby 1991:27-32
14. Vaughan DE, Schafer AI, Loscalzo J. Normal mechanisms of hemostasis and fibrinolysis. In Loscalzo J, Creager MA, Dzau VJ (Eds): Vascular Medicine. Boston, Little Brown 1992:233-247
15. Nachman RL. Thrombosis and atherogenesis: molecular connections. Blood 1992;79:1897-1906
16. Meyer D, Girma JP. von Willebrand factor: structure and function. Thromb Haemost 1993;70:99-104
17. Wagner DD. The Weibel-Palade body: the storage granule for von Willebrand factor and p-selectin. Thromb Haemost 1993;70:105-110
18. Grabowski EF, Zuckerman DB, Nemerson Y. The functional expression of tissue factor by fibrinoblasts and endothelial cells under flow conditions. Blood 1993;81:3265-3270
19. Sprengers ED, Kluft C. Plasminogen activator inhibitors. Blood 1987;69:381-387

20. Rodgers GM. Hemostatic properties of normal and perturbed vascular cells. FASEB J 1988;2:116-123
21. Dewey CF Jr, Bussolari SR, Gimbrone MA Jr, Davies PF: The dynamic response of vascular endothelial cells to fluid shear stress. J Biomech Eng 1981;103:177-185
22. Bevilacqua MP, Gimbrone MA. Inducible endothelial functions in inflammation and coagulation. Sem Thromb Haemost 1987;13:425-433
23. Stein PD, Sabbah HN. Hemorheology of turbulence. Biorheology 1980;17:301-319
24. Yoganathan AP, Wick TM, Reul H. The influence of flow characteristics of prosthetic valves on thrombus formation. In Butchart EG, Bodnar E:Current Issues in Heart Valve Disease: Thrombosis, Embolism and Bleeding. London, ICR Publishers 1992:123-148
25. Davies PF. Endothelium as a signal transduction interface for flow forces: cell surface dynamics. Thromb Haemost 1993;70:124-128
26. Badimon L, Badimon JJ, Chesbro JH, Fuster V. von Willebrand factor and cardiovascular disease. Thromb Haemost 1993;70:111-118
27 Penny WF, Weinstein M, Salzman EW, Ware JA. Correlation of circulating von Willebrand factor levels with cardiovascular hemodynamics. Circulation 1991;83:1630-1636
28. Harrison DG, Minor RL, Guerra R, Wuillen JE, Sellke FW. Endothelial dysfunction in atherosclerosis. In Rubanyi GM (Ed): Cardiovascular Significance of Endothelium-Derived Vasoactive Factors. Mount Kisco, Futura 1991:263-280
29. Burrig KF. The endothelium of advanced arteriosclerotic plaques in humans. Arteriosclerosis Thromb 1991;11:1678-1689
30. Meade TW, Ruddock V, Stirling Y, Chakrabarti R, Miller GJ. Fibrinolytic activity, clotting factors and long term incidence of ischaemic heart disease in the Northwick Park Heart Study. Lancet 1993;342:1076-1079
31. Vague IJ, Alessi MC, Vague P. Increased plasma plasminogen activator inhibitor one levels;a possible link between insulin resistance and atherothrombosis. Diabetologia 1991;34:457-462
32. Stehouwer CDA, Nauta JJP, Zeldenrust GC, Hackeng WHI, Donker AJM, den Ottolander GJH. Urinary albumin excretion, cardiovascular disease and endothelial dysfunction in non-insulin-dependent diabetes mellitus. Lancet 1992;340:319-323
33. Landin K, Tengborn L, Smith U. Elevated fibrinogen and plasminogen activator inhibitor (PAI-1) in hypertension are related to metabolic risk factors for cardiovascular disease. J Intern Med 1990;273-278
34. Winther K, Gleerup G, Hedner T:Enhanced risk of thromboembolic disease in hypertension from platelet hyperfunction and decreased fibrinolytic activity: has antihypertensive therapy any influence? J Cardiovasc Pharmacol 1992;19(Suppl 3):521-524
35. Luscher TF, Vanhoutte PM, Boulanger C, Dohi Y, Buhler FR. Endothelial dysfunction in hypertension. In Rubanyi GM (Ed): Cardiovascular Significance of Endothelium-Derived Vasoactive Factors. Mount Kisco, Futura 1991:199-221
36. Torbjorn K, Nillson J, Jannson H. Hemostatic variables of the endothelial cells as predictors of mortality: a five year prospective study (Abstract). Thromb Haemost 1993;69:1203
37. Magarey FR. Pathogenesis of mitral stenosis. Br Med J 1951;1:856-857
38. Tweedy PS. The pathogenesis of valvular thickening in rheumatic heart disease. Br Heart J 1956;18:173-185
39. Burrig KF, Schulte-Terhausen J, Hort W. Special role of the endocardium in the pathogenesis of endocarditis. In Horstkotte D, Bodnar E: Current Issues in Heart Valve Disease: Infective Endocarditis. London, ICR Publishers 1991:3-9
40. Drake TA, Pang M. Staphylococcus aureus induces tissue factor expression in cultured human cardiac valve endothelium. J Inf Dis 1988;157:749-756
41. Dvorak HF. Thrombosis and cancer. Hum Pathol 1987;18:275-284
42. Zacharski LR, Wojtukiewicz MZ, Costantini V, Ornstein DL, Memoli VA. Pathways of coagulation/fibrinolysis activation in malignancy. Semin Thromb Haemost 1992;18:104-116
43 Deppisch LM, Fayemi AO. Non-bacterial thrombotic endocarditis: clinicopathologic correlations. Am Heart J 1976;92:723-729
44. Straaton KV, Chatham WW, Reveille JD, Koopman WJ, Smith SH. Clinically significant valvular heart disease in systemic lupus erythematosus. Am J Med 1988;85:645-650
45. Ford SE, Lillicrap D, Brunet D, Ford P. Thrombotic endocarditis and lupus anticoagulant. Arch Pathol Lab Med 1989;113:350-353
46. Ginsberg JS, Demers C, Brill-Edwards P et al. Increased thrombin generation and activity in patients with systemic lupus erythematosus and anticardiolipin antibodies: evidence for a prothrombotic state. Blood 1993;81:2958-2963
47. Oosting JD, Derksen RHWM, Bobbink IWG, Hackeng TM, Bouma BN, de Groot PG. Antiphospholipid antibodies directed against a combination of phospholipids with prothrombin, protein C, or protein S: an explanation for their pathogenetic mechanism? Blood 1993;81:2618-2625
48. Stein PD, Sabbah HN, Pitha JV. Continuing disease process of calcific aortic stenosis: role of microthrombi

and turbulent flow. Am J Cardiol 1977;30:159-163

49. Salzman EW, Merrill EW. Interaction of blood with artificial surfaces. In Colman RW, Hirsh J, Marder VJ, Salzman EW (Eds). Hemostasis and Thrombosis, Basic Principles and Clinical Practice, 2nd Edition. Philadelphia, JB Lippincott 1987:1335-1347

50. Anderson JM, Schoen FJ. Interations of blood with artificial surfaces. In Butchart EG, Bodnar E. Current Issues in Heart Valve Disease: Thrombosis, Embolism and Bleeding. London, ICR Publishers 1992:160-171

51. Dewanjee MK, Trastek VF, Tago M, Torianni M, Kaye MP. Noninvasive radioisotopic technique for detection of platelet deposition on bovine pericardial mitral valve prostheses and in vitro quantification of visceral microembolism in dogs. Trans Am Soc Artif Intern Organs 1983;29:188-193

52. Stoddard MF, Dawkins PR, Longaker RA. Mobile strands are frequently attached to the St. Jude Medical mitral valve prosthesis as assessed by two-dimensional transoesophageal echocardiography. Am Heart J 1992;124:671-674

53. Isada L, Klein AL, Torelli J, Nemec J, Stewart WJ. Strands on mitral valve prostheses by transoesophageal echocardiography - another potential embolic source (Abstract). J Am Coll Cardiol 1992;(Suppl A)19:32A

54. Iung B, Cormier B, Dadez E et al. Small abnormal echoes after mitral valve replacement with bileaflet mechanical prostheses: predisposing factors and effect on thromboembolism. J Heart Valve Dis 1993;2:259-266

55. Berger K, Sauvage LF, Wood SJ, Wesolowski SA. Sewing ring healing of cardiac valve prostheses. Surgery 1967;61:102-117

56. Butchart EG. Thrombogenicity, thrombosis and embolism. In Butchart EG, Bodnar E: Current Issues in Heart Valve Disease: Thrombosis, Embolism and Bleeding. London, ICR Publishers 1992:172-205

57. Planinc D, Jeric M, Mihatov S, Omcikus M, Pagon L, Rudar M. Doppler evaluation of prosthetic mitral valves. Acta Cardiol 1991;46:79-83

58. Cleveland JC, Lebenson IM, Dague JR. Early postoperative development of aortic regurgitation related to pannus ingrowth causing incomplete disc seating of a Bjork-Shiley prosthesis. Ann Thorac Surg 1982;33:496-498

59. Bortolotti U, Galluci V, Casarotto D, Thiene G. Fibrous tissue overgrowth on Hancock mitral xenograft: a cause of late prosthetic stenosis. Thorac Cardiovasc Surgeon 1979;27:316-318

60. Marbarger JP, Clark RE. The clinical life history of explanted prosthetic heart valves. Ann Thorac Surg 1982;34:22-33

61. Yoganathan AP, Corcoran WH, Harrison EC, Carl JR. The Bjork-Shiley aortic prosthesis: flow characteristics, thrombus formation and tissue overgrowth. Circulation 1978;58:70-76

62. Bonchek LI, Braunwald NS. Modification of thrombus formation on prosthetic heart valves by the administration of low molecular weight dextran. Ann Surg 1967;165:200-205

63. Hannah H, Bull B, Braunwald NS. Development of an autogenous tissue covering on prosthetic heart valves: effect of warfarin and dextran. Ann Surg 1968;168:1075-1078

64. Polednak AP. Connective tissue responses in negroes in relation to disease. Am J Phys Anthropol 1974;41:49-58

65. Spray TL, Roberts WC. Structural changes in porcine xenografts used as substitute cardiac valves. Am J Cardiol 1977;40:319-330

66. Thiene G, Bortolotti U, Panizzon G, Milano A, Gallucci V: Pathological substrates of thrombus formation after heart valve replacement with the Hancock bioprosthesis. J Thorac Cardiovasc Surg 1980;80:414-423

67. Hassoulas J, Rose AG. Experimental evaluation of the Mitroflow pericardial heart valve prosthesis. Part II: pathologic examination. Angiology 1988;39:733-741

68. Murphy SK, Rogler WC, Fleming WH, McManus BM. Retraction of bioprosthetic heart valve cusps: a cause of wide-open regurgitation in right-sided heart valves. Hum Pathol 1988;19:140-147

69. Deviri E, Sareli P, Wisenbaugh T, Cronje SL. Obstruction of mechanical heart valve prostheses: clinical aspects and surgical management. J Am Coll Cardiol 1991;17:646-650

70. Ferrans VJ, Spray TL, Billingham ME, Roberts WC. Structural changes in glutaraldehyde-treated porcine heterografts used as substitute cardiac valves. Am J Cardiol 1978;41:1159-1184

71. Riddle JM, Magilligan DJ, Stein PD. Surface morphology of degenerated porcine bioprosthetic valves four to seven years following implantation. J Thorac Cardiovasc Surg 1981;81:279-287

72. Ishihara T, Ferrans VJ, Jones M, Boyce SW, Roberts WC. Occurrence and significance of endothelial cells in implanted porcine bioprosthetic valves. Am J Cardiol 1981;48:443-454

73. Gavin JB, Herdson PB, Monro JL, Barratt-Boyes BG. Pathology of antibiotic-treated human heart valve allografts. Thorax 1973;28:473-481

74. Gavin JB, Barratt-Boyes BG, Hitchcock GC, Herdson PB. Histopathology of 'fresh' human aortic valve allografts. Thorax 1973;28:482-487

75. Aparicio SR, Donnelly RJ, Dexter F, Watson DA. Light and electron microscopy studies on homograft and heterograft heart valves. J Pathol 1975;115:147-162

76. Ishihara T, Ferrans VJ, Jones M, Boyce SW, Roberts WC. Structure of bovine pericardium and of

unimplanted Ionescu-Shiley pericardial valvular bioprostheses. J Thorac Cardiovasc Surg 1981;81:747-757

77. Ferrans VJ, Tomita Y, Hilbert SL, Jones M, Roberts WC. Pathology of bioprosthetic cardiac valves. Hum Pathol 1987;18:586-595
78. Magilligan DJ, Oyama C, Klein S, Riddle JM, Smith D. Platelet adherence to bioprosthetic cardiac valves. Am J Cardiol 1984;53:945-949
79. Platt MR, Mills LJ, Estrera AS, Hillis LD, Buja LM, Willerson JT. Marked thrombosis and calcification of porcine heterograft valves. Circulation 1980;62:862-869
80. Hetzer R, Hill DJ, Kerth WJ, Wilson AJ, Adappa MG, Gerbode F. Thrombosis and degeneration of Hancock valves: clinical and pathological findings Ann Thorac Surg 1978;26:317-322
81. Schoen FJ, Hobson CE. Anatomic analysis of removed prosthetic heart valves: causes of failure of 33 mechanical valves and 58 bioprostheses, 1980 to 1983. Hum Pathol 1985;16:549-559
82. Croft CH, Buja LM, Floresca MZ, Nicod P, Estrera A. Late thrombotic obstruction of aortic porcine bioprostheses. Am J Cardiol 1986;57:355-356
83. Baciewicz PA, del Rio C, Goncalves MA, Lattouf OM, Guyton RA, Morris DC. Catastrophic thrombosis of porcine aortic bioprostheses. Ann Thorac Surg 1990;50:817-819
84. Jones M, Eidbo EE. Doppler color flow evaluation of prosthetic mitral valves:experimental epicardial studies. J Am Coll Cardiol 1989;13:234-240
85. Angell WW, Angell JD. Porcine valves. Prog Cardiovasc Dis 1980;23:141-166
86. Prandoni P, Pengo V, Boetto P, Zambon G, Menozzi L. Do malfunctioning bioprosthetic heart valves represent a potential thrombogenic focus? Haemostasis 1985:15:337-344
87. Lee G, Joye JA, Rose A, DeNardo S, Kozina JA, Mason DT. Evaluation of platelet kinetics following porcine and mechanical valve replacement. Clin Cardiol 1981;4:11-14
88. Dudczak R, Niessner H, Thaler E, Lechner K, Kletter K, Frischauf H, Domanig E, Aicher H. Plasma concentration of platelet-specific proteins and fibrinopeptide A in patients with artificial heart valves. Haemostasis 1981;10:186-194
89. Turpie AGG, de Boer AC, Giroux M et al. Platelet survival and betathromboglobulin after heterograft mitral valve replacement: effect of suloctidil (Abstract). Thromb Haemost 1983;50:63
90. Harker LA, Slichter SS. Studies of platelets and fibrinogen kinetics in patients with prosthetic heart valves. N Engl J Med 1970;283:1302-1305
91. Manohitharajah SM, Rahman AN, Donnelly RJ, Deverall PB, Watson DA: Platelets survival in patients with homograft and prosthetic valves. Thorax 1974;29:639-642
92. Turitto VT. Platelet rheology. In Lowe GDO (Ed): Clinical Blood Rheology Vol I. Boca Raton, CRC Press 1988:111-128
93. Lowe GDO, Barbenel JC. Plasma and blood viscosity. In Lowe GDO (Ed): Clinical Blood Rheology, Vol. I. Boca Raton, CRC Press 1988:11-44
94. Slack SM, Cui Y, Turitto VT. The effects of flow on blood coagulation and thrombosis. Thromb Haemostat 1993;70:129-134
95. Beppu S. Hypercoagulability in the left atrium, Part I: Echocardiography. J Heart Valve Dis 1993;2:18-24
96. Lowe GDO. Blood viscosity and cardiovascular disease. Thromb Haemost 1992;67:494-498
97. Hawiger J. The interaction of platelets and other cellular elements with the vessel wall. In Loscalzo J, Creager MA, Dzau VJ (Eds): Vascular Medicine. Boston, Little Brown, 1992:205-231
98. Yasaka M, Beppu S. Hypercoagulability in the left atrium, Part II: Coagulation factors. J Heart Valve Dis 1993;2:25-34
99. Stein PD, Sabbah HN. Turbulent blood flow in the ascending aorta of humans with normal and diseased aortic valves. Circ Res 1976;39:58-65
100. Reimers RC, Sutera SP, Joist JH. Potentiation by red blood cells of shear-induced platelet aggregation: relative importance of chemical and physical mechanisms. Blood 1984;64:1200-1206
101. Wurzinger LJ, Opitz R, Blasberg P, Schmid-Schonbein H. Platelet and coagulation parameters following millisecond exposure to laminar sheer stress. Thromb Haemost 1985;54:381-386
102. Ruggeri ZM. Mechanisms of shear-induced platelet adhesion and aggregation. Thromb Haemost 1993;70:119-123
103. Alkhamis TM, Beissinger RL, Chediak J. Artificial surface effect on red blood cells and platelets in laminar shear flow. Blood 1990;75:1568-1575
104. Mustard JF, Packham MA, Kinlough-Rathbone RL. Mechanisms in thrombosis. In Bloom AL, Thomas DP (Eds): Haemostasis and Thrombosis. Edinburgh, Churchill Livingstone 1987;618-650
105. Vermylen J, Verstraete M, Fuster V. Role of platelet activation and fibrin formation in thrombogenesis. J Am Coll Cardiol 1986;8:2B-9B
106. Francis JL. The detection and measurement of factor XIII activity: a review. Med Lab Sci 1980;37:137-147
107. McDonagh J. Structure and function of factor XIII. In Colman RW, Hirsh J, Marder VJ, Salzman EW (Eds): Hemostasis and Thrombosis. Philadelphia, JB Lippincott, 1987;289-300
108. Davidson CJ, Skelton TN, Kisslo KB et al. The risk of systematic embolization associated with

percutaneous balloon valvuloplasty in adults. Ann Intern Med 1988;108:557-560
109. Scotten LN, Tacca RG, Walker DK, Brownlee RT. New tilting disc cardiac prostheses: in vitro comparison of the hydrodynamic performance in the mitral position. J Thorac Cardiovasc Surg 1981;82:136-146
110. Fisher J, Rees IJ, Wheatley DJ. In vitro evaluation of six mechanical and six bioprosthetic valves. Thorac Cardiovasc Surgeon 1986;34:157-162
111. Gibbs JL, Wharton GA, Williams GJ. Doppler ultrasound of normally functioning mechanical mitral and aortic valve prostheses
112. Grunkemeier GL, Starr A, Rahimtoola SH. Prosthetic heart valve performance:long term follow up. Curr Prob Cardiol 1992;17:331-406
113. Yoganathan AP, Raemar HH, Corcoran WH, Harrison EC, Shulman IA, Parnassus W. The Starr-Edwards aortic ball valve: flow characteristics, thrombus formation and tissue overgrowth. Artif Organs 1981;5:6-17
114. Fananapazir L, Clarke DB, Dark JF, Lawson RAM, Moussalli H. Results of valve replacement with the Omniscience prosthesis. J Thorac Cardiovasc Surg 1983;86:621-625
115. Hall KV, Kaster RL. Woien A. An improved pivotal disc-type prosthetic heart valve. J Oslo City Hosp 1979;29:3-21
116. Bjork VO, Lindblom D. The monostrut Bjork-Shiley heart valve. J Am Coll Cardiol 1985;6:1142-1148
117. Nunez L, Iglesias A, Sotillo J. Entrapment of leaflet of St Jude Medical cardiac valve prosthesis by miniscule thrombus: report of two cases. Ann Thorac Surg 1980;29:567-569
118. Gabbay S, Kresh JY. Bioengineering of mechanical and biologic heart valve substitutes. In Morse D, Steiner RM, Fernandez J (Eds): Guide to Prosthetic Cardiac Valves. New York, Springer-Verlag 1985:239-256
119. Smith JR, Landaw SA. Smokers polycythemia. N Engl J Med 1978;298:6-10
120. Ernst E, Matria A, Schmolzl C, Magyarosy I. Dose-effect between smoking and blood rheology. Br J Haematol 1987;65:485-487
121. Yarnell JWG, Sweetnam, Rogers S et al. Some long term effects of smoking on the haemostatic system: a report from the Caerphilly and Speedwell Collaborative Surveys. J Clin Pathol 1987;40:909-913
122. Kannell WB, D'Agostino RB, Belanger AJ. Fibrinogen, cigarette smoking and the risk of cardiovascular disease: insights from the Framingham study. Am Heart J 1987;113:1006-1010
123. Herman AG. Platelet activation and aggregation: rationale for combining antithrombotic drugs. In Herman AG (Ed): Antithrombotics: Pathophysiological Rationale for Pharmacological Interventions. Dordrecht, Kluwer Acadamec Publishers 1991:1-26
124. Siess W. Molecular mechanisms of platelet activation. Physiol Rev 1989;69:58-178
125. Nurden AT. Human platelet membrane glycoproteins. In Bloom AL, Forbes CD, Thomas DP, Tuddenham EDG (Eds): Haemostasis and Thrombosis. Edinburgh, Churchill Livingstone 1994:115-165
126. Gewitz AM. Developmental biology of megakaryocytes and platelets. In Adamson JW (Ed): Current Opinion in Hematology. Philadelphia, Current Science 1993:256-264
127. Martin JF, Bath PMW. Platelets and megakaryocytes in vascular disease. In Herman AG (Ed): Antithrombotics: Pathophysiological Rationale for Pharmacological Interventions. Dordrecht, Kluwer Academic Publishers 1991:49-62
128. Martin JF, Daniel TD, Trowbridge EA. Acute and chronic changes in platelet volume and count after cardiopulmonary bypass induced thrombocytopenia in man. Thromb Haemost 1987;57:55-58
129. Harker LA. Thrombokinetics in idiopathic thrombocytopenic purpura. Br J Haematol 1970;19:95-104
130. Sharpe PC, Trinick T. Mean platelet volume in diabetes mellitus. Quart J Med 1993;86:739-742
131. Wedzicha JA, Cotter FE, Empey DW. Platelet size in patients with chronic airflow obstruction with and without hypoxaemia. Thorax 1988;43:61-64
132. Lanze F, Beretz A, Stierle A, Hanau D, Kubina M, Cazenave JP. Epinephrine potentiates human platelet activation but is not an aggregating agent. Am J Physiol 1988;255:H1276-H1288
133. Grignani G, Pacchiarini L, Zucchella M et al. Effect of mental stress on platelet function in normal subjects and in patients with coronary artery disease. Haemostasis 1992;22:138-146
134. Landolfi R, De Cristofaro R, DeCandida E, Rocca B, Bizzi B: Effect of fibrinogen concentration on the velocity of platelet aggregation. Blood 1991;78:377-381
135. Renaud S, Morazain R, Godsey F et al. Nutrients, platelet function and composition in nine groups of French and British farmers. Atherosclerosis 1986;60:37-48
136. Beswick AD, Fehily AM, Sharp DS, Renaud S, Giddings J. Long term diet modification and platelet activity. J Intern Med 1991;229:511-515
137. Renaud S, Godu J. Induction of large thrombi in hyperlipaemic rats by epinephrine and endotoxin. Lab Invest 1969;21:512-518
138. Renaud S, Kinlough RL, Mustard JF. Relationship between platelet aggregation and the thrombotic tendency in rats fed hyperlipaemic diets. Lab Invest 1970;22:339-343
139. Ciavatti M, Renaud S. Oxidative status and oral contraceptive;its relevance to platelet abnormalities and

cardiovascular risk. Free Radical Biol Med 1991;10:325-338

140. Trip MD, Cats VM, van Capelle FJL, Vreekin J. Platelet hyperreactivity and prognosis in survivors of myocardial infarction. N Engl J Med 1990;322:1549-1554

141. Bauer KA, Rosenberg RD. The pathophysiology of the prethrombotic state in humans: insights gained from studies using markers of hemostatic system activation. Blood 1987;70:343-350

142. Miller GJ, Meade TW. Hypercoagulability. In Butchart EG, Bodnar E: Current Issues in Heart Valve Disease: Thrombosis, Embolism and Bleeding. London, ICR Publishers 1992;81-92

143. Mosesson MW. The roles of fibrinogen and fibrin in hemostasis and thrombosis. Semin Hematol 1992;29:177-188

144. Okwusidi JI, Anvari N, Ofosu FA. Modulation of intrinsic prothrombin activation by fibrinogen and fibrin I. J Lab Clin Med 1993;121:64-70

145. Lee AJ, Lowe GDO, Woodward M, Tunstall-Pedoe H. Fibrinogen in relation to personal history of prevalent hypertension, diabetes, stroke, intermittent claudication, coronary heart disease and family history: the Scottish Heart Health Study. Br Heart J 1993;69:338-342

146. Ernst E, Resch KL. Fibrinogen as a cardiovascular risk factor: a meta-analysis and review of the literature. Ann Intern Med 1993;118:956-963

147. Qizilbash N, Jones L, Warlow C, Mann J. Fibrinogen and lipid concentrations as risk factors for transient ischaemic attacks and minor ischaemic strokes. Br Med J 1991;303:605-609

148. Gustafson C, Blomback M, Britton M, Hamsten A, Svensson J. Coagulation factors and increased risk of stroke in non-valvular atrial fibrillation. Stroke 1990;21:47-51

149. Schafer AI. The hypercoagulable states. Ann Intern Med 1985;102:814-828

150. Fuller JH, Keen H, Jarrett RJ et al. Haemostatic variables associated with diabetes and its complications. Br Med J 1979;2:964-966

151. Stirling Y, Woolf L, North WRS, Seghatchian MJ, Meade TW: Haemostasis in normal pregnancy. Thromb Haemost 1984;52:176-182

152. Gris JC, Schved JF, Feugeas O et al. Impact of smoking, physical training and weight reduction on factor VII, PAI-1 and haemostatic markers in sedentary men. Thromb Haemost 1990;64:516-520

153. Meade TW, Mellows S, Brozovic M et al. Haemostatic function and ischaemic heart disease: principal results of the Northwick Park Heart Study. Lancet 1986;2:533-537

154. Connelly JB, Cooper JA, Meade TW. Strenuous exercise, plasma fibrinogen and factor VII activity. Br Heart J 1992;67:351-354

155. Rubin DB, Wiener-Krosnish JP, Murray JF et al. Elevated von Willebrand antigen is an early plasma predictor of acute lung injury in nonpulmonary sepsis syndrome. J Clin Invest 1990;86:474-480

156. Chignard M, Balloy V, Renesto P. Leucocyte elastase-mediated release of von Willebrand factor from cultured endothelial cells. Eur Respir J 1993;6:791-796

157. Jansson JH, Nilsson TK, Johnson O. von Willebrand factor in plasma: a novel risk factor for recurrent myocardial infarction and death. Br Heart J 1991;66:351-353

158. Cortellaro M, Boschetto C, Cofrancesco E et al. The PLAT study: hemostatic function in relation to atherothrombotic ischaemic events in vascular disease patients;principal results. Arterioscler Thromb 1992;12:1063-1070

159. Folsom AR, Wu KK, Shahar E, Davis CE. Association of hemostatic variables with prevalent cardiovascular disease and asymptomatic carotid artery atherosclerosis. Arterioscler Thromb 1993;13:1829-1836

160. Greaves M, Pickering C, Knight G et al. Changes in the factor VIII complex in diabetic ketoacidosis: evidence of endothelial cell damage? Diabetologia 1987;30:160-165

161. Brenner B, Zwang E, Bronshtein M, Seligsohn U. von Willebrand factor multimer patterns in pregnancy-induced hypertension. Thromb Haemost 1989;62:715-717

162. Buller HR, ten Cate JW. Acquired antithrombin III deficiency: laboratory diagnosis, incidence, clinical implications and treatment with antithrombin III concentrate. Am J Med 1989;87(Suppl 3B):44S-48S

163. Fukuda Y, Kuroiwa Y, Okumiya K et al. Hypercoagulability in patients with mitral stenosis. Jpn Circulation J 1980;44:867-874

164. Hathaway WE. Clinical aspects of antithrombin III deficiency. Semin Hematol 1991;28:19-23

165. Schipper HG, Roos J, van den Meulen F, ten Cate JW. Antithrombin III deficiency in surgical intensive care patients. Thromb Res 1981;21:73-80

166. Butchart EG. Prosthesis-specific and patient-specific anticoagulation. In Butchart EG, Bodnar E: Current Issues in Heart Valve Diseaes: Thrombosis, Embolism and Bleeding. London, ICR Publishers 1992;293-317

167. Lidbury PS, Korbut R, Vane JR. Sodium nitroprusside modulates the fibrinolytic system in the rabbit. Br J Pharmacol 1990;101:527-530

168. Drummer C, Ludke S, Spannagl M, Schramm W, Gerzer R. The nitric oxide donor SIN-1 is a potent inhibitor of plasminogen activator inhibitor release from stimulated platelets. Thromb Res 1991;63:553-556

169. Andreotti F, Davies GJ, Hackett DR et al. Major carcadian fluctuations in fibrinolytic factors and possible relevance to time of onset of myocardial infarction, sudden cardiac death and stroke. Am J Cardiol 1988;62:635-637

170. Andreotti F, Kluft C. Circadian variation of fibrinolytic activity in blood. Chronobiol Int 1991;8:336-351

171. ECAT Angina Pectoris Study Group. ECAT angina pectoris study: baseline associations of hemostatic factors with extent of coronary arteriosclerosis and other coronary risk factors in 3000 patients with angina pectoris undergoing coronary angiography. Eur Heart J 1993;14:8-17

172. Ferrannini E, Buzzigoli G, Bonadonna R et al. Insulin resistance in essential hypertension. N Engl J Med 1987;317:350-357

173. Vague P, Vague JI, Aillaud MF et al. Correlation between blood fibrinolytic activity, plasminogen activator inhibitor level, plasma insulin level and relative body weight in normal and obese subjects. Metabolism 1986;35:250-253

174. Vague P, Vague JI, Alessi MC, Badier C, Valadier J. Metformin decreases the high plasminogen activator inhibition capacity, plasma insulin and triglyceride levels in non-diabetic obese subjects. Thromb Haemost 1987;57:326-328

175. Imataka K, Nakaoka H, Kitahara Y, Fujii J, Ishibashi M, Yamaji T: Blood haematocrit changes during paroxysmal atrial fibrillation. Am J Cardiol 1987;59:172-173

176. Petersen P. Thromboembolic complications in atrial fibrillation. Stroke 1990;21:4-13

177. Asakura H, Hifumi S, Jokahi H et al. Prothrombin fragment F1+2 and thrombin-antithrombin III complex are useful markers of the hypercoagulable state in atrial fibrillation. Blood Coag Fibrinol 1992;3:469-473

178. Uno M, Tsuji H, Sawada S, Toyoda T, Nakagawa M. Fibrinopeptide A (FPA) levels in atrial fibrillation and the effects of heparin administration. Jpn Circ J 1988;52:9-12

179. Gough SCL, Smyllie J, Berkin KE, Grant PJ, Davies JA. Relationship of haemostatic and fibrinolytic function to left atrial thrombi in patients with non-valvular atrial fibrillation (Abstract). Thromb Haemost 1991;65:991

180. Yasaka M, Miyatake K, Mitani M et el. Intracardiac mobile thrombus and D-dimer fragment of fibrin in patients with mitral stenosis. Br Heart J 1991;66:22-25

181. Levine B, Kalman J, Mayer L, Fillit HM, Packer M. Elevated circulating levels of tumor necrosis factor in severe chronic heart failure. N Engl J Med 1990;323:236-241

182. Naworth P, Stern D. Modulation of endothelial cell hemostatic properties by tumor necrosis factor. J Exp Med 1986;163:740-745

183. Edwards RL, Rickles FR. The role of leukocytes in the activation of blood coagulation. Semin Hematol 1992;29:202-212

184. Stroke Prevention in Atrial Fibrillation Investigators: Predictors of thromboembolism in atrial fibrillation: I. Clinical features of patients at risk. Ann Intern Med 1992;116:1-5

185. Koppensteiner R, Moritz A, Schlick W et al. Blood rheology after cardiac valve replacement with mechanical prostheses or bioprostheses. Am J Cardiol 1991;67:79-83

186. Pengo V, Peruzzi P, Baca M et al. The optimal therapeutic range for oral anticoagulant treatment as suggested by fibrinopeptide A levels in patients with heart valve prostheses. Eur J Clin Invest 1989;19:181-184

187. Wolf PA, Abbott RD, Kannel WB. Atrial fibrillation: a major contributor to stroke in the elderly. The Framingham Study. Arch Intern Med 1987;147:1561-1564

188. Halperin JL, Hart RG. Atrial fibrillation and stroke: new ideas, persisting dilemmas. Stroke 1988;19:937-941

189. Lundstrom T, Ryden L. Hemorrhagic and thromboembolic complications in patients with atrial fibrillation on anticoagulant prophylaxis. J Intern Med 1989;225:137-142

190. Petersen P, Boysen G, Godtfredsen J, Andersen ED, Andersen B: Placebo-controlled, randomised trial of warfarin and aspirin for prevention of thromboembolic complications in chronic atrial fibrillation. The Copenhagen AFASAK study. Lancet 1989;1:175-179

191. Stroke Prevention in Atrial Fibrillation Study Group Investigators: Preliminary report of the Stroke Prevention in Atrial Fibrillation Study. N Engl J Med 1990;322:863-868

192. Connolly SJ, Laupacis A, Gent M, Roberts RS, Cairns JA, Joyner C. Canadian Atrial Fibrillation Anticoagulation (CAFA) Study. J Am Coll Cardiol 1991;18:349-355

193. Stroke Prevention in Atrial Fibrillation Investigators: Predictors of thromboembolism in atrial fibrillation: II. Echocardiographic features of patients at risk. Ann Intern Med 1992;116:6-12

194. Wolf PA, Kannel WB, McGee DL, Meeks SL, Bharucha NE, McNamara PM. Duration of atrial fibrillation and imminence of stroke: the Framingham Study. Stroke 1983;14:664-667

195. Sanfilippo AJ, Abascal VM, Sheehan M et al. Atrial enlargement as a consequence of atrial fibrillation. Circulation 1990;82:792-797

196. Bailey GWH, Braniff BA, Hancock EW, Cohn KE. Relation of left atrial pathology to atrial fibrillation in mitral valvular disease. Ann Intern Med 1968;69:13-20

197. Daley R, Mattingley TW, Holt CL, Bland EF, White PD. Systemic arterial embolism in rheumatic heart disease. Am Heart J 1951;42:566-581
198. Wolf PA, Dawber TR, Thomas HE, Kannel WB. Epidemiologic assessment of chronic atrial fibrillation and risk of stroke: the Framingham Study. Neurology 1978;28:973-977
199. Szekely P. Systemic embolism and anticoagulant prophylaxis in rheumatic heart disease. Br Med J 1964;1:1209-1212
200. Wood P. Chronic rheumatic heart disease. In Wood P: Diseases of the Heart and Circulation, 2nd Edition. London, Eyre and Spottiswoode 1956;502-604
201. Coulshed N, Epstein EJ, McKendrick CS, Galloway RW, Walker E: Systemic embolism in mitral valve disease. Br Heart J 1970;32:26-34
202. Butchart EG, Moreno de la Santa P, Rooney SJ, Lewis PA. The role of risk factors and trigger factors in cerebrovascular events after mitral valve replacement: implications for antithrombotic management. J Card Surg 1994;9(Suppl):228-236
203. Sherrid MV, Clark RD, Cohn K. Echocardiographic analysis of left atrial size before and after operation in mitral valve disease. Am J Cardiol 1979;43:171-178
204. Burchfiel CM, Hammermeister KW, Krause-Steinrauf H, et al: Left atrial dimension and risk of systemic embolism in patients with a prosthetic heart valve. J Am Coll Cardiol 1990;15:32-41
205. Caplan LR, DCruz I, Hier DB, Reddy H, Shah S. Atrial size, atrial fibrillation and stroke. Ann Neurol 1986;19:158-161
206. Feinberg WM, Seeger JF, Carmody RF, Anderson DC, Hart RG, Pearce LA. Epidemiologic features of asymptomatic cerebral infarction in patients with nonvalvular atrial fibrillation. Arch Intern Med 1990;150:2340-2344
207. Mournier-Vehier F, Leys D, Rondpierre P, Godefroy O, Pruvo JP: Silent infarcts in patients with ischaemic stroke are related to age and size of the left atrium. Stroke 1993;24:1347-1351
208. Somerville W, Chambers RJ. Systemic embolism in mitral stenosis: relation to the size of the left atrial appendix. Br Med J 1964;2:1167-1171
209. Fraser AG. Ultrasonic detection of increased embolic risk. In Butchart EG, Bodnar E (Eds): Current Issues in Heart Valve Disease: Thrombosis, Embolism and Bleeding. London, ICR Publishers, 1992;233-244
210. Manyari D, Patterson C, Johnson D et al. An echocardiographic study on resting left ventricular function in healthy elderly subjects. J Clin Exp Gerontol 1982;4:403-420
211. Manyari DE, Patterson C, Johnson D, Melendez L, Kostuk WJ, Cape RDT. Atrial and ventricular arrhythmias in asymptomatic active elderly subjects: correlation with left atrial size and left ventricular mass. Am Heart J 1990;119:1069-1076
212. Haus E, Cusulos M, Sackett-Lundeen L, Swoyer J. Circadian variations in blood coagulation parameters, alpha-antitrypsin antigen and platelet aggregation and retention in clinically healthy subjects. Chronobiol Int 1990;7:203-216
213. Jovicic A, Mandic S. Circadian variations of platelet aggregability and fibrinolytic activity in healthy subjects. Thromb Res 1991;62:65-74
214. Willich SN, Tofler GH, Brezinski DA et al. Platelet alpha2 adrenoceptor characteristics during the morning increase in platelet aggregability. Eur Heart J 1992;13:550-555
215. Winther K, Hillegas W, Tofler GH et al. Effects on platelet aggregation and fibrinolytic activity during upright posture and exercise in healthy men. Am J Cardiol 1992;70:1051-1055
216. Haus E, Lakatua D, Swoyer J, Sackett-Lundeen L. Chronobiology in hematology and immunology. Am J Anat 1983;168:467-517
217. Seaman GV, Engel R, Swank EL, Hissen W. Circadian periodicity in some physicochemical parameters of circulating blood. Nature 1965;207:833-835
218. Bridges AB, Scott NA, NcNeill GP, Pringle TH, Belch JF. Circadian variation of white blood cell aggregation and free radical indices in men with ischaemic heart disease. Eur Heart J 1992;13:1632-1636
219. Labrecque G, Soulban G. Biological rhythms in the physiology and pharmacology of blood coagulation. Chronobiol Int 1991;8:361-372
220. Decousus H, Boissier C, Perpoint B et al. Circadian dynamics of coagulation and chronopathology of cardiovascular events. Ann N Y Acad Sci 1991;618:159-165
221. Marler JR, Price TR, Clark GL et al. Morning increase in onset of ischemic stroke. Stroke 1989;20:473-476
222. Pasqualetti P, Natali G, Casale R, Colantonio D. Epidemiological chronorisk of stroke. Acta Neurol Scand 1990;81:71-74
223. Wroe SJ, Sandercock P, Bamford J, Dennis M, Slattery J, Warlow C. Diurnal variation in incidence of stroke:Oxfordshire community stroke project. Br Med J 1992;304:155-157
224. Ridker PM, Willich SN, Muller JE, Hennekens CH. Aspirin, platelet aggregation and the circadian variation of acute thrombotic events. Chronobiol Int 1991;8:327-335
225. Muller JE, Ludmer PL, Willich SN et al. Circadian variation in the frequency of sudden cardiac death. Circulation 1987;75:131-138

226. Dewar HA, Weightman D. A study of embolism in mitral valve disease and atrial fibrillation. Br Heart J 1983;49:133-140
227. Cederblad G, Hahn L, Korsan-Bengtsen K, Pehrsson NG, Rybo G. Variations in blood coagulation, fibrinolysis, platelet function and various plasma proteins during the menstrual cycle. Haemostasis 1977;6:294-302
228. Yamazaki H, Motomiya T, Kikutani N et al. Platelet aggregation during mentrual cycle and pregnancy. Thromb Res 1979;14:333-340
229. Meade TW, Haines AP, Imeson JD, Stirling Y, Thompson SG. Menopausal status and haemostatic variables. Lancet 1983;1:22-24
230. Lee AJ, Lowe GDO, Smith WCS, Tunstall-Pedoe H. Plasma fibrinogen in women:relationships with oral contraception, the menopause and hormone replacement therapy. Br J Haematol 1993;83:616-621
231. Lindoff C, Petersson F, Lecander I, Martinsson G, Astedt B. Passage of the menopause is followed by haemostatic changes. Maturitas 1993;17:17-22
232. Meade TW, Dyer S, Howarth DJ, Imeson JD, Stirling Y. Antithrombin III and procoagulant activity: sex differences and effects of the menopause. Br J Haematol 1990;74:77-81
233. Tait RC, Walker ID, Islam SIAM, McCall F, Conkie JA, Mitchell R. Influence of demographic factors on antithrombin III activity in a healthy population. Br J Haematol 1993;84:476-480
234. Gordon T, Kannel WB, Hjortland MC, McNamara P. Menopause and coronary heart disease. Ann Intern Med 1978;89:157-161
235. Lowe GDO. Blood rheology, haemostasis and vascular diesase. In Bloom AL, Forbes CD, Thomas DP, Tuddenham EGD (Eds): Haemostasis and Thrombosis, 3rd Edition. Edinburgh, Churchill Livingstone 1994;1169-1188
236. Sullivan JL. The iron paradigm of ischemic heart disease. Am Heart J 1989;117:1177-1188
237. Salonen JT, Nyyssonen K, Korpela H, Tuomilehto J, Seppanen R, Salonen R. High stored iron levels are associated with excess risk of myocardial infarction in eastern Finnish men. Circulation 1992;86:803-811
238. Sullivan JL. Stored iron and ischemic heart disease;empirical support for a new paradigm. Circulation 1992;86:1036-1037
239. Stout RW, Crawford V. Seasonal variations in fibrinogen concentrations among elderly people. Lancet 1991;338:9-13
240. Woodhouse PR, Khaw KT, Plummer M, Foley A, Meade TW. Seasonal variations of plasma fibrinogen and factor VII activity in the elderly: winter infections and death from cardiovascular disease. Lancet 1994;343:435-439
241. Elwood PC, Beswick A, OBrien JR et al. Temperature and risk factors for ischaemic heart disease in the Caerphilly prospective study. Br Heart J 1993;70:520-523
242. Bull GM, Morton J. Environment, temperature and death rates. Age Ageing 1978;7:210-224
243. Ricci S, Celani MG, Vitali R, La Rosa F, Righetti E, Duca E: Diurnal and seasonal variations in the occurrence of stroke: a community based study. Neuroepidemiology 1992;11:59-64
244. Rooney SJ, Moreno de la Santa P, Lewis PA, Butchart EG. Sudden death in a large prosthetic valve series: experience with the Medtronic Hall valve. J Heart Valve Dis. 1994;3:5-9
245. Keatinge WR, Coleshaw SRK, Cotter F, Mattock M, Murphy M, Chelliah R. Increases in platelet and red cell counts, blood viscosity and arterial pressure during mild surface cooling: factors in mortality from coronary and cerebral thrombosis in winter. Br Med J 1984;289:1405-1408
246. Lowe GDO. Rheology of disease. In Lowe GDO (Ed): Clinical Blood Rheology, Volume II. Boca Raton, CRC Press 1988;89-111
247. Cermak J, Key NS, Balla J, Jacob HS, Vercellotti GM. C-reactive protein induces human peripheral blood monocytes to synthesise tissue factor. Blood 1993;82:513-520
248. Dinerman JL, Mehta JL. Endothelial, platelet and leukocyte interactions in ischemic heart disease: insights into potential mechanisms and their clinical relevance. J Am Coll Cardiol 1990;16:207-222
249. Bazzoni G, Dejana E, Maschio AD. Platelet-neutrophil interactions. Possible relevance in the pathogenesis of thrombosis and inflammation. Haematologica 1991;76:491-499
250. Cerletti C, Evangelista V, De Gaetano G. Polymorphonuclear leucocyte-dependent modulation of platelet function: relevance to the pathogenesis of thrombosis. Pharmacol Res 1992;26:261-268[
251. Renesto P, Chignard M. Enhancement of cathepsin G-induced platelet activation by leukocyte elastase: consequence for the neutrophil-mediated platelet activation. Blood 1993;82:139-144
252. Lowe GDO, Rumley A, Lee AJ, Crilly A, Madhok R, Tunstall-Pedoe H. Correlation of plasma fibrinogen, plasminogen activator inhibitor and red cell aggregation with interleukin-6 levels in a population study. (Abstract). Thromb Haemost 1993;69:763
253. Packham MA, Kinlough-Rathbone RL. Mechanisms of atherogenesis and thrombosis. In Bloom AL, Forbes CD, Thomas DP, Tuddenham EGD (Eds): Haemostasis and Thrombosis, 3rd Edition. Edinburgh, Churchill Livingstone 1994;1107-1138
254. Kennedy PS, Ware JA, Horak JK, Solis RT. The effect of acute changes in arterial pH and pO2 on platelet

aggregation. Microvasc Res 1981;22:324-330

255. Wedzicha JA, Syndercombe-Court D, Tan KC. Increased platelet aggregation formation in patients with chronic airflow obstruction and hypoxaemia. Thorax 1991;46:504-507

256. Kweider M, Lowe GDO, Murray GD, Kinane DF, McGowan DA. Dental disease, fibrinogen and white cell count;links with myocardial infarction? Scot Med J 1993;38:73-74

257. Yarnell JWG, Baker IA, Sweetnam PM et al. Fibrinogen, viscosity and white cell count are major risk factors for ischaemic heart disease;the Caerphilly and Speedwell Collaborative Heart Disease Studies. Circulation 1991;83:836-844

258. Lowe GDO, Fowkes FGR, Dawes J, Donnan PT, Lennie SE, Housley E: Blood viscosity, fibrinogen and activation of coagulation and leukocytes in peripheral arterial disease and the normal population in the Edinburgh Artery Study. Circulation 1993;87:1915-1920

259. Belch J. White cells, free radicals and scavengers. In Bloom AL, Forbes CD, Thomas DP, Tuddenham EGD (Eds): Haemostasis and Thrombosis, 3rd Edition. Edinburgh, Churchill Livingstone 1994:1089-1106

260. Syrjanen J, Valtonen VV, Iivanainen M, Kaste M, Huttunen JK. Preceding infection as an important risk factor for ischaemic brain infarction in young and middle aged patients. Br Med J 1988;296:1156-1160

261. Radomski MW, Moncada S. Regulation of vascular homeostasis by nitric oxide. Thromb Haemost 1993;70:36-41

262. Cadwgan T, Benjamin N. Reduced platelet nitric oxide synthesis in essential hypertension (Abstract). J Vasc Biol 1991;3:455A

263. Kjeldsen SE, Lande K, Gjesdal K et al. Increased platelet release reaction in 50-year-old men with essential hypertension: correlation with atherogenic cholesterol fractions. Am Heart J 1987;113:151-155

264. Nyrop M, Zweifler AJ. Platelet aggregation in hypertension and the effects of antihypertensive treatment. J Hypertens 1988;6:263-269

265. Fetkovska N, Amstein R, Ferracin F, Regenass M, Buhler FR, Pletscher A:-5-hydroxytryptamine kinetics and activation of blood platelets in patients with essential hypertension. Hypertension 1990;15:267-273

266. Letcher RL, Chien S, Pickering TG, Sealey JE, Laragh JH. Direct relationship between blood pressure and blood viscosity in normal and hypertensive subjects;role of fibrinogen and concentration. Am J Med 1981;70:1195-1202

267. Fowkes FGR, Lowe GDO, Rumley A, Lennie SE, Smith FB, Donnan PT. The relationship between blood viscosity and blood pressure in a random sample of the population aged 55 to 74. Eur Heart J 1993;14:597-601

268. Wolf PA, Kannel WB, Cupples LA, DAgostino RB. Risk factor interaction in cardiovascular and cerebrovascular disease. In Furlan AJ (Ed):The Heart and Stroke. London, Springer-Verlag 1987:331-355

269. MacMahon S, Peto R, Cutler J et al. Blood pressure, stroke and coronary heart disease;part 1, prolonged differences in blood pressure: prospective observational studies corrected for the regression dilution bias. Lancet 1990;335:765-774

270. Seneviratne BI, Reimers J. Nonvalvular atrial fibrillation associated with cardioembolic stroke: the role of hypertensive heart disease. Aust NZ J Med 1990;20:127-134

271. Moulton AW, Singer DE, Haas JS. Risk factors for stroke in patients with non rheumatic atrial fibrillation: a case-control study. Am J Med 1991;91:156-161

272. Wolf PA, D'Agostino RB, Kannel WB, Bonita R, Belanger AJ. Cigarette smoking as a risk factor for stroke. J Am Med Ass 1988;259:1025-1029

273. Butchart EG, Moreno de la Santa P, Rooney SJ, Lewis PA. Arterial risk factors and cerebrovascular events following aortic valve replacement. J Heart Valve Dis 1995;4:1-8

274. Tortorice KL, Carter BL. Stroke prophylaxis; hypertension management and antithrombotic therapy. Ann Pharmacother 1993;27:471-479

275. Meade TW. The epidemiology of atheroma, thrombosis and ischaemic heart disease. In Bloom AL, Forbes CD, Thomas DP, Tuddenham EGD (Eds): Haemostasis and Thrombosis, 3rd edition. Edinburgh, Churchill Livingstone 1994:1199-1227

276. Elwood PC, Renaud S, Sharp DS, Beswick AD, OBrien JR, Yarnell JWG. Ischaemic heart diesase and platelet aggregation. The Caerphilly Collaborative Heart Disease Study. Circulation 1991;83:38-44

277. Terres W, Weber K, Kupper W, Bleifeld W. Age, cardiovascular risk factors and coronary heart disease as determinants of platelet function in men;a multivariate approach. Thromb Res 1991;62:649-661

278. Ribeiro PA, Al Zaibag M, Idris M et al. Antiplatelet drugs and the incidence of thromboembolic complications of the St Jude Medical aortic prosthesis in patients with rheumatic heart disease. J Thorac Cardiovasc Surg 1986;91:92-98

279. Myers ML, Lawrie GM, Crawford ES et al. The St. Jude valve prosthesis: analysis of the clinical results in 815 implants and the need for systemic anticoagulation. J Am Coll Cardiol 1989;13:57-62

280. Barnes AJ. Rheology of diabetes mellitus. In Lowe GDO: Clinical Blood Rheology, Volume II. Boca Raton, CRC Press 1988:163-187

281. Mayne EE, Bridges JM, Weaver JA. Platelet adhesiveness, plasma fibrinogen and factor VIII levels in

diabetes mellitus. Diabetologia 1970;6:436-440

282. Reizenstein P. The haematological stress syndrome. Br J Haematol 1979;43:329-334

283. Kendall AG, Lohmann RC: Nephrotic syndrome, a hypercoagulable state. Arch Intern Med 1971;127:1021-1027

284. Vaziri ND, Gonzales E, Barton CH, Chen HT, Nguyen Q, Arquilla M. Factor XIII and its substrates, fibronectin, fibrinogen and alpha 2-antiplasmin in plasma and urine of patients with nephrosis. J Lab Clin Med 1990;117:152-156

285. Editorial. Antibodies to endothelial cells. Lancet 1991;337:649-650

286. Shatos MA, Doherty JM, Hoak JC. Alterations in human vascular endothelial cell function by oxygen free radicals: platelet adherence and prostacyclin release. Arteriosclerosis Thromb 1991;11:594-601

287. Meade TW, Stirling Y, Thompson SG et al. An international and interregional comparison of haemostatic variables in the study of ischaemic heart disease. Int J Epidemiol 1986;15:331-336

288. Merskey C, Gordon H, Lackner H. Blood coagulation and fibrinolysis in relation to coronary heart disease: a comparative study of normal white men, white men with overt coronary heart disease and normal Bantu men. Br Med J 1960;1:219-227

289. Miller GJ. Ethnicity, lipoproteins and haemostatic factors. In Cruickshank JK, Beevers DG (Eds): Ethnic Factors in Health and Disease. London, Wright 1989;280-288

290. de Simone G, Devereux RB, Chien S, Alderman MH, Atlas SA, Laragh JH. Relation of blood viscosity to demographic and physiologic variables and to cardiovascular risk factors in apparently normal adults. Circulation 1990;81:107-117

291. Iso H, Folsom AR, Wu KK et al. Hemostatic variables in Japanese and caucasian men. Plasma fibrinogen, factor VIIc, factor VIIIc and von Willebrand factor and their relations to cardiovascular disease risk factors. Am J Epidemiol 1989;130:925-934

292. Visudhiphan S, Poolsuppasit S, Piboonnukarintr O, Tumliang S. The relationship between high fibrinolytic activity and daily capsicum ingestion in Thais. Am J Clin Nutr 1982;35:1452-1458

293. Kantha SS. Dietary effects of fish oils on human health: a review of recent studies. Yale J Biol Med 1987;60:37-44

294. Gorelick PB. The status of alcohol as a risk factor for stroke. Stroke 1989;20:1607-1610

295. Balarajan R. Ethnic differences in mortality from ischaemic heart disease and cerebrovascular disease in England and Wales. Br Med J 1991;302:560-564

296. Francis RB Jr, Johnson CS. Vascular occlusion in sickle cell disease: current concepts and unanswered questions. Blood 1991;77:1405-1414

297. Bamford J, Warlow CP. Stroke and TIA in the general population. In Butchart EG, Bodnar E (Eds): Current Issues in Heart Valve Disease: Thrombosis, Embolism and Bleeding. London, ICR Publishers 1992:3-15

298. Shi F, Hart RG, Sherman DG, Tegeler CH. Stroke in the People's Republic of China. Stroke 1989;20:1581-1585

299. John S, Prasad KMS, Krishnaswami S. Early and long term results following valve replacements in the young with advanced rheumatic heart disease. In Bodnar E (Ed): Surgery for Heart Valve Disease. London, ICR Publishers 1990:44-53

300. Williams MA. Anticoagulation in developing countries. In Butchart EG, Bodnar E (Eds): Current Issues in Heart Valve Disease: Thrombosis, Embolism and Bleeding. London, ICR Publishers 1992:362-368

301. Simpson HCR, Mann JI, Meade TW, Chakrabarti R, Stirling Y, Woolf L. Hypertriglyceridemia and hypercoagulability. Lancet 1983;1:786-790

302. Davenport WD, Ball CR. Diet-induced atrial endothelial damage. Atherosclerosis 1981;40:145-152

303. Tarallo P, Henry J, Gueguen R, Siest G. Reference limits of plasma fibrinogen. Eur J Clin Chem Clin Biochem 1992;30:745-751

304. Le Devehat C, Khodabandehlou T, Dougny M. Hemorheological parameters in isolated obesity. Diabet Metabol 1992;18:43-47

305. Batist G, Bothe A, Bern M, Bistrian BR, Blackburn GL. Low antithrombin III in morbid obesity: return to normal with weight reduction. J Parenteral Enteral Nutr 1983;7:447-449

306. Stratton JR, Chandler WL, Schwartz RS et al. Effects of physical conditioning on fibrinolytic variables and fibrinogen in young and old healthy adults. Circulation 1991;83:1692-1697

307. Chandler WL, Levy WC, Veith RC, Stratton JR. A kinetic model of the circulatory regulation of tissue plasminogen activator during exercise, epinephrine infusion and endurance training. Blood 1993;81:3293-3302

308. Elwood PC, Yarnell JWG, Pickering J, Fehily AM, OBrien JR. Exercise, fibrinogen, and other risk factors for ischaemic heart disease. Caerphilly Prospective Heart Disease Study. Br Heart J 1993;69:183-187

309. Primrose JN, Davies JA, Prentice CR, Hughes R, Johnston D. Reduction in factor VII, fibrinogen and plasminogen activator inhibitor-1 activity after surgical treatment of morbid obesity. Thromb Haemost 1992;68:396-399

310. Davis JW, Shelton L, Eigenbery DA, Hignite CE, Watanabe IS. Effects of tobacco and non-tobacco cigarette

smoking on endothelium and platelets. Clin Pharmacol Ther 1985;37:529-533

311. Erikssen J, Hellem A, Stormorken H. Chronic effect of smoking on platelet count and platelet adhesiveness in presumabily healthy middle-aged men. Thromb Haemost 1977;38:606-611

312. Rival J, Riddle JM, Stein PD. Effects of chronic smoking on platelet function. Thromb Res 1987;45:75-85

313. Levine PH. An acute effect of cigarette smoking on platelet function: a possible link between smoking and arterial thrombosis. Circulation 1973;48:619-623

314. Bierenbaum ML, Fleischman AI, Stier A, Somol H, Watson PB. Effect of cigarette smoking upon in vivo platelet function in man. Thromb Res 1978;12:1051-1057

315. Davis JW, Shelton L, Watanabe IS, Arnold J. Passive smoking affects endothelium and platelets. Arch Intern Med 1989;149:386-389

316. Burghuber OC, Punzengruber C, Sinzinger H, Haber P, Silberauer K. Platelet sensitivity to prostacyclin in smokers and non-smokers. Chest 1986;90:34-38

317. Doteval A, Kutti J, Teger-Nilsson AC, Wadenvik H, Wilhelmsen L. Platelet reactivity, fibrinogen and smoking. Eur J Haematol 1987;38:55-59

318. Foo LC, Roshidah I, Aimy MB. Platelets of habitual smokers have reduced susceptibility to aggregating agents. Thromb Haemost 1991;65:317-319

319. Beswick A, Renaud S, Yarnell JWG, Elwood PC. Platelet activity in habitual smokers. Thromb Haemost 1991;66:739

320. Renaud S, Dumont E, Baudier F, Ortchanian E, Symington IS. Effect of smoking and dietary saturated fats on platelet functions in Scottish farmers. Cardiovasc Res 1985;19:155-159

321. Modesti PA, Abbate R, Gensini GF, Colella A, Serneri GGN. Platelet thromboxane A2 receptors in habitual smokers. Thromb Res 1989;55:195-201

322. Facchini FS, Hollenbeck CB, Jeppesen J, Chen YDI, Reaven GM. Insulin resistance and cigarette smoking. Lancet 1992;339:1128-1130

323. Shinton R, Beevers G. Meta-analysis of relation between cigarette smoking and stroke. Br Med J 1989;298:789-794

324. McBride PE. The health consequences of smoking: cardiovascular diseases. Med Clin N Am 1992;76:333-353

325. Neilson GH, Galea EG, Hossack KF. Thromboembolic complications of mitral valve disease. Aust NZ J Med 1978;8:372-376

326. Sturtevant FM. Smoking, oral contraceptives and thromboembolic disease. Int J Fertil 1982;27:2-13

327. Karasek RA, Theorell TGT, Schwartz J, Pieper C, Alfredsson L. Job, psychological factors and coronary heart disease. Adv Cardiol 1982;29:62-67

328. Maschewsky W. The relation between stress and myocardial infarction: a general analysis. Soc Sci Med 1982;16:455-462

329. Markowe HJL, Marmot MG, Shipley MJ et al. Fibrinogen: a possible link between social class and coronary heart disease. Br Med J 1985;291:1312-1314

330. Ernst E, Baumann M, Matrai A. Prolonged psychoemotional stress decreases blood fluidity. Clin Hemorheol 1984;4:423-429

331. Dintenfass L, Zador I. Blood rheology in patients with depressive and schizoid anxiety. Biorheology 1976;13:33-36

332. Ryder SJ, Bradley H, Brannan JJ, Turner MA, Bain WH. Thrombotic obstruction of the Bjork-Shiley valve: the Glasgow experience. Thorax 1984;487-492

333. Shetty HGM, Woods F, Routledge PA. The pharmacology of oral anticoagulants: implications for therapy. J Heart Valve Dis 1993;2:53-62

334. Siffert W, Gengenbach S, Scheid P. Inhibition of platelet aggregation by amiloride. Thromb Res 1986;44:235-240

335. Teger-Nilsson AC, Larsson PT, Hjemdahl P, Olsson G. Fibrinogen and plasminogen activator inhibitor-1 levels in hypertension and coronary heart diseases: potential effects of beta-blockade. Circulation 1991;84(Suppl VI):72-77

336. Winther K. The effect of beta-blockade on platelet function and fibrinolytic activity. J Cardiovasc Pharmacol 1987;10 (Suppl 2):94-98

337. Weisdorf DJ, Jacob HS. Beta-adrenergic blockade: augmentation of-neutrophil-mediated inflammation. J Lab Clin Med 1987;109:120-126

338. Tannous R. Beta blockers and the neutrophil. J Lab Clin Med 1987;109:109-110

339. Opie LH. Lipid-lowering and antiatherosclerotic drugs. In Opie LH (Ed): Drugs for the Heart, 3rd Edition. Philadelphia, WB Saunders Co 1991;247-261

340. Jansson JH, Johansson B, Boman K, Nilsson TK. Effects of doxazosin and atenolol on the fibrinolytic system in patients with hypertension and elevated serum cholesterol. Eur J Clin Pharmacol 1991;40:321-326

341. Lacoste LL, Lam JYT, Hung J, Waters D. Oral verapamil inhibits platelet thrombus formation in humans.

Circulation 1994;89:630-634
342. Amrani DL. Regulation of fibrinogen biosynthesis: glucocorticoid and interleukin-6 control. Blood Coag Fibrinol 1990;1:443-446
343. Zbinden G. Evaluation of thrombogenic effect of drugs. Annu Rev Pharmacol Toxicol 1976;16:177-188
344. Bush TL, Barrett-Connor E. Noncontraceptive estrogen use and cardiovascular disease. Epidemiol Rev 1985;7:80-104
345. Kaplan NM. Cardiovascular complications of oral contraceptives. Ann Rev Med 1978;29:31-40
346. Meade TW, Chakrabarti R, Haines AP, Howarth DJ, North WRS, Stirling Y. Haemostatic, lipid and blood pressure profiles of women on oral contraceptives containing 50μg and 30μg oestrogen. Lancet 1977;2:948-951
347. Lidegaard O. Oral contraception and risk of a cerebral thromboembolic attack:results of a case-control study. Br Med J 1993;306:956-963
348. Goldman L, Tosteson ANA. Uncertainty about postmenopausal estrogen: time for action, not debate. N Engl J Med 1991;325:800-802
350. Stampfer MJ, Colditz GA, Willett WC et al. Postmenopausal estrogen therapy and cardiovascular disease. Ten-year follow up from the Nurses Health Study. N Engl J Med 1991;325:756-762
351. Wilson PWF, Garrison RJ, Castelli WP. Postmenopausal estrogen use, cigarette smoking and cardiovascular morbidity in women over 50. The Framingham Study. N Engl J Med 1985;313:1038-1043
352. Roberts WC, Morrow AG. Mechanisms of left atrial thrombosis after mitral valve replacement: pathologic findings indicating obstruction to left atrial emptying. Am J Cardiol 1966;18:497-503
353. Blackstone EH, Kirklin JW. Death and other time-related events after valve replacement. Circulation 1985;72:753-767
354. Hylen JC. Mechanical malfunction and thrombosis of prosthetic heart valves. Am J Cardiol 1972;30:396-404
355. Renzulli A, De Luca L, Caruso A, Verde R, Galzerano D, Cotrufo M. Acute thrombosis of prosthetic valves: a multivariate analysis of the risk factors for a life threatening event. Eur J Cardiothorac Surg 1992;6:412-421
356. Messmer BJ, Okies, JE, Hallman GL, Cooley DA. Aortic valve replacement: two years experience with the Bjork-Shiley tilting disc prosthesis. Surgery 1972;72:772-779
357. Butchart EG, Moreno de la Santa P, Lewis PA. Risk factors and trigger factors for valve thrombosis with the Medtronic Hall valve. J Heart Valve Dis 1995;4:1-8
358. Cohn LH, Allred EN, DiSesa VJ, Sawtelle K, Shemin RJ, Collins J J Jr. Early and late risk of aortic valve replacement: a 12 years concomitant comparison of the porcine bioprosthetic and tilting disc prosthetic aortic valves. J Thorac Cardiovasc Surg 1984;88:695-705
359. Butchart EG, Lewis PA, Grunkemeier GL, Kulatilake N, Breckenridge IM. Low risk of thrombosis and serious embolic events despite low-intensity anticoagulation: experience with 1,004 Medtronic Hall valves. Circulation 1988;78(Suppl I):66-77
360. Grunkemeier GL, Starr A, Rahimtoola SH. Prosthetic heart valve performance: long term follow up. Curr Prob Cardiol 1992;17:331-406
361. Moulton AL, Singleton RT, Oster WF, Bosley J, Mergner W. Fatal thrombosis of an aortic St. Jude Medical valve despite adequate anticoagulation: anatomic and technical considerations. J Thorac Cardiovasc Surg 1982;83:472-473
362. Lindblom D. Long term clinical results after aortic valve replacement with the Bjork-Shiley prosthesis. J Thorac Cardiovasc Surg 1988;95:658-667
363. Kontos GJ, Schaff HV, Orszulak TA, Puga FJ, Pluth JR, Danielson GK: Thrombotic obstruction of disc valves: clinical recognition and surgical management. Ann Thorac Surg 1989;48:60-65
364. Massad M, Fahl M, Slim M et al. Thrombosed Bjork-Shiley standard disc mitral valve prosthesis. J Cardiovasc Surg 1989;30:976-980
365. Silber H, Khan SS, Matloff JM, Chaux A, De Robertis M, Gray R: The St. Jude valve: thrombolysis as the first line of therapy for cardiac valve thrombosis. Circulation 1993;87:30-37
366. Copans H, Lakier JB, Kinsley RH, Colsen PR, Fritz VU, Barlow JB: Thrombosed Bjork-Shiley mitral prostheses. Circulation 1980;61:169-174
367. Kinsley RH, Antunes MJ, Colsen PR. St Jude Medical valve replacement;an evaluation of valve performance. J Thorac Cardiovasc Surg 1986;92:349-360
368. Butchart EG, Lewis PA, Kulatilake ENP, Breckenridge IM. Anticoagulation variability between centres: implications for comparative prosthetic valve assessment. Eur J Cardiothorac Surg 1988;2:72-81
369. Cannegieter SC, Rosendall FR, Briet E. Thromboembolic and bleeding complications in patients with mechanical heart valve prostheses. Circulation 1994;89:635-641
370. Turpie AGG, Gunstensen J, Hirsh J, Nelson H, Gent M. Randomised comparison of two intensities of oral anticoagulation therapy after tissue heart valve replacement. Lancet 1988;1:1242-1245
371. Saour JN, Sieck JO, Mamo LAR, Gallus AS. Trial of different intensities of anticoagulation in patients with

prosthetic heart valves. N Engl J Med 1990;322:428-432

372. Altman R, Rouvier J, Gurfinkel E et al. Comparison of two levels of anticoagulation therapy in patients with substitute heart valves. J Thorac Cardiovasc Surg 1991;101:427-431

373. Turpie AGG, Gent M, Laupacis A et al. A comparison of aspirin with placebo in patients treated with warfarin after heart valve replacement. N Engl J Med 1993;329:524-529

374. Bamford J, Sandercock P, Dennis M, Burn J, Warlow C. Classification and natural history of clinically identifiable subtypes of cerebral infarction. Lancet 1991;337:1521-1526

375. Hart RG. Prevention and treatment of cardioembolic stroke. In Furlan AJ (Ed):The Heart and Stroke. London, Springer-Verlag 1987:117-138

376. Grunkemeier GL, London MR. Reliability of comparative data from different sources. In Butchart EG, Bodnar E (Eds): Current Issues in Heart Valve Disease: Thrombosis, Embolism and Bleeding. London, ICR Publishers 1992:464-475

377. Bodnar E. A critical assessment of thrombosis and embolism reporting methods. In Butchart EG, Bodnar E (Eds): Current Issues in Heart Valve Disease: Thrombosis, Embolism and Bleeding. London, ICR Publishers 1992:476-484

378. Sadowski JA, Bovill EG, Mann KG. Warfarin and the metabolism and function of Vitamin K. Poller L (Ed): Recent Advances in Blood Coagulation No.5. Edinburgh, Churchill Livingstone 1991:93-118

379. Vermeer C, Hamulyak K. Pathophysiology of vitamin K deficiency and oral anticoagulants. Thromb Haemost 1991;66:153-159

380. Hirsh J, Dalen JE, Deykin D, Poller L. Oral anticoagulants: mechanism of action, clinical effectiveness and optimal therapeutic range. Chest 1992;102(Suppl):312S-326S

381. Conway EM, Bauer KA, Barzegar S, Rosenberg RD. Suppression of hemostatic system activation by oral anticoagulants in the blood of patients with thrombotic diatheses. J Clin Invest 1987;80:1535-1544

382. Quick AJ, Stanley-Brown M, Bancroft FW. A study of the coagulation defect in hemophilia and in jaundice. Am J Med Sci 1935;190:501-511

383. Bussey HI, Force RW, Bianco TM, Leonard AD. Reliance on prothrombin time ratios causes significant errors in anticoagulation therapy. Arch Intern Med 1992;152:278-282

384. Ansell JE. Imprecision of prothrombin time monitoring of oral anticoagulation. Am J Clin Pathol 1992;98:237-239

385. van den Besselaar AMHP. International standardization of laboratory control of oral anticoagulation therapy: a survey of thromboplastin reagents used for prothrombin time testing. J Heart Valve Dis 1993;2:42-52

386. Duckert F. Standardisierungsbemuhungen auf dem gebiete der thromboplastinzeit. Schweiz Rundschau Med 1981;70:110-113

387. Ng VL, Levin J, Corash L, Gottfried EL. Failure of the International Normalised Ratio to generate consistent results within a local medical community. Am J Clin Pathol 1993;99:689-694

388. Furie B, Diuguid CF, Jacobs M, Diuguid DL, Furie BC. Randomized prospective trial comparing the native prothrombin antigen with the prothrombin time for monitoring oral anticoagulant therapy. Blood 1990;75:344-349

389. Hemker HC. Thrombin generation, an essential step in hemostasis and thrombosis. In Bloom AL, Forbes CD, Thomas DP, Tuddenham EGD (Eds): Haemostasis and Thrombosis, 3rd Edition. Edinburgh, Churchill Livingstone, 1994;477-490

390. Boisclair MD, Ireland H, Lane DA. Assessment of hypercoagulable states by measurements of activation fragments and peptides. Blood Rev 1990;4:25-40

391. Millenson MM, Bauer KA, Kistler JP, Barzegar S, Tulin L, Rosenberg RD. Monitoring mini-intensity anticoagulation with warfarin: comparison of the prothrombin time using a sensitive thromboplastin with prothrombin fragment F1+2 levels. Blood 1992;79:2034-2038

392. van Wersch JWJ, van Mourik-Alderliesten CH, Coremans A. Determination of markers of coagulation activation and reactive fibrinolysis in patients with mechanical heart valve prosthesis at different intensities of oral anticoagulation. Blood Coag Fibrinol 1992;3:183-186

393. Kistler JP, Singer DE, Millenson MM et al. Effects of low intensity anticoagulation on level of activity of the hemostatic system in patients with atrial fibrillation. Stroke 1993;24:1360-1365

394. Bloom AL. Physiology of blood coagulation. Hemostasis 1990;(Suppl I)20:14-29

395. Inauen W, Bombeli T, Baumgartner HR, Haeberli A, Straub PW. Effects of the oral anticoagulant phenprocoumon on blood coagulation and thrombogenesis induced by rabbit aorta subendothelium exposed to flowing human blood: role of dose and shear rate. J Lab Clin Med 1991;118:280-288

396. Turitto VT, Muggli R, Baumgartner HR. Surface reactivity and thrombus formation: subendothelium versus artifical surfaces. Trans Am Soc Artif Intern Organs 1978;24:568-572

397. Rams JJ, Davis DA, Lolley DM, Berger MP, Spencer M. Detection of microemboli in patients with artificial heart valves using transcranial Doppler: preliminary observations. J Heart Valve Dis 1993;2:37-41

398. Hirsh J. Effectiveness of anticoagulants. Sem Thromb Haemost 1986;12:21-37

399. Cortelazzo S, Finazzi G, Viero P et al. Thrombotic and hemorrhagic complications in patients with mechanical heart valve prosthesis attending an anticoagulation clinic. Thromb Haemost 1993;69:316-320
400. Fihn SD, McDonell M, Martin D et al. Risk factors for complications of chronic anticoagulation. Ann Intern Med 1993;118:511-520
401. Schachner A, Deviri E, Shabat S. Patient-regulated anticoagulation. In Butchart EG, Bodnar E (Eds): Current Issues in Heart Valve Disease: Thrombosis, Embolism and Bleeding. London, ICR Publishers 1992;318-324
402. Landefeld CS, Rosenblatt MW, Goldman L. Bleeding in outpatients treated with warfarin: relation to the prothrombin time and important remediable lesions. Am J Med 1989;87:153-159
403. Landefeld CS, Beyth RJ. Anticoagulant-related bleeding: clinical epidemiology, prediction and prevention. Am J Med 1993;95:315-328
404. Shetty HGM, Routledge PA. The use of computers in anticoagulation management. In Butchart EG, Bodnar E (Eds): Current Issues in Heart Valve Disease: Thrombosis, Embolism and Bleeding. London, ICR Publishers 1992:331-336
405. Pedersen FM, Hamberg O, Hess K, Ovesen L. The effect of dietary vitamin K on warfarin-induced anticoagulation. J Intern Med 1991;229:517-520
406. Sixty Plus Reinfarction Study Research Group: Risk of long term oral anticoagulant therapy in elderly patients after myocardial infarction. Lancet 1982;1:64-68
407. European Atrial Fibrillation Trial Study Group: Secondary prevention in-non-rheumatic atrial fibrillation after transient ischaemic attack or minor stroke. Lancet 1993;342:1255-1262
408. Loeliger EA, van Duk-Wierda CA, van den Besselaar AMHP, Broekmans AW, Roos J: Anticoagulant control and the risk of bleeding. In Meade TW (Ed): Anticoagulants and Myocardial Infarction: a Reappraisal. Chichester, John Wiley 1984:135-177
409. Lowe GDO, Walker ID. Anticoagulant-related bleeding. In Butchart EG, Bodnar E (Eds): Current Issues in Heart Valve Disease: Thrombosis, Embolism and Bleeding. London, ICR Publishers 1992:425-436
410. Shetty HGM, Backhouse G, Bentley DP, Routledge PA. Effective reversal of warfarin induced excessive anticoagulation with low dose vitamin K. Thromb Haemost 1992;67:13-15
411. Francis CW, Marder VJ, Evarts CM, Yaukoolbodi S. Two-step warfarin therapy: prevention of postoperative venous thrombosis without excessive bleeding. J Am Med Ass 1983;249:374-378
412. MacCallum PK, Thomson JM, Poller L. Effects of fixed minidose warfarin on coagulation and fibrinolysis following major gynaecological surgery. Thromb Haemost 1990;64:511-515
413. Forfar JC. A 7-year analysis of hemorrhage in patients on long term anticoagulant treatment. Br Heart J 1979;42:128-132
414. Miller DC, Oyer PE, Mitchell RS et al. Performance characteristics of the Starr-Edwards model 1260 aortic valve prosthesis beyond 10 years. J Thorac Cardiovasc Surg 1984;88:193-207
415. Kase CS, Robinson RK, Stein RW et al: Anticoagulant related intracerebral hemorrhage. Neurology 1985;35:943-948
416. Mattle H, Kohler S, Huber P, Rohner M, Steinsiepe KF. Anticoagulation-related intracranial extracerebral hemorrhage. J Neurol Neurosurg Psych 1989;52:829-837
417. Kase CS. Intracerebral hemorrhage: non-hypertensive causes. Stroke 1986;17:590-595
418. Radberg JA, Olsson JE, Radberg CT. Prognostic parameters in spontaneous intracerebral hematomas with special reference to anticoagulant treatment. Stroke 1991;22:571-576
419. Franke CL, de Jonge J, van Swieten JC, Op de Coul AAW, van Gijn J. Intracerebral hematomas during anticoagulant treatment. Stroke 1990;21:726-730
420. Feldman E. Intracerebral hemorrhage. Stroke 1991;22:684-691
421. Coon WW, Willis PW. Hemorrhagic complications of anticoagulant therapy. Arch Intern Med 1974;133:386-392
422. Landefeld CS, Goldman L. Major bleeding in outpatients treated with warfarin: incidence and prediction by factors known at the start of outpatient therapy. Am J Med 1989;87:144-152
423. Gurwitz JH, Goldberg RJ, Holden A, Knapic N, Ansell J. Age-related risks of long term oral anticoagulant therapy. Arch Intern Med 1988;148:1733-1736
424. Gohlke-Bärwolf C, Acar J, Burckhardt D et al. Guidelines for prevention of thromboembolic events in valvular heart disease. J Heart Valve Dis 1993;2:398-410
425. Miller VT, Rothrock JF, Pearce LA, Feinberg WM, Hart RG, Anderson DC. Ischemic stroke in patients with atrial fibrillation: effect of aspirin according to stroke mechanism. Neurology 1993;43:32-36
426. Boston Area Anticoagulation Trial for Atrial Fibrillation Investigators. The effect of low-dose warfarin on the risk of stroke in patients with non-rheumatic atrial fibrillation. N Engl J Med 1990;323:1505-1511
427. Yasaka M, Yamaguchi T, Miyashita T, Tsuchiya T. Regression of intracardiac thrombus after cardioembolic stroke. Stroke 1990;21:1540-154
428. Butchart EG, Lewis PA, Bethel JA, Breckenridge IM. Adjusting anticoagulation to prosthesis thrombogenicity and patient risk factors: recommendations for the Medtronic Hall valve. Circulation

1991;84(Suppl III):61-69

429. Horstkotte D, Schulte H, Bircks W, Strauer B. Unexpected findings concerning thromboembolic complications and anticoagulation after complete 10 year follow up of patients with St. Jude Medical prostheses. J Heart Valve Dis 1993;2:291-301

430. Moggio RA, Hammond GL, Stansel HC Jr, Glen WWL. Incidence of emboli with cloth covered Starr-Edwards valve without anticoagulation and with varying forms of anticoagulation. J Thorac Cardiovasc Surg 1978;75:296-299

431. Mok DK, Boey J, Wang R et al. Warfarin versus dipyridamole-aspirin and pentoxifyllin-aspirin for the prevention of prosthetic heart valve thromboembolism: a prospective randomized clinical trail. Circulation 1985;82:1059-1063

432. Dale J, Myhre E. Can acetylsalicylic acid alone prevent arterial thromboembolism? A pilot study in patients with aortic ball valve prostheses. Acta Med Scand Suppl 1981;645:73-78

433. Nunez L, Aguado GM, Larrea JL, Celemin D, Oliver J. Prevention of thromboembolism using aspirin after mitral valve replacement with porcine bioprostheses. Ann Thorac Surg 1984;37:84-87

434. Antiplatelet Trialists Collaboration. Collaborative overview of randomised trials of antiplatelet therapy - III: Reduction in venous thrombosis and pulmonary embolism by antiplatelet prophylaxis among surgical and medical patients. Br Med J 1994;308:235-246

435. Cazenave JP, Gachet C, Lanza F. Pharmacological inhibition of the ADP-GP IIb/IIIa-fibrinogen pathway of platelet aggregation. In Herman AG (Ed): Antithrombotics. Dordrecht, Kluwer Academic Publishers 1991;83-97

436. Fuster V, Israel DH. Platelet inhibitor drugs after prosthetic heart valve replacement. In Butchart EG, Bodnar E (Eds): Current issues in Heart Valve Disease: Thrombosis, Embolism and Bleeding. London, ICR Publishers 1992:247-262

437. Buchanan MR, Brister SJ. Antithrombotics and the lipoxygenase pathway. In Herman AG (Ed): Antithrombotics. Dordrecht, Kluwer Academic Publishers 1991:159-179

438. Moake JL, Turner NA, Stathopoulos NA, Nolasco L, Hellums JD. Shear-induced platelet aggregation can be mediated by vWF released from platelets, as well as by exogenous large or unusually large vWF multimers, requires adenosine diphosphate, and is resistant to aspirin. Blood 1988;71:1366-1374

439. Harker LA, Hanson SR, Kirkman TR. Experimental arterial thromboembolism in baboons: mechanisms, quantitation and pharmacologic prevention. J Clin Invest 1979;64:559-569

440. Vane JR. Inhibition of prostaglandins as a mechanism of action for aspirin-like drugs. Nature (New Biol) 1971;231:232-235

441. Tohgi H, Konno S, Tamura K, Kimura B, Kawano K. Effects of low-to-high doses of aspirin on platelet aggregability and metabolities of thromboxane A2 and prostacyclin. Stroke 1992;23:1400-1403

442. Clarke RJ, Mayo G, Price P, Fitzgerald GA. Suppression of thromboxane A2 but not of systemic prostacyclin by controlled-release aspirin. N Engl J Med 1991;325:1137-1141

443. Kyrle PA, Eichler HG, Jager U, Lechner K. Inhibition of prostacyclin and thromboxane A2 generation by low-dose aspirin at the site of plug formation in man in vivo. Circulation 1987;75:1025-1029

444. Moncada S, Korbut R. Dipyridamole and other phosphodiesterase inhibitors act as antithrombotic agents by potentiating endogenous prostacyclin. Lancet 1978;1:1286-1289

445. Lorenzet R, Niemetz J, Marcus AJ, Broekman MJ. Enhancement of mononuclear procoagulant activity by platelet 12-hydroxyeicosatetraenoic acid. J Clin Invest 1986;78:418-423

446. Altman R, Boullon F, Rouvier J, Raca R, de la Fuente L, Favaloro R. Aspirin and prophylaxis of thromboembolic complications in patients with substitute heart valves. J Thorac Cardiovasc Surg 1976;72:127-129

447. Dale J, Myrhe E, Storstein O, Stormorken H, Efskind L. Prevention of arterial thromboembolism with acetylsalicyclic acid: a controlled clinical study in patients with aortic ball valves. Am Heart J 1977;94:101-111

448. Chesebro JH, Fuster V, Elveback LR et al. Trial of combined warfarin plus dipyridamole or aspirin therapy in prosthetic heart valve replacement: danger of aspirin compared with dipyridamole. Am J Cardiol 1983;51:1537-1541

449. Meade TW, Roderick PJ, Brennan PJ, Wilkes HC, Kelleher CC. Extracranial bleeding and other symptoms due to low dose aspirin and low intensity oral anticoagulation. Thromb Haemost 1992;68:1-6

450. Steele PM, Weily HS, Davies H, Pappas G, Genton E. Platelet survival time following aortic valve replacement. Circulation 1975;51:358-362

451. Martin W, Smith JA, White DG. The mechanisms by which hemoglobin inhibits the relaxation of rabbit aorta induced by nitrovasodilators, nitric oxide or bovine retractor penis inhibiting factor. Br J Pharmacol 1986;89:563-571

452. Gerzer R, Karrenbrock B, Siess W, Heim JM. Direct comparison of the effects of nitroprusside, SIN 1 and various nitrates on platelet aggregation and soluble guanylate cyclase activity. Thromb Res 1988;52:11-21

453. Groves PH, Lewis MJ, Cheadle HA, Penny WJ. SIN-1 reduces platelet adhesion and platelet thrombus

formation in a porcine model of balloon angioplasty. Circulation 1993;87:590-597

454. Drummer C, Ludke S, Spannagl M, Schramm W, Gerzer R. The nitric oxide donor SIN-1 is a potent inhibitor of plasminogen activator inhibitor release from stimulated platelets. Thromb Res 1991;63:553-556

455. Fitzgerald GA. Dipyridamole. N Engl J Med 1987;316:1247-1257

456. Stein B, Fuster V. Clinical pharmacology of platelet inhibitors. In Fuster V, Verstraete M (Eds). Thrombosis in Cardiovascular Disorders. Philadelphia, WB Saunders 1992;99-119

457. Bult H, Fret HRL, Jordaens FH, Herman AG. Dipyridamole potentiates platelet inhibition by nitric oxide. Thromb Haemost 1991;66:343-349

458. Saniabadi AR, Fisher TC, McLaren M, Belch JF, Forbes CD. Effect of dipyridamole alone and in combination with aspirin on whole blood platelet aggregation, PGI2 generation and red cell deformability ex vivo in man. Cardiovasc Res 1991;25:177-183

459. Defreyn G, Bernat A, Delebassee D, Maffrand JP. Pharmacology of ticlopidine: a review. Sem Thromb Haemost 1989;15:159-166

460. McTavish D, Gaulds D, Goa KL. Ticlopidine. an updated review of its pharmacology and therapeutic use in platelet-dependent disorders. Drugs 1990;40:238-259

461. Installe E, Gonzalez M, Schoevaerdts JC, Tremouroux J. Prevention by ticlopidine of platelet consumption during extracorporeal circulation for heart surgery and lack of effect on operative and postoperative bleeding. J Cardiovasc Pharmacol 1981;3:1174-1183

462. Goldman M, Auckland A, Hall C, Hawker RJ, McCollum CN. Antithrombotic effect of ticlopidine and aspirin plus dipyridamole compared (Abstract). Thromb Haemost 1983;50:62

463. Palareti G, Poggi M, Torricelli P, Balestra V, Coccheri S. Long term effects of ticlopidine on fibrinogen and haemorheology in patients with peripheral vascular disease. Thromb Res 1988;52:621-629

464. Finelli C, Palareti G, Poggi M et al. Ticlopidine lowers plasma fibrinogen in patients with polycythaemia rubra vera and additional thrombotic risk factors. Acta Haematol 1991;85:113-118

465. Antiplatelet Trialists Collaboration: Collaborative overview of randomised trials of antiplatelet therapy - I: Prevention of death, myocardial infarction, and stroke by prolonged antiplatelet therapy in various categories of patients. Br Med J 1994;308:81-106

466. Delorme MA, Burrows RF, Ofosu FA, Andrew A. Thrombin regulation in mother and fetus during pregnancy. Sem Thromb Haemost 1992;18:81-90

467. Bremme K, Ostlund E, Almqvist I, Heinonen K, Blomback M. Enhanced thrombin generation and fibrinolytic activity in normal pregnancy and the puerperium. Obst Gynaecol 1992;80:132-137

468. Buchan PC. Rheology of normal and abnormal pregnancy. On Lowe GDO (Ed). Clinical Blood Rheology, Vol II. Boca Raton, CRC Press 1988:203-212

469. Louden KA, Pipkin F, Heptinstall S, Fox SC, Mitchell JRA, Symonds EM. A longitudinal study of platelet behaviour and thromboxane production in whole blood in normal pregnancy and the puerperium. Br J Obst Gynaecol 1990;97:1108-1114

470. Bonnar J, Daly L, Sheppard BL. Changes in the fibrinolytic system during pregnancy. Sem Thromb Haemost 1990;16:221-229

471. McColgin SW, Martin JN, Morrison JC. Pregnant women with prosthetic heart valves. Clin Obst Gynecol 1989;32:76-88

472. Oakley CM. Anticoagulation during pregnancy. In Butchart EG, Bodnar E (Eds). Current Issues in Heart Valve Disease: Thrombosis, Embolism and Bleeding. London, ICR Publishers 1992:339-345

473. Sbarouni E, Oakley CM. Outcome of pregnancy in women with valve prostheses. Br Heart J 1994;71:196-201

474. Iturbe-Alessio I, Fonseca MC, Mutchinik O, Santos MA, Zajarias A, Salazar E. Risks of anticoagulant therapy in pregnant women with artificial heart valves. N Engl J Med 1986;315:1390-1393

475. Wang RYC, Lee PK, Chow JSF, Chen WWC. Efficacy of low dose, subcutaneously administered heparin in treatment of pregnant women with artificial heart valves. Med J Aust 1983;2:126-128

476. Bonnar J. Long term self-administered heparin therapy for prevention and treatment of thromboembolic complications of pregnancy. In Kakkar VV, Thomas DP (Eds): Heparin: Chemistry and Clinical Usage. London, Academic Press 1976:247-260

477. Whitfield LR, Lele AS, Levy G. Effect of pregnancy on the relationship between concentration and anticoagulant action of heparin. Clin Pharmacol Ther 1983;34:23-28

478. Kaplan KL, Owen J. Plasma levels of platelet secretory proteins. Crit Rev Oncol Hematol 1986;5:235-255

479. Chen J, Karlberg KE, Sylven C. Heparin and low molecular weight heparin but not hirudin stimulate platelet aggregation in whole blood from acetylsalicylic acid treated healthy volunteers. Thromb Res 1991;63:319-329

480. Hall JG, Pauli RM, Wilson KM. Maternal and fetal sequelae of anticoagulation during pregnancy. Am J Med 1980;68:122-140

481. Dahlman TC. Osteoporotic fractures and the recurrence of thromboembolism during pregnancy and the

puerperium in 184 women undergoing thromboprophylaxis with heparin. Am J Obst Gynecol 1993;168:1265-1270

482. Cotrufo M, de Luca TSL, Calabro R, Mastrogiovanni G, Lama D. Coumarin anticoagulation during pregnancy in patients with mechanical valve prostheses. Eur J Cardiothorac Surg 1991;5:300-305

483. Sareli P, England MJ, Berk MR et al. Maternal and fetal sequelae of anticoagulation during pregnancy in patients with mechanical heart valve prostheses. Am J Cardiol 1989;63:1462-1465

484. Stein PD, Alpert JS, Copeland J, Dalen JE, Goldman S, Turpie AGG. Antithrombotic therapy in patients with mechanical and biological prosthetic heart valves. Chest 1992;102(Suppl):445S-455S

485. Katholi RE, Nolan SP, McGuire LB. Living with prosthetic heart valves: subsequent noncardiac operations and the risk of thromboembolism or hemorrhage. Am Heart J 1976;92:162-167

486. Carter SA, McDevitt E, Gatje BW, Wright IS. Analysis of factors affecting the recurrence of thromboembolism off and on anticoagulation therapy. Am J Med 1958;25:43-51

487. Grip L, Blomback M, Chulman S. Hypercoagulable state and thromboembolism following warfarin withdrawal in post-myocardial infarction patients. Eur Heart J 1991;12:1225-1233

488. McIntyre H. Management, during dental surgery, of patients on anticoagulants. Lancet 1966;2:99-100

489. Robinson GA, Nylander A. Warfarin and cataract extraction. Br J Ophthal 1989;73:702-703

490. Rustad H, Myrhe E. Surgery during anticoagulant treatment: the risk of increased bleeding on oral anticoagulant treatment. Acta Med Scand 1963;173:115-119

491. Fraser AG, Angelini GD, Ikram S, Butchart EG. Left atrial ball thrombus: echocardiographic features and clinical implications. Eur Heart J 1988;9:672-677

492. Beppu S, Park YD, Sakakibara H, Nagata S, Nimura Y. Clinical features of intracardiac thrombus based on echocardiographic observations. Jpn Circ J 1984;48:75-82

493. Calandre L, Ortega JF, Bermejo F. Anticoagulation and hemorrhagic infarction in cerebral embolism secondary to rheumatic heart disease. Arch Neurol 1984;41:1152-1154

494. Hart RG. Cardiogenic embolism to the brain. Lancet 1992;339:589-594

495. Vitale N, Renzulli A, Cerasuolo F et al. Prosthetic valve obstruction: thrombolysis versus operation. Ann Thorac Surg 1994;57:365-370

496. Hausmann D, Mugge A, Daniel WG. Valve thrombosis: diagnosis and management. In Butchart EG, Bodnar E: Current Issues in Heart Valve Replacement: Thrombosis, Embolism and Bleeding. London, ICR Publishers 1992:387-401

497. Graver LM, Gelber PM, Tyras DH. The risks and benefits of thrombolytic therapy in acute aortic and mitral prosthetic valve dysfunction: report of a case and review of the literature. Ann Thorac Surg 1988;46:85-88

498. Butchart EG, Breckenridge IM. The timing of prosthetic valve reoperations based on an analysis of risk factors. Z Kardiol 1986;(Suppl 2)75:155-159

499. Sobel BE. Thrombolysis in the treatment of acute myocardial infarction. In Fuster V, Verstraete M (Eds): Thrombosis in Cardiovascular Disorders. Philadelphia, WB Saunders 1992;289-326

500. Efstratiadis T, Munsch C, Crossman D, Taylor KM. Aprotinin therapy after thrombolytic treatment. Ann Thorac Surg 1991;52:1320-1321

501. Wardlaw JM, Warlow CP. Thrombolysis in acute ischaemic stroke: does it work? Stroke 1992;23:1826-1839

502. Yamaguchi T, Hayakawa T, Kiuchi H. Intravenous tissue plasminogen activator ameliorates the outcome of hyperacute embolic stroke. Cerebrovasc Dis 1993;3:269-273.

Subject Index

Compiled by Dr. Peter Rea

A

I